NURSE'S REFERENCE LIBRARY®

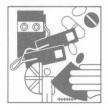

Treatments

Nursing88 Books™
Springhouse Corporation
Springhouse, Pennsylvania

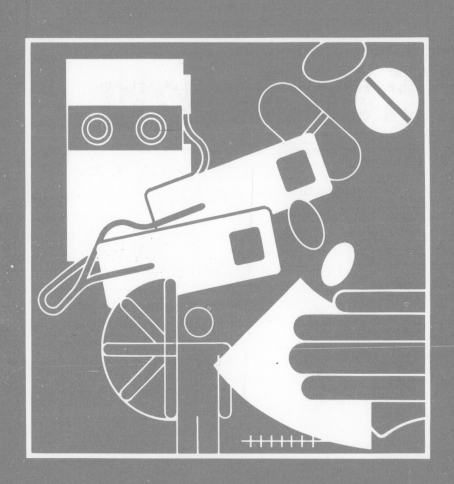

NURSE'S REFERENCE LIBRARY ®

Treatments

Nursing88 Books™
Springhouse Corporation
Springhouse, Pennsylvania

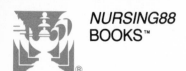

NURSING88
BOOKS™

Springhouse Corporation Book Division

CHAIRMAN
Eugene W. Jackson

VICE-CHAIRMAN
Daniel L. Cheney

PRESIDENT
Warren R. Erhardt

VICE-PRESIDENT AND DIRECTOR
William L. Gibson

VICE-PRESIDENT, BOOK OPERATIONS
Thomas A. Temple

VICE-PRESIDENT, CORPORATE OPERATIONS
Bacil Guiley

PROGRAM DIRECTOR, REFERENCE BOOKS
Stanley E. Loeb

NURSE'S REFERENCE LIBRARY®

Staff for this volume

EXECUTIVE EDITOR
Matthew Cahill

CLINICAL DIRECTOR
Barbara McVan, RN

ART DIRECTOR
John Hubbard

Clinical Editor: Joanne Patzek DaCunha, RN, BS

Contributing Clinical Editors: June E. Breit, RN; Margaret Worthington Brennan, RN; Merilee Jensen Grimes, RN, BSN, MS; Jo-Ann Kamencik, RN, MSN; Anne Doyle McClure, RN, BA, MSN; Camille Marano Morrison, RN, MSN; Rebecca Sass Olivet, RN, BA, BSN; Julie N. Tackenberg, RN, MA, CNRN; Eileen M. Wenckus, RN, MSN

Book Editors: Michael Boyette, Catherine Harold, June Norris, Patricia M. Shinehouse

Contributing Editors: Andrea F. Barrett, Barbara Hodgson, Roberta Kangilaski, Kevin J. Law, Virginia Peck, Vince Rause

Drug Information Manager: Larry Neil Gever, RPh, PharmD

Editorial Services Manager: David R. Moreau

Copy Editors: Diane M. Labus, Doris Weinstock, Debra Young

Production Coordinator: Susan Hopkins Rodzewich

Senior Designer: Matie Anne Patterson

Designers: Lorraine Carbo, Linda Franklin, Carol Cameron-Sears, Mary Wise

Illustrators: Dimitrios Bastas, Maryanne Buschini, David Christiana, Steve Cusano, Design Management, Stephen Early, Len Epstein, Dan Fione, Jean Gardner, John Gist, Linda Gist, Robin Heller, Tom Herbert, Polly Krumbhaar-Lewis, Robert Neumann, Taylor Oughton, Robert Phillips, George Retseck, Eileen Rudnick, Dennis Schofield, Lauren Simeone, Bruce VanPatter, Robert Walsh

Art Production Manager: Robert Perry

Art Assistants: Anna Brindisi, Loretta Caruso, Donald Knauss, Mark Marcin, Lisa Rich, Robert Wieder

Director of Composition/Editorial Services: David C. Kosten

Assistant Typography Manager: Diane Paluba

Typographers: Elizabeth DiCicco, Nancy Wirs

Senior Production Manager: Deborah C. Meiris

Assistant Production Manager: Timothy A. Landis

Assistants: Maree E. DeRosa, Denine M. Lichtfuss

Special thanks to Nancy Holmes and Marlene C. Rosensweig, who assisted in the preparation of this volume.

NURSING88 BOOKS™

NURSE'S REFERENCE LIBRARY®

This volume is part of a series conceived by the publishers of *Nursing88®* magazine and written by hundreds of nursing and medical specialists. This series, the NURSE'S REFERENCE LIBRARY, is the most comprehensive reference set ever created exclusively for the nursing profession. Each volume brings together the most up-to-date clinical information and related nursing practice. Each volume informs, explains, alerts, guides, educates. Taken together, the NURSE'S REFERENCE LIBRARY provides today's nurse with the knowledge and the skills that she needs to be effective in her daily practice and to advance in her career.

Other volumes in the series:

Diseases	Drugs	Procedures	Practices	Signs & Symptoms
Diagnostics	Assessment	Definitions	Emergencies	Patient Teaching

Other publications:

NEW NURSING SKILLBOOK™ SERIES

Giving Emergency Care Competently
Monitoring Fluid and Electrolytes Precisely
Assessing Vital Functions Accurately
Coping with Neurologic Problems Proficiently
Reading EKGs Correctly

Combatting Cardiovascular Diseases Skillfully
Nursing Critically Ill Patients Confidently
Dealing with Death and Dying
Managing Diabetes Properly
Giving Cardiovascular Drugs Safely

NURSING PHOTOBOOK™ SERIES

Providing Respiratory Care
Managing I.V. Therapy
Dealing with Emergencies
Giving Medications
Assessing Your Patients
Using Monitors
Providing Early Mobility
Giving Cardiac Care
Performing GI Procedures
Implementing Urologic Procedures

Controlling Infection
Ensuring Intensive Care
Coping with Neurologic Disorders
Caring for Surgical Patients
Working with Orthopedic Patients
Nursing Pediatric Patients
Helping Geriatric Patients
Attending Ob/Gyn Patients
Aiding Ambulatory Patients
Carrying Out Special Procedures

***Nursing88* DRUG HANDBOOK™**

NURSING YEARBOOK88

NURSING PHOTOBOOK ANNUAL

CLINICAL POCKET MANUAL™ SERIES

Diagnostic Tests	Cardiovascular Care	Surgical Care	Assessment
Emergency Care	Respiratory Care	Medications and I.V.s	Drug Interactions
Fluids and Electrolytes	Critical Care	Ob/Gyn Care	Documentation
Signs and Symptoms	Neurologic Care	Pediatric Care	

NURSE REVIEW™ SERIES

Cardiac Problems
Respiratory Problems
Gastrointestinal Problems
Neurologic Problems
Vascular Problems

Genitourinary Problems
Endocrine Problems
Musculoskeletal Problems
Metabolic Problems
Hematologic Problems

Contents

1 Reviewing Treatment Fundamentals

2 Treating Cardiovascular Dysfunction

3 Treating Respiratory Dysfunction

4 Treating Gastrointestinal Dysfunction

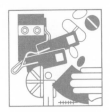

Advisory Board

At the time of publication, the advisors, clinical consultants, and contributors held the following positions.

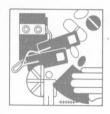

Clinical Consultants

Reza R. Azar, MD, Medical Director, Buxmont Pain Treatment Center, Doylestown, Pa.

Gregory D. Borowski, MD, Endocrinologist, Moses Taylor Hospital, Scranton, Pa.

Sander M.Z. Cohen, MD, Chief Resident, Wills Eye Hospital, Philadelphia

T. Forcht Dagi, MD, MPH, FACS, Staff Neurologist, Walter Reed Army Medical Center, Washington, D.C.; Assistant Professor of Surgery, Uniformed Services University of the Health Sciences, Washington, D.C.

Armando deMoya, MD, AASECT, Assistant Clinical Professor, Georgetown University Hospital, Washington, D.C.; President, Washington Reproductive Associates, P.C., Washington, D.C.

Brian B. Doyle, MD, Acting Director, Psychiatry Residency Program, Georgetown University School of Medicine, Washington, D.C.

Bethany C. Jackson, PhD, RD, LD, Clinical Assistant Professor, Emory University School of Medicine, Division of Nutrition, Atlanta

Kathleen A. Kucer, MD, Dermatologist, Grand View Hospital, Sellersville, Pa.

Daniel Edward McGunegle, MD, Associate Professor and Director of Ob/Gyn Services, Truman Medical Center East, Kansas City, Mo.

Robin L. Miller, MD, Senior Scientist, Biological Response Modifiers Program, National Cancer Institute, Frederick, Md.

Frank N. Ritter, MD, Clinical Professor of Otolaryngology, University of Michigan Medical Center, Ann Arbor

Gizell Maria Rossetti, MD, Staff Neurologist, Nicolet Clinic, Neenah, Wis.

Harrison J. Shull, Jr., MD, FACP, Clinical Professor of Medicine, Vanderbilt University, Nashville, Tenn.

Eric Z. Silfen, MD, FACEP, FACP, Chairman, Department of Emergency Medicine, Reston (Va.) Hospital Center

Michael I. Sorkin, MD, Associate Professor of Medicine, and Director, Peritoneal Dialysis Program, University of Pittsburgh School of Medicine, Renal-Electrolyte Division, Department of Medicine; Associate Director, Renal Section, Veterans Administration Medical Center, Pittsburgh

Alan G. Stern, MD, FACC, Attending Cardiologist, Helene Fuld Medical Center, Trenton, N.J.

Barry L. Tonkonow, MD, Doylestown (Pa.) Hospital

Peter G. Tuteur, MD, FACP, Associate Professor of Medicine, Pulmonary Disease Division, Washington University School of Medicine, St. Louis

William M. Valenti, MD, Associate Professor of Medicine—Infectious Diseases, University of Rochester (N.Y.) School of Medicine and Dentistry

Joan E. Watson, RN, PhD, Director, Graduate Programs, Nursing Administration and Nursing Education, University of Pittsburgh School of Nursing

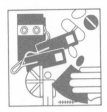

Contributors

Susan A. Albrecht, RN, PhD, Assistant Professor, University of Pittsburgh School of Nursing

Ruth-Ellen Blauer, RN, MA, Chairperson, Department of Nursing, Castleton (Vt.) College

Barbara Gross Braverman, RN, MSN, CS, Psychotherapist, The Counseling Program, Pennsylvania Hospital, Philadelphia

David Chaussard, CURN, BSN, MBA, Head Nurse, Urology and ENT, Kansas University Medical Center, Kansas City

Mary Elesha-Adams, RN, MSN, AASECT, Health Educator, East Carolina University, Greenville, N.C.

Marcia Jo Hill, RN, MSN, Manager, Dermatologic Therapeutics, Methodist Hospital, Houston

Sande Jones, RN, C, MS, Inservice Coordinator, Nursing Education, Mount Sinai Medical Center, Miami Beach

Christina Algiere Kasprisin, RN, MS, Quality Attainment Coordinator (Nursing), Saint Francis Hospital, Tulsa, Okla.; Assistant Clinical Professor (Nursing), University of Oklahoma, Oklahoma City

Pamela Peters Long, RN, BSN, Director, Institute for Cancer Control, Atlanta

Mary M. Lutz, RN, BSN, RRT, Respiratory Nurse Specialist, National Jewish Center for Immunology and Respiratory Medicine, Denver

Anne Doyle McClure, RN, BA, MSN, Biomedical Writer, Lansdale, Pa.

Kay McCoy, RN, Ophthalmic Nurse Consultant, Drake, Colo.

Nina Hubej Olesinski, RN, MSN, Clinical Nurse Consultant, Ophthalmology and Otolaryngology, University of Illinois Eye and Ear Infirmary, Chicago; Faculty, University of Illinois College of Nursing, Chicago

Martha Burgess Page, RN, C, MSN, Assistant Program Director, Pain Management Program, Shaughnessy Rehabilitation Hospital, Salem, Mass.

Frances W. Quinless, RN, PhD, CCRN, Chairperson, Department of Nursing Education and Services, University of Medicine and Dentistry of New Jersey, School of Health Related Professions, Newark

Grace M. Redheffer, RN, MSN, CEN, Emergency Nursing Consultant, Norristown, Pa.

Marilyn Sawyer Sommers, RN, MA, CCRN, Director, Critical Care Nursing, University of Cincinnati Medical Center

Linda A. Spencer, RN, MPH, Assistant Professor of Nursing and Community Health Medicine, Nell Hodgson Woodruff School of Nursing, Emory University, Atlanta

Audrey Stephan, RN, MSN, Assistant Professor of Nursing, Bergen Community College, Paramus, N.J.

Julie N. Tackenberg, RN, MA, CNRN, Clinical Specialist, Intermediate Neurosensory Care Unit, Thomas Jefferson Medical Center, Philadelphia

Joseph B. Warren, RN, BSN, Director, Clinical Research, Kinetic Concepts, Inc., San Antonio, Tex.

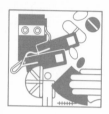

Foreword

Today more than ever, you need an informed, practical guide to all types of treatments. The reason? Well, besides keeping current with some dramatic therapeutic advances, such as cerebellar implants for cerebral palsy and bone growth stimulators for unmending fractures, you need to know what's in store for your patient—no matter whether he's receiving a drug or special diet, about to undergo surgery, or a candidate for a whole host of other treatments. You also need a clear understanding of your responsibilities: how to prepare your patient for a particular treatment, how to care for him after it, and perhaps most important of all, how to spot complications early. What's more, if a treatment regimen requires long-term compliance, you'll need to spell out for the patient just what he has to do—and why.

In *Treatments*, the latest volume in the Nurse's Reference Library, you'll find this information and more. You'll discover more than 300 drug regimens, surgeries, diets, behavior modification techniques, pain control measures, and other treatments.

This rich source of information is logically organized for easy use. Chapter 1 serves as a tablesetter for the book, focusing on such broad issues as drug selection and action, measures to promote good nutrition, and advances in treatments. This chapter also details such broad nursing responsibilities as how to encourage compliance with treatment, how to perform preoperative and postoperative assessments, and how to reduce the risk of postoperative complications.

Chapters 2 to 20, the body of the book, center on specific treatments. Conveniently organized by body system or health problem, each chapter begins with a brief introduction outlining key issues, trends, and nursing responsibilities. After this introduction, you'll find a discussion of drug therapy. For the sake of economy, pharmacologically or therapeutically related drugs are considered as a class. Each class, in turn, is covered in a standard format.

First, an introduction identifies the drugs within the class and summarizes their indications, effects, and cautions. The next section, *Purpose and action*, succinctly explains the drugs' mechanism of action and therapeutic aim. Then *Monitoring* discusses such concerns as drug interactions, administration precautions and tips, and notable side effects and corrective measures. In *Home care instructions*, the concluding section, you'll find important teaching directions to help the patient comply with therapy and ward off any unintended effects.

After the section on "Drug Therapy," you'll typically find sections on surgery and, when appropriate, other forms of treatment, such as special diets, balloon catheter treatments, inhalation therapies, counseling, and sex therapy. Each treatment in these sections is again organized according to a standard format. After a brief introduction defines and characterizes the treatment, *Purpose* identifies the therapeutic aim. Next, *Preparation* discusses specific steps you'll take to prepare the patient physically and psychologically for the treatment. The following section, *Procedure*, summarizes how the treatment is performed. Or, if the treatment can be performed by nurses, it provides step-by-step directions. *Monitoring and aftercare* emphasizes nursing care during and after treatment. *Home care instructions* focuses on measures to improve compliance or hasten recovery.

Throughout this book, special graphic symbols signal important features. *Complications*, for instance, alerts you to measures that can help prevent, detect, or manage the untoward effects of a treatment. Another feature, *Question-and-answer guides*, provides clear answers to questions patients commonly ask about treatments. *Advanced equipment* sheds light on new or complex equipment, and *Patient-teaching aids* provide directions for measures the patient must follow at home. In the sections on drug therapy, the feature *Comparing drugs* outlines the similarities and differences among drugs within a class. Depending on the drug class, it may focus on mechanism of action, route of administration, side effects, interactions, teaching pointers, or other topics. *Interactions* points out life-threatening drug interactions and why they occur.

The book closes with two helpful appendices. The first appendix summarizes selected treatments not found in the body of the book. The second appendix, organized by disorder, outlines appropriate treatment for more than 600 conditions.

As you can readily see, *Treatments* is an impressive volume. It should prove a valuable reference for hospital, clinic, and home health nurses. I recommend it.

Frances J. Storlie, RN, PhD, CANP

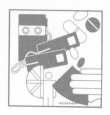

Overview

A skeptical nurse once asked, "Why should I learn about treatments? After all, doctors perform most of them."

Well, like many skeptics, our misguided nurse took a short-sighted view of her own situation. True, doctors do *perform* most treatments. But nurses certainly have their share of responsibility. For instance, we're responsible for preparing a patient mentally and physically for a treatment. At times, we assist with (and even perform) the treatment itself. After the treatment, we help assess the patient's response and monitor for any complications. And we pave the way for compliance and recovery by providing clear, thorough directions for home care.

As you can readily see, we do play a major role in treatments. But before we can carry it out effectively, we need a sound grasp of current treatments, their benefits, and their potential pitfalls. And we need a clear understanding of today's professional climate.

Increasing professional demands

Today, we need to make the commitment to update and apply our knowledge of treatments. That's because the demand for skilled nursing care is perhaps greater than ever before. At a time when many nursing staffs are at an all-time low, we're faced with a higher percentage of acutely ill patients than ever before. We're also required to teach more patients in less time, partly because of rapid growth in outpatient procedures. And in certain treatments, such as milieu therapy and some pain control measures, we're called upon to be primary therapists.

With these increased demands, we need to be able to quickly anticipate the treatment a patient needs, help prepare him for it, and assess the quality of his response to it. An accident victim, for example, may require a number of treatments—autotransfusion, administration of vasopressors, reduction of fractures, and others—all of which we need to anticipate before a doctor orders them. A patient undergoing portal-systemic shunting requires clear teaching about the surgery's risks and unwavering emotional support. A patient receiving penicillin needs close monitoring to promptly detect and correct adverse, even life-threatening, reactions. Only with a firm grasp of these and many other treatments can we hope to keep up with our growing professional demands.

Advances in treatments

Another reason for learning about treatments is simply to keep pace with technology. Interferons, laser surgery, genetic engineering, new cholesterol-lowering drugs—these are but a few of the recent therapeutic advances. As the primary coordinators of our patients' care, we're responsible for gaining a working knowledge of these new treatments.

Certainly, advances in treatments have opened new avenues of care for many patients; however, they've also spawned a disturbing trend. With the growing use of sophisticated machines like lasers and ultrasonic lithotriptors comes the risk of shifting our focus from patient care to a fascination with these modern tools of the trade. By keeping in mind that these devices are intended to serve the patient, we'll more readily provide the humane care each patient needs—and deserves.

Litigation on the rise

Unfortunately, yet another reason to improve our knowledge of treatments is a legal one. Health care professionals everywhere have become concerned over the continuing rise in malpractice litigation. For nurses, a thorough application of sound knowledge represents our best defense. Not only must we carry out our independent nursing actions correctly, but we're bound to recognize and oppose incorrect or inappropriate orders. When a drug dosage seems unusually high, for example, we must be ready to check and double-check the order, making sure it's correct. And, as always, we must be sure to carefully document pertinent details of each patient's care.

Our professional calling

Surely, any of the reasons mentioned here should convince our skeptical nurse that we do indeed need to learn about treatments. But just in case she still isn't convinced, let me remind her of our professional calling: to provide every patient with the best nursing care possible. And that requires us to be knowledgeable about all types of treatments.

Ruth Blauer, RN, MS

1 Reviewing Treatment Fundamentals

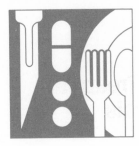

Reviewing Treatment Fundamentals

Introduction

Treatments. You're involved with them daily to help patients combat or prevent disease. At times, you're responsible for planning and initiating treatments, such as bladder training for the patient with spinal cord injury. Other times, you're responsible for assisting with them. Regardless of the role you take, you'll often be called upon to help evaluate the outcome of treatments. What's more, you'll need to provide thorough teaching to reduce the patient's anxiety and encourage his compliance.

CHOOSING A TREATMENT PROTOCOL

Many factors influence the choice of a treatment protocol: the patient's age, his current diagnosis and medical history, his personal—or his doctor's—preference, his financial resources and, of course, his perception of health. Added to these factors are the availability of equipment and the proximity of specialists.

Patient's age
Age often affects a patient's ability to tolerate treatment. For example, an in-

fant's more vulnerable to complications because of his immature body systems. An elderly patient's also at risk, as aging may increase his susceptibility to chronic or debilitating disorders.

Current diagnosis
The patient's current diagnosis influences treatment choice. Research studies help determine the recommended treatment by tracking how effectively different treatments cure a disorder or relieve its symptoms. As a result, a "tried and true" treatment is often the first choice. For example, when cancer involves the tail or body of the pancreas, radiation has proved to be the most successful palliative treatment. However, when cancer involves the head of the pancreas and common bile duct, Whipple's procedure is the better choice.

Medical history
Suppose the patient's history reveals long-term liver disease. This, too, may help determine a treatment protocol. For example, a drug metabolized by the liver wouldn't be recommended since its metabolism—and effectiveness—would be unpredictable. What's more, the drug might also aggravate liver disease. Likewise, if the patient has renal disease, a drug excreted by the kidneys wouldn't be recommended;

its delayed excretion would increase the risk of nephrotoxicity.

Whose preference wins out?

While the doctor may prefer one treatment over another, the patient's preference prevails when there's a choice. For example, the patient with Stage I breast cancer may be treated by lumpectomy with radiation or by mastectomy. Since the patient knows the family support she can depend on and her coping mechanisms, self-image, and health expectations, she's best able to decide between the treatment choices.

A matter of convenience

The availability of equipment and specialists can also influence treatment choice. For example, if the patient lives a great distance from a medical center that offers hemodialysis, he may opt to perform peritoneal dialysis at home.

Weighing risks and benefits

For certain disorders, a number of treatments are available—some conservative, some radical, and many in between. Weighing the risks and benefits of each is a must. Typically, evaluating the factors discussed above will help define these risks and benefits. For example, if an elderly patient with severely compromised cardiopulmonary function has a hip fracture, the doctor may elect to treat the fracture with traction rather than risk general anesthesia to do an open reduction. However, if the patient's cardiopulmonary function improves, the doctor may reconsider surgery.

ity to independently maintain their activities of daily living.

Typically, the patient's diagnosis determines whether a conservative or more radical treatment is the first step toward restoring health. For example, drug therapy for chronic arthritis pain is usually initiated before more radical—and more expensive—joint replacement. Likewise, antacids and antihistamines should be tried before gastrectomy for peptic ulcer disease.

At times, though, more radical treatment is necessary to avoid jeopardizing the patient's life. For example, in pheochromocytoma, surgical excision of the tumor is the only treatment that can prevent potentially life-threatening hypertensive crisis.

The role of rest

Whether the patient undergoes a conservative or a radical treatment, rest often helps restore his health. How? By decreasing basal metabolic rate, rest lowers the body's oxygen demands. It also reduces temperature, blood pressure, and respiratory rate as well as sympathetic and parasympathetic stimulation of gastric secretions.

As a primary treatment, rest helps relieve lower back pain and promotes bone and ligament healing. As an adjunctive treatment, it reduces stress and promotes healing.

DRUG THERAPY

Restoring Health: Treatment's Goal

Restoring health is easier for some patients than for others, partly because definitions of health vary greatly. However, most people see health as the abil-

Drug Selection

After determining that a patient should receive drug therapy, the doctor must evaluate several factors before selecting a drug. These include the drug's classification, its action and side effects, and the availability of trade or generic brands. The doctor's experience with the drug and the patient's medical history and ability to comply with therapy are also key considerations.

Drug classification

To select a specific drug, the doctor may first narrow his choice to a group of drugs that share the same therapeutic and pharmacologic characteristics. For example, if the patient has a seizure disorder, the doctor may examine the drugs within the class of anticonvulsants. Then, he may select the pharmacologic class of benzodiazepine anticonvulsants as the most effective. Next, he can compare the drugs within that class to determine which one would be best for treating seizures.

Suppose the patient has an infection, though. Before selecting an antibiotic, the doctor must identify the causative organism. Only then can he select among the antibiotics effective against it. That's because some organisms are resistant to certain antibiotics.

Is drug action easily measured?

One factor that may recommend one drug over another is the drug's action on a target organ. Consider the use of warfarin to impede coagulation. Here, the target organ is the liver, where the drug depresses the synthesis of Factors II, VII, IX, and X, thereby interfering with the role of vitamin K in the clotting process. The drug's action can be directly evaluated by testing prothrombin time.

Do side effects outweigh benefits?

As a nurse, you know that a drug can produce side effects that may seem to the patient as bad as (or even worse than) the disorder it aims to treat. The alopecia, weight loss, and nausea that so often accompany chemotherapy are classic examples of hard-to-tolerate side effects.

When selecting a drug, the doctor must determine whether potential side effects are unacceptable enough to out-weigh the drug's benefit. Fortunately, many side effects lessen or disappear when dosage is reduced. Others subside after continued therapy.

You'll need to clearly warn the patient about potential side effects. Otherwise, if they occur, he may not comply with therapy. Also, monitor him closely to promptly detect and manage any side effects. For example, if the patient gets severe diarrhea while receiving antibiotics, he's at risk for fluid and electrolyte imbalance and perianal skin breakdown. Your next step may be administration of fluids or an antidiarrheal drug, if ordered.

Trade or generic?

When the doctor selects a trade brand, you'll need to warn the patient not to use a generic substitute without the doctor's approval. Doing so may mean sacrificing drug efficacy. For example, suppose the seizure patient is stabilized on a trade brand anticonvulsant. Switching to a generic brand may cause seizure activity to recur. Why? Because quality control may not be as precise with a generic brand; as a result, the patient may have fluctuating blood levels of the drug.

When past experience counts

Because a doctor can't be familiar with every drug on the market, he may choose among those drugs with which he's familiar. Beyond that, he may base his drug choice on being more comfortable with the side effects of a specific drug or more satisfied with its efficacy.

Medical history: A crucial guide

After considering the characteristics of the drug as well as his experience with it, the doctor must review the patient's history. For example, a history of liver or kidney disease or allergy to a drug or class of drugs often influences drug selection. Allergic reactions may range from rash, fever, or urticaria with pruritus to life-threatening anaphylactic shock. Such reactions are unpredictable in antimicrobial therapy because the patient may become sensitized to an antimicrobial drug without having previously received it. A patient with a history of penicillin hypersensitivity may also have hypersensitivity to a cephalosporin because of cross-allergenicity. By questioning a patient about his known and suspected drug allergies, you can help the doctor make a wise drug choice.

THE FIVE RIGHTS OF DRUG ADMINISTRATION

Before administering any drug, be sure to observe these five "rights."

Right patient. Check the patient's name against his hospital identification number. Try to place patients with similar names on different units or floors to avoid errors in drug administration.

Right drug. Call the pharmacist to validate generic and trade name equivalents. Call the doctor to clarify the order, if necessary. *Do not* assume that the nurse who transcribed the order did so correctly.

Right time. Learn the hospital's standard administration times for o.d., b.i.d., and t.i.d. Be aware that certain drugs, such as antiarrhythmics, must be administered on a 24-hour schedule.

Right route. Call the doctor to clarify the route of drug administration, if necessary. Do not confuse "I.V. push" with "I.V. piggyback" or substitute one route for another, to avoid cardiac and respiratory complications.

Right dose. Be familiar with the recommended and therapeutic doses for the drug you're giving. If you're unsure, don't hesitate to ask the pharmacist or consult a drug reference book. Remember, as the one who administers the drug, you have the ultimate responsibility.

After administering any drug, you'll need to monitor the patient's response. For example, after administering a diuretic, you'll need to monitor urine output. After giving a cardiac glycoside, such as digoxin, you'll need to monitor heart rate.

Can the patient comply?

Because compliance is key to successful treatment, the doctor must evaluate the patient's ability to comply when selecting a drug. For example, if the patient has no medical insurance and a low income, ordering an expensive drug may result in noncompliance.

Drug Action

To monitor therapy, you'll need to understand how the drug is absorbed, distributed, metabolized, and excreted. This will help you identify adverse reactions and any problems with drug efficacy. You'll also need to be familiar with the patient's history of rashes, fever, or respiratory disorders, which may mimic an adverse reaction.

Absorption

Except for drugs that act locally, every drug must be absorbed into the bloodstream before it can act within the body. *Absorption* depends on the administration route (enteral or parenteral) and on conditions at the administration site, such as circulation. Rotating injection sites for heparin and insulin helps prevent tissue necrosis, which could decrease absorption. Drug concentration and dosage also affect absorption; the higher the concentration or dosage, the more rapidly the drug's absorbed.

A urine pH between 4.6 and 8.2 affects drug absorption by passive diffusion in the renal tubules. In aspirin or phenobarbital overdose, alkalinizing the urine can reduce absorption, thus increasing drug excretion.

Distribution

As a drug starts to be absorbed, it moves from the bloodstream into body fluids and tissues—a process called *distribution*. Drugs are distributed or transported from the administration site to receptor sites largely by binding with plasma proteins, such as albumin. Because of this, a patient with hypoproteinemia may require parenteral albumin replacement to promote drug distribution.

A drug's ability or inability to cross a lipid membrane affects its distribution to body sites. For example, penicillin and its derivatives can't pass through the blood-brain barrier.

Through absorption and distribution, a drug reaches its site of action and combines with cell receptors. Storage reservoirs—namely, subcutaneous and intramuscular tissues—have an affinity for certain drugs. Debilitated patients, though, may absorb and distribute medications more effectively via I.V. administration, since their storage reservoirs are inadequate and excessive injections may break down tissue.

Metabolism

Some drugs are excreted virtually unchanged. Most, however, are *metabolized* by the liver into a less active, more water-soluble form for excretion by the kidneys. Although the liver is the primary site of drug metabolism, the lungs, kidneys, and intestines may also be involved in this process.

Drugs absorbed from the GI tract travel first to the liver's portal system and are taken up by hepatic cells for metabolism. Certain drugs, like propranolol, undergo a "first-pass effect" in the liver. That is, they're extensively metabolized before entering systemic circulation; therefore, only a fraction of the unmetabolized drug remains to produce the desired effect. As a result, oral doses of such drugs need to be higher than parenteral doses.

Excretion

The kidneys excrete most drugs unchanged or as a metabolite. However, the lungs are primarily responsible for excreting volatile anesthetics, such as halothane. Negligible drug excretion also occurs through perspiration, saliva, tears, breast milk, and feces.

Impaired renal or hepatic function can hinder drug excretion. For example, because gentamicin is excreted almost completely unchanged by the kidneys, renal impairment can lead to especially high blood levels, or drug toxicity.

Drug Toxicity

Broadly defined, *toxicity* refers to drug effects that are deleterious rather than therapeutic. It may be predictable, as with side effects and an overdose, or unpredictable, as with a drug allergy or an idiosyncratic response.

Toxicity may occur during short- or long-term therapy. For example, a patient receiving penicillin may go into anaphylactic shock after an initial dose. Or an arthritis patient who regularly takes aspirin may have GI bleeding.

How is toxicity measured? By the patient's symptoms, such as headache and GI upset, and by laboratory data, such as drug blood levels.

Recognizing—and avoiding—toxicity

Several factors can determine whether a drug will have a toxic effect.

• *Drug interactions.* A drug interaction occurs when one drug administered in combination with or shortly after another drug alters the effect of one or both drugs. It may result from altered absorption, distribution, metabolism, or excretion of one drug by another or from a combination of the drugs' actions or effects. For example, probenecid inhibits renal excretion of penicillin, thus raising blood levels of this drug. One drug may displace another from plasma-protein binding sites, as warfarin does with tolbutamide. By altering the body's electrolyte balance, one drug may indirectly influence the effect of another. For example, certain thiazide diuretics can cause hypokalemia, increasing the risk of toxicity in a patient taking a cardiac glycoside.

Combining certain drugs with food may also trigger an interaction. For example, taking tetracycline with dairy products interferes with its absorption.

Frequently, drug interactions can be prevented by modifying drug dose, schedule, or route. If the patient is taking drugs that may interact, teach him about reportable symptoms.

• *Physiologic function.* How well organs are functioning can affect drug absorption, metabolism, or excretion, influencing the risk of toxicity. For example, when renal function is impaired, drugs excreted by the kidneys remain in the body for a prolonged period, increasing the risk of toxicity.

When hepatic function is impaired, drugs metabolized by the liver are metabolized erratically, ineffectively, or not at all.

• *Nutrition.* Poor nutrition can upset electrolyte balance. If it causes hypokalemia in a patient who's taking a cardiac glycoside, toxicity is a threat.

• *Patient's age.* In an infant or young child, the drug dose must be carefully calculated to avoid toxicity. The elderly patient is also at risk for toxicity. He's more likely to suffer from impaired kidney or liver function, poor circulation, and malnutrition—all of which may contribute to toxicity.

• *Compliance.* How well a patient complies with a specific drug therapy can influence toxicity, especially if he fails to take the prescribed dose or follow the correct schedule.

Modifying Drug Therapy

When the patient's a child or an elderly adult, expecting a baby, or breast-feeding, you'll need to observe certain precautions when administering drugs.

Adjusting drug dosage and route in children

During development, a child's ability to absorb, distribute, metabolize, and excrete drugs changes dramatically. So, you'll need to pay special attention to drug dosage and administration route. When calculating dosages, don't use formulas that modify adult dosages. Instead, calculate dosages on the basis of body weight (mg/kg) or body surface area (mg/square meter).

If the patient's under age 18 months, use the vastus lateralis for I.M. injection instead of the gluteus maximus to avoid sciatic nerve damage. Do likewise in older children who are unable to ambulate independently because of cerebral palsy or any other physical retardation affecting size, muscle mass, and ambulation.

Safeguarding mother and child

Almost all drugs cross the placenta to some extent. During the first trimester, the fetus is especially vulnerable to damage from maternal drug use. Of course, the safest rule is to avoid all drugs during pregnancy. However, if a drug does need to be given, its risk to the fetus must be weighed against its benefit to the mother.

Most drugs a nursing mother takes appear in breast milk. Drug levels in breast milk tend to be highest shortly after taking each dose. As a result, advise the nursing mother to breast-feed before taking any drug, not after. Also make sure she checks with her doctor first; he may want her to replace breast-feeding with bottle-feeding during drug therapy.

Avoiding toxicity in the elderly

When an elderly patient is receiving drug therapy, you'll need to focus on avoiding toxicity. Why? First, the elderly consume more drugs than any other age group—primarily because they have a greater variety of diseases and often require more than one drug. They may also suffer liver dysfunction, which alters drug metabolism; kidney dysfunction, which alters drug excretion; malabsorption, which alters drug absorption and distribution (because of low plasma protein levels); and poor circulation, which also alters drug distribution. What's more, total body mass and lean body mass tend to decrease with age, while the proportion of body fat tends to increase. Therefore, drug dosage typically needs to be adjusted.

Toxicity can stem from noncompliance. For example, an elderly patient may fail to take the prescribed dose or follow the correct schedule, or he may prematurely stop his medication. He may consume medications prescribed for a previous disorder or indiscriminately take medications ordered p.r.n.

To improve compliance, make sure the patient can open his medication bottles easily. If he has arthritis, he should ask the pharmacist for standard caps instead of childproof ones. Find out if he's on a fixed income. If so, he may try to make his medications last longer. Warn against decreasing or stopping his medication.

If he skips meals, he may miss doses scheduled at mealtimes. If he has difficulty swallowing pills, suggest crushing them (unless contraindicated) and mixing them with pureed food.

Teaching Patients about Drug Therapy

Typically, you'll be responsible for teaching the patient about his prescribed drug. First, you'll need to note the name of the drug, including trade and generic brands, and its purpose. That way, the patient can judge whether the drug is working. Also describe drug characteristics, such as its size and shape (for tablets and capsules), consistency (for liquids), color, and taste, if applicable, so he'll be sure he's taking the correct drug. Review the dose, schedule, and administration route and any special precautions or instructions to follow when taking the drug. Teach him what adverse reactions to report to his doctor. Finally, mention any specific tips for storing the drug. See *Taking Medications Correctly*, pages 8 and 9, for more information.

DIETARY THERAPY

Promoting Good Nutrition

Good nutrition supports cellular growth and reproduction and helps the body resist infection and recover from trauma or disease.

To make good nutrition part of your patient's life-style, teach him to eat a well-balanced diet. Have him select from the four food groups daily, following these guidelines:
- milk group (milk and dairy products, such as yogurt, cheese, and ice cream): 2 to 3 cups daily for children under age 9; 3 or more cups for ages 9 to 12; 4 or more cups for teenagers; and 2 or more cups for adults.
- meat group (including poultry, fish, legumes, eggs, beef, pork, and lamb): 2 or more servings daily. If the patient is a vegetarian, have him substitute dry beans, peas, or nuts for meat.
- bread and cereal group (including whole grain and enriched breads, rice, cereal, and pasta): no recommended daily amount. Typically, servings from this group account for up to 50% of calories in the American diet and up to 90% in some other countries.
- fruit and vegetable group (including all fruits and vegetables): four or more servings daily.

The government has also developed

TAKING MEDICATIONS CORRECTLY

Dear Patient:

Your doctor has prescribed medication for you to help treat your condition. In order for your medication to be beneficial, however, you must take it *as prescribed*.

Safety tips
• Keep your medication in its original container or in a properly labeled prescription bottle. If you're taking more than one medication, do *not* mix them together in a pillbox.
• Store your medication in a cool, dry place or as directed by your pharmacist. *Don't* keep it in the bathroom medicine cabinet, where heat and humidity may cause it to lose its effectiveness. All containers should have childproof caps and should be kept out of the reach of children. (The top shelf of a closet is a good storage place.)
• Always take your medication in a well-lit room. Read the label to make sure you're taking the right medication. If you don't understand the directions, ask your pharmacist or doctor for clarification.
• Don't take medication whose expiration date has passed. Not only will it be ineffective, but it may be harmful. Discard the medication by flushing it down the toilet.

• If you miss a dose or several doses, ask your doctor or pharmacist for further directions (unless you were given specific instructions beforehand.)
• Refill all prescriptions promptly so you don't run out of medication when the pharmacy is closed.
• Have all prescriptions filled at the same store so that the pharmacist can keep a complete record of your medications. Inform him of any medication allergies and any nonprescription drugs you're taking.
• Don't start taking any nonprescription drugs without first checking with your pharmacist about potential interactions with other drugs you're taking. (Remember, nonprescription drugs can be harmful, too, if not taken correctly.) If you're taking a nonprescription drug, call your doctor if your condition doesn't improve after a few days.
• If you're pregnant or breast-feeding, speak to your doctor before taking any medication or home remedy. Some drugs may be harmful to the fetus.
• Your medication has been prescribed specifically for you. Do *not* share it with other members of your family or with friends; they could have a serious allergic reaction.

Administration tips

- Make a medication calendar. To do this, use a calendar with enough space to write in the names of the drugs and the times you should take them each day. Then put a check mark next to the drug when you take it.
- Set your alarm clock to go off when it's time to take your medication. Or ask a friend or relative to remind you.
- Write down the following information about each of your medications on index cards or on a chart: its name, its purpose, its appearance, directions for taking it, special cautions or side effects, and when to take it.
- Don't forget that most drugs cause side effects. Make sure you know the potential side effects that your medication can cause, especially those that must be reported to your doctor or pharmacist. If you have any questions about symptoms you're experiencing while taking your medication, call your doctor immediately.

Additional information for your prescribed medication

_____

_____

_____

_____

_____

_____

_____

_____

_____

_____

_____

a list of recommended daily allowances (RDAs), which can help the patient plan his meals. RDAs specify the recommended daily consumption of many essential nutrients. However, by eating a well-balanced diet from the four food groups, a person should receive a sufficient amount of essential nutrients. RDAs are intended as guidelines only for healthy people. Pregnancy, chronic disease, infection, or trauma will increase nutritional requirements.

Combating disease with proper nutrition

Many diseases result or can worsen from a deficiency or an excess of essential nutrients. As a result, dietary modifications often serve as a curative—and preventive—treatment. For example, reducing dietary cholesterol and saturated fats can reduce the risk of coronary artery disease. Reducing carbohydrates and fats, coupled with exercise, can promote weight loss and ease cardiac work load. Restricting sodium can lower blood pressure.

In electrolyte deficiency, dietary supplements can restore and maintain normal serum levels.

Monitoring Dietary Therapy

To evaluate the effectiveness of dietary therapy, you'll need to record the patient's daily weight and monitor his laboratory tests.

Tracking daily weight

One of the most objective ways of monitoring dietary therapy, weight helps evaluate the balance between caloric intake and energy expenditure. It also reflects changes in hydration, helping you assess fluid retention or the effectiveness of diuretic therapy or dialysis.

If possible, weigh the patient at the same time each day on the same type of scale. Also, be sure that he's wearing similar clothing each time.

Warn the patient about the hazards of popular weight-loss diets. For example, nutritional deficiencies can stem from eliminating foods or by restricting intake to one food, such as grapefruit. Emphasize the importance of maintaining dietary protein to preserve muscle strength and tone and to allow tissue healing. However, advise against liquid protein drinks. Although high in protein and devoid of carbohydrates and fats, these drinks predispose a person to ketosis.

Recognize that those who diet without supervision are also prone to electrolyte imbalances. Two of the most common are hypokalemia, caused by indiscriminate use of diuretics and abstinence from potassium-rich foods, and hypernatremia, caused by overreliance on low-calorie, high-sodium frozen dinners.

What laboratory tests reveal

Laboratory tests evaluate nutritional status and monitor dietary therapy. These blood and urine tests evaluate nutrients absorbed from the GI tract or products for cellular use; waste products en route to the kidneys, lungs, or liver; and blood components. For example, serum levels of cholesterol and triglycerides help determine if the patient is ingesting too much fat. Blood glucose levels determine if the body's insulin supply is adequate to digest dietary sugars. Nitrogen balance compares nitrogen intake and output; a negative balance indicates inadequate intake of protein or calories.

Encouraging Compliance

No matter what the goal of dietary therapy, you can help encourage the patient's compliance by adapting therapy as much as possible to his food preferences and daily routine. When helping the patient find substitutes for foods he must avoid, consider his income and life-style. Does he typically eat "on the run" or does he enjoy spending time in the kitchen? Are his favorite foods highly spiced or bland? Emphasize that even if the patient must follow a special diet, it must be a well-balanced one to avoid new nutritional problems.

SURGERY

Surgery may range from minor to major, from conservative to radical. This treatment can be classified as elective, required, urgent, or emergency.

Elective surgery is primarily a matter of choice. Although the patient can survive without it, the surgery may improve his comfort or self-esteem. Examples include dermatologic surgery, such as scar removal, or plastic surgery, such as breast reduction or augmentation.

Required surgery is recommended by the doctor, and the patient may eagerly comply because of discomfort. This surgery may be delayed even though it's inevitable. Examples include herniorrhaphy (without incarceration) and removal of impacted wisdom teeth.

Urgent surgery is also inevitable but shouldn't be delayed. This surgery aims to restore health or prevent the patient's condition from deteriorating. Examples include repair of perforated peptic ulcer and incarcerated hernia.

A dramatic or sudden change in the patient's condition may demand *emergency* surgery. Preoperative preparation may be abbreviated or omitted to get the patient into the operating room as quickly as possible. Examples include emergency open-heart surgery and repair of a traumatic amputation.

Performing a Preoperative Assessment

A thorough preoperative assessment helps systematically identify and correct problems before surgery and establishes a baseline for postoperative comparison. When performing this assessment, focus on problem areas suggested by the patient's history and on any body system that will be directly affected by the surgery.

Assess cardiovascular status

Begin by inspecting the chest for any abnormal pulsations. Then auscultate at the fifth intercostal space over the left midclavicular line. If you can't hear an apical pulse, ask the patient to turn onto his left side; the heart may shift closer to the chest wall. Note the rate and quality of the apical pulse. Next, auscultate heart sounds. If you hear thrills, suspect mitral valve regurgitation or stenosis. Remember that murmurs you hear on the right side of the heart are more likely to change with respiration than left-sided murmurs. Diminished breath sounds may point to emphysema. Or the patient may have an unusually thick chest wall.

Palpate radial and pedal pulses bilaterally and note any differences in quality, rate, or rhythm. Also, check for extremity coolness or edema. Compare blood pressure bilaterally, using a cuff two-thirds the length of the patient's arm. A difference greater than 15 mm Hg in systolic or diastolic pressure may indicate unilateral arterial compression or obstruction. Remember that preoperative anxiety may spuriously elevate systolic pressure.

Check the chest and lungs

First, inspect the patient's chest for scars suggesting previous surgery.

Next, assess his respiratory rate and pattern. Check for asymmetrical chest expansion and use of accessory muscles. Auscultate the lungs for diminished breath sounds and crackles or rhonchi. Differentiate crackles from rhonchi by asking the patient to cough; crackles will not clear with coughing.

Now check for circumoral and nailbed pallor, which may indicate recent hypoxia. Clubbing of the fingers, barrel chest, and cyanotic earlobes indicate the chronic hypoxia and hypercapnia that are characteristic of chronic obstructive pulmonary disease. Be sure to chart any shortness of breath or cough (note with or without sputum).

An alternative to inhalation anesthesia, such as a spinal block, may be required if the patient has questionable pulmonary status.

Perform a GI assessment

After inspecting abdominal contour and symmetry, auscultate bowel sounds in each quadrant. Then palpate the abdomen for any tenderness or distention; percuss for air and fluid. Don't palpate before auscultating to avoid stimulating peristalsis.

Chart intake and output, if ordered. Also assess the patency and function of any ostomy appliances.

Assess the genitourinary system

First, palpate above the symphysis pubis for any bladder distention. Then obtain a sample for urinalysis and, if it smells foul, for cultures. If ordered, monitor urinary output and try to correlate any excess or deficit with blood urea nitrogen or creatinine levels. If urinary output falls, first assess catheter patency, if applicable. Also check for pedal edema and bibasilar crackles, which may signal impending congestive heart failure.

Assess neurologic function

Begin by evaluating the patient's orientation to person, place, and time. However, recognize that anxiety may make him slightly disoriented. Note whether his pupils are uniform in size and shape.

Assess the patient's gross motor function (for example, how he walks) and fine motor function (how he writes). Look for any neurologic changes, such as slurred speech. Of course, check first whether the patient has removed his dentures. Inform the doctor of any behavorial changes, from lethargy to agitation, which may herald increased intracranial pressure.

Appraise psychological status

Psychological barriers like depression can significantly interfere with recovery from surgery. Preparing the patient psychologically for surgery is just as important as preparing him physically. Set aside plenty of time to allow him to discuss his feelings about the impending surgery. Give him the option of seeing a clergyman. Be understanding if he displays regressive behavior; any patient, regardless of his age, may show regression when placed in the same stressful situation. Expect some anxiety. However, if the patient seems inappropriately relaxed or unconcerned, consider the possibility that he's suppressing his fears. Such a patient may cope poorly with surgical stress.

Encourage the patient to draw support from his family or friends. If possible, allow them to visit with the patient preoperatively. Also, include them in your nursing care plan. If they feel as calm and confident as possible, they can provide invaluable emotional support for the patient.

Finally, make sure the patient doesn't have any lingering questions about the surgery. Typically, the doctor will answer most of his questions, but you should evaluate the patient's understanding and clear up any misconceptions. Remember, before the patient can sign an informed consent for surgery, he must be aware of the procedure and the risks involved. Never have a patient sign a consent form if his understanding is questionable.

Preparing the Patient for Surgery

Among your other key responsibilities before surgery are patient teaching, coordinating and charting the results of diagnostic tests, and giving preoperative medications.

Patient teaching about coughing and deep-breathing exercises, positioning, and monitoring or supportive equipment (such as a nasogastric tube) can improve compliance and decrease the risk of postoperative complications.

Charting the results of diagnostic tests provides a baseline for postoperative assessment. Typically, the patient will have had a chest X-ray to screen for pulmonary and cardiac problems, and laboratory tests, such as a complete blood count and serum electrolyte and blood urea nitrogen studies, to evaluate basic body functions.

If the patient's scheduled for morning surgery, the doctor will usually order a sedative the night before to ensure a good night's sleep. Keep these tips in mind: never mix more than two medications in a syringe; always give diazepam alone; and select an injection site that's suited to the patient's age and development.

A final check before surgery

The morning of surgery, follow these important steps:
- Verify that the patient has been NPO since midnight. Ensure that he has signed a consent form.
- Be sure the results of ordered diagnostic tests appear on the chart.
- Tell the patient to remove jewelry, makeup, or nail polish. Ask the patient to shower with antimicrobial soap, if ordered, and to perform mouth care. Warn against swallowing water.
- Instruct him to remove any dentures or partial plates. Note on the chart if the patient has dental crowns, caps, or braces. Also have him remove contact lenses, glasses, prostheses (such as an artificial eye), or hearing aids.
- Tell the patient to void and to put on a surgical cap and gown.
- Take and record his vital signs.
- Give preoperative medication.

Variations for same-day surgery

When the patient's scheduled for same-day surgery, he'll have preoperative tests performed before admission. Also, he'll usually bring a signed consent form with him. Be sure to check when the tests were performed as well as when he signed the consent form. Keep in mind that a signed consent form older than 24 hours isn't legally binding.

As before, you'll need to prepare the patient physically and psychologically, but you'll have limited time to do so. Your teaching about postoperative care is crucial since you'll have few, if any, opportunities for reinforcement.

Performing a Postoperative Assessment

The patient's recovery largely depends on the care he receives postoperatively. When assessing him, be systematic yet sensitive to his needs. Compare your findings with the preoperative assessment and report any significant changes immediately. (See *Recognizing and Managing Common Postoperative Complications*, pages 14 and 15.)

Check vital signs

Begin by verifying that the patient has a patent airway and by checking his *respiratory rate, rhythm, and depth*. Excessive sedation from analgesics or a general anesthetic can cause respiratory depression.

Observe for tracheal deviation from

RECOGNIZING AND MANAGING COMMON POSTOPERATIVE COMPLICATIONS

Despite your best efforts to prepare the patient for surgery and its aftermath, complications sometimes still occur. Fortunately, though, by knowing how to recognize and manage them, you can limit their effect. Common postoperative complications include hypovolemia, septicemia, septic shock, atelectasis, pneumonia, thrombophlebitis, and pulmonary embolism.

HYPOVOLEMIA

Characterized by decreased blood volume, hypovolemia may result from blood loss, severe dehydration, third-space fluid sequestration (as in burns, peritonitis, intestinal obstruction, or acute pancreatitis), or abnormal fluid loss (as in excessive vomiting or diarrhea). This complication develops when the patient loses from 15% to 25% of his total blood volume.

To detect hypovolemia, check for hypotension and a rapid, feeble pulse. You'll also find cool, clammy, and perhaps slightly mottled skin; rapid, shallow respirations; oliguria or anuria; and lethargy.

To treat hypovolemia:
• Administer I.V. crystalloids, such as normal saline solution or Ringer's lactate, to increase blood pressure.
• To restore urinary output and fluid volume, administer colloids, such as plasma, albumin, or dextran.

SEPTICEMIA AND SEPTIC SHOCK

Septicemia, a severe systemic infection, may result from a break in asepsis during surgery or wound care or from peritonitis (as in ruptured appendix or ectopic pregnancy). The most common causative organism in postoperative septicemia is *Escherichia coli.*

Septic shock occurs when bacteria release endotoxins into the bloodstream. The endotoxins decrease vascular resistance, resulting in dramatic hypotension.

To detect septicemia, check for fever, chills, rash, abdominal distention, prostration, pain, headache, nausea, or diarrhea.

To detect septic shock, watch for these additional symptoms: a drastic fall in blood pressure, tachycardia, tachypnea, flushed skin, confusion, and perhaps coma. An elevated white blood cell count is also characteristic in septic shock.

To treat septicemia:
• Obtain specimens (blood, wound, and urine) for culture and sensitivity tests to verify the cause of septicemia and guide treatment. Then administer antibiotics, as ordered.
• Monitor vital signs and level of consciousness to detect septic shock.

To treat septic shock:
• Administer I.V. antibiotics, as ordered. Monitor serum peak and trough levels to help ensure effective therapy.
• Give I.V. fluids and blood or blood products to restore circulating blood volume.

ATELECTASIS AND PNEUMONIA

In atelectasis, incomplete lung expansion causes the distal alveoli to collapse. After surgery, this complication usually results from excessive retained secretions, which provide an excellent medium for bacterial growth and set the stage for stasis pneumonia. In this acute inflammation, the alveoli and bronchioles become plugged with a fibrous exudate, making them firm and inelastic.

---

midline. As you auscultate the lungs, note any chest asymmetry, unequal lung expansion, or use of accessory muscles. Diminished breath sounds at the lung bases commonly occur in the patient who has inhaled the anesthetic and in those with chronic obstructive pulmonary disease (COPD) or heavy smoking habits. Encourage coughing and deep breathing to promote excre-

tion of the anesthetic and optimal gas exchange and acid-base balance. This will also help you assess the patient's level of consciousness by testing his ability to follow commands.

Next, assess the patient for cyanosis. Circumoral, nail bed, or sublingual cyanosis denotes an arterial oxygen saturation less than 80%. Earlobe cyanosis, usually accompanying COPD,

To detect atelectasis, auscultate for diminished or absent breath sounds over the affected area and note flatness on percussion. Observe for decreased chest expansion and mediastinal shift toward the side of collapse. Also, assess for fever, restlessness or confusion, worsening dyspnea, and increased blood pressure, pulse, and respiratory rate.

To detect pneumonia, watch for sudden onset of shaking chills with high fever and headache. Again, auscultate for diminished breath sounds or for telltale crackles over the affected lung area. Assess the patient for dyspnea, tachypnea, and sharp chest pain that's exacerbated by inspiration. He may also develop a productive cough with pinkish or rust-colored sputum. Observe for cyanosis with hypoxemia, confirmed by arterial blood gas measurement. Chest X-rays demonstrate patchy infiltrates or areas of consolidation.

To treat atelectasis or pneumonia:
• Encourage the patient to cough and deep-breathe every 1 to 2 hours while he's awake. Show him how to use an incentive spirometer to facilitate deep breathing.
• Perform chest physiotherapy, if ordered.
• Administer antibiotics, if ordered.
• Administer humidified air or oxygen to loosen secretions, as ordered.
• Elevate the head of the patient's bed to reduce pressure on the diaphragm and to encourage optimal lung expansion.
• Reposition the patient at least every 2 hours to prevent pooling of secretions.

THROMBOPHLEBITIS AND PULMONARY EMBOLISM

Postoperative venous stasis associated with immobility predisposes the patient to thrombophlebitis—an inflammation of a vein, usually in the leg, accompanied by clot formation. If a clot breaks away, it may become lodged in the lung, causing a pulmonary embolism. This obstruction of a pulmonary artery interrupts blood flow, thereby decreasing gas exchange in the lungs.

To detect thrombophlebitis, watch for telltale signs along the length of a superficial vein. For example, the vessel will feel hard and thready or cordlike and will be extremely sensitive to pressure; the surrounding area may be red, swollen, and warm. Also note any swelling along the affected leg, especially at the ankle, as well as pale, cold skin. Recognize that deep vein thrombophlebitis is characterized by aching or cramping pain, especially in the calf, when the patient walks or dorsi-flexes the foot (Homans' sign).

To detect a pulmonary embolism, assess for sudden anginal or pleuritic chest pain; dyspnea; rapid, shallow respirations; cyanosis; restlessness; and possibly a thready pulse. Auscultate for fine to coarse crackles over the affected lung area.

To treat thrombophlebitis:
• Elevate the affected leg and apply warm compresses and antiembolism stockings.
• Offer analgesics, as ordered.
• Administer I.V. heparin, if ordered, to hinder clot formation. During this therapy, monitor prothrombin and partial thromboplastin times daily.

To treat a pulmonary embolism:
• Administer oxygen by face mask or nasal cannula, as ordered, to improve tissue perfusion.
• Administer an analgesic and I.V. heparin, as ordered.
• Elevate the head of the patient's bed to relieve dyspnea.

---

may be exacerbated by anesthesia. Also assess for other signs of respiratory distress, including nasal flaring, inspiratory or expiratory grunts, changes in posture to ease breathing, and progressive disorientation.

After assessing respiratory rate, take the patient's *blood pressure.* Systolic pressure shouldn't vary more than 15% from the preoperative reading. (An exception is the patient who is hypotensive preoperatively.) Administration of I.V. fluids and blood products during surgery can increase both systolic and diastolic pressures. Also, be aware of any drugs given during surgery, so you can evaluate their potential vasodilative or vasoconstrictive effects.

Typically, the patient is placed in a supine position. Remember that rapid changes in position may cause ortho-static hypotension associated with lingering vasodilative effects of the anesthetic. Conversely, postoperative pain may increase systolic pressure by causing sympathetic and parasympathetic stimulation.

After checking blood pressure, take the patient's *temperature*. The route will vary with the patient's age and the type of surgery he's had. Rectal temperature is preferred over axillary temperature for infants and young children. In the adult cardiac patient, though, rectal temperature can cause vagal stimulation; therefore, oral or axillary temperature is preferred. Oral temperature is contraindicated if the patient is still groggy from the effects of anesthesia. Recognize, too, that slowing of basal metabolism associated with anesthesia may cause postoperative hypothermia. Provide blankets, as necessary. Also be aware that a slight fever is equally likely—the result of the body's response to the trauma of surgery. Fever may also signal infection or dehydration.

After assessing temperature, count the patient's *heart rate* for 1 minute. An irregular rhythm may reflect the effects of anesthesia or may be a pre-existing arrhythmia, such as atrial fibrillation. Assess the rate and quality of radial and pedal pulses, and note any dependent edema. Compare this data against the preoperative assessment to confirm any significant changes. An overly rapid pulse rate may signal bleeding, dehydration, or shock. Correlate pulse rate with blood pressure, urine output, and overall clinical status to verify any of the above.

Record intake and output

Postoperative intake measures food and oral fluids, including ice chips, as well as I.V. fluids and blood products. If the patient is receiving peritoneal dialysis or three-way bladder irrigation after surgery, you'll probably keep a separate flow sheet to identify positive or negative fluid balance.

A minimum output of 30 ml/hour is acceptable for an adult. Many patients have difficulty voiding after surgery, though, because of decreased parasympathetic stimulation. Palpate the patient's bladder regularly to assess the need for catheterization. Because anesthesia slows peristalsis, fecal output isn't usually measured until bowel sounds return.

Other sources of output include nasogastric contents and wound drainage. With Hemovac and Jackson Pratt drainage devices, you can measure drainage precisely because both devices are secured through the suture line into the operative site. Wound drainage can also be estimated by observing the amount of staining on dressings.

When documenting output, note the source of output; its quantity, color, and consistency; and the duration over which the output occurred. Notify the doctor of significant changes, such as a change in the color and consistency of nasogastric contents from dark green to "coffee grounds."

Provide comfort measures

All too often following surgery, the patient may be unable to assume a comfortable position because of activity restrictions, immobilization devices, or an array of tubes and monitoring lines. As a result, assess the patient's level of comfort and offer analgesics, as ordered. Although most patients will complain when they experience severe pain, some may suffer silently. Their only signs may be increased pulse rate and blood pressure. Recognize that emotional support can do much to relieve pain. Physical measures, such as positioning, back rubs, and creating a comfortable environment in the patient's room, can also promote comfort and decrease the need for analgesics or, at least, enhance their effectiveness.

After administering an analgesic, always document the dose, administration site, and patient's response. Note positioning that may have enhanced the drug's effectiveness as well as specific safety measures, such as raising side rails, to protect the patient's welfare.

Examine the surgical wound

No matter where the patient's incision is located, you'll need to closely examine it. First, note the wound's location and describe its length, width, and type (horizontal, transverse, or puncture). Next, document the type of dressing, if any. Is the dressing stained by drainage? If so, estimate its quantity and note its color and odor. Or, if the patient has a drainage device, record the amount of drainage. Make sure the device is secure. If the patient has a colostomy, note any fecal output. Describe the number of any sutures, staples, or Steri-strips used to close the wound and assess approximation of wound edges.

Assess the abdomen

For postoperative abdominal assessment, you'll rely on the skills of observation and auscultation. First, observe for changes in abdominal contour. Abdominal dressings and tubes or other devices may distort this contour. To detect abdominal asymmetry, stand at the foot of the patient's bed to view the abdomen.

Next, measure abdominal girth for a baseline to help promptly identify intraabdominal bleeding. Also, observe for Cullen's sign—a bluish hue around the umbilicus that often accompanies intraabdominal or peritoneal bleeding.

Auscultate bowel sounds in all four quadrants for at least 1 minute per quadrant. Typically, you won't be able to detect bowel sounds for at least 6 hours after surgery, since the anesthetic (except local) slows peristalsis. Repeat auscultation every 2 hours.

If the patient has a nasogastric tube, regularly check its patency. If you suspect tube displacement, try to aspirate gastric contents. Or confirm proper tube placement by instilling air with a bulb syringe while you auscultate over the epigastric area.

Reducing the Risk of Postoperative Complications

To avoid extending the patient's hospital stay and to speed his recovery, perform the following measures to prevent postoperative complications.

Turn and reposition the patient

Turning and repositioning the patient every 2 hours promotes circulation, thereby reducing the risk of skin breakdown—especially over bony prominences. When the patient's in a lateral recumbent position, tuck pillows under bony prominences to reduce friction and promote comfort. Each time you turn the patient, carefully inspect the skin to detect redness or other signs of breakdown.

Keep in mind that turning and repositioning may be contraindicated in some patients, such as those who've undergone neurologic or musculoskeletal surgery that demands immobilization postoperatively.

Encourage coughing and deep breathing

This promotes lung expansion, which helps clear anesthetics from the body. Coughing and deep breathing also decrease the risk of pulmonary and fat emboli and of hypostatic pneumonia associated with secretion buildup in the airways.

Encourage the patient to cough and deep-breathe at least every 2 hours (except after craniotomy, to avoid increasing intracranial pressure). Show him how to use an incentive spirometer.

Monitor nutrition and fluids

Adequate nutrition and fluids are essential to ensure proper hydration, promote healing, and provide energy to match the increased basal metabolism

HOW TO APPLY DRY DRESSINGS

Dear Patient:

As directed by the doctor, you'll need to change your dressing _____ times a day. Here's how.

1

First, gather several 4" × 4" gauze pads, cleansing solution (such as povidone-iodine), and sterile lukewarm water (boiled for 5 minutes) to wet the gauze pads. Also collect a sterile bowl (washed, rinsed, and immersed in boiling water for 5 minutes), baby oil, surgical tape, scissors, a plastic bag, and rubber gloves.

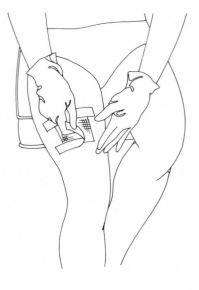

2

Wash your hands, and put on rubber gloves. Then, to remove the tape, hold your skin taut and pull the old tape strips toward the wound (as shown at the top of the next column). Remove *all* the old tape. If the tape sticks, soften it with baby oil.

3

Now, slowly remove the old dressing. Does it stick to the wound? If so, stop and moisten the dressing with sterile lukewarm water. When the dressing's loose, remove it. Then discard it in the plastic bag.

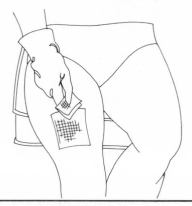

4

Before you clean the wound, examine it carefully for any changes since the last dressing change, especially an increase in swelling, redness, drainage or pus, or odor. If you think the wound looks worse, contact your doctor.

5

Take one of the gauze pads and saturate it with sterile water and cleansing solution. Then fold the pad into quarters. Holding the pad as shown, gently wipe from the top of the wound to the bottom in one motion. Then discard this pad in the plastic bag.

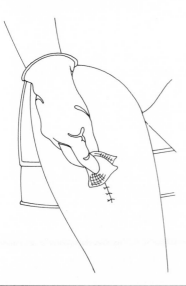

6

Saturate another gauze pad, fold it into quarters, and wipe the wound again, this time on one side first and then on the other. Do this several times to clean the entire wound area that the dressing will cover. Then use another clean gauze pad to pat the wound dry. Remove the rubber gloves and discard them in the plastic bag.

7

Next, apply a clean gauze pad over the area. Depending on the amount of drainage, use several layers of pads. As the nurse has demonstrated, secure the pads with tape or with

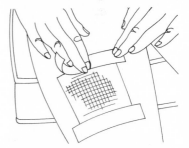

Montgomery straps (lengths of adhesive tape used in place of taping directly to the skin to make dressing changes easier). Be sure you've collected all soiled material in the plastic bag. Tie the bag, and dispose of it properly.

associated with surgery. If the patient has a protein deficiency or compromised immune function preoperatively, expect to deliver supplemental protein via hyperalimentation to promote healing. If he has renal failure, this treatment would be contraindicated. Why? The patient's inability to break down protein could lead to dangerously high blood nitrogen levels.

Because carbohydrates supply the body's major source of energy, provide a diet high in carbohydrates and calories but low in polysaccharides. If the patient will be immobilized for a prolonged period, also make sure he receives added high-density lipoproteins (such as vegetable fats) to counteract the breakdown of subcutaneous fat stores and provide extra energy.

Meticulously record intake and output, watch for signs of dehydration and edema, and monitor serum electrolyte levels. Keep in mind the type of surgery the patient has had. For example, after GI surgery, the patient's at risk for potassium, hydrogen, and chloride imbalance. Why? These electrolytes are concentrated in the stomach and may be lost via postoperative suctioning or vomiting. Learn to recognize signs of electrolyte imbalances; for example, arrhythmias may signal potassium imbalance, whereas thirst and decreased skin turgor may signal sodium imbalance. To avoid or correct an electrolyte imbalance, administer supplemental electrolytes, as ordered.

Provide wound care

This three-step process involves assessing, cleansing, and redressing the patient's surgical wound. Always observe sterile technique during wound care to reduce the risk of nosocomial infection. When assessing the wound, first note its location. Then describe the number and condition of any sutures or staples. Is the skin around the wound red or warm to the touch? Have any sutures or staples pulled out? Are they tearing the skin?

If the wound is draining, describe the amount, color, odor, and consistency of the drainage. Record any topical ointments applied as well as the number, type, and size of dressings. On the tape securing the dressing, note the date and time of each dressing change. If the patient is allergic to tape or has a bulky dressing, use Montgomery straps to reduce skin irritation associated with frequent removal and reapplication of tape.

Promote exercise and ambulation

Early postoperative exercise and ambulation can significantly reduce the risk of thromboembolism as well as improve ventilation and brighten the patient's outlook.

Perform passive range-of-motion exercises—or better yet, encourage active range-of-motion exercises—to prevent joint contractures and muscle atrophy and to promote circulation. These exercises can also help you assess the patient's strength and tolerance.

Before encouraging ambulation, have the patient dangle at the side of the bed and perform deep-breathing exercises. How well the patient tolerates this step is often a key factor in predicting out-of-bed tolerance.

Begin ambulation by helping the patient walk a few feet from his bed to a sturdy chair. Then have him gradually progress each day from ambulating in his room to ambulating in the hallway, with or without assistance, as necessary. Document the frequency of ambulation and the patient's tolerance, including his use of analgesics.

Discharge Planning

Effective discharge planning begins at admission. To individualize discharge planning and promote compliance, you'll need to identify goals for the patient and evaluate his success in achieving them. For example, if the patient will be injecting insulin himself, you'll need to allow sufficient time for teaching, demonstration, and return demonstration.

Another way to increase compliance is to give the patient an index card listing each medication that he must take at home as well as its dose and schedule. If the patient has had surgery, you'll need to teach him about changing his wound dressing and reporting any complications. (See *How to Apply Dry Dressings*, pages 18 and 19.) Also, outline any postoperative activity restrictions, such as refraining from sexual intercourse for several weeks after cardiac surgery.

through the urinary tract. Another treatment, percutaneous transluminal coronary angioplasty, can now replace more risky coronary artery bypass grafting in some patients with occluded coronary arteries.

Besides being less risky than many traditional treatments, these alternatives—and many others like them—typically cost less and entail a shorter hospital stay. At times, they can be performed on an outpatient basis. What's more, they're less disruptive to the patient's life since recovery time is faster and associated disability occurs less commonly.

TREATMENT ALTERNATIVES

A LOOK AHEAD

Although drug and dietary therapy and surgery are among the main treatment choices for a patient, other treatments fall outside these categories. Some serve as alternatives to more traditional surgery. For example, where kidney stones were once removed by surgery, they can now be pulverized by shock waves in a treatment called extracorporeal shock wave lithotripsy, then easily passed

Scientific and technological breakthroughs continue to expand the range and effectiveness of treatments. This trend, of course, is likely to continue. And with it will come increased nursing responsibilities. Keeping current with emergent trends (plus perfecting your traditional duties) will enhance your skills and make you an increasingly valuable member of the health care team.

Selected References

Beyers, Marjorie, et al. *The Clinical Practice of Medical-Surgical Nursing*, 2nd ed. Boston: Little, Brown & Co., 1984.

Brunner, Lillian, and Suddarth, Doris. *Textbook of Medical-Surgical Nursing*, 5th ed. Philadelphia: J.B. Lippincott Co., 1984.

Cataldo, Corrine, and Whitney, Eleanor. *Nutrition and Dietary Therapy: Principles and Practice*. St. Paul: West Publishing Co., 1985.

Hahn, Anne, et al. *Pharmacology in Nursing*, 16th ed. St. Louis: C.V. Mosby Co., 1985.

Nursing88 Drug Handbook. Springhouse, Pa.: Springhouse Corp., 1988.

Potter, Patricia, and Perry, Anne. *Fundamentals of Nursing: Concepts, Process and Practice*. St. Louis: C.V. Mosby Co., 1985.

Scipien, Gladys, and Barnard, M. *Comprehensive Pediatric Nursing*, 3rd ed. New York: McGraw-Hill Book Co., 1983.

2 Treating Cardiovascular Dysfunction

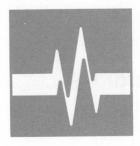

Treating Cardiovascular Dysfunction

Introduction

The ancients believed that the heart was the seat of the soul, the center of a person's being. That notion has since been replaced by a less romantic view, but the heart is just as important to modern medicine as it was to the philosophers of old—and, in its own way, just as mysterious.

The heart is a seemingly simple organ, and yet millions of dollars and years of research haven't yielded a workable mechanical replacement. It's perhaps the most intensively studied and best understood organ in the body, and still heart disease remains the leading cause of death in the United States.

But in recent years the heart has at last begun to yield its secrets, and the result has been a wave of new treatments. Long gone are the days when an MI survivor was sent home from the hospital with a bottle of pills and a prayer. Now he may have thousands of dollars worth of electronic equipment implanted in his chest, a Holter monitor strapped to his waist, or an appointment for cardiac catheterization clutched in his hand.

Much of this progress sounds almost like science fiction: the near-successes that have been achieved with the artificial heart or the discovery of cyclosporine, which has made heart transplants possible for hundreds of patients. Less dramatic, but far more significant for your patients, are the here-and-now advances that have already saved hundreds of thousands of lives: beta blockers and calcium channel blockers, which can prevent MI and help cardiac patients live virtually normal lives; percutaneous transluminal coronary angioplasty, which offers some patients a nonsurgical alternative to coronary artery bypass surgery; streptokinase and tissue-plasminogen activator, which can dissolve clots in coronary arteries and restore perfusion to an ischemic heart muscle in minutes; and cardioassistive devices, which can buy time for a failing heart and perhaps permit it to recover.

Nursing on center stage

Amid all these high-tech advances, you'll find nursing in the spotlight. The new technology has created expanded nursing roles—for example, the operation of intraaortic balloon pumps and ventricular assist devices. But as the treatments in this chapter show, traditional nursing skills continue to remain important, as close patient monitoring, prompt action at the bedside, and patient education have all taken on new dimensions. Indeed, today more than ever before, good nursing care is at the heart of good cardiac care.

DRUG THERAPY

Sympatholytic Antihypertensives

This pharmacologic class includes *clonidine, guanabenz, guanadrel, guanethidine, methyldopa,* the *reserpine derivatives,* and *trimethaphan.* Except for trimethaphan, all these drugs are typically given orally. In hypertensive crisis, though, trimethaphan or the reserpine derivatives are given I.V.

For maintenance therapy, the sympatholytics pose the same obstacle to patient compliance as do many other antihypertensives: their common side effects, such as fatigue and drowsiness, *seem worse* than living with untreated hypertension. The reserpines especially produce severe side effects, such as persistent depression. What's more, many of these drugs interact with other prescribed or over-the-counter (OTC) medications, making safe, long-term therapy difficult. And close patient monitoring is required early in therapy to establish the correct dosage. (See *Comparing Sympatholytic Antihypertensives* for further information on indications, interactions, and related nursing care.)

Purpose and action
To lower blood pressure by blocking adrenergic stimulation of blood vessels.

Monitoring
When the patient begins therapy, monitor his response to the drug and its dosage. Check for common side effects, such as postural hypotension. To do so, take his blood pressure while he's lying down and after he has been standing for at least 10 minutes. (The doctor will also probably evaluate his blood pressure after exercise.) Ideally, his blood pressure while he's standing will be in the normal range, and he won't experience any faintness, dizziness, fatigue, or weakness. Also, check the patient's legs and feet for edema caused by fluid retention.

Review the patient's medication regimen for possible interactions.

Home care instructions
• Reinforce the importance of taking the prescribed medication even though the patient may be asymptomatic. Reassure him that side effects should diminish within 4 to 6 weeks. However, if they persist, he should notify his doctor so that the dosage can be adjusted. Warn him not to discontinue the drug without consulting his doctor.
• To minimize postural hypotension, tell the patient to avoid standing in one position for a prolonged period, to use an air conditioner in hot weather, and to avoid alcohol and hot showers and baths. Teach him to lie down or place his head between his knees if he feels dizzy, weak, or faint.
• Warn him that side effects may also include drowsiness and nasal congestion. If he's taking guanadrel, instruct him not to use nasal decongestants without a doctor's order since they can precipitate a hypertensive reaction.
• To relieve dry mouth, suggest hard candy, ice chips, chewing gum, or frequent rinsing of his mouth with water. Also recommend using a soft toothbrush and waxed dental floss. If your patient wears dentures, he can remove them and rinse them two or three times a day to keep his gums moistened. Tell him to avoid mouthwashes containing alcohol, since they can further dry his mouth. What's more, suggest that he tell his dentist about his medication regimen since dry mouth can promote tooth demineralization.
• Advise the patient to watch for signs of fluid retention, such as swollen ankles. Tell him to weigh himself every

COMPARING SYMPATHOLYTIC ANTIHYPERTENSIVES

DRUG AND INDICATIONS	INTERACTIONS	SPECIAL CONSIDERATIONS
Clonidine Used for essential, renal, and malignant hypertension	Alcohol, barbiturates, and other sedatives increase hypotensive effects; monoamine oxidase (MAO) inhibitors, tolazoline, and tricyclic antidepressants reduce these effects. Paradoxical hypertension may occur with propranolol.	• Check patient's blood pressure and pulse frequently, especially during dosage adjustment period. • Teach patient ways to avoid postural hypotension. Monitor for dry mouth, sedation, and constipation. In a patient with a history of depression, watch for depressive episodes. • Withdraw drug slowly to prevent rebound hypertension.
Guanabenz Used for mild or moderate hypertension	Alcohol, barbiturates, benzodiazepines, and phenothiazines increase hypotensive effects; tricyclic antidepressants and tolazoline diminish them. Cardiac glycosides, propranolol, and guanethidine cause bradycardia.	• Monitor patient for dry mouth, fatigue, constipation, and depression. • Watch for postural hypotension (even though this side effect occurs less commonly with guanabenz than with other sympatholytics). • Withdraw drug slowly to prevent rebound hypertension.
Guanadrel Used for mild or moderate hypertension	MAO inhibitors, phenothiazines, tricyclic antidepressants, and antihistamines reduce guanadrel's effects. Alcohol and alpha- and beta-adrenergic blockers worsen postural hypotension. Cardiac glycosides may cause bradycardia. Sympathomimetic ingredients in over-the-counter (OTC) cough and cold medications may bring on hypertension.	• Contraindicated in pheochromocytoma or frank congestive heart failure. • Monitor blood pressure during dosage adjustment period. • Teach patient ways to minimize postural hypotension. • Inform doctor of persistent diarrhea, sudden weight gain, or edema. • Watch diabetic patient for signs of hypoglycemia; guanadrel can have additive hypoglycemic effects. • Warn patient not to use OTC cough and cold medications. • Discontinue drug 2 to 3 days before elective surgery to reduce the risk of vascular collapse during anesthesia.
Guanethidine Used for moderate or severe hypertension	Alcohol, levodopa, rauwolfia derivatives, and diuretics enhance hypotensive effects; tricyclic antidepressants, MAO inhibitors, oral contraceptives, phenothiazines, dopamine, and catecholamines diminish these effects. Sympathomimetic ingredients in OTC cough and cold medications may bring on hypertension.	• Contraindicated in pheochromocytoma. • Teach patient ways to minimize postural hypotension. • Can cause transient urinary retention; advise patient to report any hesitancy with urination. • Discontinue drug 2 to 3 days before elective surgery to reduce risk of vascular collapse during anesthesia. • Warn patient to avoid OTC cough and cold medications.

(continued)

COMPARING DRUGS

COMPARING SYMPATHOLYTIC ANTIHYPERTENSIVES *(continued)*

DRUG AND INDICATIONS	INTERACTIONS	SPECIAL CONSIDERATIONS
Methyldopa Used for sustained mild to severe hypertension	Tricyclic antidepressants, phenothiazines, amphetamines, and norepinephrine may cause hypertensive effects. Sympathomimetics in OTC cough and cold preparations may produce similar effects.	• Contraindicated in renal disease. • Draw serum sample before treatment begins to provide baseline hematologic status. Continue to monitor during therapy to detect hemolytic anemia. • Watch for fever and hepatic changes, which could indicate a hypersensitivity reaction; if they occur, stop drug and call doctor. • Monitor patient for sedative effects and signs of postural hypotension. • Watch for signs of fluid retention. Give a diuretic, if ordered. • Warn patient to avoid OTC cough and cold medications.
Reserpine derivatives Used for mild or moderate hypertension	MAO inhibitors may cause excitability and hypertension. Catecholamines may prolong reserpine's action.	• Reserpine derivatives are seldom used because of their severe side effects. • Monitor patient carefully for drug-induced depression. Look for anorexia, insomnia, despondency; stop drug and notify doctor if symptoms occur. Depression can persist for months after drug discontinuation. • Give drug with food or milk to decrease GI upset. • Monitor for sedative effects. • Watch for signs of fluid retention. • Discontinue drug 2 to 3 weeks before elective surgery to reduce risk of vascular collapse during anesthesia.
Trimethaphan Used to reduce blood pressure quickly in hypertensive crisis	Prolonged effects may occur with neuromuscular blockers. Decreased effects may occur with sympathomimetics and anti-inflammatory analgesics; additive hypotension may occur with diuretics, preanesthetics, anesthetics, and vasodilators.	• Contraindicated in anemia and respiratory insufficiency. • Give only I.V., using an infusion pump. Give oxygen during treatment. • Monitor blood pressure frequently for severe hypotension. If it occurs, discontinue drug and call doctor. • Be alert for respiratory distress, especially with high doses. • Elevate the head of patient's bed to enhance hypotensive effect; don't elevate it more than 30 degrees to prevent cerebral anoxia. • Watch for and report decreased drug effect; tolerance can develop quickly.

day at the same time and on the same scale, and to call his doctor if he gains 3 lb or more. If his doctor has recommended a salt-restricted diet, explain how sodium contributes to hypertension and fluid retention.

Angiotensin-Converting-Enzyme Inhibitors

The newest class of antihypertensive drugs, angiotensin-converting-enzyme (ACE) inhibitors have rapidly gained popularity among clinicians. These drugs, *captopril* and *enalapril*, can be used alone or in combination with other drugs—especially thiazide diuretics—as the first step of antihypertensive therapy in patients with normal renal function. They're also used for severe congestive heart failure in patients who don't respond to cardiac glycosides and diuretics.

However, because ACE inhibitors can cause severe side effects, they're generally reserved for patients who experience intolerable side effects from other antihypertensive drugs or fail to respond to them. These drugs commonly produce renal dysfunction, such as insufficiency and nephrotic syndrome, and thus are contraindicated in renal impairment. In addition, neutropenia may develop several weeks after initiation of therapy. For this reason, ACE inhibitors should be used cautiously in patients with autoimmune disease (especially systemic lupus erythematosus) or immunosuppression. Because these drugs can cause severe hypotension, they should be given carefully to patients with volume depletion or severe hyponatremia.

Purpose and action
By inhibiting angiotensin-converting enzyme, these drugs prevent pulmonary conversion of angiotensin I to angiotensin II. This lessens arterial resistance and afterload, decreasing cardiac work load, and curtails aldosterone secretion, reducing fluid retention. The net effect: lower blood pressure.

Monitoring
Before starting ACE inhibitor therapy, evaluate the results of hematologic and renal and liver function tests. If you detect any abnormalities, such as proteinuria or an elevated white blood cell (WBC) count, hold the drug and notify the doctor; he may need to reconsider the desirability of ACE inhibitor therapy.

Check the patient's drug regimen for possible interactions. For example, use of ACE inhibitors with other antihypertensives, ganglionic blocking agents, nitroglycerin, or probenecid increases the effects of ACE inhibitors and may cause additive hypotension, requiring careful blood pressure monitoring. Potassium-sparing diuretics and potassium supplements, which increase renin activity and decrease aldosterone secretion, may cause hyperkalemia in combination with ACE inhibitors. When combining these drugs, carefully monitor the patient's serum potassium levels. Indomethacin and salicylates can decrease the antihypertensive effect of ACE inhibitors; patients taking these drugs may require increased dosages of ACE inhibitors.

If the patient is taking a diuretic or adhering to a sodium-restricted diet, watch for a precipitous drop in blood pressure about 3 hours after receiving his initial dose of an ACE inhibitor. If this occurs, place the patient in a supine position and infuse normal saline solution, as ordered.

During ACE inhibitor therapy, monitor the patient's pulse rate and blood pressure frequently and assess him often for edema. Also check his WBC count and differential periodically for changes.

Several weeks after initiation of therapy, watch for the development of neutropenia, marked by mild symptoms of infection.

Home care instructions
• Instruct the patient never to interrupt or discontinue his prescribed medication regimen without consulting his doctor.
• Tell him to take a missed dose as soon as possible, but warn him never to double-dose.
• Because food interferes with ACE inhibitor absorption, instruct the patient to take the drug on an empty stomach 1 hour before meals.
• Tell him to watch for and immediately report any signs of infection (such as fever and sore throat) or swollen hands or feet.
• Also instruct him to report excessive sweating, vomiting, or diarrhea. Explain that the resultant volume deficit may lead to severe hypotension.
• Teach the patient to minimize orthostatic hypotension by rising slowly from a sitting or lying position.
• Advise him to avoid potassium-containing salt substitutes and to limit intake of foods with a high potassium content, such as bananas.

Vasodilator Antihypertensives

The vasodilators *hydralazine* and *minoxidil* treat severe hypertension that proves unmanageable with maximum therapeutic doses of diuretics and adrenergic blocking agents. Oral hydralazine, used alone or with other antihypertensives, treats essential hypertension. When given parenterally, hydralazine lowers blood pressure rapidly.

Because hydralazine usually lowers diastolic pressure more than systolic pressure, it isn't considered a primary treatment for essential hypertension. It should be used cautiously in patients with a hypersensitivity to other antihypertensives, rheumatic heart disease, cerebrovascular accident (CVA), coronary artery disease, aortic aneurysm, renal failure, mitral valve disease, or MI.

The potent vasodilator minoxidil treats severe refractory hypertension. This drug directly dilates arteriolar vessels, thereby decreasing peripheral vascular resistance and profoundly lowering both systolic and diastolic pressures. Because minoxidil spurs adrenal secretion of catecholamines, it's contraindicated in pheochromocytoma. It's also contraindicated in pulmonary hypertension associated with mitral stenosis, CVA, malignant hypertension, drug hypersensitivity, pericardial effusion, renal failure, and coronary insufficiency. Generally, minoxidil isn't given to patients who've recently experienced MI because it precipitates angina and tachycardia.

Purpose and action
These vasodilators directly relax arteriolar smooth muscle (the force opposing ventricular ejection), producing a reflex increase in cardiac output. Minoxidil also causes a reflex increase in heart rate.

Monitoring
If the patient's taking hydralazine, observe him closely for side effects, especially if he's receiving a daily dose exceeding 200 mg. Mild effects include headache, nausea, palpitations, flushing, anxiety, sweating, rapid or irregular heartbeat, depression, and dry mouth. Severe effects, which may require discontinuation of therapy, include numbness and tingling in the extremities, dependent edema, lymphadenopathy, and a lupus erythematosus–like syndrome marked by weakness, joint pain, pruritus, blisters, rash, sore throat, and fever.

Check the patient's drug regimen for concurrent use of diuretics, monoamine oxidase (MAO) inhibitors, or epinephrine. Use of hydralazine with diuretics (particularly diazoxide) or MAO inhibitors can increase hypotensive effects; if you do give these drugs together, carefully monitor the patient's blood pressure. When hydralazine is used with epinephrine, tachycardia and hypotension may result.

During long-term therapy, periodically monitor the patient's complete blood count, lupus erythematosus cell preparation, and antinuclear antibody determinations.

If the patient's taking minoxidil, frequently check his apical pulse and blood pressure. Fluid retention occurs in almost all patients receiving the drug; give loop diuretics, if ordered. Observe for dependent edema and enforce a sodium-restricted diet, as ordered. Weigh the patient daily and report any rapid gain of 3 lb or more.

Note and report other side effects, including flushing or skin redness, chest pain, pruritus, and rash. Keep in mind that up to 80% of patients receiving minoxidil develop hypertrichosis: the elongation, thickening, and darkening of hair on the temples, eyebrows, forehead, and sideburn areas. This extra hair typically appears within the first 6 weeks of therapy but disappears 1 to 6 months after discontinuation of the drug.

Check the patient's drug regimen for possible interactions. Concurrent use of minoxidil with diuretics and other antihypertensives may produce profound hypotension; guanethidine is especially dangerous and should be discontinued before beginning therapy, if possible. Epinephrine or norepinephrine may cause excessive cardiac stimulation, resulting in tachycardia, angina, and congestive heart failure. If the patient's taking either of these drugs, frequently check his blood pressure and pulse.

Home care instructions
• Warn the patient not to discontinue taking his medicine without consulting his doctor.

• Instruct him to take his pulse for 1 minute every morning before getting out of bed. He should call his doctor if he notes a rate above 100 or below 60, if he detects an abnormal rhythm, or if he experiences pain.
• Tell the patient to call the doctor immediately if he experiences dyspnea, dizziness, fainting, swollen feet or hands, chest pain, easy bruising, joint pain, or a rash.
• Instruct him to weigh himself weekly at the same time of day, on the same scale, and wearing the same amount of clothing. If he gains 3 lb or more, he should call his doctor.
• Instruct the patient to take the drug with food to increase absorption.
• Tell him to limit salt intake, as prescribed by the doctor.
• If the patient experiences hypertrichosis from minoxidil, explain that this side effect will disappear once therapy is stopped, although it may take several months. Tell the female patient to use depilatory creams to remove unwanted hair.
• Instruct the patient to change position slowly and not to stand in one position for longer than a minute. Also tell him to avoid hot baths and showers, strenuous exercise, and alcohol consumption.

Beta-Adrenergic Blockers
[Beta blockers]

By inhibiting the sympathetic response to beta-adrenergic stimulation and depressing renin output, beta-adrenergic blockers decrease heart rate, conduction velocity, cardiac output, and myocardial contractility. These powerful drugs are used primarily to control hypertension, either alone or in combination with other drugs (such as diuretics) in the second step of stepped-care antihypertensive therapy. They may also be used to reduce the frequency of angina attacks, to control tachycardia and other arrhythmias, and to minimize damage (and possibly lower mortality) in acute myocardial infarction. They may be given prophylactically to lower the risk of reinfarction.

Beta blockers can be classified into two groups, based on the type of beta-receptors they affect. The selective beta blockers—*acebutolol, atenolol*, and *metoprolol*—act primarily on beta receptors in the heart (beta$_1$-receptors). In contrast, the nonselective beta blockers—*nadolol, pindolol, propranolol*, and *timolol*—inhibit both beta$_1$-receptors and beta$_2$-receptors, which are found in skeletal muscle, blood vessels, and bronchioles. Beta blockers can be further classified by their ability to stimulate beta-adrenergic receptors, an ability known as intrinsic sympathomimetic activity (ISA), or beta-agonist activity. In general, the higher a drug's ISA, the less it lowers cardiac output and produces dangerous side effects, such as bradycardia and bronchoconstriction. Pindolol has the highest ISA of all beta blockers, followed by acebutolol and timolol; the other beta blockers possess low ISAs.

Typically, both selective and nonselective beta blockers are contraindicated in patients with heart block, cardiogenic shock, or congestive heart failure (CHF) and in patients with a hypersensitivity to one of the drugs. Because nonselective beta blockers may inhibit bronchodilation from beta$_2$ stimulation, they shouldn't be given to patients with obstructive respiratory disorders, such as bronchial asthma, allergic rhinitis or other respiratory allergies, chronic obstructive pulmonary disease, or bronchospasm. All beta blockers—but particularly acebutolol, atenolol, and pindolol—should be administered carefully to patients with impaired renal or hepatic function; generally, such patients should receive reduced dosages. Beta blockers can

mask signs of hypoglycemia, such as reduced blood pressure and tachycardia, and so should be used cautiously in diabetes mellitus. Because these drugs can reduce the heart's ability to respond to reflex stimuli, beta blocker therapy should be withdrawn before surgery.

Common side effects of beta blockers include cardiovascular disturbances, such as bradycardia, hypotension, and CHF; and CNS disturbances, such as fatigue, lethargy, and dizziness. These CNS effects occur most commonly with propranolol and metoprolol, because these drugs have moderate lipid solubility and thus can more readily penetrate into the CNS.

The side effects of beta blockers can be so severe that the patient may feel worse during therapy than before it. As a result, noncompliance with the prescribed drug regimen may be one of the foremost problems you face when caring for a patient on beta blocker therapy.

Purpose and action
Beta blockers inhibit the sympathetic response to stress by interfering with the effects of catecholamines on beta-receptors. (See *How Beta Blockers Affect the Sympathetic Nervous System.*) The resultant decrease in cardiac contractility, increase in sympathetic vasoconstriction, and depression of renin secretion help lower blood pressure. In addition, reduced myocardial oxygen requirements help prevent angina and infarction, and reduced adrenergic stimulation helps control arrhythmias.

Monitoring
Always check the patient's apical pulse for 1 minute before administering beta blockers. If you detect a rate below 60 or over 100, withhold the drug and notify the doctor. Monitor the patient's blood pressure frequently throughout therapy and report severe hypotension immediately: the doctor may need to alter the dosage or change drugs.

Also monitor the patient for signs of

HOW BETA BLOCKERS AFFECT
THE SYMPATHETIC NERVOUS SYSTEM

To fully understand what happens when you administer a beta blocker, you need to understand how the sympathetic nervous system works.

A division of the autonomic nervous system, the sympathetic nervous system originates in the thoracic (T1) to lumbar (L2) segments of the spinal cord. Impulses from the brain travel from these nerves to various vital organs, such as the heart, blood vessels, lungs, liver, kidneys, bladder, and intestines, and regulate their activity.

When stimulated, sympathetic nerves secrete norepinephrine and epinephrine, which in turn stimulate receptor sites on the innervated organ. Two major types of receptors exist: alpha and beta. Alpha-receptors are located in blood vessels throughout the body and control vasoconstriction. Beta-receptors are classified according to location: beta$_1$ (heart), which influence heart rate and cardiac contractility, and beta$_2$ (peripheral blood vessels, skeletal muscle, and bronchioles), which control dilation and relaxation in these structures.

Although there are subtle differences in the way each beta blocker influences beta receptors, all of them block the action of norepinephrine and epinephrine at beta$_1$- and beta$_2$-receptor sites. By doing so, they help combat the sympathetic response to beta stimulation and produce opposing physiologic effects.

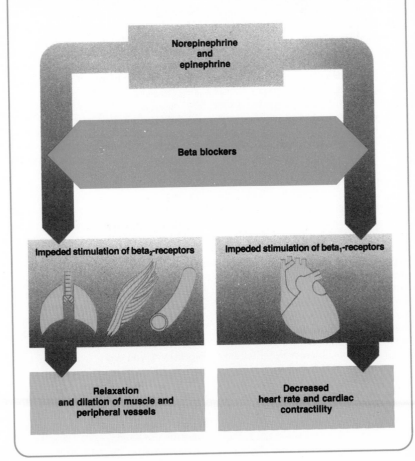

Norepinephrine
and
epinephrine

Beta blockers

Impeded stimulation of beta$_2$-receptors

Impeded stimulation of beta$_1$-receptors

Relaxation
and dilation of muscle and
peripheral vessels

Decreased
heart rate and cardiac
contractility

developing CHF: pulmonary congestion, dyspnea, unexplained weight gain, peripheral edema, and distended neck veins. Weigh the patient daily to assess for fluid retention.

If the patient has a history of respiratory disorders, watch him closely for adverse pulmonary effects, such as airway constriction and dyspnea. Report any such effects to the doctor immediately.

If the patient has diabetes, assess him regularly for symptoms of hypoglycemia that aren't masked by beta blockers, such as diaphoresis, hunger, and fatigue. Because the combined effects of insulin and beta blockers may promote hypoglycemia, the diabetic patient may need readjustment of his medication or dietary regimen.

Check the patient's drug regimen for possible interactions. For example, concurrent use of beta blockers and catecholamine-depleting drugs, such as reserpine, can cause severe hypotension, so monitor blood pressure and heart rate in a patient taking both drugs. Interactions with cardiac glycosides or verapamil can depress cardiac conduction and possibly lead to heart block; watch for and immediately report significant EKG changes. Aminophylline and beta blockers have antagonistic effects; watch the patient for bronchospasm and regulate doses carefully.

To minimize withdrawal symptoms, beta blocker therapy should be discontinued gradually, if possible—ideally, over 1 to 2 weeks. As the drug is discontinued, watch the patient for withdrawal symptoms. Notify the doctor if the patient develops diaphoresis, palpitations, severe headache, chest pain, malaise, or tremors.

Home care instructions

• Teach the patient about his disease and how beta blocker therapy works. Stress the importance of taking the drug exactly as prescribed, even if he feels worse. Emphasize that he should never change the dosage or stop the drug without consulting his doctor. Explain that abrupt withdrawal may cause angina, rebound hypertension, or other side effects.

• If the patient takes one dose daily, instruct him to take a missed dose if he remembers within 8 hours of the scheduled administration time. If he takes two or more doses a day, tell him to take a missed dose as soon as he remembers. Warn him never to double-dose.

• If the patient's receiving propranolol or metoprolol, tell him to take the drug with food to increase absorption. Other beta blockers can be taken without regard to meals.

• Instruct the patient to check his pulse for 1 minute before taking his prescribed dosage. Explain that if his pulse rate is below 60 or above 100, he should call his doctor immediately and not take the drug until the doctor instructs him to do so.

• Tell the patient to weigh himself at least once a week at the same time of day, on the same scale, and while wearing the same amount of clothing. Have him notify the doctor if he gains 3 lb or more.

• Also tell him to report difficulty breathing, wheezing, coughing, depression, dizziness, rash, fever, or swollen hands or feet.

• If the patient develops symptoms of an allergic reaction, such as rash, fever, sore throat or pharyngitis, reassure him that these symptoms are usually mild and transient.

• If the patient has diabetes, explain to him that beta blockers can mask some signs of hypoglycemia, including lowered blood pressure and tachycardia. As a result, he should be alert for symptoms that aren't masked by beta blockers, such as hunger, sweating, and fatigue.

• Because beta blockers may cause dizziness, weakness, and fatigue, warn the patient to avoid overexertion or known sources of stress until his response to the drug has been established.

• If the patient experiences visual disturbances or CNS effects, tell him to avoid driving or performing other tasks that require visual acuity, mental alertness, and coordination and to notify the doctor.

• To prevent orthostatic hypotension, remind him to avoid prolonged standing or sudden rising.

• Explain that beta blockers may produce symptoms of peripheral vascular insufficiency, such as numbness, tingling, and coldness in his fingers and toes. To minimize these symptoms, tell him to avoid prolonged exposure to cold temperatures.

• Instruct the patient to limit his salt intake, as ordered, to minimize fluid retention.

• Warn him to limit his alcohol consumption. Explain that heavy drinking can raise his blood pressure.

• If the patient smokes, encourage him to stop. Tell him that tobacco use, through as-yet-unclear mechanisms, can reduce the effectiveness of beta blockers.

Diuretics

Diuretics represent the mainstay in pharmacologic management of hypertension. In fact, diuretics satisfactorily control mild hypertension in about one third of all patients. Because of their safety, effectiveness, and reasonable cost, they're often the first choice for treating hypertension and congestive heart failure (CHF).

Diuretics also prove valuable in managing fluid overload, especially in pulmonary edema, ascites, cirrhosis, peripheral edema, or anasarca. The four types of diuretics—thiazide, thiazide-like, potassium-sparing, and loop—possess somewhat different indications and mechanisms of action. (See *Comparing Diuretics*, pages 34 and 35.)

Typically, diuretics are contraindicated in patients with anuria, hepatic coma, severe fluid and electrolyte depletion, and hypersensitivity to another diuretic. They should be used cautiously in patients with renal or hepatic failure, in pregnant women, and in children. They should also be used cautiously in elderly patients, who are most likely to experience side effects and fluid and electrolyte imbalances.

Intravenous doses of diuretics should be given slowly over several minutes. Rapid or excessive diuresis can cause hypovolemia, hypotension, and vascular collapse.

Purpose and action
Diuretics affect the renal tubular absorption and excretion of water, sodium, chloride, and potassium. By causing sodium and water excretion as well as by altering peripheral vascular resistance through dilation of the smooth muscle of blood vessels, diuretics help control hypertension and reduce fluid volume.

Monitoring
During therapy, regularly assess the patient's vital signs, intake and output, and weight. If you're giving a diuretic I.V., check blood pressure frequently and be alert for pain and irritation at the insertion site, possibly indicating drug extravasation. If you detect severe hypotension, hematuria, diarrhea, or hypovolemia, discontinue the drug and notify the doctor.

Throughout therapy, check levels of serum electrolytes, serum creatinine, and blood urea nitrogen (BUN). Levels of serum electrolytes, especially potassium, can be altered with diuretic use. Elevated levels of serum creatinine and BUN may indicate renal damage; exceedingly high levels can decrease the effectiveness of diuretics. If the patient has a history of gout, watch for elevated serum uric acid levels.

If the patient has diabetes, carefully monitor his blood and urine glucose levels when administering diuretics; he may require an adjustment in his ther-

COMPARING DIURETICS

DRUG AND MECHANISM OF ACTION	INDICATIONS
Loop diuretics	
Furosemide Inhibits reabsorption of sodium, chloride, and water in the ascending loop of Henle, with a weak diuretic effect in the proximal and distal tubules. Causes excretion of potassium, hydrogen, calcium, magnesium, ammonium, and bicarbonate.	Used to treat edema associated with congestive heart failure (CHF), cirrhosis, and renal disease. Less ototoxic than ethacrynic acid.
Ethacrynic acid Inhibits sodium and chloride reabsorption in the proximal tubule and loop of Henle, promoting potassium and hydrogen ion excretion. Hypotensive effects result from hypovolemia and decreased vascular resistance.	Used to treat severe edema associated with CHF, cirrhosis, and renal disease. Because of severe side effects, generally used after furosemide for these applications.
Bumetanide Inhibits reabsorption of sodium and chloride in the ascending loop of Henle; may have additional activity in the proximal tubule to promote phosphate excretion.	Used to treat edema associated with CHF, cirrhosis, and renal disease. May be less ototoxic than furosemide. Can be safely prescribed for patients allergic to furosemide.
Thiazide diuretics	
Chlorothiazide and hydrochlorothiazide Reduce sodium reabsorption and increase potassium secretion in the distal tubule. Promote sodium, bicarbonate, and potassium excretion and renal retention of calcium and uric acid.	Used alone or with other drugs in step 1 treatment of hypertension. Also used to treat edema associated with CHF, cirrhosis, renal disease, and corticosteroid therapy.
Thiazide-like diuretics	
Chlorthalidone Structurally related to the thiazides with a similar mechanism of action.	Used alone or with other drugs to treat essential hypertension. Also used to treat edema associated with CHF.
Metolazone Structurally related to the thiazides with a similar mechanism of action.	Used in severe hypertension; more effective than thiazides in severe renal failure.
Potassium-sparing diuretics	
Spironolactone Competes with aldosterone for cellular receptor sites in the distal tubule. Promotes sodium, chloride, and water excretion without potassium loss.	Moderate diuretic action (less than that of thiazides); used to potentiate actions of other diuretics and to spare potassium.
Triamterene Promotes excretion of sodium and carbonate with little or no excretion of potassium. Blocks potassium excretion by direct action on the distal tubule.	Weak diuretic action; used with other diuretics because of potassium-sparing ability.
Amiloride Inhibits sodium reabsorption and potassium excretion by direct action on the distal tubule.	Used for adjunctive treatment of hypertension when a potassium-sparing diuretic is needed.

SPECIAL CONSIDERATIONS

• Advise the patient to eat plenty of potassium-rich foods to avoid hypokalemia.
• Tell the patient to avoid eating natural black licorice; the glycyrrhizic acid it contains can cause hypokalemia.

• Watch for swelling or pain in the joints, which may indicate gout. Monitor uric acid levels.
• Tell the patient to report ototoxic signs: vertigo, tinnitus, or hearing loss.

• Same as for furosemide.

• Same as for furosemide.
• Use with antimuscarinics can increase GI irritability.

• Use with corticotropin or with sodium bicarbonate or insulin infusion can decrease serum potassium levels.

• Advise the patient to eat plenty of potassium-rich foods to avoid hypokalemia. Tell him to avoid eating natural black licorice.
• Monitor calcium and uric acid levels.
• Before surgery, notify the anesthetist that the patient is receiving thiazides; they enhance the action of muscle relaxants.
• Can cause photosensitivity; avoid excessive sun exposure.

• Same as for thiazide diuretics.

• Same as for thiazide diuretics.

• Watch for signs of hyperkalemia, such as weakness, confusion, and paresthesias or heaviness in the legs.

• Tell the patient to limit potassium intake.
• Can cause breast swelling and tenderness, and menstrual abnormalities.

• Watch for signs of hyperkalemia (see Spironolactone, above).
• Tell the patient to limit potassium intake.
• Can cause gout. Check for swollen or painful joints. Monitor uric acid levels.
• Withdraw drug over several days to avoid excessive rebound potassium excretion.

• Watch for signs of hyperkalemia (see Spironolactone, above).
• Tell the patient to limit potassium intake.
• Can cause CNS disturbances. Advise the patient to use caution when driving a car or operating machinery.

apeutic regimen. A patient on insulin may need to increase the dosage.

Check the patient's drug regimen for possible interactions. Concurrent use of cardiac glycosides commonly leads to hypokalemia. If you're giving the two drugs concurrently, monitor the patient closely for signs of toxicity: fatigue, weakness, arrhythmias, blurred vision, anorexia, and nausea.

Home care instructions

• Tell the patient to notify his doctor immediately if he experiences tinnitus, abdominal pain, diarrhea, sore throat, or fever—especially if he's taking furosemide. GI side effects commonly develop after 1 or 2 months of treatment.
• Tell him to expect an increase in the frequency and amount of urination.
• Instruct him to take the drug in the morning and afternoon to avoid nocturia. Advise him to take it with meals or a snack to reduce GI upset.
• Teach him how to recognize symptoms of hypokalemia or hyperkalemia (depending on the type of diuretic he's taking). Instruct him to report any of these symptoms to his doctor. Stress the importance of keeping appointments for serum potassium determinations.
• Tell him to weigh himself every week at the same time of day, on the same scale, and wearing similar clothing. Have him notify the doctor of any weight loss or gain exceeding 3 lb.

Nitrates

The oldest and most commonly used vasodilators, nitrates help treat and prevent acute angina. In fact, they effectively treat both angina pectoris and Prinzmetal's angina. They're also used to reduce cardiac work load in congestive heart failure and acute MI.

Available in various forms, the nitrates include *erythrityl tetranitrate, isosorbide dinitrate, nitroglycerin,* and *pentaerythritol tetranitrate.* Choice of drug and form depends on the patient's angina. For example, sublingual nitroglycerin and sublingual or chewable isosorbide dinitrate provide relief of acute angina pectoris. The long-acting nitrates and topical, transdermal, transmucosal, and extended-release oral nitroglycerin provide prophylaxis and long-term management of recurrent angina. Intravenous nitroglycerin is used during the critical phase of unstable angina or in preinfarction angina. It must be prepared only in glass containers and delivered through special nonabsorbent tubing. That's because up to 80% of the drug can be absorbed into regular plastic I.V. containers or tubing.

Nitrates are contraindicated in patients with hypersensitivity to one of the drugs, severe anemia, profound hypotension, increased intracranial pressure, glaucoma, head trauma, or cerebral hemorrhage. They should be used cautiously during early MI and in hepatic or renal insufficiency and hyperthyroidism.

Purpose and action

To relieve or prevent angina by reducing cardiac oxygen demands through relaxation of all smooth muscle. This decreases left ventricular end-diastolic pressure and systemic vascular resistance. Nitrates also increase blood flow through collateral coronary vessels.

Monitoring

At the beginning of therapy, monitor the patient's blood pressure and the intensity and duration of his response to the medication. Note relief of pain and reduction in the frequency of attacks.

Be alert for serious side effects, such as circulatory collapse, seizures, coma, and respiratory failure. Notify the doctor immediately of such effects and begin emergency treatment. Also watch for other side effects: headache, dizziness, flushing, blurred vision, dry mouth, postural hypotension, palpitations, and syncope. Provide acetaminophen to relieve headaches until their incidence decreases (usually after several days).

Check the patient's drug regimen for possible interactions. For example, taking nitroglycerin with an antihypertensive may potentiate orthostatic hypotension. Combining nitroglycerin and tricyclic antidepressants may cause hypotension.

If you must defibrillate a patient who's wearing a transdermal nitroglycerin patch, be sure to remove the patch first. The reason? The patch, which has an aluminum backing, may explode if it comes in contact with the defibrillator's electric current.

Home care instructions

• Tell the patient to take his medication as prescribed, even if he isn't experiencing anginal pain. Explain that taking the drug on schedule will help prevent this pain. Reassure him that the drug isn't habit-forming.

• Instruct him to call the doctor immediately if he develops symptoms of possible toxicity: blue lips, palms, or fingernails; syncope or extreme dizziness; a feeling of pressure in the head; dyspnea; weakness or fatigue; weak, rapid heartbeat; fever; or seizures.

• Tell the patient to store the drug in a cool, dark place in a tightly closed container and to replace his supply every 3 months.

• Warn him to avoid alcohol, which may lower blood pressure when taken with nitrates.

• If he's taking oral tablets, instruct him to take them on an empty stomach 30 minutes before or 1 to 2 hours after meals. Unless they're chewable tablets, tell him to swallow them whole. Instruct him to keep a record of the number of tablets he takes and to bring this record with him on follow-up doctor's visits.

• If the patient is taking sublingual tablets, tell him to take a tablet as soon as he feels anginal pain. Teach him to wet the tablet with saliva, to place it under his tongue, and then to sit or lie down and relax. Tell him to allow the pill to dissolve naturally and not swallow until it has done so, then to relax for 15 minutes after the pain goes away to prevent dizziness. Explain that if one tablet doesn't relieve the pain after 5 minutes, he should take a second one; if he does so but gets no relief after another 5 minutes, he should take a third tablet. If he doesn't get relief after another 5 minutes, he should notify the doctor immediately. Warn the patient never to take more than three tablets.

• If ordered, tell the patient to take an additional dose of the short-acting oral or sublingual form 5 to 10 minutes before a stressful situation or strenuous exercise. Remind him that the drug effects will last up to 30 minutes.

• If the doctor has prescribed topical nitroglycerin ointment, teach the patient how to apply it. Show him how to spread it in a uniform, thin layer on any hairless area (without rubbing it in), then cover it with plastic film to aid absorption and protect his clothing. If he's using the Tape-Surrounded Appli-Ruler (TSAR) system, tell him to keep the TSAR on the skin to protect his clothing and ensure that the ointment remains in place.

• If the patient's using the transdermal patch, show him how to apply it. Explain that he can use any hairless area except the distal parts of his arms or legs (absorption is poorer at these sites). Also warn him to avoid prolonged proximity to microwave ovens. Explain that a radiation leak may heat the patch's aluminum backing, causing burns.

Calcium Channel Blockers

Calcium channel blockers—*diltiazem*, *nifedipine*, and *verapamil*—treat vasospastic angina (also known as Prinzmetal's or variant angina) and classic, stable angina pectoris. They're especially useful because their negative inotropic effects (decreased force of contraction) are minor (with diltiazem), masked by a reflex increase in heart rate (with nifedipine), or countered by reduced afterload (with verapamil). What's more, verapamil's antiarrhythmic actions, which slow impulse conduction and prolong the refractory period in the atrioventricular node, make it the drug of choice for treating atrial fibrillation and flutter. This drug may also be used prophylactically for atrial tachyarrhythmias and essential hypertension.

Calcium channel blockers are contraindicated in patients with impaired cardiac contractility, impulse conduction, or impulse formation. Such disorders include sick sinus syndrome, severe hypotension, second- or third-degree heart block, advanced congestive heart failure (CHF), extreme bradycardia, cardiogenic shock, or severe left ventricular dysfunction. These drugs should be used cautiously in impaired hepatic or renal function. Side effects tend to occur most commonly with nifedipine and verapamil.

Purpose and action

Calcium channel blockers inhibit the influx of calcium ions into myocardial cells, resulting in reduced force of cardiac contraction, depressed sinoatrial and atrioventricular nodal conduction (except nifedipine), and relaxation of coronary artery smooth muscle. These actions combat angina by increasing myocardial perfusion and lowering oxygen requirements.

Monitoring

During I.V. infusion of calcium channel blockers, frequently monitor the patient's EKG, pulse rate, and blood pressure and auscultate his lungs. Keep emergency equipment readily available. Also check regularly for edema and weight gain.

Watch for serious side effects of calcium channel blockers: dyspnea, coughing or wheezing, chest pain, syncope, irregular or rapid heartbeat, hypotension, peripheral edema, and bradycardia. Also note minor effects, such as dizziness, headache, nausea, fatigue, constipation, flushing, or rash.

Review the patient's drug regimen for possible interactions. Concurrent use of digitalis, beta-adrenergic blockers, or quinidine causes severe effects (see *Hazards of Using Calcium Channel Blockers with Other Cardiac Drugs*). Nitrates may accentuate hypotension, and disopyramide may aggravate CHF symptoms. As a precaution, don't administer disopyramide for 48 hours before or 24 hours after I.V. infusion of verapamil.

Home care instructions

• If the patient's taking diltiazem or verapamil, instruct him to count his pulse rate for 1 minute before each dose and to notify his doctor if the rate is less than 50. If he's taking verapamil, warn him to avoid alcohol, which may aggravate CHF symptoms.

• Tell the patient to watch for and report early signs of CHF: swollen hands or feet, lung congestion, or dyspnea.

• Instruct him to weigh himself once a week at the same time of day, on the same scale, and wearing the same amount of clothes. Advise him to notify his doctor of an overall weight gain of 3 lb or more.

• Tell him to swallow oral medication whole, without crushing or chewing it.

• Instruct the patient to take a missed dose as soon as he remembers, unless he doesn't remember until near the time for the next scheduled dose. In this case, he should skip the missed dose and resume his schedule with the next dose. He should never double-dose.

• If a calcium channel blocker is prescribed for a patient on nitrate therapy for angina, instruct him to continue complying with his nitrate schedule. Explain that he may experience worsened anginal attacks for a few days. If he's taking nitroglycerin, he may increase its use during this period, as ordered.

HAZARDS OF USING CALCIUM CHANNEL BLOCKERS WITH OTHER CARDIAC DRUGS

INTERACTING DRUG	EFFECT	NURSING ACTIONS
Beta blockers	Severe bradycardia, increased atrioventricular (AV) conduction block, congestive heart failure (CHF)	• Because of additive myocardial depressant effects, don't give I.V. verapamil and beta blockers within 4 hours of each other. • To decrease the risk of CHF, gradually discontinue beta blockers before beginning nifedipine therapy, if possible. Carefully monitor patients taking diltiazem or verapamil concurrently with beta blockers. Watch for peripheral or pulmonary edema, dyspnea, wheezing, and cough.
Cardiac glycosides	Severe bradycardia, increased AV conduction block, digitalis toxicity	• Monitor serum cardiac glycoside levels carefully; verapamil and nifedipine raise these levels by 50% to 70%. (The degree of increase relates directly to the dose of calcium channel blocker.) • Assess for signs of cardiac glycoside toxicity: irregular rhythm, headache, blurred vision, halos around lights, green or yellow flashes, confusion, hallucinations, and GI upset.
Quinidine	Severe hypotension, ventricular tachycardia	• Carefully monitor blood pressure and pulse rate.

• Tell him to take his medication with food to prevent GI upset.

• Explain to the patient that he can help prevent constipation, a possible side effect, by eating plenty of vegetables and fresh or dried fruits. He may also take a mild laxative, if recommended by his doctor.

Cardiac Glycosides

Extracted from dried leaves of the plant *Digitalis purpurea*, the cardiac glycosides include *deslanoside, digitoxin,* and *digoxin.* Because these drugs increase cardiac output while slowing the ventricular rate, they're used for congestive heart failure (CHF), cor pulmonale, right-sided heart failure resulting from pulmonary hypertension, chronic obstructive pulmonary disease, and atrial tachyarrhythmias. In fact, digoxin is the drug of choice for maintenance therapy in CHF. Deslanoside, by contrast, has only a single use: it's employed for loading doses in adults.

All the cardiac glycosides produce similar cardiovascular effects; however, they differ in rates of absorption, metabolism, and excretion. The choice of drug and method of administration depends on the disorder and the desired onset of activity. For example, digoxin, the most commonly prescribed cardiac glycoside, requires several I.V. loading doses over a 24- to 48-hour pe-

RECOGNIZING DIGITALIS TOXICITY

Digoxin and digitoxin, two commonly prescribed cardiac glycosides, have a narrow range between therapeutic and toxic blood levels. As a result, toxicity is a common problem. In infants and young children, the first symptoms are usually arrhythmias. In older children and adults, GI symptoms usually herald toxicity.

Detecting toxicity
To detect toxicity, watch for extracardiac symptoms: anorexia, nausea, vomiting, abdominal pain, diarrhea, headache, fatigue, and weakness. The patient may also experience visual disturbances, such as blurring, halos around lights, or diplopia.
  Be alert for signs of heart failure. And check the pulse for bradycardia or tachycardia. Monitor the EKG for premature ventricular contractions, atrial fibrillation, accelerated junctional nodal rhythm, atrioventricular dissociation, or heart block.

Confirming toxicity
Draw serum samples for measuring drug levels at least 6 hours after an oral dose, the duration necessary for the serum and tissues to reach equilibrium levels. The therapeutic level for digoxin ranges from 0.5 to 2.0 ng/ml; levels greater than 2.5 ng/ml cause toxicity. The therapeutic level for digitoxin ranges from 14 to 26 ng/ml; levels greater than 35 ng/ml cause toxicity.

riod to reach therapeutic serum levels for CHF maintenance.

Because cardiac glycosides have a narrow range between therapeutic and toxic blood levels, they carry a high risk of toxicity. In fact, toxicity occurs in nearly one third of patients who undergo therapy, possibly causing life-threatening arrhythmias, hypotension, or severe CHF. These effects may result from overdosage or altered absorption, changes in serum electrolyte levels (especially hypokalemia), renal or hepatic dysfunction, drug interactions, or other factors. In a patient with sensitivity to cardiac glycosides, toxicity can develop even with normally therapeutic doses.

Contraindications to therapy include ventricular tachycardia and fibrillation and hypersensitivity reactions. These drugs should be used cautiously in the elderly and in patients with renal or hepatic insufficiency, hypothyroidism, severe pulmonary disease, acute MI, atrioventricular (AV) block, constrictive pericarditis, or idiopathic hypertrophic subaortic stenosis.

Purpose and action
The cardiac glycosides' precise mechanism of action is unknown. However, these drugs seem to promote movement of calcium from extracellular to intracellular myocardial cytoplasm and increase intracellular sodium by inhibiting adenosine triphosphatase, the enzyme that regulates potassium and sodium concentrations in myocardial cells. These two mechanisms decrease conduction velocity through the AV node, thereby prolonging the refractory period, slowing the firing rate of the sinoatrial node, and increasing the force of cardiac contraction.

Monitoring
Before administering the first dose of a cardiac glycoside, obtain baseline heart rate and rhythm, blood pressure, and serum electrolyte levels. Before giving each subsequent dose, monitor the patient's apical-radial pulse for 1 minute. If you note any sudden increase or decrease in rate or new irregularities, withhold the drug and call the doctor. Also monitor serum potassium levels carefully, and notify the doctor of falling levels; he'll want to take corrective action before hypokalemia occurs.

Throughout therapy, carefully monitor the patient for symptoms of toxicity (see *Recognizing Digitalis Toxicity*). Be sure to notify the doctor immediately of any early symptoms; he will order measurement of serum electrolyte and drug levels.

To prevent toxicity from drug interactions, closely review the patient's drug regimen. Be on the lookout for beta-adrenergic blockers, thiazide-like and loop diuretics, calcium channel blockers, quinidine, and cimetidine since these drugs may raise serum levels of cardiac glycosides. Antacids, kaolin-pectin mixtures, or neomycin may decrease absorption of cardiac glycosides and should be given as far apart as possible. Amphotericin B, carbenicillin, ticarcillin, corticosteroids, and diuretics can cause hypokalemia, and parenteral calcium and thiazides can produce hypercalcemia and hypomagnesemia. These electrolyte imbalances can increase the risk of digitalis toxicity.

Also check the patient's regimen for phenylbutazone, phenytoin, phenobarbital, and rifampin, which can speed hepatic metabolism and shorten the therapeutic duration of cardiac glycosides. Similarly, check for propranolol, reserpine, succinylcholine, epinephrine, and isoproterenol, which may increase the risk of arrhythmias.

Home care instructions
• Instruct the patient to take his medication at the same time each day. Or, if the patient's an infant or young child, tell his parents to give the drug in divided doses, as ordered.
• Tell the patient or his parents to count the pulse for 1 minute before each dose. Emphasize the importance of notifying the doctor if the rate is less than 60 or greater than 100 or if skipped beats or new irregularities are detected.
• Instruct the patient or his parents to watch for and immediately report early symptoms of toxicity, such as anorexia, nausea, or a bloated feeling. Other symptoms include weakness, blurred vision, and halos around lights.
• Also emphasize the importance of reporting signs of fluid retention, such as lung congestion, shortness of breath, or swelling.
• Tell the adult patient to weigh himself once a week on the same scale, at the same time of day, and wearing similar amounts of clothing, and to notify the doctor if he gains 3 lb or more.

• If the doctor also has prescribed a loop or thiazide diuretic, instruct the patient to take a potassium supplement or to eat foods high in potassium, as ordered.
• If diarrhea occurs, tell the patient to call the doctor, who may prescribe an antidiarrheal to prevent hypokalemia.
• If appropriate, tell the patient to follow a low-salt diet.

Inotropic Drugs

This group of emergency cardiac drugs, which increase myocardial contractility, includes *amrinone* and the adrenergic drugs *dobutamine, dopamine, epinephrine, isoproterenol,* and *norepinephrine.* Because these drugs don't stimulate all classes of adrenergic receptors (alpha, beta, and dopaminergic) equally, their effects and indications differ. For example, amrinone (which has no adrenergic action) and dobutamine provide short-term management of patients with congestive heart failure (CHF) or cardiogenic shock who fail to respond to cardiac glycosides, diuretics, and other vasodilators. Dopamine boosts blood pressure and cardiac output in patients with cardiogenic shock, refractory CHF, or cardiac arrest. Epinephrine treats asystole and ventricular fibrillation as well as anaphylaxis and bronchospasm. The cardiac stimulant isoproterenol is used in patients with heart block or severe bradycardia who fail to respond to atropine. Norepinephrine, a potent vasopressor, treats hypotension and shock.

In hypovolemic shock, the inotropic drugs aren't a substitute for blood and fluid replacement. They should be given only after whole blood or plasma expanders correct hypovolemia.

Because infiltration of inotropic drugs may lead to tissue sloughing, a central venous line or a large peripheral vein should be used. Also, a vol-

COMPARING INOTROPIC DRUGS

DRUG AND ACTION	CONTRAINDICATIONS AND CAUTIONS
Amrinone This biperiden derivative facilitates calcium influx into the cell, increasing myocardial contractility. It has no adrenergic action.	• Contraindicated in patients with severe aortic or pulmonary valvular disease. • Use cautiously in idiopathic hypertrophic subaortic stenosis (IHSS).
Dobutamine This synthetic catecholamine acts as a strong beta$_1$-stimulant and a weak beta$_2$- and alpha-stimulant. It enhances contractility and diminishes peripheral vascular resistance.	• Contraindicated in IHSS.
Dopamine This precursor to norepinephrine directly stimulates alpha-, beta-, and dopaminergic receptors. It enhances renal perfusion, increases myocardial contractility, and, in high doses, causes vasoconstriction.	• Contraindicated in uncorrected tachyarrhythmias, pheochromocytoma, and ventricular fibrillation. • Use cautiously in patients with occlusive vascular disease, cold injuries, diabetic endarteritis, or arterial embolism; in pregnant patients; and in those taking MAO inhibitors.
Epinephrine A naturally occurring catecholamine, epinephrine stimulates beta$_2$-receptors in low doses and alpha-receptors in high doses. The drug increases contractility and vasodilation.	• Contraindicated in narrow-angle glaucoma, shock (except for anaphylactic shock), organic brain damage, cardiac dilatation, and coronary insufficiency. Also contraindicated during general anesthesia with halogenated hydrocarbons or cyclopropane and during labor (may delay second stage). • Use with extreme caution in patients with chronic obstructive pulmonary disease who've developed degenerative cardiac disease. Also use cautiously in elderly patients and in those with hyperthyroidism, angina, hypertension, psychoneurosis, or diabetes.
Isoproterenol A beta-stimulant, isoproterenol acts on beta$_1$-receptors to increase contractility and conduction velocity and on beta$_2$-receptors to produce vasodilation.	• Contraindicated in digitalis-induced tachycardia, arrhythmias (especially tachyarrhythmias), and recent myocardial infarction. • Use cautiously in coronary insufficiency, diabetes, or hyperthyroidism.
Norepinephrine A naturally occurring catecholamine with potent alpha- and beta$_1$-stimulation, norepinephrine produces vasoconstriction and increased contractility.	• Contraindicated in pregnancy, mesenteric or peripheral vascular thrombosis, profound hypoxia, hypercapnia, or hypotension from blood volume deficits; or during cyclopropane or halothane anesthesia. • Use cautiously in hypertension, hyperthyroidism, or severe cardiac disease.

INTERACTIONS	ADMINISTRATION TIPS
Disopyramide: excessive hypotension *Digitalis:* increased inotropic effect	• Don't dilute drug with dextrose solutions. Instead, use normal or half-normal saline solution. Discard solutions after 24 hours.
Anesthetics: arrhythmias *Beta blockers:* diminished effect *MAO inhibitors, tricyclic antidepressants:* potentiate pressor effects	• Because dobutamine is incompatible with alkaline solutions, don't mix it with sodium bicarbonate injection.
Ergot alkaloids: hypertension *Furazolidone, phenytoin:* hypotension, bradycardia	• Don't mix drug with alkaline doses of epinephrine.
Anesthetics: arrhythmias *Digitalis, guanethidine:* severe hypertension *Tricyclic antidepressants, phentolamine:* hypotension *Propranolol:* hypertension, bradycardia	• Don't mix epinephrine with alkaline solutions. Use dextrose 5% in water, normal saline solution, or a combination of the two. Mix just before use. • Because an epinephrine solution deteriorates after 24 hours, discard it at that time or if the solution becomes discolored or contains precipitate. Store the solution in a light-resistant container until use. • Massage the site after injection to counteract possible vasoconstriction. To prevent tissue necrosis, rotate injection sites. • Avoid I.M. injection into buttocks; gas gangrene may occur. • If the patient experiences a sharp rise in blood pressure, give a rapid-acting vasodilator to counteract pressor effects.
Propranolol: antagonistic effects *Epinephrine:* additive effects *Tricyclic antidepressants:* arrhythmias	• If the patient experiences angina, stop the drug immediately and notify the doctor. • If possible, don't give this drug at bedtime because it may interrupt sleep patterns.
Guanethidine, methyldopa, tricyclic antidepressants: possible severe hypertension *MAO inhibitors:* increased pressor effects *General anesthetics:* arrhythmias	• Administer in dextrose and saline solution. Discard solutions after 24 hours. • During infusion, check blood pressure every 2 minutes until stabilized, then every 5 minutes. Also check pulse and color and temperature of extremities. Titrate infusion according to findings, using doctor's guidelines. • If prolonged I.V. therapy is necessary, change injection sites frequently. Check sites frequently for signs of extravasation. • Report decreased urinary output to the doctor immediately. • Keep emergency drugs on hand to reverse effects of norepinephrine: atropine for reflex bradycardia, propranolol for arrhythmias, and phentolamine for increased vasopressor effects. • When stopping drug, slow infusion rate gradually. Monitor for severe hypotension, even after stopping the drug.

umetric infusion pump should be used to ensure the correct infusion rate and prevent inadvertent delivery of a bolus of medication. And with some inotropic drugs—especially dopamine and dobutamine—the infusion must be tapered gradually to prevent severe hypotension.

Purpose and action
The inotropic drugs provide emergency treatment of acute cardiac conditions. See *Comparing Inotropic Drugs*, pages 42 and 43, for the specific mechanism of action for each drug.

Monitoring
During administration of an inotropic drug, monitor the patient's blood pressure and heart rate frequently (as often as every 5 minutes). Check urine output hourly.

Monitor the EKG continuously to detect arrhythmias, particularly tachyarrhythmias. Assess the need for pulmonary artery catheterization, which provides information on cardiac filling pressures, cardiac output, and peripheral resistance. This information allows adjustment of dosage to help maintain maximum cardiac contractility.

If the patient's receiving dopamine, epinephrine, or norepinephrine, regularly assess his extremities for strength and rhythm of peripheral pulses, color, capillary refill time, and skin temperature. These drugs may severely compromise peripheral circulation.

Assess the I.V. site hourly for blood return and signs of infiltration, such as continued hypotension in spite of the infusion, swelling, erythema, and coolness over the infusion site. If infiltration occurs, inject 10 to 15 ml of sodium chloride with 5 to 10 mg of phentolamine, as ordered.

Carefully review the patient's medication regimen because many drugs interact with inotropic agents.(See *Comparing Inotropic Drugs*, pages 42 and 43.)

Home care instructions
Because inotropic drugs are given I.V. in critical care and cardiac stepdown units, you needn't provide home care instructions.

Antiarrhythmics

Typically the treatment of choice for arrhythmias, these drugs primarily fall into one of four classes, with each class acting on the heart in a distinct way. (Atropine, another drug used as an antiarrhythmic, doesn't fit into any of these classes.)

Selection of the precise drug and dosage isn't always easy. For one thing, pinpointing the precise cause of the arrhythmia, and predicting how it will respond to a given drug, is often difficult. For another, patients' reactions to various drugs may differ, depending on their age, condition, and other medical problems. Some may suffer severe, even life-threatening, side effects, while others may tolerate a drug easily. And, finally, certain antiarrhythmics have a narrow therapeutic index: the toxic dose isn't much greater than the therapeutic one.

Contraindications to antiarrhythmic therapy depend on the type of arrhythmia and on the other drugs the patient may be taking. Cardiac glycosides, in particular, alter the effectiveness of many antiarrhythmics, and the combination of the two may cause severe complications—even, paradoxically, *worsening* of arrhythmias. In addition, hepatic and renal insufficiency can complicate therapy by decreasing metabolism and excretion of antiarrhythmic drugs.

Purpose and action
Antiarrhythmics fall into four different classes:
• *Class I* drugs (*disopyramide, lidocaine, phenytoin, procainamide,* and *quinidine*) stabilize the membranes of

myocardial cells, which decreases sodium transport through cardiac tissues and slows conduction through the atrioventricular (AV) node. They also prolong the refractory period and decrease automaticity.

• *Class II* drugs are beta-adrenergic blockers; the only one currently used as an antiarrhythmic is *propranolol*. It binds to beta-receptor sites, blocking adrenergic stimulation of the heart.

• *Class III* drugs include *bretylium* and *amiodarone*. Their action is complex: initially, they exert a brief adrenergic *stimulatory* effect on the cardiovascular system by causing release of norepinephrine. Eventually, however, they deplete the body's supply of norepinephrine and begin to function as adrenergic blockers.

• *Class IV* drugs are calcium channel blockers. *Verapamil*, the only one widely used for arrhythmias, inhibits the influx of calcium into myocardial cells, which in turn slows activity through the sinoatrial (SA) and AV nodes.

One drug, *atropine*, doesn't fit neatly into any of these four classes. It blocks the vagal effects on the SA node, relieving severe nodal or sinus bradycardia and AV block and accelerating the heart rate by increasing AV conduction. (See *Using Atropine as an Antiarrhythmic.*)

Monitoring

When caring for a patient receiving an antiarrhythmic, regularly check his pulse rate, rhythm, and blood pressure. Also check his drug regimen for possible interactions, and be alert for side effects (see *Comparing Antiarrhythmics,* pages 46 to 48, for details).

Home care instructions

• Caution the patient about cardiac complications, such as palpitations and changes in heart rate or rhythm. Instruct him to take his pulse every morning before getting out of bed and to call his doctor if the rate drops below 60 or exceeds 100.

USING ATROPINE AS AN ANTIARRHYTHMIC

Atropine—a derivative of the poisonous belladonna plant—is a drug of many faces. It's used as an adjunct to anesthesia; as an antispasmodic, bronchodilator, and mydriatic; and, ironically, as an antidote for certain kinds of poisoning. In cardiac care, it's given intravenously, usually to treat bradycardia, escape rhythms, and heart block accompanying acute MI.

Atropine is so versatile because it blocks parasympathetic effects throughout the body. In the heart, it blocks the action of acetylcholine on parasympathetic receptors, thereby increasing heart rate, conduction velocity, and force of contraction. In addition to its use in MI, atropine often successfully reverses first-degree atrioventricular (AV) block and Mobitz Type I block, two arrhythmias that are associated with increased vagal tone. (Mobitz Type II block, by contrast, usually isn't related to vagal tone and therefore doesn't respond to atropine.) It can sometimes also control complete AV block, but a temporary or permanent pacemaker usually offers a better solution. And, finally, atropine is often used with epinephrine and intubation to treat asystole.

Administering atropine

You need to work fast when you're giving atropine to cardiac patients, for two reasons. First, you're likely to be giving it in an emergency, when every second counts. But a less obvious reason for rapidly infusing the drug is to overcome a paradoxical effect: small doses may briefly lower rather than raise heart rate, probably as a result of central vagal stimulation. Although this effect is reversed once peripheral cholinergic blocking occurs, it can be life-threatening in a patient with bradycardia.

To a certain extent, giving atropine to a patient who has suffered an MI is a calculated risk; the drug can cause myocardial ischemia, arrhythmias (including ventricular tachycardia and fibrillation), hypertension, or hypotension. And in many cases, differentiating the drug's effects from underlying disease is difficult, even impossible. Other side effects are less serious and subside once the drug is withdrawn; these include headache, drowsiness, depression, confusion, flushed dry skin, dry mouth, urinary retention, blurred vision, photophobia, eye pain, and conjunctivitis.

COMPARING ANTIARRHYTHMICS

DRUG AND INDICATION	SPECIAL CONSIDERATIONS
Class I	
Disopyramide (Class IA) Used for premature ventricular contractions (PVCs) and ventricular tachycardia	• Contraindicated in cardiogenic shock and second- or third-degree heart block. Use cautiously in congestive heart failure (CHF), renal or hepatic disease or impairment, myasthenia gravis, narrow-angle glaucoma, and conduction abnormalities. • Check apical pulse before administering; report a rate under 60 or over 120. • Watch for hypotension, edema, and decreased urinary output. • Increase patient's fiber and fluid intake to prevent constipation. • Report depression, fatigue, weakness, dizziness, or agitation. • If the patient is receiving phenytoin, monitor for arrhythmias.
Procainamide (Class IA) Used for atrial tachycardia, junctional tachycardia, PVCs, and ventricular tachycardia	• Contraindicated in complete atrioventricular (AV) block. • Watch for severe transient hypotension during I.V. administration; monitor EKG and blood pressure continuously. • Amiodarone and cimetidine may increase blood levels of the drug; watch for signs of toxicity. • Enhanced muscle relaxation may occur when drug is combined with neomycin, kanamycin, or sodium bicarbonate. • Rash, itching, or pain with breathing may indicate lupuslike reaction or allergy.
Quinidine (Class IA) Used for atrial tachycardia	• Contraindicated in cardiac glycoside toxicity when AV conduction is grossly impaired, unless the patient has a pacemaker. Use with caution in myasthenia gravis. • I.V. route is used only to treat acute arrhythmias, since it can cause severe cardiovascular reactions. • Check for possible interactions. Acetazolamide, antacids, or sodium bicarbonate may raise quinidine blood levels; barbiturates, phenytoin, rifampin, and nifedipine decrease quinidine's effect. Verapamil may cause hypotension; monitor blood pressure. • Monitor complete blood count for signs of hemolytic anemia, thrombocytopenia, and agranulocytosis. • Watch for vertigo, headache, and light-headedness. Restrict ambulation if necessary; report symptoms. • Call doctor if signs of toxicity—diarrhea, nausea, fever, cinchonism, abnormal liver function tests, or tinnitus—develop. • Watch for PVCs, severe hypotension, sinoatrial (SA) or AV block, ventricular fibrillation, tachycardia, aggravation of CHF, and EKG changes (especially widening of QRS complex, notched P waves, widened QT interval, and ST-segment depression).
Lidocaine (Class IB) Used for ventricular fibrillation, ventricular tachycardia, and PVCs	• Given only in hospital, since continuous monitoring is required. • Contraindicated in patients with Stokes-Adams syndrome or heart block. Use cautiously in patients with Wolff-Parkinson-White syndrome, CHF, or renal or hepatic impairment. • Compare EKGs with baseline throughout therapy. • Watch for signs of overdose, such as blurred or double vision, nausea, vomiting, tinnitus, and tremors; call doctor if they occur. Monitor blood levels.

DRUG AND INDICATION	SPECIAL CONSIDERATIONS
Mexiletine (Class IB) Used for PVCs and ventricular tachycardia	• Monitor pulse rate and rhythm and EKGs for worsening of arrhythmias; drug has paradoxical action in some patients. Also watch for hypotension, heart block, and Torsades de Pointes. • Watch for and report CNS, musculoskeletal, and visual disturbances.
Phenytoin (Class IB) Used for glycoside-induced arrhythmias; relatively ineffective against other arrhythmias	• Contraindicated in patients with phenacemide or hydantoin hypersensitivity, bradycardia, SA or AV block, or Stokes-Adams syndrome. Use cautiously in presence of hepatic or renal dysfunction, hypotension, myocardial insufficiency, or respiratory depression; in elderly or debilitated patients; and in those receiving other hydantoin derivatives. • Watch for interactions: phenytoin's effects are diminished by alcohol, antacids, antihistamines, barbiturates, antineoplastics, CNS depressants, oxacillin, and reserpine; they're increased by aspirin, anticoagulants, anticonvulsants, cimetidine, phenothiazines, and sulfonamides. Lidocaine and propranolol cause additive cardiac depressant effects. • To prevent precipitation of drug, do not mix with dextrose 5% in water, and do not administer I.M. without adjusting dosage. • To prevent "purple glove syndrome," do not administer phenytoin via I.V. push into veins in the patient's hand. • To minimize nausea, give divided doses with or after meals. But don't administer phenytoin with tube feedings; decreased absorption may result. • Adverse reactions include ventricular fibrillation, CNS effects (such as slurred speech and confusion), blood dyscrasias, hypocalcemia, toxic hepatitis, exfoliative dermatitis, hirsutism, and toxic epidermal necrolysis.
Tocainide (Class IB) Used for PVCs and ventricular tachycardia	• Tocainide is similar to lidocaine but may be given orally. Contraindicated in patients who are hypersensitive to lidocaine or amide-type local anesthetics. • Watch for interactions: allopurinol increases blood levels of tocainide; propranolol may cause paranoia. • See also special considerations for lidocaine.
Encainide (Class IC) Used for atrial fibrillation, atrial flutter, atrial and ventricular tachycardia, PVCs, and Wolff-Parkinson-White syndrome	• Use cautiously in patients with sustained ventricular tachycardia or ventricular fibrillation. Monitor such patients continuously, and keep resuscitation equipment readily available. • Review EKGs regularly and compare with baseline. • Report CNS, musculoskeletal, and visual disturbances; dosage may require adjustment. • Allopurinol may increase blood levels; propranolol may cause paranoia.
Flecainide (Class IC) Used for atrial and ventricular tachycardia and Wolff-Parkinson-White syndrome	• Assess for side effects: transient blurred vision, dizziness, and light-headedness; dosage may need adjustment. • When given with propranolol, expect a slight increase in blood levels of both drugs.

(continued)

COMPARING ANTIARRHYTHMICS *(continued)*

DRUG AND INDICATION	SPECIAL CONSIDERATIONS

Class II (beta-adrenergic blockers)

Propranolol
Used for atrial fibrillation, atrial tachycardia, ventricular tachycardia, and Wolff-Parkinson-White syndrome

- Contraindicated in patients with AV block; may cause asystole.
- When Wolff-Parkinson-White syndrome is complicated by atrial fibrillation, propranolol may worsen arrhythmias; monitor EKGs.
- Also watch for CHF, bronchospasm, hypotension, and bradycardia.
- See "Beta-Adrenergic Blockers," in this chapter, for more information.

Class III

Amiodarone
Used for atrial fibrillation, atrial flutter, atrial tachycardia, PVCs, ventricular tachycardia, and Wolff-Parkinson-White syndrome

- Often effective for arrhythmias that are resistant to other drug therapy; however, side effects limit its use. Side effects are more prevalent at high doses; they disappear gradually after drug is discontinued but may linger for as long as 4 months. Photosensitivity is the most common one; others include corneal microdeposits, altered liver and thyroid functions, pneumonitis, and fibrosis (most prevalent in patients taking more than 600 mg daily). Recommend sunscreen and methylcellulose ophthalmic solution.
- To prevent nausea, divide loading dosage into three doses and give with meals. If necessary, divide maintenance dosage into two doses and give with meals.
- Watch for interactions: bradycardia may occur with beta blockers, lidocaine, and calcium channel blockers.

Bretylium
Used for PVCs, ventricular fibrillation, and ventricular tachycardia

- Severe postural hypotension, the most common side effect, limits drug use to emergencies in which immediate control of life-threatening arrhythmias is required and in which monitoring and resuscitation equipment is at hand. Contraindicated in cardiac glycoside toxicity. Monitor blood pressure, heart rate, and rhythm frequently; notify doctor of any significant change.
- To minimize postural hypotension, keep patient supine until tolerance develops and avoid sudden postural changes while patient is receiving bretylium. If patient's supine diastolic pressure falls below 75 mm Hg, administer prescribed norepinephrine, dopamine, or volume expanders.
- Watch for potentiation of antihypertensive medications.
- For ventricular fibrillation, give I.V. injections as rapidly as possible. Follow dosage directions carefully to minimize GI effects.
- When giving bretylium I.M., rotate injection sites to prevent tissue damage, and inject no more than 5 ml at any one site.

Class IV (calcium channel blockers)

Verapamil
Used for atrial fibrillation, atrial flutter, and atrial tachycardia

- Contraindicated in sick sinus syndrome, AV conduction disturbances, cardiogenic shock, and advanced CHF (unless it's secondary to atrial tachyarrhythmias).
- See "Calcium Channel Blockers," in this chapter, for more information.
- Not usually effective against ventricular arrhythmias but may slow ventricular response to atrial fibrillation or flutter.

• Warn him about possible neurologic side effects (confusion, dizziness, and fatigue), especially if he's taking amiodarone or disopyramide. Tell him to call his doctor if such symptoms occur and to avoid driving or other activities requiring coordination and alertness.
• Advise him to call his doctor if he experiences other hypersensitivity reactions, such as blurred vision, photophobia, rash, dyspnea, cough, pleuritic chest pain, fever, edema, or weakness.

Anticoagulants

By interrupting the normal clotting process, the anticoagulant drugs *heparin* and *warfarin* prevent or inhibit thrombus formation. However, these drugs don't affect circulating thrombin; this action requires a thrombolytic drug, such as streptokinase.

Anticoagulants help prevent and treat pulmonary emboli and deep vein thrombosis, and reduce thrombus formation during MI or after cardiovascular surgery. In addition, heparin provides anticoagulant effects in patients with disseminated intravascular coagulation or atrial fibrillation and in those undergoing such procedures as dialysis and cardiopulmonary bypass. Warfarin, used for rheumatic heart disease with valvular damage, may also be used for atrial arrhythmias that disrupt normal hemodynamics.

Occasionally, anticoagulants are given prophylactically in low doses after major abdominal or thoracic surgery. Most commonly, they're given to patients with a history of thromboembolism or with prolonged bed-rest restrictions to prevent venous thrombosis or pulmonary embolism. This practice remains controversial, however.

The onset and duration of the two drugs varies. Heparin, given parenterally only, acts immediately, with peak effects occurring within minutes and residual effects lasting up to 6 hours. Warfarin, given orally only, has a more cumulative and prolonged action and generally requires several days to reach therapeutic levels. Because of this delay, heparin is often combined with warfarin during the first stage of anticoagulant therapy. Once warfarin reaches therapeutic levels, heparin is discontinued and the patient remains on warfarin for the duration of therapy.

Because anticoagulants carry a high risk of bleeding, they're usually contraindicated in patients with blood dyscrasias, open wounds, suspected intracranial hemorrhage, bacterial endocarditis, GI ulcers, severe hepatic or renal disease, threatened abortion, or recent surgery involving the eye, brain, or spinal cord. In addition, warfarin is contraindicated in patients with vitamin K deficiency.

Anticoagulants should be used cautiously in female patients during menses and immediately postpartum, and in patients with a drainage tube, hepatic or renal disease, alcoholism, hypertension, allergies, asthma, GI ulcers, or any other condition that increases the risk of hemorrhage.

Purpose and action
Heparin blocks the conversion of prothrombin to thrombin and of fibrinogen to fibrin. Warfarin indirectly interferes with coagulation by depressing hepatic synthesis of vitamin K–dependent clotting factors. (See *How Anticoagulants Inhibit Clotting*, page 50.)

Monitoring
During heparin therapy, monitor the patient's complete blood count frequently to detect possible thrombocytopenia (which can cause arterial thrombosis). Also regularly check partial thromboplastin time (PTT): values 1.5 to 2 times higher than the control value indicate good anticoagulant action.

Whenever possible, administer I.V. heparin using an infusion pump, and

HOW ANTICOAGULANTS INHIBIT CLOTTING

Damage to the endothelium of a blood vessel sets in motion a chain of biochemical reactions—the coagulation cascade—that leads to formation of a clot. As shown in this diagram, the cascade consists of intrinsic and extrinsic pathways. Activation of the intrinsic pathway begins when Factor XII comes in contact with collagen; activation of the extrinsic pathway, when tissue factor (or thromboplastin) acts on Factor VII. Both pathways ultimately activate Factor X. Coagulation then proceeds along a common pathway and ends with the formation of an insoluble fibrin clot at the injury site.

Normally, clot formation activates the body's fibrinolytic system to keep the clot from enlarging and to dissolve further clots as they form. But if the fibrinolytic system fails to work correctly, anticoagulant drugs may be needed to reverse or head off the clotting mechanism.

How do these drugs work? Heparin accelerates the activity of antithrombin III, a circulating plasma protein that neutralizes the activity of thrombin and other proteins involved in the coagulation cascade by acting on Factors II (prothrombin), V, IX, and X. Warfarin antagonizes vitamin K, which is responsible for hepatic formation of Factors II, VII, IX, and X, and so inhibits the liver's activation of these factors.

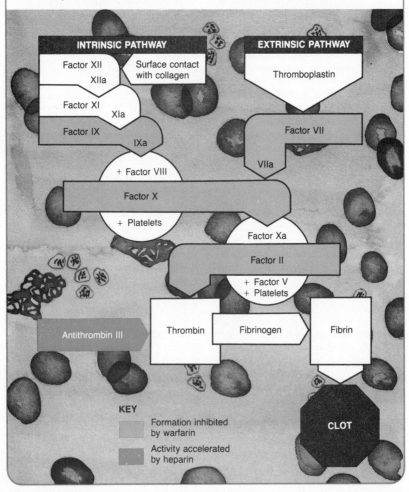

check the rate frequently. If the patient's receiving a continuous infusion, you can obtain a serum sample for PTT measurement 8 hours after therapy begins. If he's receiving intermittent infusion, obtain a sample at least 30 minutes before the next scheduled infusion to prevent falsely elevated PTT. For the same reason, be sure to obtain any sample from the *unaffected* arm. To minimize bleeding, apply pressure dressings over venipuncture sites and avoid I.M. injections of other drugs.

If the patient's taking warfarin, frequently check prothrombin time (PT). Look for a PT of 1.5 to 2 times the control value; notify the doctor if PT exceeds 2.5 times the control, which may indicate an increased risk of bleeding. Also be alert for serious GI effects, including anorexia, nausea or vomiting, diarrhea, and paralytic ileus.

Throughout anticoagulant therapy, regularly observe the patient for bleeding gums, bruises, petechiae, epistaxis, melena, tarry stools, hematuria, or hematemesis. Notify the doctor if you detect any of these signs of bleeding; he may alter or discontinue anticoagulant therapy. In addition, he may order protamine sulfate to reverse the effects of heparin or vitamin K to counteract the effects of warfarin.

Investigate the patient's drug regimen for possible interactions (see *Anticoagulant Alert*).

Home care instructions

Because heparin is administered parenterally and almost exclusively in the hospital, it doesn't require home care instructions. However, warfarin therapy requires these directions:
• Instruct the patient to take the prescribed dose at the same time each day.
• Stress the importance of regular follow-up tests to monitor warfarin levels.
• Instruct the patient and his family to watch for and immediately report signs of bleeding, including hematuria, tarry stools, bleeding from the nose or gums, bruises and petechiae, hematemesis, or increased menstrual flow.

ANTICOAGULANT ALERT

Both heparin and warfarin interact with a large number of other drugs. Typically, the result is an increased risk of bleeding, diminished anticoagulant action, or ulcerogenic effects.

HAZARDS OF HEPARIN USE

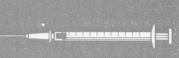

The risk of bleeding increases when heparin is given with dextrans, dipyridamole, piperacillin, and valproic acid. It also increases when given with aspirin, carbenicillin, cefamandole, chloroquine, hydroxychloroquine, moxalactam, nonsteroidal anti-inflammatory agents, or plicamycin. In contrast, heparin's anticoagulant effect diminishes when used with antihistamines, cardiac glycosides, oral contraceptives, protamine, or tetracycline.

WARINESS ABOUT WARFARIN

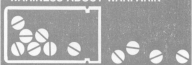

The risk of bleeding rises when warfarin is given with amiodarone, chloramphenicol, clofibrate, diflunisal, thyroid drugs, heparin, anabolic steroids, cimetidine, disulfiram, glucagon, inhalation anesthetics, metronidazole, quinidine, influenza vaccine, sulindac, sulfinpyrazone, or sulfonamides. The risk also rises with concurrent, prolonged acetaminophen therapy. What's more, fatal hemorrhage can occur several weeks after cessation of barbiturate therapy unless the warfarin dosage is reduced.

The risk of ulcerogenic effects increases when warfarin is used with ethacrynic acid, indomethacin, mefenamic acid, oxyphenbutazone, phenylbutazone, or salicylates.

Warfarin's effectiveness decreases when carbamazepine, ethchlorvynol, griseofulvin, haloperidol, paraldehyde, or rifampin is given concurrently. Similarly, its effectiveness diminishes when used with laxatives or diuretics.

• To minimize bleeding, instruct the patient to brush his teeth gently, using a soft-bristled toothbrush; to floss gently with waxed floss; and to shave with an electric razor instead of a blade. Also instruct him to tell his dentist that he's taking warfarin before undergoing any dental work.

• Warn the patient to avoid over-the-counter drugs containing aspirin or other salicylates. Tell him never to take any other drug without first consulting his doctor.

• Because vitamin K can interfere with warfarin's anticoagulant action, advise the patient to eat roughly the same amounts of vitamin K–containing foods each day to prevent altered drug effects. Explain that leafy green vegetables contain the highest amounts of vitamin K and that fruits, cereals, dairy products, and meats supply lower amounts.

• Warn him to avoid excessive alcohol consumption, which can increase the risk of bleeding.

• Advise him to carry a Medic Alert card specifying his prescribed drug and dosage.

Thrombolytics

The thrombolytic enzymes *streptokinase* and *urokinase* along with a promising new investigational drug, *tissue plasminogen activator,* provide rapid correction of acute and extensive thrombotic disorders. For example, streptokinase or urokinase infusion can serve as an alternative to surgery in massive pulmonary emboli. Streptokinase, which has replaced urokinase as the drug of choice for most thrombotic disorders, also helps dissolve acute deep-vein and arterial thrombi. And when given via intracoronary infusion early in acute MI, it can open an occluded coronary artery and prevent primary or secondary thrombus formation in the vessels surrounding the necrotic area, minimizing myocardial damage.

But streptokinase isn't without drawbacks. Because the drug is derived from hemolytic streptococci, it may trigger an allergic reaction, especially in a patient with a previous streptococcal infection. Such a patient also may develop streptokinase resistance, requiring dangerously high doses to produce therapeutic effects. (For this patient, urokinase may be a better choice.) And because streptokinase counteracts coagulation systemically, it puts the patient at high risk for bleeding.

For this reason, streptokinase is contraindicated in patients with ulcerative wounds, recent internal injuries, visceral or intracranial malignancy, ulcerative colitis or diverticulitis, severe hypertension, hepatic or renal insufficiency, uncontrolled hypocoagulation, chronic pulmonary disease with cavitation, subacute bacterial endocarditis or rheumatic disease, or recent cerebral embolism, thrombosis, or hemorrhage. It's also contraindicated for at least 10 days after any surgery or intraarterial diagnostic procedure. It should be used carefully when treating arterial emboli originating in the left side of the heart because of the risk of cerebral infarction.

Purpose and action
These drugs work by promoting formation of plasmin, a proteolytic enzyme that dissolves a clot's fibrin threads. Urokinase reacts directly with plasminogen to create plasmin, whereas streptokinase joins with plasminogen in a complex that then reacts with additional plasminogen to form plasmin.

Monitoring
Before beginning streptokinase or urokinase therapy, draw serum samples for blood typing and cross matching and for determination of prothrombin time and partial thromboplastin time. Also obtain a baseline EKG and electrolyte, arterial blood gas, blood urea

nitrogen, creatinine, and cardiac enzyme levels. Check subsequent findings against these baselines regularly throughout therapy.

At the start of streptokinase therapy, watch for signs of hypersensitivity: hypotension, shortness of breath, wheezing, a feeling of tightness and pressure in the chest, and angioedema. Keep emergency resuscitation equipment readily available. Throughout therapy, continuously monitor the EKG and compare it with baseline readings to detect possible arrhythmias. Inform the doctor of any abnormalities and be prepared to administer lidocaine or procainamide, as ordered.

Carefully assess the patient for signs of bleeding. Monitor him every 15 minutes for the first hour, every 30 minutes for the next 7 hours, and then once every 8 hours thereafter. If you detect bleeding, stop therapy and notify the doctor. Ensure that packed red blood cells and whole blood, as well as aminocaproic acid, are readily available to treat possible hemorrhage.

Check the patient's vital signs frequently, and monitor pulses, color, and sensory function in the extremities every hour. If the patient develops fever (a common effect of streptokinase), administer acetaminophen rather than aspirin. Also avoid giving the patient other drugs that could precipitate bleeding, such as indomethacin and phenylbutazone.

Because the patient is prone to bruising during his course of thrombolytic therapy, handle him gently and as little as possible. Keep invasive procedures and venipunctures to a minimum, and pad the side rails of his bed to prevent injury.

After discontinuing thrombolytic therapy, expect to administer anticoagulants to prevent recurrence of thromboses.

Home care instructions

Because thrombolytics are given only in the hospital, they don't require home care instructions.

AN ALTERNATIVE THROMBOLYTIC

An exciting new drug known as tissue plasminogen activator (TPA), although used investigationally at present, promises to be a more effective and less risky alternative to streptokinase. In fact, TPA dissolves blood clots three times as rapidly as streptokinase and has several other advantages. Because TPA is more fibrin-specific than streptokinase, it's less likely to cause systemic anticoagulant effects. It's also less antigenic (since it's a naturally occurring human serum protease) and produces fewer and milder reactions. Unlike streptokinase, which is most effective when administered through time-consuming and risky cardiac catheterization, TPA begins working almost immediately after I.V. injection. What's more, TPA's effects last about 10 minutes, allowing prompt performance of any invasive procedures, such as coronary artery bypass grafting, without a high risk of hemorrhage. (Streptokinase infusion, in contrast, contraindicates invasive procedures for at least 2 hours after discontinuation of therapy.)

SURGERY

Heart Transplant

This complex and controversial procedure involves the replacement of a diseased heart with a healthy one from a brain-dead donor. (Alternatively, the diseased heart may be replaced with an artificial one—an even more controversial procedure.) Limited to patients with end-stage cardiac disease, heart transplant offers a last hope for survival after more conservative medical or surgical therapies have failed. Most candidates for this surgery have severe coronary artery disease with widespread left ventricular dysfunction caused by MI and associated fibrosis. Others suffer from idiopathic hypertrophic subaortic stenosis, myotonic muscular dystrophy, or cardiomyopathy caused by viral infection.

Typically, heart transplant is contraindicated in patients with irreversible pulmonary hypertension, severe peptic ulcers, unresolved pulmonary embolism, acute infection, carcinoma, severe hepatic or renal dysfunction, or insulin-dependent diabetes. Relative contraindications include advanced age, extreme cachexia, and mental instability.

Heart transplants are performed infrequently despite continued improvements in technique and antirejection drugs. In fact, the 1-year survival rate is 70% to 90%, and the 5-year rate is about 50%. The surgery's frequency is limited by its high cost and the scarcity of suitable donor hearts.

Although transplantation may represent the only means available to prolong a patient's life, it is by no means a certain cure. Serious postoperative complications include infection and tissue rejection; most patients can expect to experience one or both complications. Rejection, caused by the patient's immune response to foreign antigens from the donor heart, usually occurs within the first 6 weeks after surgery. It's treated with potent immunosuppressive drugs, such as azathioprine, corticosteroids, and cyclosporine—sometimes in massive doses. (See *Reviewing Antirejection Drugs*, pages 56 and 57.) However, the resulting immunosuppression leaves the patient vulnerable to potentially life-threatening infection.

A patient undergoing a heart transplant needs special nursing care before and after surgery. This care focuses on thorough preoperative preparation and, most important, on comprehensive postoperative measures to help prevent infection and tissue rejection. Your role in transplantation surgery covers more than physical care measures, however. For, when faced with the many uncertainties of this overwhelmingly complex and frightening surgery, the patient and his family will need not only your expert nursing care but also your strong emotional support.

Purpose
To replace a diseased heart with a healthy one in patients with end-stage cardiac disease.

Preparation
The patient awaiting heart transplantation faces many difficult questions and often overwhelming fears. Begin to address them by meeting with the patient and his family to discuss the procedure, possible complications, and the impact on their lives of transplantation and a prolonged recovery period. Remember that this surgery affects the entire family, not just the patient. Encourage them to express their concerns and to ask questions; if necessary, refer them for psychological counseling.

Discuss the prospects of a successful transplant and of postoperative complications, including tissue rejection. Make sure they understand that transplantation doesn't guarantee a life free from medical problems and that it requires lifelong follow-up care.

Explain what to expect before surgery, including food and fluid restrictions and the need for intubation and mechanical ventilation. Prepare them for the sights and sounds of the recovery room and intensive care unit. If possible, arrange for them to tour these facilities and meet the staff. Describe postoperative isolation measures, if ordered, and the tests used to detect tissue rejection and other complications. Explain the expected immunosuppressive drug regimen necessary to combat rejection.

Ensure that the patient or a responsible family member has signed a consent form.

Procedure
First, the surgeon performs a medial sternotomy and incises the pericar-

UNDERSTANDING THE ARTIFICIAL HEART

The Jarvik 7 total artificial heart (TAH) consists of two mechanical ventricles attached to Dacron sleeves, which are stitched to the patient's aorta, pulmonary artery, and atria. The TAH is powered by compressed air, which activates internal diaphragms and valves to pump blood. The TAH may be used in place of a human donor heart as a permanent transplant or as a temporary measure to sustain life until a suitable donor heart becomes available.

Possible complications associated with the TAH include infection, thrombus formation, embolization, calcification, and mechanical failure.

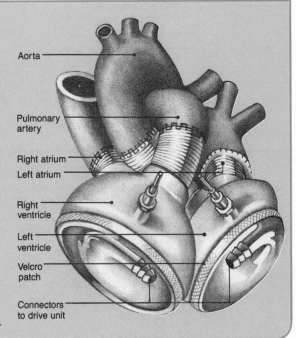

Aorta

Pulmonary artery

Right atrium

Left atrium

Right ventricle

Left ventricle

Velcro patch

Connectors to drive unit

dium to expose the diseased heart. He then orders the patient heparinized to reduce the risk of clotting, clamps the ascending aorta, and initiates cardiopulmonary bypass. He then excises the diseased heart, leaving intact the posterior walls of the left and right atria—known as the atrial cuff—to serve as a protective shell for the donor heart. Meanwhile, the donor heart, which is infused with a cold cardioplegic solution to protect it from deterioration, is kept immersed in an ice-saline solution in a cooler.

After removing the diseased heart, the surgeon inspects and trims the donor heart to fit the recipient's atrial cuff, being especially careful not to damage the sinoatrial node. He anastomoses the left and right atria, then the great ves-

sels. Next, he aspirates air from the cardiac chambers and unclamps the ascending aorta to restore cardiac perfusion and circulation. If the heart doesn't beat spontaneously, he applies an electric shock until it does so.

Finally, the surgeon checks for and repairs any small vascular leaks, removes the patient from the cardiopulmonary bypass machine, reverses heparinization, and places temporary pacing wires and chest drains. After closing the sternum, fascia, and subcutaneous tissue, he or an assistant sutures the incision and covers the wound with a dry sterile dressing.

Monitoring and aftercare

Following surgery, maintain reverse isolation for 4 weeks or follow your hos-

REVIEWING ANTIREJECTION DRUGS

DRUG	MECHANISM OF ACTION	SIDE EFFECTS
Azathioprine	Decreases or inhibits tissue rejection by interfering with synthesis of DNA and RNA	Bone marrow depression, leukopenia, thrombocytopenia, anemia, hepatotoxicity, nausea, vomiting
Cyclosporine	A fungal metabolite that selectively suppresses T lymphocytes without depressing bone marrow; long-term effects are unknown	Hirsutism, hypertension, myocardial fibrosis, tremors (especially with high doses; may resolve spontaneously), hepatic dysfunction, nephrotoxicity
Lymphocyte immune globulin; antithymocyte globulin (ATG or ATGAM)	A highly controversial drug derived from inoculating animals (rabbits, horses) with human thymocytes and harvesting the antibodies; evidently acts by selectively depleting lymphocytes responsible for cell-mediated immunity	Chills and fever, leukopenia, thrombocytopenia, rash, pruritus, arthralgia, chest and back pain, headache, nausea, vomiting, diarrhea, peripheral thrombophlebitis, stomatitis, dyspnea, hypotension, night sweats, pain at infusion site
Muromonab-CD3	A mouse-derived monoclonal antibody to human T cells that blocks the generation and function of T-effector cells; used investigationally in heart transplantation	Fever, chills, tremors, dyspnea, wheezing, chest pain, nausea, vomiting, diarrhea
Prednisone	A glucocorticoid that inhibits intracellular enzymes and RNA and DNA synthesis; has anti-inflammatory properties	Edema, weight gain, psychosis, congestive heart failure, glucose intolerance

pital's protocol. Administer immunosuppressive drugs, as ordered. Remember that these drugs typically mask obvious signs of infection. Watch for more subtle signs, such as fever above 100° F. (37.8° C.). Expect to administer prophylactic antibiotics and maintain strict asepsis when caring for incision and drainage sites.

Assess the patient for signs of hemodynamic compromise, such as severe hypotension, decreased cardiac output, and shock. Check and record vital signs every 15 minutes until the patient's condition stabilizes.

Monitor the EKG for disturbances in heart rate and rhythm, such as bradycardia, ventricular tachycardia, and heart block. Such disturbances may result from myocardial irritability or ischemia, fluid and electrolyte imbalance, hypoxemia, or hypothermia. If you detect serious abnormalities, notify the doctor and assist with epicardial pacing.

To ensure adequate myocardial perfusion, maintain arterial pressure within the guidelines set by the doctor. Usually, mean arterial pressure below 70 mm Hg results in inadequate tissue perfusion. Also monitor pulmonary artery, central venous, and left atrial

SPECIAL CONSIDERATIONS

- Ensure measurement of white blood cells (WBCs), hemoglobin, and platelets once a month. If WBC count is less than 3,000/mm³, discontinue drug.

- Monitor liver function tests closely.
- To minimize GI upset, give in divided doses or after meals.

- Carefully monitor blood pressure, urine output, and blood urea nitrogen and serum creatinine levels.
- Monitor liver function tests; dosage

adjustment may be necessary.
- Tell the female patient to use a depilatory cream to remove excess hair, if necessary.

- During administration, carefully watch the patient for signs of hypersensitivity reaction; before administration, skin testing for sensitivity is recommended.
- Regularly monitor complete blood count.
- Assess the patient's skin for disruptions, and compare baseline to assessment results; report any changes.
- Assess and report headache and joint, chest, and back pain.
- Closely monitor intake and output; report abnormalities as well as episodes of

nausea, vomiting, or diarrhea.
- Assess extremities for redness, warmth, and pain.
- Examine oral mucosa for stomatitis.
- Assess respiratory status regularly; report any abnormalities.
- Carefully monitor blood pressure during therapy.
- If the patient develops night sweats, provide for his comfort and notify the doctor.
- Assess the infusion site for redness and swelling. Report any changes.

- Contraindicated in hypersensitivity.
- Monitor for side effects, which usually occur during the first 2 days of treatment.

- Withhold drug if the patient's temperature exceeds 100° F. (37.8° C.).

- Watch for and report edema.
- Weigh the patient regularly and compare results to his baseline weight.
- Monitor for fatigue, tachycardia, and

dyspnea.
- Observe closely for mental changes.
- Check blood glucose levels frequently and compare them to baseline values.

pressure, as ordered.

Frequently evaluate peripheral pulses, capillary refill time, and skin temperature and color, and auscultate heart sounds. Notify the doctor of any abnormalities. Evaluate tissue oxygenation by assessing breath sounds, chest excursion, and symmetry of chest expansion. Check arterial blood gas levels every 2 to 4 hours and adjust ventilator settings as needed to maintain them within prescribed limits.

Maintain chest tube drainage at the prescribed negative pressure (usually −10 to −40 cmH₂O). Milk chest tubes every hour to maintain patency, and

regularly assess for hemorrhage, excessive drainage (greater than 200 ml/hour), or sudden decrease or cessation of drainage.

Continuously assess the patient for signs of tissue rejection. Be alert for decreased electrical activity on EKG, right axis shift, atrial arrhythmias, conduction defects, ventricular gallop, ventricular failure, jugular vein distention, malaise, lethargy, weight gain, and increased T cell count. Report any of these signs immediately.

As ordered, administer antiarrhythmic, inotropic, pressor, and analgesic medications, as well as I.V. fluids and blood products. Monitor intake and output and assess for hypokalemia or other electrolyte imbalances.

Evaluate for the effects of denervation. Look for an elevated resting heart rate or a sinus rhythm that's unaffected by respirations. A lack of heart rate variation in response to changes in position, Valsalva's maneuver, or a carotid massage indicates complete denervation. Remember that atropine, anticholinergics, and edrophonium may have no effect on a denervated heart and that the effects of quinidine, digoxin, and verapamil may vary.

Throughout the patient's recovery period, assess carefully for complications. Watch especially for symptoms of cerebrovascular accident (altered level of consciousness, pupillary changes, weakness and loss of movement in the extremities, ataxia, aphasia, dysphagia, sensory disturbances), pulmonary embolism (dyspnea, cough, hemoptysis, chest pain, pleural friction rub, cyanosis, hypoxemia), and impaired renal perfusion (decreased urine output, elevated blood urea nitrogen and serum creatinine levels).

After weaning the patient from the ventilator and removing the endotracheal tube, promote chest physiotherapy. Start him on incentive spirometry and encourage him to cough, turn frequently, and deep-breathe. Also assist him with range-of-motion exercises, as ordered, to enhance peripheral circulation and prevent thrombus formation and other complications of prolonged immobility.

Home care instructions
• Explain that the doctor will schedule frequent (weekly to monthly) myocardial biopsies to check for signs of tissue rejection. Stress the importance of keeping these appointments, and reassure the patient that biopsy doesn't require hospitalization.
• Instruct the patient to immediately report any signs of rejection (fever, weight gain, dyspnea, lethargy, weakness) or infection (chest pain; fever;

sore throat; or redness, swelling, or drainage from the incision site).
• Explain that postpericardiotomy syndrome often develops after open-heart surgery. Tell him to call his doctor if he experiences its characteristic symptoms: fever, muscle and joint pain, weakness, and chest discomfort.
• If the patient shows signs of denervation, advise him to rise slowly from a sitting or lying position to minimize orthostatic hypotension.
• Make sure he knows the dose, schedule, and effects of prescribed drugs.
• Encourage him to follow his prescribed diet, especially noting sodium and fat restrictions.
• Instruct the patient to maintain a balance between activity and rest. Tell him to try to sleep at least 8 hours a night, to rest briefly each afternoon, and to take breaks when he's engaging in tiring physical activity. As appropriate, tell him he can climb stairs, engage in sexual activity, take baths and showers, and do light housework and other chores. Tell him to avoid lifting heavy objects (greater than 20 lb or so), driving, or doing heavy work (such as mowing the lawn or vacuuming) until his doctor grants permission. If the doctor has prescribed an exercise program, urge him to follow it.

Ventricular Assist Device

A temporary life-sustaining treatment for a failing heart, the ventricular assist device (VAD) diverts systemic blood flow from a diseased ventricle into a centrifugal pump. Used most commonly to assist the left ventricle, this device may also be used to assist the right ventricle or both ventricles. (See *VAD: A Step Removed from the Artificial Heart.*)

Candidates for a VAD include patients with massive MI, irreversible

V.A.D.: A STEP REMOVED FROM THE ARTIFICIAL HEART

Ventricular assist devices (VADs) have much in common with artificial hearts. The most important difference is that VADs *assist* the heart rather than replace it. And in most cases, they're temporary, whereas the artificial heart is intended as a permanent substitute. These differences mean that the VAD doesn't have to be as compact as the artificial heart (in fact, the pumping chambers themselves usually aren't implanted in the patient) and can be used to aid one or both ventricles.

A new VAD

One type of VAD (shown here) bridges the gap between temporary VADs and the artificial heart. Like the artificial heart, it's implanted permanently in the chest cavity, but it doesn't entirely replace the patient's own heart. The permanent VAD is powered through the skin by a belt of electrical transformer coils surrounding the patient's waist; in addition, it can run off an implanted

rechargeable battery for up to an hour at a time. Most commonly, the permanent VAD is used for patients awaiting heart transplants or those with end-stage cardiac disease who aren't transplant candidates.

An old problem

Both VADs and artificial hearts attempt to duplicate the seemingly simple task of the heart: pumping blood through the body. Designing a pump is fairly straightforward, but researchers still haven't solved the riddle of how blood swirls through the pulsing chambers of the heart without clotting. Despite the use of anticoagulants and special Dacron linings, both the artificial heart and the VAD often cause formation of thrombi, leading to pulmonary embolism, cerebrovascular accident, and other ominous complications. That's why the artificial heart hasn't yet proved successful and why VADs are used only when less dramatic measures have failed.

PERMANENT LEFT VENTRICULAR ASSIST DEVICE

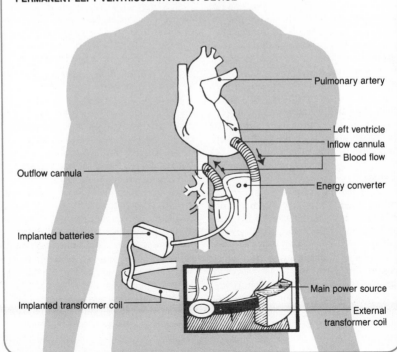

cardiomyopathy, acute myocarditis, inability to wean from cardiopulmonary bypass, valvular disease, bacterial endocarditis, or rejection of a heart transplant. In addition, the device is sometimes used for patients awaiting a heart transplant.

The VAD carries a high risk of complications. For example, the device damages blood cells, creating the risk of thrombus formation and subsequent pulmonary embolism or cerebrovascular accident. As a result, if ventricular function hasn't improved in 96 hours, the doctor may consider a heart transplant.

Purpose

To temporarily reduce ventricular work, allowing the myocardium to rest and contractility to improve.

Preparation

Reinforce the doctor's explanation of the procedure and answer any questions that the patient or his family may have. Be sure that informed consent has been obtained and that the patient understands the risks of the treatment.

Explain that food and fluids will be restricted before surgery and that the patient's cardiac function will be monitored continuously, using an EKG, a pulmonary artery catheter, and an arterial line. If time allows, the surgeon may order that the patient's chest be shaved and scrubbed with an antiseptic solution.

Procedure

In the operating room, the patient will be prepared and given a general anesthetic. Then the surgeon will make an incision in the chest. If the patient will be receiving a left VAD, the surgeon places the cannulas in the left atrium and aorta. For a right VAD, he places them in the right atrium and pulmonary artery. After suturing the cannulas in place, the surgeon connects them to tubing that runs to the pump head of the VAD. In most cases, the surgeon will leave the pump itself outside the body, with Dacron tubing entering the chest through the incision.

Finally, he'll turn on and adjust the pump, check that it's working properly and that the sutures aren't leaking, and apply an occlusive dressing over the operative site.

Monitoring and aftercare

After the operation, the patient is returned to an intensive care unit. Before he arrives, place an air mattress or sheepskin on his bed; it will help you position him and avoid skin breakdown.

Expect the patient to still be under the effects of the general anesthetic when he arrives; usually the anesthetic isn't reversed, as a sedative measure. As the anesthetic wears off, administer analgesics, as ordered.

Keep the patient immobilized while the VAD is in place to prevent accidental extubation, contamination, or disconnection of the device. Use soft restraints on both of the patient's hands.

If you've been trained to adjust the device's pump, maintain cardiac output at 5 to 8 liters/minute, pulmonary capillary wedge pressure at 10 to 20 mm Hg, central venous pressure at 8 to 16 mm Hg, mean blood pressure above 60 mm Hg, and left atrial pressure at 4 to 12 mm Hg. Also monitor the patient for signs of poor perfusion and ineffective pumping. Such signs include arrhythmias, hypotension, cool skin, slow capillary refill, oliguria or anuria, confusion, restlessness, and anxiety.

Administer heparin, as ordered, to prevent clotting in the pump head and thrombus formation. Be sure to check for bleeding, especially at the operative sites. Every 4 hours monitor prothrombin time, partial thromboplastin time, and hemoglobin and hematocrit levels. Notify the doctor of abnormal findings.

Because of your patient's debilitated state, be on guard for infection. Assess incisions and the cannula insertion site for signs of infection, and culture any suspicious exudate. Monitor the patient's white blood cell count and differential daily, and take rectal or core temperatures every 4 hours. Using aseptic technique, change the dressing over the cannula insertion sites daily.

Provide supportive care, such as lubricating the skin every 4 hours. Perform passive range-of-motion exercises every 2 hours.

Home care instructions
Because a VAD serves as short-term therapy for critically ill patients, it doesn't entail home care instructions.

Coronary Artery Bypass Grafting

Coronary artery bypass grafting (CABG) circumvents an occluded coronary artery with an autogenous graft (usually a segment of the saphenous vein or internal mammarian artery), thereby restoring blood flow to the myocardium. CABG techniques vary according to the patient's condition and the number of arteries being bypassed; the most common procedure, aorto-coronary bypass, involves suturing one end of the autogenous graft to the ascending aorta and the other end to a coronary artery distal to the occlusion.

More than 100,000 Americans (most of them male) undergo CABG each year, making it one of the most common cardiac surgeries. Prime candidates for CABG include patients with severe angina from atherosclerosis and others with coronary artery disease who are at high risk for MI. If successful, CABG can relieve anginal pain, improve cardiac function, and possibly enhance the patient's quality of life. But although the surgery relieves pain in about 90% of patients, its long-term effectiveness is uncertain. Its benefits may be only temporary; problems such as graft closure and development of atherosclerosis in other coronary arteries sometimes necessitate repeat surgery.

What's more, no clear evidence exists that CABG reduces the risk of MI.

Besides patient preparation, your role focuses on careful postoperative monitoring to ensure adequate ventilation and cardiac output and to promptly detect complications, such as arrhythmias, hypertension or hypotension, cardiac tamponade, thromboembolism, and MI.

Purpose
To bypass one or more narrowed or occluded coronary arteries, thereby improving myocardial perfusion and relieving anginal pain.

Preparation
Begin by reinforcing the doctor's explanation of the surgery. Next, explain the complex equipment and procedures used in the intensive care or recovery unit. If possible, arrange a tour of the unit for the patient and his family before surgery. Tell him that he'll awaken from surgery with an endotracheal tube in place and be connected to a mechanical ventilator. He'll also be connected to a cardiac monitor and have in place a nasogastric tube, a chest tube, an indwelling catheter, arterial lines, epicardial pacing wires, and possibly a pulmonary artery catheter. Reassure him that this equipment should cause him little discomfort and will be removed as soon as possible. Ensure that he or a responsible family member has signed a consent form.

The evening before surgery, have the patient shower with antiseptic soap and shave him from his chin to his toes. Restrict food and fluids after midnight and provide a sedative, if ordered. On the morning of surgery, also provide a sedative, as ordered, to help him relax.

Before surgery, assist with pulmonary artery catheterization and insertion of arterial lines. Then begin cardiac monitoring.

Procedure
Surgery begins with graft harvesting: the surgeon makes a series of incisions

BYPASSING CORONARY OCCLUSIONS

In this example of coronary artery bypass grafting, the surgeon has used saphenous vein segments to bypass occlusions in three sections of coronary artery.

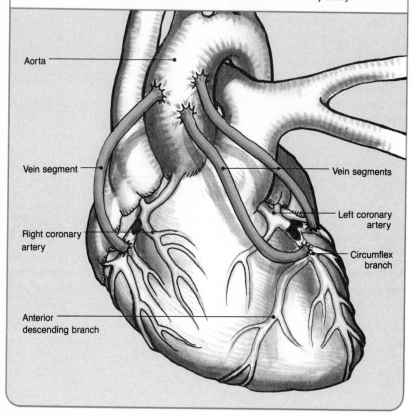

Aorta

Vein segment

Vein segments

Left coronary artery

Right coronary artery

Circumflex branch

Anterior descending branch

in the patient's thigh or calf, and removes a saphenous vein segment for grafting. (As an alternative, the surgeon may use a segment of the internal mammarian artery.)

Once the grafts are obtained, the surgeon performs a medial sternotomy and exposes the heart. He then initiates cardiopulmonary bypass (see *Understanding Cardiopulmonary Bypass,* pages 64 and 65). To reduce myocardial oxygen demands during surgery and to protect the heart, he induces cardiac hypothermia and standstill by injecting a cold cardioplegic solution (potassium-enriched saline solution)

into the aortic root.

After the patient is fully prepared, the surgeon sutures one end of the venous graft to the ascending aorta and the other end to a patent coronary artery distal to the occlusion. (He sutures the graft in a reversed position to promote proper blood flow.) He repeats this procedure for each artery he bypasses. Once the grafts are in place, he flushes the cardioplegic solution from the heart and discontinues cardiopulmonary bypass. He then implants epicardial pacing electrodes, inserts a chest tube, closes the incision, and applies a sterile dressing.

Monitoring and aftercare

Following CABG, assess the patient for signs of hemodynamic compromise, such as severe hypotension, decreased cardiac output, and shock. Check and record vital signs every 15 minutes until the patient's condition stabilizes. Monitor the EKG for disturbances in heart rate and rhythm. If you detect serious abnormalities, notify the doctor and be prepared to assist with epicardial pacing or, if necessary, cardioversion or defibrillation.

To ensure adequate myocardial perfusion, maintain arterial pressure within the guidelines set by the doctor. Usually, mean arterial pressure below 70 mm Hg results in inadequate tissue perfusion; pressure above 110 mm Hg can cause hemorrhage and graft rupture. Also monitor pulmonary artery, central venous, and left atrial pressure, as ordered.

Frequently evaluate the patient's peripheral pulses, capillary refill time, and skin temperature and color, and auscultate for heart sounds. Notify the doctor of any abnormalities. Also evaluate tissue oxygenation by assessing breath sounds, chest excursion, and symmetry of chest expansion. Check arterial blood gas (ABG) results every 2 to 4 hours, and adjust ventilator settings as needed to maintain ABG values within prescribed limits. Monitor the patient's intake and output and assess him for electrolyte imbalance, especially hypokalemia.

Maintain chest tube drainage at the prescribed negative pressure (usually -10 to -40 cmH$_2$O). Milk chest tubes every hour to maintain patency and assess regularly for hemorrhage, excessive drainage (greater than 200 ml/hour), and sudden decrease or cessation of drainage.

As the patient's incisional pain increases, give an analgesic, as ordered. Give other drugs, as ordered.

Throughout the recovery period, assess for symptoms of cerebrovascular accident (altered level of consciousness, pupillary changes, weakness and loss of movement in extremities, ataxia, aphasia, dysphagia, sensory disturbances), pulmonary embolism (chest pain, dyspnea, hemoptysis, pleural friction rub, cyanosis, hypoxemia), and impaired renal perfusion (decreased urine output, elevated blood urea nitrogen and serum creatinine levels).

After weaning the patient from the ventilator and removing the endotracheal tube, promote chest physiotherapy. Start him on incentive spirometry and encourage him to cough, turn frequently, and deep-breathe. Assist him with range-of-motion exercises, as ordered, to enhance peripheral circulation and prevent thrombus formation.

Home care instructions

• Instruct the patient to watch for and immediately notify the doctor of any signs of infection (fever; sore throat; or redness, swelling, or drainage from the leg or chest incisions) or possible arterial reocclusion (angina, dizziness, dyspnea, rapid or irregular pulse, or prolonged recovery time from exercise).
• Explain that postpericardiotomy syndrome often develops after open-heart surgery. Tell the patient to call his doctor if such symptoms as fever, muscle and joint pain, weakness, or chest discomfort occur.
• Prepare the patient for the possibility of postoperative depression, which may not develop until weeks after discharge. Reassure him that this depression is normal and should pass quickly.
• Make sure the patient understands the dose, frequency of administration, and possible side effects of all prescribed medications.
• Encourage the patient to follow his prescribed diet, especially noting any sodium and cholesterol restrictions. Explain that this diet can help reduce the risk of recurrent arterial occlusion.
• Instruct him to maintain a balance between activity and rest. Tell him to try to sleep at least 8 hours a night, to schedule a short rest period for each

afternoon, and to rest frequently when engaging in tiring physical activity. As appropriate, tell him he can climb stairs, engage in sexual activity, take baths and showers, and do light chores. Tell him to avoid lifting heavy objects (greater than 20 lb or so), driving a car, or doing heavy work (such as lawn mowing or vacuuming) until his doctor grants permission. If the doctor has prescribed an exercise program, encourage the patient to follow it.

● Refer the patient to a local chapter of the Mended Hearts Club and the American Heart Association for information and support.

ADVANCED EQUIPMENT

UNDERSTANDING CARDIOPULMONARY BYPASS

Open-heart surgery often involves a technique known as cardiopulmonary bypass to divert blood from the heart and lungs to an extracorporeal circuit with a minimum of hemolysis and trauma. As shown in this simplified diagram, the cardiopulmonary bypass (or "heart-lung") machine uses a mechanical pump to provide ventricular pumping action, an oxygenator to perform gas exchange, and a heat exchanger to cool the blood and lower the metabolic rate during surgery.

To perform this procedure, the surgeon inserts cannulas into the right atrium or the inferior or superior vena cava for blood removal, and into the ascending aorta,

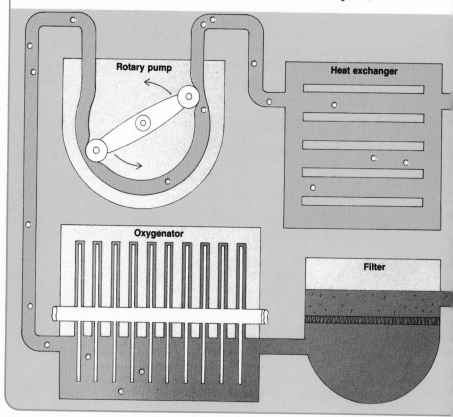

Valve Replacement

Severe valvular stenosis or insufficiency often requires excision of the affected valve and replacement with a mechan- ical or biological prosthesis. The mitral and aortic valves are affected most commonly because of the high pressure generated by the left ventricle during contraction.

Indications for valve replacement de- pend on the patient's symptoms and on the affected valve. For example, if the

femoral artery, or iliac artery for blood re- turn. He may also insert a vent into the left ventricle to aspirate blood.

After heparinizing the patient and priming the pump with fluid to replace diverted venous blood, the surgeon switches on the machine. The pump draws blood from the vena cava cannulas into the machine, where it passes through a filter, oxygenator, heat exchanger, and another filter and bubble trap before being returned to arterial circulation. During cardiopulmonary bypass, an anesthesiologist or perfusionist maintains mean arterial pressure by adjusting the rate of perfusion or by infusing fluids or vasopressor drugs.

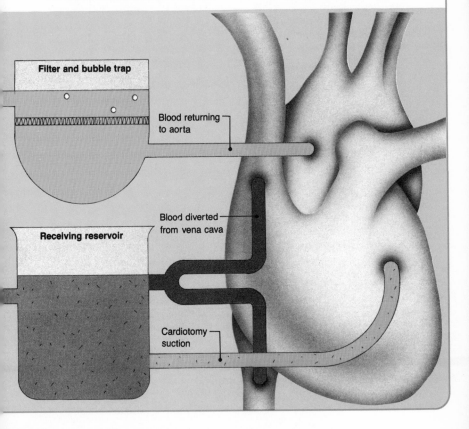

Filter and bubble trap

Blood returning to aorta

Blood diverted from vena cava

Receiving reservoir

Cardiotomy suction

patient has severe symptoms that can't be managed with drugs and dietary restrictions, valve replacement (or commissurotomy) must be performed to prevent life-threatening congestive heart failure. In aortic insufficiency, valve replacement is usually done once symptoms—palpitations, dizziness, dyspnea on exertion, angina, and murmurs—have developed or if the chest X-ray and EKG reveal left ventricular hypertrophy. In aortic stenosis, which may be asymptomatic, valve replacement may be performed if cardiac catheterization reveals significant stenosis. In mitral stenosis, it's indicated if the patient develops fatigue, dyspnea, hemoptysis, arrhythmias, pulmonary hypertension, or right ventricular hypertrophy. In mitral insufficiency, surgery is usually done when the patient's symptoms—dyspnea, fatigue, and palpitations—interfere with his activities or if insufficiency is acute, as in papillary muscle rupture.

Although valve replacement surgery carries a low mortality, it can cause serious complications. Hemorrhage may result from unligated vessels, anticoagulant therapy, or coagulopathy resulting from cardiopulmonary bypass during surgery. Cerebrovascular accident may result from thrombus formation due to turbulent blood flow through the prosthetic valve or from poor cerebral perfusion during cardiopulmonary bypass. Bacterial endocarditis can develop within days of implantation or months later. Valve dysfunction or failure may occur as the prosthetic device wears out.

Purpose
To excise a diseased or incompetent valve and replace it with a mechanical or biological prosthesis.

Preparation
As necessary, reinforce and supplement the doctor's explanation of the procedure. Listen to the patient's concerns and encourage him to ask questions. Tell him that he'll awaken from surgery in an intensive care unit or recovery room. Mention that he'll be connected to a cardiac monitor and have I.V. lines, an arterial line, and possibly a pulmonary artery or left atrial catheter in place. Explain that he'll breathe through an endotracheal tube that's connected to a mechanical ventilator, and that he'll have a chest tube in place.

Before surgery, expect to assist with insertion of an arterial line and possibly a pulmonary artery catheter. As ordered, initiate cardiac monitoring. Ensure that the patient has signed a consent form and that necessary laboratory studies and blood typing and cross matching have been performed.

Procedure
After performing a medial sternotomy and initiating cardiopulmonary bypass (see *Understanding Cardiopulmonary Bypass*, pages 64 and 65), the surgeon cannulates the coronary arteries and perfuses them with a cold cardioplegic solution. For aortic valve replacement, he clamps the aorta above the right coronary artery; for mitral valve replacement, he incises the left atrium to expose the mitral valve.

After excising the diseased valve, the surgeon sutures around the margin of the valve annulus (the ring or encircling structure, which is left intact after valve excision). He then threads the suture material through the sewing ring of the prosthetic valve and, using a valve holder, positions the prosthesis and secures the sutures. Once he's satisfied with prosthetic placement, he removes the patient from the bypass machine. As the heart fills with blood, the surgeon vents the aorta and ventricle for air. Finally, he places epicardial pacemaker leads, inserts a mediastinal chest tube, closes the incision, and applies a sterile dressing.

Monitoring and aftercare
After surgery, closely monitor the patient's hemodynamic status for signs of compromise. Watch especially for severe hypotension, decreased cardiac

COMPARING PROSTHETIC VALVES

Commonly used mechanical prosthetic valves include the Starr-Edwards caged-ball valve and the Bjork-Shiley tilting disk. Although these durable valves can withstand considerable stress, they have several disadvantages. For instance, their large size makes them sometimes difficult to fit. And because blood flow is turbulent through these valves, long-term anticoagulant therapy is necessary to prevent thrombus formation.

Biological prosthetic heart valves consist of either porcine xenograft, such as the Carpentier-Edwards valve, or bovine pericardium, such as the Ionescu-Shiley valve. Because biological prosthetic valves don't obstruct blood flow, they don't require anticoagulant therapy. However, they're difficult to insert and less durable (prone to degeneration or calcification) than their mechanical counterparts.

STARR-EDWARDS VALVE

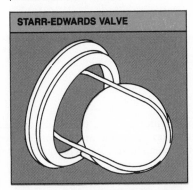

BJORK-SHILEY VALVE

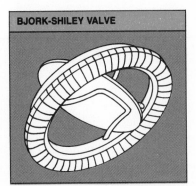

CARPENTIER-EDWARDS VALVE

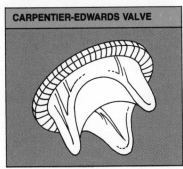

IONESCU-SHILEY VALVE

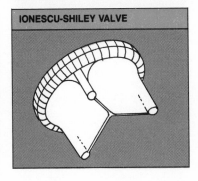

output, and shock. Check and record vital signs every 15 minutes until his condition stabilizes. Frequently assess heart sounds; report distant heart sounds or new murmurs, which may indicate prosthetic valve failure.

Monitor the EKG for disturbances in heart rate and rhythm, such as bra-dycardia, ventricular tachycardia, and heart block. Such disturbances may point to injury of the conduction system, which may occur during valve replacement because of the proximity of the atrial and mitral valves to the atrioventricular node. Arrhythmias also may result from myocardial irritability or ischemia, fluid and electrolyte imbalance, hypoxemia, or hypothermia. If you detect serious abnormalities, notify the doctor and be prepared to assist with temporary epicardial pacing.

To ensure adequate myocardial perfusion, maintain mean arterial pressure within the guidelines set by the doctor. For adults, this range is usually between 70 and 100 mm Hg. Also monitor pulmonary artery and left atrial pressure, as ordered.

Frequently assess the patient's peripheral pulses, capillary refill time, and skin temperature and color, and auscultate for heart sounds. Evaluate tissue oxygenation by assessing breath sounds, chest excursion, and symmetry of chest expansion. Report any abnormalities. Check arterial blood gas (ABG) levels every 2 to 4 hours, and adjust ventilator settings as needed.

Maintain chest tube drainage at the prescribed negative pressure (usually -10 to -40 cmH$_2$O for adults). Milk chest tubes every hour to maintain patency, and assess regularly for hemorrhage, excessive drainage (greater than 200 ml/hour), and sudden decrease or cessation of drainage.

As ordered, administer analgesic, anticoagulant, antibiotic, antiarrhythmic, inotropic, and pressor medications, as well as I.V. fluids and blood products. Monitor intake and output and assess for electrolyte imbalances, especially hypokalemia. Once anticoagulant therapy begins, evaluate its effectiveness by monitoring prothrombin time daily.

Throughout the patient's recovery period, observe him carefully for complications. Watch especially for symptoms of cerebrovascular accident (altered level of consciousness, pupillary changes, weakness and loss of movement in the extremities, ataxia, aphasia, dysphagia, sensory disturbances), pulmonary embolism (dyspnea, cough, hemoptysis, chest pain, pleural friction rub, cyanosis, hypoxemia), and impaired renal perfusion (decreased urinary output and elevated blood urea nitrogen and serum creatinine levels).

After weaning the patient from the ventilator and removing the endotracheal tube, promote chest physiotherapy. Start him on incentive spirometry, and encourage him to cough, turn frequently, and deep-breathe. Gradually increase his activities.

Home care instructions
• Tell the patient to immediately report chest pain, fever, or redness, swelling, or drainage at the incision site.
• Explain that postpericardiotomy syndrome—fever, muscle and joint pain, weakness, and chest discomfort—often develops after open-heart surgery. Tell the patient to notify the doctor if these symptoms occur.
• Make sure the patient understands the dose, schedule, and side effects of all prescribed drugs.
• Advise him to wear a Medic Alert bracelet and carry a card with information and instructions on his anticoagulant and antibiotic therapy.
• Encourage him to follow his prescribed diet, noting especially sodium and fat restrictions.
• Provide tips for maintaining a balance between activity and rest. Tell him to try to sleep at least 8 hours a night, to schedule a short rest period for each afternoon, and to rest frequently when engaging in tiring physical activity. As appropriate, tell him he can climb stairs, engage in sexual activity, take baths and showers, and do light housework and other chores. Tell him to avoid lifting heavy objects (greater than 20 lb or so), driving a car, or doing heavy work (such as lawn mowing or vacuuming) until his doctor grants permission. If the doctor has prescribed an exercise program, encourage the patient to follow it carefully.
• Instruct the patient to inform his dentist or any of his other doctors that he has a prosthetic valve before undergoing any surgery or extensive dental work. He'll probably need to take prophylactic antibiotics.

Repair of Congenital Heart Defects

Occurring in 8 to 10 of every 1,000 live births, congenital heart defects are classified as *acyanotic* or *cyanotic*. Common acyanotic defects include ventricular septal defect (VSD), atrial septal defect (ASD), coarctation of the aorta, and patent ductus arteriosus (PDA). Common cyanotic defects include tetralogy of Fallot and transposition of the great arteries.

The timing of corrective surgery depends on the type and extent of the defect. For instance, surgery to repair transposition of the great arteries is typically performed when the patient is between ages 3 months and 3 years. Repair of coarctation of the aorta is usually delayed until ages 4 to 8 unless severe complications develop earlier. Surgical repair may even occur during adulthood if a small defect has gone undetected until then.

Surgical repair of heart defects can cause severe complications, such as cardiogenic shock, congestive heart failure, hypoxemia, hypercapnia, arrhythmias, hypotension, hemorrhage, cardiac tamponade, and cardiac arrest. As in any surgical procedure, infection poses a constant threat. In addition, neonates are particularly susceptible to alterations in thermoregulation following surgery.

Purpose

To surgically correct cardiac defects resulting from congenital anomalies.

Preparation

Help the child and his family cope with their anxieties by providing comprehensive preoperative teaching and emotional support. Before surgery, carefully explain all treatment and diagnostic procedures to the child (if he's old enough to understand) and his family. Be sure to tailor your explanations to the child's level of understanding. For instance, you may tell a preschooler that the doctor is going to fix his heart, whereas you may offer a more detailed explanation to a school-age child.

To help decrease postoperative anxiety, prepare the child and his family for the sights and sounds of the intensive care unit (ICU). Tell them about expected I.V. lines, monitoring equipment, and endotracheal and chest tubes. If possible, arrange for them to meet the ICU staff. Encourage them to ask questions and express their concerns. Ensure that the parents have signed a consent form.

Before surgery, expect to assist with insertion of an arterial line and possibly a pulmonary artery catheter. Begin cardiac monitoring as ordered.

Procedure

The surgical procedure depends on the type, size, and location of the defect (see *Reviewing Common Congenital Heart Defects*, pages 70 and 71). For most defects, the surgeon performs a medial sternotomy or a thoracotomy. If the procedure requires cardiopulmonary bypass, he inserts cannulas into the heart and great vessels and attaches them to a bypass machine (see *Understanding Cardiopulmonary Bypass*, pages 64 and 65). He then repairs the defect, discontinues cardiopulmonary bypass, puts a chest tube in place, closes the incision, and applies a sterile dressing.

Monitoring and aftercare

Expect the child awakening from anesthesia to be anxious when confronted with the tubes, monitors, and alarms of the ICU. Help decrease his anxiety by speaking in a soft, soothing voice and by touching him gently. Encourage his parents to visit as much as possible.

Following surgery, closely monitor the child's hemodynamic status. Watch particularly for severe hypotension, decreased cardiac output, and shock. Check and record vital signs every 15

REVIEWING COMMON CONGENITAL HEART DEFECTS

DEFECT		PATHOPHYSIOLOGY
Ventricular septal defect (VSD)	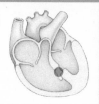	One or more abnormal openings in the ventricular septum allow shunting of blood from the left to the right ventricle. Results from incomplete closure of the ventricular septum by the 8th week of gestation. Varies in size from a pinhole to absence of entire septum.
Atrial septal defect		One or more openings between the left and right atria (includes ostium secundum, ostium primum, and sinus venosus) allow shunting of blood between the chambers. Results from delayed or incomplete closure of the foramen ovale or atrial septum. Small defects are often asymptomatic and may go undetected in childhood; they lead to CHF and pulmonary vascular disease in adulthood.
Patent ductus arteriosus (PDA)		A PDA between the pulmonary artery bifurcation and the descending aorta allows left-to-right shunting of blood from the aorta to the pulmonary artery, resulting in recirculation of arterial blood through the lungs. Caused by failure of the ductus to close after birth. May produce no clinical effects initially, but over time can precipitate pulmonary vascular disease and infective endocarditis.
Coarctation of the aorta	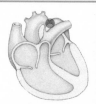	Constriction of the aorta, usually below the left subclavian artery near the junction of the ligamentum arteriosum and pulmonary artery. Often classified as preductal (occurring above the ligamentum arteriosum) or postductal (occurring below it). May result from spasm and constriction of smooth muscle in ductus arteriosus during normal closure or from abnormal development of the aortic arch.
Tetralogy of Fallot		A complex of four defects: VSD, overriding aorta, pulmonary stenosis, and right ventricular hypertrophy. Blood shunts from right to left through the VSD, permitting mixing of unoxygenated and oxygenated blood and resulting in cyanosis. Results from incomplete development of ventricular septum and pulmonary outflow tract.
Transposition of the great arteries		Reversal of normal position of the great arteries; the aorta arises from the right ventricle and the pulmonary artery from the left ventricle, producing two noncommunicating circulatory systems. Unoxygenated blood flows through the right atrium and ventricle and out the aorta to systemic circulation; oxygenated blood circulates back to the lungs. Results from faulty embryonic development (exact mechanism unknown).

TREATMENT	PROGNOSIS
Medical: For small VSD, conservative management; many close spontaneously. For medium to large VSD, bed rest, oxygen, digoxin, diuretics, and fluid restrictions for acute congestive heart failure (CHF); prophylactic antibiotics to prevent infective endocarditis; and monitoring for pulmonary artery hypertension. *Surgical:* For medium to large VSD, closure or patch graft, usually during preschool years.	Good for small defects that close spontaneously or are surgically correctable, but poor for extremely large, irreparable, or untreated defects
Medical: Usually unnecessary, except in ostium primum with accompanying CHF (see medical management for VSD above). *Surgical:* Direct closure or patch graft during preschool or early school-age years.	Excellent in asymptomatic persons, but poor in those with cyanosis and severe untreated defects
Medical: CHF regimen; catheterization to deposit a plug in the ductus to prevent shunting; indomethacin to induce ductus spasm and closure. *Surgical:* Ductal ligation in infants who fail to respond to medical management; ligation and division of ductus in all patients after age 1.	Good for small or surgically corrected defects, but poor if PDA advances to intractable CHF
Medical: In infants with preductal coarctation, CHF regimen and possibly balloon angioplasty to force open the area of coarctation. *Surgical:* For children between ages 4 and 8 (or for younger children or infants with unmanageable CHF), resection with anastomosis of aorta or insertion of a prosthetic graft.	Depends on the severity of associated defects, such as VSD or aortic stenosis; often good if corrective surgery is done before degenerative changes occur
Medical: Relief of cyanosis with knee-chest positioning and administration of oxygen, morphine, and possibly propranolol; prophylactic antibiotics to prevent infective endocarditis. *Surgical:* Palliative surgery, such as Blalock-Taussig, Potts-Smith-Gibson, or Waterston procedures, to enhance pulmonary circulation and relieve hypoxia; corrective surgery to relieve pulmonary stenosis and close VSD; usually done by age 2.	Generally good
Medical: Balloon septotomy to enlarge the foramen ovale and improve oxygenation; CHF regimen; administration of alprostadil to maintain open ductus arteriosus in neonates. *Surgical:* Mustard or Senny procedure to redirect venous return to the appropriate ventricle; usually done between ages 3 months and 3 years.	Generally good with prompt corrective surgery

minutes until the child's condition stabilizes and then every 30 minutes to 1 hour thereafter.

Monitor the EKG for disturbances in heart rate and rhythm, such as bradycardia, ventricular tachycardia, and heart block. Such disturbances may result from myocardial irritability or ischemia, fluid and electrolyte imbalance, hypoxemia, or hypothermia. If you detect serious abnormalities, notify the doctor and prepare to assist with epicardial pacing.

To ensure adequate myocardial perfusion, maintain arterial pressure within the guidelines set by the doctor. Also monitor pulmonary artery and left atrial pressure.

Frequently evaluate the child's peripheral pulses, capillary refill time, and skin temperature and color, and auscultate his heart sounds. Notify the doctor of any abnormalities. Also evaluate tissue oxygenation by assessing breath sounds, chest excursion, and symmetry of chest expansion. Check the child's arterial blood gas levels every 2 to 4 hours and adjust ventilator settings as needed.

Maintain chest tube drainage at the prescribed negative pressure. Milk chest tubes every hour to maintain patency. In addition, assess the child regularly for hemorrhage and excessive or insufficient drainage.

As ordered, administer antiarrhythmic, inotropic, and pressor medications, as well as I.V. fluids and blood products. Carefully monitor intake and output and assess for electrolyte imbalances, especially hypokalemia.

As the child's incisional pain increases, provide analgesics, as ordered. Because an infant or young child may not be able to express the degree of pain he's experiencing, watch for physiologic clues, such as diaphoresis, pallor, tachycardia, elevated blood pressure, and chest splinting on inspiration.

Throughout the child's recovery period, watch for developing complications. Be especially alert for symptoms of cerebrovascular accident (altered level of consciousness, pupillary changes, weakness and loss of movement in the extremities, ataxia, aphasia, dysphagia, sensory disturbances), pulmonary embolism (dyspnea, cough, hemoptysis, chest pain, pleural friction rub, cyanosis, hypoxemia), and impaired renal perfusion (decreased urinary output and elevated blood urea nitrogen and serum creatinine levels).

After weaning the child from the ventilator and removing the endotracheal tube, promote chest physiotherapy. Start him on incentive spirometry and encourage him to cough, turn frequently, and deep-breathe. Also assist him with range-of-motion exercises, as ordered, to enhance peripheral circulation and to prevent thrombus formation.

Home care instructions

● Instruct the parents to immediately notify the doctor if their child develops chest pain, fever, muscle or joint pain, or weakness.
● Warn the parents that prolonged hospitalization may cause behavioral changes in their child and that separation anxiety and changes in dietary habits and sleep patterns may persist for some time after discharge. Encourage them to relate to their child in a loving, consistent manner and to offer him opportunities to express his feelings through conversation and play.
● Make sure the parents understand the dose, schedule, administration technique, and possible side effects of all prescribed medications. If the doctor has prescribed a cardiac glycoside, emphasize the importance of reporting early signs of toxicity promptly.
● Instruct the parents on how best to meet any special nutritional needs their child may have.
● Advise them of any rest requirements or activity restrictions for their child.
● Stress the importance of regular checkups to assess their child's condition.

Vascular Repair

Surgical repair often represents the treatment of choice for vessels damaged by arteriosclerotic or thromboembolic disorders (such as aortic aneurysm or arterial occlusive disease), trauma, infections, or congenital defects. It may also be used for patients with obstructions that severely compromise circulation or for patients with vascular disease that doesn't respond to drug therapy or nonsurgical treatments, such as balloon catheterization. Emergency surgery is typically required for life-threatening dissecting or ruptured aortic aneurysms or limb-threatening acute arterial occlusion.

Vascular repair includes aneurysm resection, grafting, embolectomy, interruption of vena cava blood flow, and vein stripping. The specific surgery used depends on the type, location, and extent of vascular occlusion or damage (see *Understanding Types of Vascular Repair*, pages 74 and 75). However, in all vascular surgeries the potential for serious complications—such as vessel trauma, emboli, hemorrhage, and infection—exists. Grafting carries added risks: the graft may occlude, narrow, dilate, or rupture.

When caring for a patient awaiting vascular repair, your responsibilities include careful preoperative assessment and patient preparation. After surgery, they include steps to maintain circulatory status, prevent infection and other complications, and promote a return to normal functioning.

Purpose
To restore vessel patency by bypassing vascular obstructions or by replacing, removing, or reinforcing portions of a diseased vessel.

Preparation
If the patient requires emergency surgery, briefly explain the procedure to him, if possible. If he doesn't require immediate surgery, make sure that he and his family understand the doctor's explanation of the surgery and its possible complications.

If the patient's undergoing vein stripping, tell him that he'll receive a local anesthetic before the procedure. If the patient's undergoing other vascular surgery, inform him that he'll receive a general anesthetic. Mention that he'll awaken from the anesthetic in the intensive care or recovery unit. Explain that he'll have an I.V. line in place to provide access for fluids and drugs, EKG electrodes for continuous cardiac monitoring, and an arterial line or a pulmonary artery catheter to provide continuous pressure monitoring. He may also have a urinary catheter in place to allow accurate output measurement. If appropriate, explain that he'll be intubated and placed on mechanical ventilation. Also explain that his vital signs and incision site will be checked regularly.

On the day before scheduled surgery, perform a complete vascular assessment. Take vital signs to provide a baseline. Evaluate the strength and sound of the blood flow and the symmetry of the pulses, and note any bruits. Record the temperature of the extremities, their sensitivity to motor and sensory stimuli, and any pallor, cyanosis, or redness. Rate peripheral pulse volume and strength on a scale of 0 (pulse absent) to 4 (bounding, strong) and check capillary refill time by blanching the fingernail or toenail (normal refill time is under 3 seconds).

As ordered, instruct the patient to restrict food and fluids for at least 12 hours before surgery. Tell him that he probably will receive a sedative to help him relax and sleep the night before surgery. Ensure that he has signed a consent form.

If the patient's awaiting surgery for aortic aneurysm repair, be on guard for symptoms of acute dissection or rupture. Note especially sudden severe pain in the chest, abdomen, or lower

UNDERSTANDING TYPES OF VASCULAR REPAIR

AORTIC ANEURYSM REPAIR

Purpose
To reinforce the wall of the aorta or to remove an aneurysmal segment

Procedure
The surgeon first makes an incision to expose the aneurysm site. If necessary, he places the patient on a cardiopulmonary bypass machine; then he clamps the aorta above the aneurysm. Depending on the severity of the aneurysm—and on whether it's ruptured—he wraps the weakened arterial wall with Dacron to reinforce it (right) or replaces the damaged portion with a Dacron graft.

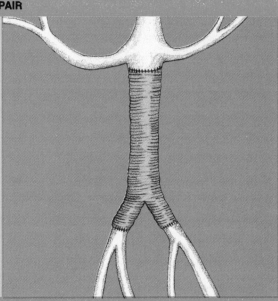

BYPASS GRAFTING

Purpose
To bypass an arterial obstruction resulting from arteriosclerosis

Procedure
After exposing the affected artery, the surgeon anastomoses a synthetic or autogenous graft to divert blood flow around the occluded arterial segment. The graft may be synthetic, or it may be a vein harvested from elsewhere in the patient's body.
   The illustration at right shows a femoropopliteal bypass.

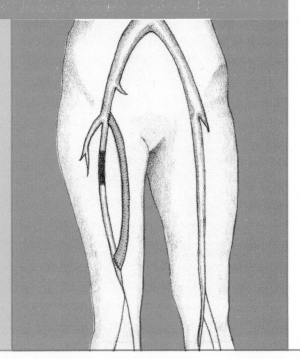

EMBOLECTOMY

Purpose
To remove an embolism from an artery

Procedure
The surgeon inserts a balloon-tipped Fogarty catheter into the artery and passes it through the thrombus (top). He then inflates the balloon and withdraws the catheter to remove the thrombus (bottom).

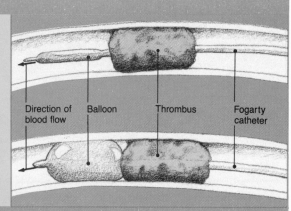

Direction of blood flow   Balloon   Thrombus   Fogarty catheter

SURGICAL INTERRUPTION OF THE INFERIOR VENA CAVA

Purpose
To block circulation through the vena cava

Procedure
The surgeon makes a flank incision. Then he uses a catheter to insert a clip, a filter, a balloon, or an umbrella device (shown at right) into the vein.

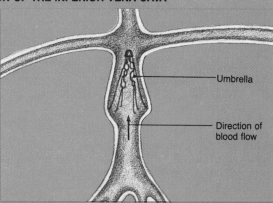

Umbrella

Direction of blood flow

VEIN STRIPPING

Purpose
To remove the saphenous vein and its branches to treat varicosities

Procedure
The surgeon ligates the saphenous vein. He then threads the stripper into the vein, secures it, and pulls it back out, bringing the vein with it.

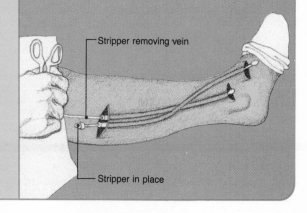

Stripper removing vein

Stripper in place

back; severe weakness; diaphoresis; tachycardia; or a precipitous drop in blood pressure. If any such symptoms occur, call the doctor immediately; he may need to perform emergency surgery to save the patient's life.

Procedure

See *Understanding Types of Vascular Repair,* pages 74 and 75, for a description of the different surgeries.

Monitoring and aftercare

Check and record the patient's vital signs every 15 minutes until his condition stabilizes and every 30 minutes to 1 hour thereafter. Monitor the EKG for abnormalities in heart rate or rhythm. Also monitor other pressure readings and carefully record intake and output. Check the patient's dressing regularly for excessive bleeding. Position the patient as ordered, and instruct him on recommended levels of activity during early stages of recovery. Provide analgesics, as ordered, for the patient's incisional pain.

Frequently assess peripheral pulses, using Doppler ultrasonography if palpation proves difficult. Check all extremities for muscle strength and movement, color, temperature, and capillary refill time.

Throughout the patient's recovery period, assess him often for signs of complications. Fever, cough, congestion, or dyspnea may indicate pulmonary infection. Low urine output and elevated blood urea nitrogen and serum creatinine levels may point to renal dysfunction. Severe pain and cyanosis in a limb may indicate occlusion. Hypotension, tachycardia, restlessness and confusion, shallow respirations, abdominal pain, and increased abdominal girth may signal hemorrhage; report any of these signs immediately. In addition, frequently check the incision site for drainage and signs of infection.

As the patient's condition improves, help wean him from the ventilator, if appropriate. To promote good pulmo-

nary hygiene, encourage him to cough, turn, and deep-breathe frequently. As ordered, assist him with range-of-motion exercises in his legs to help prevent thrombus formation.

Home care instructions

• If appropriate, instruct the patient to check his pulse in the affected extremity before rising from bed each morning. If the patient can't check his own pulse, teach a family member to do it for him. Tell the patient to notify the doctor if he can't palpate his pulse or if he develops coldness, pallor, or pain in the extremity.

• Explain the importance of strict compliance with any prescribed medication regimen. Make sure the patient understands the schedule and the expected side effects of all prescribed medications.

• Also stress the importance of regular checkups to monitor his condition.

Pacemaker Insertion

Pacemakers are battery-operated generators that emit timed electrical signals, triggering contraction of the heart muscle and controlling the heart rate. Whether temporary or permanent, they're used when the heart's natural pacemaker fails to work properly.

Temporary pacemakers may be used in emergency situations—for example, when drug therapy fails to correct dangerous bradycardia or heart block and time or the patient's condition doesn't permit implantation of a permanent pacemaker—or during open-heart surgery. They're also used for observing pacing's effects on cardiac function, so that an optimum rate can be selected before a permanent pacemaker is implanted.

Permanent pacemakers are used when the heart's natural pacemaker is

UNDERSTANDING PACEMAKER VOCABULARY

"The firing loss seems to be caused by undersensing. The threshold needs to be increased to be sure the heartbeat's captured." A patient who overhears comments such as these may find them confusing or even frightening. Like any specialized field, cardiac pacing has its own jargon, which can seem overwhelming if you don't know what's being said. To help you convert this jargon into plain English, here's a quick primer.

Artifact The spike recorded on the EKG depicting the electrical energy discharged from the pulse generator.

Capture Contraction of the heart muscle in response to discharge from the pulse generator.

Electrode The thin, electrically conductive wire that's enclosed within the lead wire of the system. It comes in direct contact with the heart and sends signals to the pulse generator.

Failure to pace Absence of an artifact on the EKG when the pacemaker, according to program, should be firing.

Failure to sense A condition in which the pulse generator doesn't respond at all to the heart's signals (see *Undersensing*, below).

Firing loss Combined failure to sense and capture, caused by mechanical failure of the unit.

Lead The wire surrounding the electrode, which delivers the electrical energy from the pulse generator to the heart and receives the sensing in-

formation. Leads can be unipolar (single terminal) or bipolar (double terminal).

Noncapture (failure to capture) The failure of the heart to respond to a correctly synchronized pacing stimulus.

Oversensing A condition in which the pulse generator responds too readily to signals for impulse generation.

Pulse generator The device that includes the power source and circuitry for transmitting pacing signals as well as for sensing the heart's intrinsic activity.

Sensing The ability to recognize the electrical signal that stimulates (or inhibits) the discharge of electrical energy by the pulse generator.

Threshold The amount of electrical energy necessary to consistently cause depolarization.

Undersensing A condition in which the pulse generator occasionally fails to respond to the heart's signals (see *Failure to sense*, above).

irreversibly disrupted. Indications include symptomatic bradycardia, advanced symptomatic atrioventricular (AV) block, sick sinus syndrome, sinus arrest, sinoatrial block, Stokes-Adams syndrome, tachyarrhythmias, and ectopic rhythms caused by antiarrhythmic drugs.

Permanent pacemaker implantation is a common procedure; worldwide, about 100,000 people undergo it every year. More than 300 types of pacemakers exist, and many of them are programmable to perform varied functions. Pacemakers are categorized according to their capabilities (see

Reviewing Pacemaker Codes, page 80). Choice of a pacemaker depends on the patient's age and condition, the doctor's preference and, increasingly, the device's cost, which can be several thousand dollars.

Nursing care—particularly postoperative monitoring—is vital for patients receiving a permanent pacemaker. Early complications include serous or bloody drainage from the insertion site, swelling, ecchymosis, incisional pain, and impaired mobility; less common complications include venous thromboses, embolism, infection, pneumothorax, pectoral or diaphragmatic

REVIEWING TYPES OF
TEMPORARY PACEMAKERS

Temporary pacemakers come in four types: transcutaneous, transvenous, transthoracic, and epicardial. They're used to pace the heart after cardiac surgery, during cardiopulmonary resuscitation, and when sinus arrest, symptomatic sinus bradycardia, or complete heart block occurs. Temporary pacing may also correct tachyarrhythmias that fail to respond to drug therapy.

Transcutaneous pacemaker

Completely noninvasive and easily applied, this pacemaker proves especially useful in an emergency. To perform pacing with this device, the doctor places electrodes on the skin directly over the heart and connects them to a pulse generator.

Transthoracic pacemaker

Transthoracic pacing involves needle insertion of leads into the heart. Used in emergencies, it rarely stimulates the heart and commonly causes complications.

Transvenous pacemaker

This device, a balloon-tipped pacing catheter, is inserted via the subclavian or jugular vein into the right ventricle. The procedure can be done at the bedside or in the cardiac catheterization laboratory. Transvenous pacemakers offer better control of the heartbeat than either transcutaneous or transthoracic pacemakers, but electrode insertion takes longer, thus limiting its usefulness in emergencies.

Epicardial pacemaker

Implanted during open-heart surgery, the epicardial pacemaker permits rapid treatment of postoperative complications. During surgery, the doctor attaches the leads to the heart and runs them out through the chest incision. Afterward, they're coiled on the patient's chest, insulated, and covered with a dressing. If pacing is needed, the leads are simply uncovered and attached to a pulse generator. When pacing is no longer needed, the leads can simply be pulled out under a local anesthetic.

---

muscle stimulation from the pacemaker, arrhythmias, cardiac tamponade, congestive heart failure, and abnormal pacemaker operation with lead dislodgment. Late complications (up to several years) include failure to capture, failure to sense, firing loss, and pacemaker rejection.

Purpose
To control the heart rate by delivering timed electrical impulses to the myocardium.

Preparation
If pacing is done in an emergency, briefly explain the procedure to the patient, if possible. (See *Reviewing Types of Temporary Pacemakers* for details on insertion or application.)

If the patient's scheduled for permanent implantation, ensure that he and his family understand the doctor's explanation of the need for an artificial pacemaker, the potential complications, and the alternatives. Obtain baseline vital signs and record a 12-lead EKG or rhythm strip. Evaluate radial and dorsalis pedis pulses and assess the patient's mental status.

Restrict food and fluids for 12 hours before the procedure. Explain to the patient that he may receive a sedative before the procedure and will probably have his upper chest shaved and scrubbed with an antiseptic solution. Inform him that when he arrives in the operating room, his hands may be restrained so that they don't inadvertently touch the sterile area, and his chest will be draped with sterile towels. Unless he's scheduled to undergo a thoracotomy, explain that he'll receive a local, rather than a general, anesthetic. Tell him that he'll be in the operating room for about an hour.

Check that the patient or a responsible family member has signed a consent form.

Procedure

Insertion or application of a temporary pacemaker varies, depending on the device (see *Reviewing Types of Temporary Pacemakers*).

Permanent pacemakers can be implanted through a thoracotomy (which requires a general anesthetic), but the transvenous endocardial approach is more commonly used. With this method, which is done under a local anesthetic, the patient's sedated and his chest is prepared. Then the surgeon makes a 3- to 4-inch incision in the subcutaneous tissue of the chest, inserts the electrode catheter through a vein, and uses fluoroscopy to guide it into the appropriate chamber of the heart (depending on the type of pacemaker). After inserting the leads, he uses a pacing system analyzer to set the pulse generator to the proper stimulating and sensing thresholds, and then attaches the pulse generator to the leads and implants it into a pocket of muscle in the patient's chest wall. He uses nonabsorbable sutures to tie the connection, leaving extra lengths of leads coiled under the pulse generator to decrease tension on the leads and to simplify subsequent replacement of the pulse generator, if necessary. He then closes the incision and applies a tight occlusive dressing.

Monitoring and aftercare

After pacemaker insertion, provide continuous EKG monitoring. Chart the type of insertion, lead system, pacemaker mode, and pacing guidelines. Take vital signs every 30 minutes until the patient stabilizes, and watch the EKG for signs of pacemaker problems.

Be on guard for signs of a perforated ventricle, with resultant cardiac tamponade. Ominous signs include persistent hiccups, distant heart sounds, pulsus paradoxus, hypotension accompanied by narrow pulse pressure, increased venous pressure, bulging neck veins, cyanosis, decreased urinary output, restlessness, and complaints of fullness in the chest. Report any of these signs immediately and prepare the patient for emergency surgery.

If your patient's condition worsens dramatically and he requires defibrillation, follow these guidelines to avoid damaging the pacemaker: place the paddles at least 4 inches (10 cm) from the pulse generator and avoid anterior/posterior paddle placement. Have a backup temporary pacemaker available. If your patient has an external pacemaker, turn it off. Finally, keep the current under 200 joules, if possible.

Assess the area around the incision for swelling, tenderness, and hematoma, but don't remove the occlusive dressing for the first 24 hours without a doctor's order. When you do remove it, check the wound for drainage, redness, and unusual warmth or tenderness.

After the first 24 hours, begin passive range-of-motion (ROM) exercises for the affected arm, if ordered. Progress to active ROM in 2 weeks.

Home care instructions

• Tell the patient to take his pulse every day before getting out of bed. Instruct him to record his heart rate, along with the date and time, to help his doctor determine whether the pacemaker requires adjustment.
• Stress the importance of calling the doctor immediately if his pulse rate drops below the minimal pacemaker setting or if it exceeds 100 beats/minute. Also have him report difficulty breathing, dizziness, fainting, or swollen hands or feet. Similarly, have him report redness, warmth, pain, drainage, or swelling at the insertion site.
• Warn the patient to avoid placing ex-

REVIEWING PACEMAKER CODES

A three-letter pacemaker code developed by the Intersociety Commission for Heart Disease provides a simple description of a pacemaker's capabilities. (Two letters can be appended to identify other functions, but they're rarely used.) Here's a summary of the codes and what they mean:
- The first letter signifies the heart chamber being paced: **A** (atrium), **V** (ventricle), or **D** (dual, or both chambers).
- The second letter identifies the heart chamber that the pacemaker senses: **A, V, D,** or **O** (none).
- The third letter indicates how the pacemaker responds to the sensed event: **T** (triggered by the event), **I** (inhibited by the event), **D** (triggered and inhibited by the event), **O** (not applicable), or **R** (reverse—that is, the pacemaker responds by *slowing* the heartbeat rather than by speeding it).

The chart below shows some common pacemaker configurations.

PACEMAKER CODE AND INDICATIONS	ADVANTAGES	DISADVANTAGES
AAI, AAT • Sick sinus syndrome with intact atrioventricular (AV) conduction	• Simplest system that provides sequential AV depolarization • Requires single lead • Easily understood function	• Won't pace ventricle if AV block develops • Inhibits atrial impulses by sensing QRS complexes
VVI, VVT • Atrial flutter or fibrillation, or multifocal atrial tachycardia with slow ventricular response • Infrequent bradycardia • Insufficient hemodynamic response to AV sequential pacing • Recurrent pacemaker-mediated tachycardia (PMT)	• Requires single lead • Relatively simple to operate	• Doesn't change rate in response to increased metabolic demands • Doesn't preserve AV synchrony • May cause retrograde AV conduction and echo beats • May cause pacemaker syndrome
VDD • Impaired AV conduction with normal sinus node function	• Maintains AV synchrony and rate responsiveness to increased metabolic demands when atrial rate stays within tracking limits	• Requires two leads • Doesn't pace atrium • May cause PMT • Lacks AV synchrony and rate responsiveness during atrial bradycardia
DVI • Atrial bradycardia • PMT in VDD and DDD modes	• Maintains AV synchrony during atrial bradycardia • Permits AV rate control to decrease myocardial oxygen demands during angina • Lack of atrial sensing may prevent PMT	• Requires two leads • Doesn't maintain AV synchrony unless pacemaker's programmed rate exceeds spontaneous atrial rate • Doesn't respond to increased metabolic demands • Lack of atrial sensing may cause competitive rhythms
DDD • Atrial bradycardia • Normal sinus node function with abnormal AV conduction	• Maintains AV synchrony • Most closely mimics normal cardiac physiology	• Requires two leads • May cause PMT • Paced rate doesn't increase to meet metabolic demands if sinus node dysfunction occurs, unless programmed to do so

cessive pressure over the insertion site, moving suddenly or jerkily, or extending his arms over his head for 8 weeks after discharge. Tell him to notify the doctor if the site drains or becomes red, painful, warm, or foul-smelling.

• Tell him that he's free to follow his normal routines, including sexual activity, and that he may bathe and shower normally. Urge him to follow dietary and exercise instructions.

• Remind the patient to carry his pacemaker identification at all times and to show his card to airline clerks when he travels; the pacemaker will set off metal detectors but won't be harmed.

• Explain the special precautions that he'll have to take to prevent disruption of the pacemaker by electrical or electronic devices. For example, he should avoid placing electric hair clippers or shavers directly over the pacemaker, maintain a distance of at least 3 feet from microwave ovens, and avoid close contact with electric motors and gasoline engines. He should also keep away from automobile antitheft devices and high-voltage electric lines. Advise him to tell any doctor of his implanted pacemaker before undergoing certain diagnostic tests, such as magnetic resonance imaging.

• Mention that the doctor may provide instructions for testing the pacemaker, using a transistor radio or the telephone.

BALLOON CATHETER TREATMENTS

Intraaortic Balloon Counterpulsation

Intraaortic balloon counterpulsation (IABC) temporarily reduces left ventricular work load and improves cor-onary perfusion. In this treatment, the doctor threads a balloon catheter through the femoral artery into the descending thoracic aorta. Once the catheter's in place, he connects its external end to a pump that automatically inflates the balloon in early diastole and deflates it just before systole. (See *Understanding the Balloon Pump*, page 82.)

IABC is used in patients with cardiogenic shock from acute MI, septic shock, intractable angina pectoris before surgery, intractable ventricular arrhythmias, or ventricular septal or papillary muscle ruptures. It's also used for patients who suffer pump failure before or after cardiac surgery. Typically performed at the bedside as an emergency procedure, balloon catheter insertion may also be performed in the operating room—for example, when a patient can't be weaned from a cardiopulmonary bypass machine.

IABC is contraindicated if the patient's aortic valve is incompetent, since blood would flow back through the valve into the left ventricle during diastole. It's also contraindicated in an aortic aneurysm (since the catheter can rupture or extend the aneurysm); in severe atherosclerosis of the aorta or the iliac or femoral arteries; and in bleeding disorders (because of the risk of bleeding from the catheterization site). Since IABC is a short-term measure, its use is controversial for patients with end-stage heart disease. Also controversial is its use for severe shock; studies have shown that it doesn't decrease mortality in these cases.

Purpose
To reduce left ventricular work load and improve coronary perfusion by augmenting aortic diastolic pressure.

Preparation
If time permits, explain to the patient that the doctor will place a special catheter in the aorta to help his heart pump more easily. Be sure that the patient or a family member has signed a

consent form and recognizes the risks and possible complications of IABC.

Explain how the catheter is inserted and that it will be connected to a large console next to his bed. Mention that the console has an alarm system, that any alarms will be answered promptly, and that the pumping sound of the console is normal and doesn't mean that his heart has stopped beating. Explain that because of the catheter, he won't be able to sit up, bend his knee, or flex his hip more than 30 degrees.

Next, attach the patient to an EKG for continuous monitoring, and make sure that he has an arterial line, a pul-

ADVANCED EQUIPMENT

UNDERSTANDING THE BALLOON PUMP

The intraaortic balloon pump consists of a single-chambered or multichambered polyurethane balloon attached to an external pump console by means of a large-lumen catheter. This external pump works in precise counterpoint to the left ventricle, inflating the balloon with helium or carbon dioxide early in diastole and deflating it just before systole. As the balloon inflates, it forces blood toward the aortic valve, thereby raising pressure in the aortic root and augmenting diastolic pressure to improve coronary perfusion. What's more, it improves peripheral circulation by forcing blood through the brachiocephalic, common carotid, and subclavian arteries arising from the aortic trunk.

The balloon deflates rapidly at the end of diastole. This reduces aortic volume and pressure, thereby decreasing the effort required by the left ventricle to open the aortic valve. This decreased work load, in turn, lowers the heart's oxygen requirements and, combined with the improved myocardial perfusion, helps prevent or diminish myocardial ischemia.

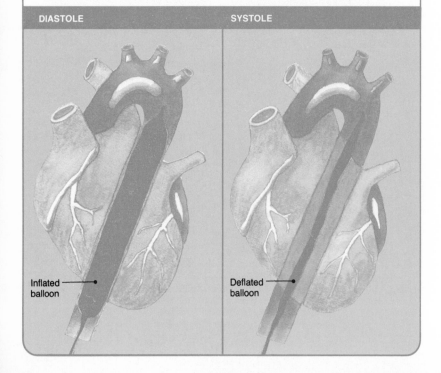

DIASTOLE

SYSTOLE

Inflated balloon

Deflated balloon

monary artery catheter, and a peripheral I.V. line in place. If the procedure's performed at bedside, gather the appropriate equipment, including a surgical tray for percutaneous catheter insertion, heparin, sterile saline solution, the IABC catheter, and the pump console. Connect the EKG monitor to the pump console. Then shave, disinfect, and drape the femoral site.

Procedure

After injecting a local anesthetic, the doctor inserts a needle with a stylet into the femoral artery. He then removes the stylet, inserts a guidewire into the artery, and advances a dilator over the guidewire to enlarge the lumen of the artery. After removing the dilator, he next inserts an introducer sheath.

Before inserting the balloon, he tests it for leaks by manually inflating and deflating it in a basin of sterile saline solution. Then he wraps the balloon tightly around the catheter, flushes the central lumen of the balloon catheter with heparinized saline, and inserts the balloon catheter through the sheath.

The balloon may rupture during insertion, which can cause a fatal gas embolism if it isn't detected before pumping begins. Ruptures may be caused by overwrapping the balloon or by the balloon snagging on the catheter, introducer, or arterial plaque. In rare cases, the catheter itself may break, which can cause clotting, gas embolism, or perforation of the artery.

Once the balloon is in place, the doctor verifies its position by fluoroscopy. If placed correctly, the upper tip of the catheter will lie in the descending thoracic aorta just below the left subclavian artery, and the base of the balloon will be above the renal artery branches of the aorta.

After the doctor has positioned the balloon, he unwraps it by turning a special handle. He then inflates the balloon and verifies that it's the proper size, sutures the sheath to the skin, bleeds air out of the system, and connects the catheter to the console. At this point, he'll watch for blood in the connecting tubing of the console—a telltale sign of balloon rupture or a broken catheter. If he detects no problems, pumping can begin.

Monitoring and aftercare

If you're responsible for monitoring the pump's console, you can select any of three signals to regulate inflation and deflation of the balloon: the EKG, the arterial waveform, or the intrinsic pump rate. If the EKG is used, the pump is set to inflate the balloon in the middle of the T wave (diastole) and deflate just before the QRS complex (systole). With the arterial waveform, the upstroke of the arterial wave triggers balloon inflation (see *Timing the Balloon Pump,* page 84). However, if neither of these signals can be used, you can also set the pump to inflate and deflate at a predetermined intrinsic rate. You're not likely to see IABC used this way at bedside, however; generally, the rate is predetermined only when the patient has no intrinsic heartbeat, such as during cardiopulmonary bypass.

You can expect to see a number of complications with IABC. The most common one, arterial embolism, stems from clot formation on the balloon's surface. Other complications include extension or rupture of an aortic aneurysm, perforation of the femoral or iliac arteries, femoral artery occlusion, and sepsis. Bleeding at the insertion site is often aggravated by pump-induced thrombocytopenia, caused by platelet aggregation around the balloon.

To help prevent complications, use strict aseptic technique, maintain the catheterized leg in good alignment and prevent hip flexion, and frequently assess the insertion site. Don't elevate the head of the bed more than 30 degrees, to prevent upward migration of the catheter and occlusion of the left subclavian artery. If the balloon does occlude the artery, you may see a diminished left radial pulse, and the patient may report dizziness. Incorrect balloon placement may also cause flank

TIMING THE BALLOON PUMP

Although IABC can be synchronized with the EKG, the arterial waveform is characteristically used to precisely adjust balloon-pump timing. The reason: the arterial waveform directly reflects diastole and systole. In contrast, the EKG shows *electrical* activity, which may not always correlate with the cardiac cycle—especially when the heart is diseased.

Ideally, balloon inflation should begin when the aortic valve closes—at the dicrotic notch on the arterial waveform. Deflation should occur just before systole. Proper timing is crucial: early inflation may damage the aortic valve by forcing it closed, whereas late inflation permits most of the blood emerging from the ventricle to flow past the balloon, reducing pump effectiveness. What's worse, late deflation increases the resistance against which the left ventricle must pump, possibly causing cardiac arrest.

The illustration directly below shows how IABC boosts peak diastolic pressure and lowers systolic and end-diastolic pressure. The four arterial waveforms below that show correctly and incorrectly timed balloon inflation and deflation.

ARTERIAL WAVEFORMS

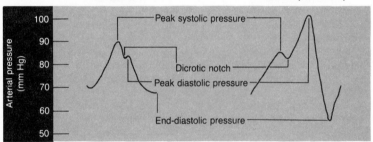

Unassisted — Assisted (with IABC)

Arterial pressure (mm Hg): 100, 90, 80, 70, 60, 50

Peak systolic pressure — Dicrotic notch — Peak diastolic pressure — End-diastolic pressure

Early inflation

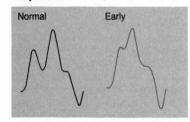

Normal — Early

Late inflation

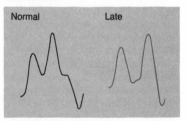

Normal — Late

Early deflation

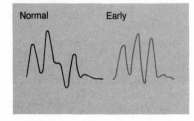

Normal — Early

Late deflation

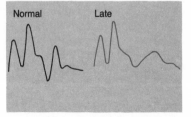

Normal — Late

pain or a sudden drop in urine output.

To forestall complications, assess distal pulses and note the color, temperature, and capillary refill of the patient's extremities. Assess the affected leg's warmth, color, and pulses, and the patient's ability to move his toes, at 30-minute intervals for the first 4 hours after insertion, then hourly for the duration of IABC. Often, arterial flow to the involved extremity diminishes during insertion, but the pulse should strengthen once pumping begins.

If your patient is receiving heparin or low-molecular-weight dextrans to inhibit thrombosis, keep in mind that he's still at risk for thrombus formation. Watch for such signs as a sudden weakening of pedal pulses, pain, and motor or sensory loss. If indicated, apply antiembolism stockings for 8 hours, remove them, and then reapply them. Encourage active range-of-motion exercises every 2 hours for the arms, the unaffected leg, and the affected ankle. Also be sure to maintain adequate hydration to help prevent thrombus formation. If bleeding occurs at the catheter insertion site, apply direct pressure over it and notify the doctor.

To discontinue IABC, the doctor will deflate the balloon, clip the sutures, and remove the catheter. Then he'll allow the site to bleed for 5 seconds to expel clots, after which you'll apply direct pressure for 30 minutes. Afterward, apply a pressure dressing and evaluate the site for bleeding and hematoma formation hourly for the next 4 hours.

Gas leaks from a damaged catheter or ruptured balloon can quickly cause gas embolism. Leaks may be detected by an alarm on the console. If the alarm sounds or if you note blood in the catheter, shut down the pump console and immediately place the patient in Trendelenburg's position to prevent the embolus from reaching the brain. Then notify the doctor.

Home care instructions

IABC is used only in the hospital for critically ill patients. As a result, there are no treatment-related directions for home care.

Percutaneous Transluminal Coronary Angioplasty

A relatively new therapy for coronary artery disease, percutaneous transluminal coronary angioplasty (PTCA) offers some patients a nonsurgical alternative to coronary artery bypass surgery. In PTCA, a tiny balloon catheter is used to dilate a coronary artery that's been narrowed by atherosclerotic plaque.

PTCA, which was first performed in 1977, has now evolved into a sophisticated radiologic technique. Performed in the cardiac catheterization laboratory under a local anesthetic, it doesn't involve a thoracotomy. With PTCA, hospitalization usually lasts 3 to 5 days, compared with a typical 2-week stay for coronary artery bypass. The patient is usually ambulatory within a day after PTCA and can often return to work within a few weeks. Another advantage of PTCA is its relatively low cost—about 20% that of coronary artery bypass.

Unfortunately, however, PTCA is an option for only about 10% of the candidates for coronary artery bypass. Usually it's indicated for patients who have myocardial ischemia documented by an EKG or thallium scan and a lesion in the proximal portion of a single coronary artery. (Recently, however, patients with multiple proximal lesions have undergone successful PTCA.) Lesions in the left main coronary artery aren't usually treated by PTCA because of higher mortality and increased risk of coronary artery spasm.

PTCA is most successful when lesions are noncalcified, concentric, discrete, and smoothly tapered. Patients with a history of less than 1 year of disabling angina are preferred since their lesions tend to be softer and more compressible.

Although PTCA avoids many of the risks of surgery, it can cause serious complications. The most dangerous, arterial dissection during dilatation, can lead to coronary artery rupture, cardiac tamponade, myocardial ischemia or infarction, or death. Other complications include coronary artery spasm, decreased coronary artery blood flow, allergic reactions to contrast medium, and arrhythmias during catheter manipulation. Infrequently, thrombi may embolize, cause a cerebrovascular accident.

Purpose

To increase the luminal diameter of a diseased coronary artery, thereby improving blood flow.

Preparation

Prepare the patient for PTCA by reinforcing the doctor's explanation of the procedure, including its risks and alternatives. Tell him that a catheter will be inserted into an artery or vein in the groin area and that he may feel pressure as the catheter moves along the vessel. Also explain that he'll be awake during the procedure and may be asked to take deep breaths to allow visualization of the radiopaque balloon catheter. He may also have to answer questions about how he's feeling during the procedure and will have to notify the cardiologist if he experiences any angina. Advise him that the entire procedure lasts from 1 to 4 hours and that he'll have to lie flat on a hard table during that time.

Explain to the patient that a contrast medium will be injected to outline the lesion's location. Warn him that during the injection he may feel a hot, flushing sensation or transient nausea. Check his history for allergies; if he's had allergic reactions to shellfish, iodine, or contrast medium, notify the doctor.

Tell the patient that an I.V. line will be inserted. Explain that the groin area of both legs will be shaved and cleansed with an antiseptic and that he'll experience a brief stinging sensation when a local anesthetic is injected.

Restrict the patient's food and fluid intake for at least 6 hours before the procedure or as ordered. Ensure that coagulation studies, complete blood count, serum electrolyte studies, and blood typing and cross matching have been performed. Also palpate the bilateral distal pulses (usually the dorsalis pedis or posterior tibial pulses) and mark them with indelible marker to help you locate them later. Take vital signs and assess the color, temperature, and sensation in the patient's extremities to serve as a baseline for posttreatment assessment. Before the patient goes to the catheterization laboratory, sedate him as ordered and put a 5-lb sandbag on the bed, to be used later for the application of direct pressure on the arterial puncture site.

Procedure

Although PTCA is performed in the cardiac catheterization laboratory, a surgical team must stand by during the procedure, in case emergency coronary artery bypass is required.

After preparing and anesthetizing the catheter insertion site, the doctor inserts a guidewire into the femoral artery by a percutaneous approach (other sites, such as the brachial artery with a cutdown approach, may be used instead). The doctor threads the catheter into the coronary artery with the help of fluoroscopy and confirms the presence of the lesion by angiography. Then he introduces a small double-lumen balloon-tipped catheter through the guidewire, positions it, and repeatedly inflates the balloon with a solution of saline and contrast medium to a pressure of 3 to 5 atmospheres. The expanding balloon compresses the atherosclerotic plaque against the arterial wall, expanding the arterial lumen.

To confirm the success of PTCA, the doctor measures the pressure gradient across the lesion and performs a repeat angiogram. After completing the procedure, he leaves the catheter in place to provide access in case coronary artery occlusion develops. Afterward, the patient is returned to the intensive care unit or recovery area for monitoring.

Monitoring and aftercare

When the patient returns from the cardiac catheterization laboratory, he may be receiving I.V. heparin or nitroglycerin. In addition, he'll have the sandbag over the cannulation site to minimize bleeding and hemorrhaging until the arterial catheter is removed. He'll require continuous arterial and EKG monitoring.

To prevent excessive hip flexion and migration of the catheter, keep the patient's leg straight and elevate the head of the bed no more than 15 degrees; at mealtimes, elevate the head of the bed 15 to 30 degrees. For the first hour, monitor vital signs every 15 minutes, then every 30 minutes for 2 hours, and then hourly for the next 5 hours. If vital signs are unstable, notify the doctor and continue to check them every 5 minutes.

When you take vital signs, assess the peripheral pulses distal to the catheter insertion site and the color, temperature, and capillary refill time of the extremity. If pulses are difficult to palpate because of the size of the arterial catheter, use a Doppler stethoscope to hear them. Notify the doctor if pulses are absent.

Assess the catheter insertion site for hematoma formation, ecchymosis, or hemorrhage. If an expanding ecchymotic area appears, mark the area to determine the rapidity of expansion. If bleeding occurs, apply direct pressure and notify the doctor.

Monitor cardiac rate and rhythm continuously and notify the doctor of any changes or if the patient reports chest pain; it may signal vasospasm or coronary occlusion.

Give I.V. fluids at a rate of at least 100 ml/hour to promote excretion of the contrast medium, but be sure to assess the patient for signs of fluid overload (distended neck veins, atrial and ventricular gallops, dyspnea, pulmonary congestion, tachycardia, hypertension, and hypoxemia).

The doctor will remove the arterial catheter 6 to 12 hours after the procedure. Afterward, apply direct pressure over the insertion site for at least 30 minutes. Then apply a pressure dressing and assess the patient's vital signs according to the same schedule you used when he first returned to the unit.

Home care instructions

- Instruct the patient to call his doctor if he experiences any bleeding or bruising at the arterial puncture site.
- Explain the necessity of taking all prescribed medications, and ensure that the patient understands their intended effects.
- Tell the patient that he can resume normal activity. Most patients experience an increased exercise tolerance.
- Instruct him to return for a stress thallium imaging test and follow-up angiography, as recommended by his doctor.

Balloon Valvuloplasty

First performed in 1979 on children with congenital heart disease, balloon valvuloplasty has now been performed on hundreds of adults in the United States. It's used to enlarge the orifice of a heart valve that's stenotic because of a congenital defect, calcification, rheumatic fever, or aging. A doctor performs valvuloplasty in a cardiac catheterization laboratory by inserting a balloon-tipped catheter through the femoral vein or artery, threading it into the heart, and repeatedly inflating it against the leaflets of the diseased valve.

Despite valvuloplasty's benefits, the treatment of choice for valvular heart disease remains surgery—either valve replacement or commissurotomy. But for those who are considered poor candidates for surgery, valvuloplasty offers an alternative. Most valvuloplasties are successful, improving valvular function and lowering pressure across the valve to normal levels.

Balloon valvuloplasty can cause complications, however. For example, the procedure can worsen valvular insufficiency by misshaping the valve so that it doesn't close completely. Another serious complication is embolism caused by pieces of the calcified valve breaking off and traveling to the brain or lungs. In addition, valvuloplasty can cause severe damage to the delicate valve leaflets, requiring immediate surgery to replace the valve. Other complications include bleeding and hematoma at the arterial puncture site, arrhythmias, myocardial ischemia, MI, and circulatory defects distal to the catheter entry site. Fortunately, the most serious complications of valvuloplasty—valvular destruction, MI, and calcium emboli—rarely occur.

Purpose
To enlarge the valvular orifice and improve mobility of valve leaflets, thereby correcting valvular stenosis.

Preparation
Reinforce the doctor's explanation of the procedure, including its risks and alternatives, to the patient or his parents. Restrict food and fluid intake for at least 6 hours before valvuloplasty, or as ordered.

Explain that the patient will have an I.V. line inserted to provide access for any medications. Mention that the patient's groin area will be shaved and cleansed with an antiseptic and that he'll feel a brief stinging sensation when a local anesthetic is injected.

Since the procedure itself is done under a local anesthetic, it can be especially frightening to a pediatric patient.

In simple and reassuring terms, explain that the doctor will insert a catheter into an artery or vein in the groin area and that the patient may feel pressure as the catheter moves along the vessel. Also explain to the patient that he needs to be awake because the doctor may need him to take deep breaths (to allow visualization of the catheter) and to answer questions about how he's feeling. Warn him that the procedure lasts up to 4 hours and that he may feel discomfort from lying flat on a hard table during that time. Ensure that the patient or his parents have signed a consent form.

Make sure that results of routine laboratory studies and blood typing and cross matching are available. Just before the procedure, palpate the bilateral distal pulses (usually the dorsalis pedis or posterior tibial pulses) and mark them with indelible ink. Take vital signs and assess color, temperature, and sensation in the patient's extremities to serve as a baseline for post-treatment assessment. Administer a sedative, as ordered.

Once you've prepared the patient, place a 5-lb sandbag on his bed, to be used later for applying pressure over the puncture site.

Procedure
After preparing and anesthetizing the catheter insertion site, the doctor inserts a catheter into the femoral artery (for left-heart valves) or femoral vein (for right-heart valves). He then passes the balloon-tipped catheter through this catheter and, guided by fluoroscopy, slowly threads it into the heart.

Next, he positions the deflated balloon in the valve opening and repeatedly inflates it with a solution containing saline and a contrast medium. As the balloon inflates, the valve leaflets split free of one another, permitting them to open and close properly and increasing the valvular orifice.

Valvuloplasty is considered a success if hemodynamic pressure decreases across the valve after balloon inflation.

If it does, the doctor removes the balloon-tipped catheter. However, he'll leave the other catheter in place in case the patient needs to return to the laboratory for a repeat procedure.

Monitoring and aftercare

When the patient returns to the critical care unit or recovery area, he may be receiving I.V. heparin or nitroglycerin. He'll also have the sandbag placed over the cannulation site to minimize bleeding until the arterial catheter is removed, and will require continuous arterial and EKG monitoring.

To prevent excessive hip flexion and migration of the catheter, keep the affected leg straight and elevate the head of the bed no more than 15 degrees. (At mealtimes, you can elevate the head of the bed 15 to 30 degrees). For the first hour, monitor vital signs every 15 minutes, then every 30 minutes for 2 hours, and then hourly for the next 5 hours. If vital signs are unstable, notify the doctor and continue to check them every 5 minutes.

When you take vital signs, assess peripheral pulses distal to the insertion site and the color, temperature, and capillary refill time of the extremity. If pulses are difficult to palpate because of the size of the arterial catheter, use a Doppler stethoscope. Notify the doctor if pulses are absent.

Observe the catheter insertion site for hematoma formation, ecchymosis, or hemorrhage. If an expanding ecchymotic area appears, mark the area to help determine the pace of expansion. If bleeding occurs, apply direct pressure and notify the doctor.

Following the doctor's orders or your hospital's protocol, auscultate regularly for murmurs, which may indicate worsening valvular insufficiency. Notify the doctor if you detect a new or worsening murmur.

Provide I.V. fluids at a rate of at least 100 ml/hour to help the kidneys excrete the contrast medium. But be sure to assess for signs of fluid overload: distended neck veins, atrial and ventric-

ular gallops, dyspnea, pulmonary congestion, tachycardia, hypertension, and hypoxemia.

The doctor will remove the catheter 6 to 12 hours after valvuloplasty. Afterward, apply direct pressure over the puncture site for at least 30 minutes. Then apply a pressure dressing and assess vital signs according to the same schedule you used when the patient first returned to the unit.

Home care instructions

• Tell the patient (or his parents) that he can resume normal activity. Most patients with successful valvuloplasties experience increased exercise tolerance.

• Instruct him to call his doctor if he experiences any bleeding or increased bruising at the puncture site or any recurrence of symptoms of valvular insufficiency, such as breathlessness or decreased exercise tolerance.

• Stress the need for regular follow-up visits with his doctor.

ELECTROSHOCK TREATMENTS

Defibrillation

In defibrillation, a strong burst of electric current is delivered to the heart through paddles applied to the patient's chest. This brief electric shock completely depolarizes the myocardium, allowing the heart's natural pacemaker to regain control of cardiac rhythm.

Defibrillation is the treatment of choice for ventricular fibrillation and pulseless ventricular tachycardia. It's also used for asystole when ventricular fibrillation is suspected. Successful about 40% of the time, defibrillation must be performed as soon as possi-

CARDIOPULMONARY RESUSCITATION: WHY THE CONFUSION?

Cardiopulmonary resuscitation—CPR. Every nurse learns it. And, as it sometimes seems, every one learns it differently. In nursing school, for example, you may have been taught to perform chest compressions at a rate of 60 to 80 per minute. You may have practiced it that way for years, only to find that the "new" standard calls for 80 to 100 compressions per minute. And if you had learned CPR according to Red Cross standards, you might have had trouble at recertification if your instructor followed the guidelines issued by the American Heart Association.

Some 30 years after it was developed at Johns Hopkins University, CPR is still a mainstay in the treatment of cardiac and respiratory arrest. It's performed countless times every day, and it has saved thousands of lives—in hospitals, at accident sites, even on city street corners. So why does there seem to be so much disagreement about how to do it right?

The simple answer is that nobody's entirely sure which CPR technique works best. The reason? CPR's an emergency procedure. It's performed on all sorts of people, by all sorts of people, and in all sorts of circumstances. That makes it virtually impossible to set up careful, controlled studies of various techniques. And it means that many of the specific recommendations must be based on theory rather than on rigorous scientific proof of their effectiveness.

In fact, minor variations in CPR probably aren't all that important. What *is* important—and has been proved—is that CPR works, and the sooner it's initiated, the better. That's why prompt recertification and regular practice are so important—to be sure you don't have to stop and think when you need to perform CPR.

Preparation

Keep in mind that ventricular fibrillation causes cardiac output to drop to zero and leads to unconsciousness. Thus, if the EKG suggests ventricular fibrillation but your patient is responsive and awake, the EKG is wrong—probably because of electrical interference. No matter what the EKG tells you, *never defibrillate a patient who's alert*; if you do, you could trigger lethal arrhythmias or cardiac standstill.

If you've determined that defibrillation is necessary, call promptly for help and begin CPR. When the defibrillator arrives, make sure that you or another staff member continues CPR during preparation of the equipment.

If you're preparing the defibrillator, plug it in and turn it on. Then turn on the oscilloscope and attach the defibrillator's EKG leads to the patient; you'll use them to monitor the EKG throughout the procedure. Next, apply conductive gel or paste to the paddles, or place two gel pads on the patient's bare chest in the appropriate position. If you're using gel or paste, coat the entire surface of the paddles by rubbing them together. Be sure to remove any gel from your hands and the sides of the paddles, since excess conductant will provide a pathway for the electric current and cause burns. Then select the electric charge on the defibrillator control, following your hospital's policy or the doctor's orders. (The American Hospital Association recommends 200 joules for the first two attempts at defibrillation and 360 joules for any subsequent attempts.)

ble—even before intubation or drug administration. If ventricular fibrillation lasts for more than a few minutes, it causes irreparable brain damage.

Purpose

To correct ventricular tachycardia or fibrillation and allow the heart's natural pacemaker to resume initiation of the heartbeat.

Procedure

First, check the patient's monitor to be sure that it still indicates ventricular fibrillation or tachycardia. Then stop CPR for 5 to 10 seconds and palpate for a carotid pulse. *If you detect a pulse, don't defibrillate the patient.*

If the carotid pulse is absent, position the paddles. If you're using *standard paddles* on a male patient, put

A.I.C.D.: HIGH-TECH HELP
FOR FAILING HEARTS

Like many nurses, you may be seeing an increasing number of patients with a history of ventricular fibrillation. Studies show that these patients are greatly at risk for further episodes of ventricular tachyarrhythmia, making them good candidates for an automatic implantable cardiac defibrillator (AICD). An AICD can help control ventricular fibrillation even after the patient leaves the hospital; it generally supplements antiarrhythmic drugs, pacemakers, or both—or it may be used after such therapies fail. Newer AICD models can also convert such arrhythmias as ventricular tachycardia and Torsades de Pointes; these models use the absence of a true isoelectric line between QRS complexes as their discharging cue.

The doctor implants the AICD (which has three defibrillator electrodes attached to its base generator) into the patient's abdominal cavity. He inserts the apical cardiac electrode through a left thoracotomy at the fifth intercostal space. Using fluoroscopy, he inserts the second electrode via the superior vena cava, positioning it

near the right atrial junction. He positions the third electrode in the right ventricle.

When the AICD senses a ventricular tachyarrhythmia, it discharges a small shock (25 to 30 joules) to defibrillate the heart automatically. If the initial discharge doesn't end the arrhythmia, the AICD can discharge up to four more times, increasing the voltage each time. The unit usually lasts 3 years or for up to 100 discharges.

Your main responsibility for a patient with an AICD involves preoperative and postoperative care and patient teaching. Tell the patient that he'll have small incisions in the left side of his chest, right shoulder, and abdomen, and that once the unit is implanted, he'll be able to feel it discharge. (Some patients describe the sensation as a sudden blow to the chest.) Warn the patient that if ventricular arrhythmias occur, he'll probably experience sudden faintness or shortness of breath (or both), followed by the discharge and a return to a feeling of well-being. The episode usually lasts less than 30 seconds.

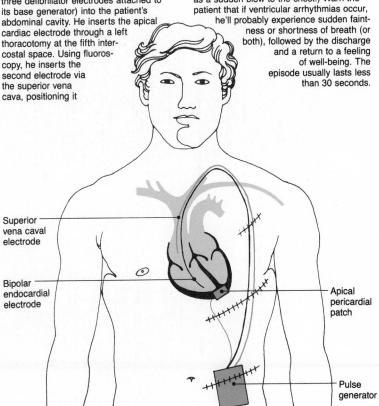

Superior vena caval electrode

Bipolar endocardial electrode

Apical pericardial patch

Pulse generator

one paddle beneath the clavicle, to the right of the upper end of his sternum; put the other on the left lateral wall of his chest, to the left of the cardiac apex. For a female patient, place the paddles at the mid- or anterior-axillary level, not over the breasts.

If you're using *A/P paddles*, place the flat one (without a discharge button) under the patient's body, behind the heart and just below the left scapula. Place the other paddle on the patient's

UNDERSTANDING SYNCHRONIZED CARDIOVERSION

Like defibrillation, synchronized cardioversion delivers an electric charge to the heart to correct arrhythmias. But there are two important differences: with cardioversion, much lower energy levels are used (typically 25 to 50 joules), and the burst of electricity is precisely timed to coincide with the peak of the R wave.

Unlike defibrillation, cardioversion can't be used to treat ventricular fibrillation since a fibrillating heart doesn't generate an R wave. But it's the treatment of choice for unstable ventricular tachycardia (accompanied by chest pain, dyspnea, and hypotension) and unstable paroxysmal atrial tachycardia that fail to respond to drug therapy.

Synchronized cardioversion can be performed as an elective or emergency procedure. In elective cases, the nurse usually assists the doctor, but in an emergency, many hospitals authorize nurses to perform the procedure.

Preparing the patient
For emergency cardioversion, you'll prepare the patient as you would for defibrillation. However, cardiac output will often still be adequate, so you won't have to initiate CPR and you'll have a bit more time to work. Consider sedating the patient unless he's profoundly hypotensive, unconscious, or showing signs of pulmonary edema. If there's time, explain the need for prompt cardioversion.

If you're assisting with elective cardioversion, explain to the patient that food and fluids will be restricted for 12 hours. Make sure that he understands the doctor's explanation of risks and complications and that he's signed a consent form. Tell the patient that an I.V. line will be inserted (if one hasn't been already) in case medications are needed and that a 12-lead EKG will be performed before cardioversion. If the patient's receiving oxygen, explain that it will be discontinued during the

procedure, as a precaution against fire, but will be reinstituted immediately after it.

Check the patient's medication history. Elective cardioversion is often contraindicated in a patient receiving a cardiac glycoside because of the risk of lethal arrhythmias. If the patient's receiving a cardiac glycoside, make sure that his potassium level is normal, since potassium plays a key role in conducting and regulating electric impulses within the heart.

Performing cardioversion
Once you've prepared the patient for cardioversion, take his vital signs and gather emergency resuscitation equipment. Connect the patient to the defibrillator's EKG leads and turn on the oscilloscope. Next, adjust the gain to create an R wave at least 3 cm high. Turn on the synchronization control and ensure that each R wave is marked. Now set the control to the proper energy level (as prescribed by the doctor or hospital protocol). Prepare and place the paddles as you would for defibrillation, then press them firmly onto the patient's chest and push the charge button until the display indicates that the proper energy level has been reached. Say "All clear!" and verify that no one is touching the patient or the bed. Then hold the discharge button down until the paddles discharge. Unlike defibrillation, the paddles will not discharge immediately; there will be a slight delay while the defibrillator synchronizes with the R wave.

After the paddles discharge, remove them from the patient's chest and evaluate the EKG to determine whether cardioversion was successful. If the arrhythmia wasn't corrected, repeat the procedure using a higher setting.

After successful cardioversion, check the patient's vital signs every 15 minutes for at least an hour or until precardioversion levels are reached.

chest, directly over his heart.

Once the paddles are properly placed, press them firmly against the patient's skin to ensure good contact. (Be sure to keep the standard paddles at least 2 cm apart at all times, to prevent arcing.) Then push the charge button until the display indicates that the proper power level has been reached, and in a loud voice, say, "All clear!" to warn everyone to step back from the bed. *Before operating the defibrillator,* ensure that no one is touching the bed or the patient. (Don't forget about yourself; you should be touching only the paddles, not the patient.)

Hold down the discharge button to deliver the electric current and then remove the paddles from the patient's chest. Check the EKG and carotid pulse to determine whether defibrillation was successful. If it wasn't, defibrillate the patient again. If the patient still doesn't respond, continue defibrillation and all resuscitation measures until the doctor ends resuscitation or the patient stabilizes. When you've finished, turn off and unplug the defibrillator. Clean the paddles with soap and water.

Monitoring and aftercare

Check the patient's vital signs every 15 minutes for at least an hour, and monitor the EKG continuously. If the cardiac rhythm worsens, notify the doctor immediately. Assess the patient's chest for burns. If burns have occurred, apply the prescribed ointment.

In some cases, the doctor may choose to surgically insert an automatic implantable cardiac defibrillator (AICD), which automatically delivers an electric current to the heart when it senses irregular rhythms (see *AICD: High-Tech Help for Failing Hearts,* page 91). If your patient is scheduled to have an AICD implanted, reinforce the doctor's explanation of the device and how it works.

Home care instructions

• Tell the patient to take his pulse for a full minute every day before getting out of bed and to notify his doctor immediately if the rate is less than 60 or greater than 100 beats/minute, or if he experiences palpitations, dizziness, or fainting.

• Emphasize the need for the patient to continue regular appointments with his doctor for routine EKGs and evaluation of his response to medication.

• If your patient will be getting an AICD, outline the special precautions he'll have to take.

FLUID ASPIRATION

Pericardiocentesis

Typically performed at bedside in a critical care unit, pericardiocentesis involves the needle aspiration of excess fluid from the pericardial sac. It may be the treatment of choice for life-threatening cardiac tamponade (except when fluid accumulates rapidly, in which case immediate surgery is usually preferred).

Pericardiocentesis may also be used to aspirate fluid in subacute conditions, such as viral or bacterial infections and pericarditis. What's more, it provides a sample for laboratory analysis to confirm diagnosis and identify the cause of pericardial effusion.

Pericardiocentesis carries some risk of potentially fatal complications, such as inadvertent puncture of internal organs (particularly the heart, lung, stomach, or liver) or laceration of the myocardium or of a coronary artery. Therefore, keep emergency equipment readily available during the procedure.

Purpose

To remove excessive pericardial fluid, thus relieving myocardial compression and increasing cardiac output.

Preparation

Before pericardiocentesis, help the patient relax by clearly explaining the procedure. Briefly discuss possible complications, such as arrhythmias and organ or artery puncture, but reassure him that such complications occur rarely. Tell him he'll have an I.V. line inserted to provide access for medications, if needed. Make sure the patient (or a family member, if appropriate) has signed a consent form.

Place the patient in a supine position in his bed, with his upper torso raised 60 degrees and his arms supported by pillows. Shave the needle insertion site on his chest, if necessary, and cleanse the area with an antiseptic solution. Then apply 12-lead EKG electrodes. If ordered, assist the doctor in attaching the pericardial needle to the precordial lead (V) of the EKG and also to a three-way stopcock.

Procedure

After starting continuous EKG monitoring and administering a local anesthetic at the puncture site, the doctor inserts the aspiration needle in one of three areas. He'll probably choose the subxiphoid approach, with needle insertion in the angle between the left costal margin and the xiphoid process, to avoid needle contact with the pleura and the coronary vessels and thus decrease the risk of damage to these structures. As an alternative, however, he may insert the needle into the fifth intercostal space next to the left side of the sternum, where the pericardium normally isn't covered by lung tissue. He may opt for a third approach, in which he inserts the needle at the cardiac apex; however, because this method poses the greatest risk of complications, such as pneumothorax, he needs to proceed cautiously.

After inserting the needle, the doctor slowly advances it into the pericardial sac to a depth of 1″ to 2″, or until he can aspirate fluid. He then clamps a hemostat to the needle at the chest wall to prevent needle movement.

The doctor aspirates pericardial fluid slowly. If he finds large amounts of fluid, he may place an indwelling catheter into the pericardial sac to allow continuous slow drainage. After he has removed the fluid, he withdraws the needle and places a dressing over the site.

Monitoring and aftercare

During pericardiocentesis, closely monitor the patient's blood pressure and central venous pressure. Check the EKG pattern continuously for premature ventricular contractions and elevated ST segments, which may indicate that the needle has touched the ventricle; elevated PR segments, which may indicate that the needle has touched the atrium; and large, erratic QRS complexes, which may indicate that the needle has penetrated the heart. Also watch for signs of organ puncture, such as hypotension, decreased breath sounds, chest pain, dyspnea, hematoma, and tachycardia.

Note and record the volume and character of any aspirated fluid. Blood that has accumulated slowly in the patient's pericardial sac usually doesn't clot after it has been aspirated; blood from a sudden hemorrhage, however, will clot.

After pericardiocentesis, check vital signs at least hourly and maintain continuous EKG monitoring. Expect the patient's blood pressure to rise as tamponade is relieved. Be alert for the development of recurring tamponade; watch for decreased blood pressure, narrowing pulse pressure, increased central venous pressure, tachycardia, muffled heart sounds, tachypnea, pleural friction rub, distended neck veins, anxiety, and chest pain. Notify the doctor of these signs; he may need to repeat pericardiocentesis or surgically drain the pericardium in the operating room.

Home care instructions

Urge the patient to keep follow-up medical appointments.

MISCELLANEOUS TREATMENTS

Valsalva's Maneuver

This easy-to-perform maneuver can help relieve angina or correct atrial arrhythmias by triggering vagal stimulation of the heart.

Initially, the maneuver raises intrathoracic pressure from its normal level of -3 to -4 mm Hg to levels of 60 mm Hg or higher. This increase in pressure is transmitted directly to the great vessels and the heart, causing decreased venous return and stroke volume and lowered systolic pressure. Within seconds, the baroreceptors respond by increasing the heart rate and causing peripheral vasoconstriction.

When the patient exhales at the end of the maneuver, blood pressure begins to rise. But peripheral vasoconstriction is still present, and the combination of rising blood pressure and vasoconstriction causes vagal stimulation, which in turn slows the heart rate.

Unfortunately, Valsalva's maneuver can cause such complications as mobilization of venous thrombi, bleeding, ventricular arrhythmias, and asystole. It's contraindicated for patients with severe coronary artery disease, acute MI, or moderate to severe hypovolemia.

Purpose
To relieve angina and to help correct atrial arrhythmias.

Preparation
Explain to the patient what Valsalva's maneuver is and, in simple terms, what it's intended to accomplish. If the patient suffers from angina, tell him that the maneuver will diminish his heart's work load and will thereby relieve the angina. For the patient with an atrial

COUGH C.P.R.: NEW WEAPON AGAINST VENTRICULAR ARRHYTHMIAS

Like Valsalva's maneuver, a simple cough may help convert potentially lethal arrhythmias to normal sinus rhythm. While Valsalva's maneuver is used for atrial arrhythmias, however, coughing can disrupt *ventricular arrhythmias*. By closing the epiglottis and strongly contracting the respiratory muscles, coughing greatly increases intrathoracic pressure. The compressive force of this pressure increase promotes coronary perfusion. Researchers believe that coronary perfusion also improves as a result of increased aortic pressure and reflex coronary vasodilation secondary to baroreceptor activation.

So far, cough CPR has been used mainly in cardiac catheterization laboratories, where doctors have found that continuous, forced coughing spurts, 1 to 3 seconds apart and beginning just before or at the onset of ventricular tachycardia or fibrillation, can help patients maintain consciousness for up to 30 seconds.

Cough CPR buys time for defibrillation by maintaining cerebral perfusion. In addition, it's a technique that heart patients can potentially use on their own, even after they've left the hospital.

arrhythmia, you can explain that the maneuver temporarily raises the blood pressure and that the heart responds by beating more slowly. Explain how the maneuver is done (you can describe it as trying to exhale while holding one's breath), and briefly demonstrate it yourself.

Warn your patient that he may feel faint or dizzy, and place him in a supine position. Start an I.V. line if one isn't running already, and take vital signs. Then attach a 12-lead EKG to the patient and gather resuscitation equipment and medications. Monitor the EKG and continue to record it throughout the entire procedure.

Procedure
Instruct the patient to take a deep breath and then to bear down as if def-

ecating. If no syncope, dizziness, or arrhythmias occur, have him continue to hold his breath and bear down for 10 seconds. Then tell him to exhale and breathe quietly. If the maneuver is successful, the patient's heart rate will begin to slow before he exhales.

Monitoring and aftercare
Assess the EKG and vital signs when the procedure is completed. You'll need to monitor the patient's EKG continuously for at least 12 hours to ensure that arrhythmias don't return. If an atrial arrhythmia doesn't resolve following the maneuver, the doctor will probably order drug therapy.

Home care instructions
If Valsalva's maneuver relieves angina or corrects the arrhythmia, teach the patient to do it at home. Tell him that if palpitations or angina occurs after he leaves the hospital, he should lie down (to prevent fainting or dizziness) and perform the maneuver for 10 seconds. Tell him that if the maneuver doesn't relieve his symptoms, he'll need to call his doctor immediately.

Carotid Sinus Massage

Carotid sinus massage (CSM) is a noninvasive method for evaluating and terminating certain tachyarrhythmias. It involves manual stimulation of pressure receptors in the carotid artery, which in turn triggers a parasympathetic response and depresses heart rate and conductivity.

Patient response to CSM differs, depending on the type of arrhythmia involved. (This difference can be used diagnostically to help distinguish ectopic tachyarrhythmias from sinus tachycardia, but it limits CSM's usefulness as a treatment.) With sinus tachycardia, the heart rate slows grad-

ually when CSM is applied, and speeds up again after it's terminated. In atrial tachycardia, the response is unpredictable; the arrhythmia may terminate or remain unaffected, or atrioventricular (AV) block may worsen. In paroxysmal atrial tachycardia, reversion to sinus rhythm occurs 20% of the time. In nonparoxysmal tachycardia and ventricular tachycardia, there's no response. In atrial fibrillation or flutter, ventricular rate slows because of increased AV block.

Depending on hospital and unit protocol, CSM may be performed by either a doctor or a nurse. Continuous EKG monitoring during the procedure is essential because of potential complications: CSM may cause ventricular standstill, ventricular tachycardia, or ventricular fibrillation. By worsening AV block, CSM can also cause junctional or ventricular escape rhythms.

Another potential complication is cerebral damage from inadequate tissue perfusion. If the carotid artery is totally occluded during CSM, decreased cerebral blood flow may cause a cerebrovascular accident (CVA). Also, compression of the carotid sinus may loosen endothelial plaque, which can migrate and cause CVA.

CSM shouldn't be used in patients with cardiac glycoside toxicity, cerebrovascular disease, or previous carotid surgery. It should be used cautiously in elderly patients, in those receiving cardiac glycosides, and in those with heart block, hypertension, coronary artery disease, diabetes mellitus, or hyperkalemia.

Purpose
• To slow the heart rate and terminate arrhythmias
• To distinguish ectopic tachyarrhythmias from sinus tachycardia.

Preparation
With the patient in bed, place a pillow behind his shoulder blades to extend his head. Insert an I.V. line and gather emergency resuscitation equipment.

Turn the patient's head away from the site being massaged; this will make the artery less likely to roll behind the trachea during massage.

Explain the procedure to the patient, and connect him to a cardiac monitor or to an EKG machine. Assess and document his cardiac rhythm and neurologic status and auscultate both carotid arteries for bruits. A bruit close to the jaw line suggests arteriosclerotic plaques in the carotid artery and is an absolute contraindication to CSM.

Procedure
Using the tips of your index and middle fingers, locate the patient's larynx, and then slide your fingers laterally into the groove between the trachea and the neck muscles. You'll know you've found the carotid artery when you feel a strong pulse. Next, follow the carotid artery to the bifurcation—the location of the carotid sinus area—by sliding your fingers to the angle of the mandible. Place four fingers medial to the pulsating artery. Press the artery against the underlying vertebrae and begin massaging it firmly in a head-to-toe direction. Massage for *no longer than 5 seconds* because of the risk of asystole. Release the artery as soon as

the EKG shows that the heart rate has begun to slow.

If massage on one side is ineffective, perform CSM on the other side, again massaging for no longer than 5 seconds. Massage only one carotid sinus at a time; never massage both simultaneously.

Monitoring and aftercare
As soon as you finish CSM, check the patient's vital signs, watching especially for hypotension and bradycardia. Continue cardiac monitoring for at least 4 hours to assess the effects of treatment and to alert you to the return of the arrhythmia. Also check your patient's neurologic status every hour for the first 4 hours to detect symptoms of CVA.

Home care instructions
• Show the patient how to take his radial pulse. Instruct him to take it for a full minute each morning before getting out of bed and whenever he experiences chest pain, palpitations, dizziness, or fainting.
• Warn him that these signs, or a heart rate of less than 60 or greater than 100 beats/minute, indicate that he should call his doctor.

Selected References

Brannon, P., and Towner, S. "Ventricular Failure: New Therapy Using the Mechanical Assist Device," *Critical Care Nurse* 6(2):70-85, March/April 1986.

Crumpley, L., and Rinkenberger, R. "An Overview of Antiarrhythmic Drugs," *Critical Care Nurse* 3(4):57-63, July/August 1983.

Elzy, P., and Marsh, L. "Artificial Heart Implantation: Nursing Protocol, Preparation, Participation," *AORN Journal* 42(2):171-78, August 1985.

Evans, N. "Clinical Assessment of Pacemaker Function: The ICHD Code," *Dimensions of Critical Care Nursing* 4(3):140-45, May/June 1985.

Gershan, J., and Jiricka, M. "Percutaneous

Transluminal Coronary Angioplasty: Implications for Nursing," *Focus on Critical Care* 11(4):28-35, August 1984.

Haak, S. "Intra-Aortic Balloon Pump Techniques," *Dimensions of Critical Care Nursing* 2(4):196-204, July/August 1983.

Kenner, C., et al. *Critical Care Nursing: Body, Mind, Spirit,* 2nd ed. Boston: Little, Brown & Co., 1985.

McCauley, K., and Brest, A. *McGoon's Cardiac Surgery: An Interprofessional Approach to Patient Care.* Philadelphia: F.A. Davis Co., 1984.

Shinn, J., and Douglas, M. *Advances in Cardiovascular Nursing.* Rockville, Md.: Aspen Systems Corp., 1985.

3

Treating Respiratory Dysfunction

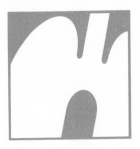

Treating Respiratory Dysfunction

Introduction

Whether acute or chronic, respiratory disorders can cause ineffective airway clearance, abnormal breathing patterns, or impaired gas exchange. To help correct these problems, drug therapy, surgery, or ventilatory support may be necessary.

Opening the airways
Drugs such as xanthine bronchodilators and adrenergics dilate bronchial passages and reduce airway resistance. This decreases the work of breathing and allows the patient to satisfy his oxygen needs. Corticosteroids decrease inflammation and increase the responsiveness of the airways to bronchodilators. When secretions or mucus plugs obstruct the airways, chest physiotherapy or bronchoscopy may improve ventilation.

Incisions and intubations
When a patent airway can't be established and endotracheal intubation is contraindicated, a tracheostomy may be performed. This surgery creates an opening into the trachea, providing an emergency airway or a means to establish mechanical ventilation.

When ventilation is impaired by blood or air accumulating in the pleural cavity, a chest tube may need to be inserted to remove the fluid or air. This permits the lungs to reinflate.

Delivering oxygen
Seriously impaired gas exchange may call for mechanical ventilation, which controls or assists the patient's breathing, or for oxygen therapy, which improves blood oxygenation in the spontaneously breathing patient. Other treatments, such as continuous positive airway pressure (CPAP) and intermittent positive-pressure breathing, may be used as mechanical ventilation modes, as weaning aids, or as prophylaxes against atelectasis.

A common calling
No matter where you practice nursing, you may be called on to explain, perform, or assist with respiratory treatments. That means you'll have to be knowledgeable about basic treatments, such as postural drainage and percussion. And you'll have to become familiar with some of the newer or more advanced therapies, such as nasal CPAP for obstructive sleep apnea.

What's more, you'll need to anticipate complications of respiratory treatments and, if possible, prevent their occurrence. For example, in the patient with a chest tube, you may be able to prevent tension pneumothorax by carefully checking tube position and function. When complications can't be prevented, you'll need to spot telltale signs and intervene promptly.

DRUG THERAPY

Xanthine Bronchodilators

Xanthine bronchodilators include theophylline; its soluble salts, aminophylline and oxtriphylline; and a related derivative, dyphylline. These drugs relax bronchiolar smooth muscle. As a result, they're used to treat bronchial asthma, chronic bronchitis, and emphysema. They also play an important role in treating acute respiratory conditions, such as status asthmaticus.

Aminophylline, the major I.V. preparation, provides rapid treatment of bronchoconstriction. *Theophylline*, in contrast, provides long-term control of asthma and other bronchospastic conditions. Both theophylline and its derivatives are available in varied oral, parenteral, and rectal forms, with different durations of action. Short-acting oral preparations may present a patient compliance problem because of the frequent doses required. However, newer sustained-release formulations can help overcome this by permitting daily or twice-daily dosing.

Chief side effects of the xanthines include GI distress and CNS stimulation. Fortunately, these can often be avoided by careful dosage titration. Unfortunately, toxicity may occur abruptly, heralded by tachycardia, ventricular arrhythmias, or seizures. Milder symptoms don't always precede these severe toxic effects.

The xanthines are contraindicated in patients with a hypersensitivity to xanthine compounds, such as caffeine and theobromine, or with severe arrhythmias. They should be used cautiously in patients with liver disease, conges-tive heart failure, pulmonary edema, viral infection, or recent viral immunization because these conditions slow the rate of drug metabolism. Because the xanthines can increase the volume and acidity of gastric secretions, they should also be used cautiously in patients with peptic ulcer disease.

Purpose and action
The xanthines relax bronchiolar smooth muscle by inhibiting phosphodiesterase, the enzyme that degrades cyclic adenosine monophosphate.

Monitoring
Evaluate therapy's effectiveness by monitoring respirations and by asking the patient if spasmodic coughing and chest tightness have subsided. Check pulmonary function studies (primarily FEV_1, the amount of air exhaled in the first second of a forced expiration after a full inspiration) for indications of increased airflow. Monitor the patient's vital signs and pulse quality.

Watch the patient carefully for GI signs of toxicity, which may include bleeding, abdominal pain, diarrhea, nausea, and vomiting (possibly bloody). Also watch for CNS signs, such as irritability, confusion, seizures, dizziness, insomnia, trembling, and headache. Is the patient's face flushed? Is he urinating more frequently? Are his respiratory and pulse rates rapid? Does he feel weak? If any of these untoward signs occur, stop the drug immediately and notify the doctor.

If you're administering aminophylline I.V., watch for rash and hives for up to 24 hours. Discontinue the drug if these signs of hypersensitivity occur. If no such signs occur, switch the patient to an oral form, when ordered. Typically, you'll give an oral dose before discontinuing the infusion.

Review the patient's medication regimen for possible interactions. Propranolol and nadolol, for example, may cause bronchospasm. Oral contraceptives, troleandomycin, erythromycin, and cimetidine decrease hepatic clearance of xanthines. Ephedrine and other bronchodilators can produce additive effects. Primidone, rifampin, barbiturates, and phenytoin reduce serum xanthine levels.

Monitor serum drug levels carefully, especially if the patient has congestive heart failure, liver disease, pulmonary edema, or another condition that can decrease drug metabolism. The doctor may need to reduce the dose, depending on serum levels. Also monitor drug levels if your patient smokes, since tobacco stimulates xanthine metabolism.

Initially evaluate serum levels at least 72 hours after the first dose. Then measure peak serum levels 8 to 12 hours after the morning dose of a 24-hour preparation; 4 to 6 hours after the morning dose of a 12-hour preparation; 2 hours after the dose of a standard, rapidly absorbed preparation; or 30 minutes after an I.V. loading dose. Serum theophylline levels should range from 10 to 20 mcg/ml.

Home care instructions

• Instruct the patient to report signs of drug toxicity. Warn him not to exceed the prescribed dosage.
• Tell the patient to take the drug with food and a full glass of water to reduce GI upset. Caution him not to eat large amounts of charcoal-broiled foods, because the hydrocarbons contained in these can lower serum xanthine levels.
• Also tell him to avoid smoking because this increases drug metabolism.
• Warn him not to dissolve, crush, or chew a continuous-release formulation.
• If the patient misses a dose, tell him to take it as soon as he remembers. However, if he doesn't remember until the next dose is due, have him skip the missed dose and return to his regular schedule. He shouldn't double-dose.
• Warn the patient not to change the drug brand or formulation (from a short-acting to a continuous-release preparation, for example) without consulting his doctor.
• Caution against ingesting large amounts of caffeinated beverages or foods because of increased CNS stimulation. Also caution against using over-the-counter drugs, such as cold and allergy remedies, that contain ephedrine and theophylline salts because of increased CNS stimulation.
• Tell the patient to notify his doctor if he develops a cold or other viral illness; his dosage may need adjustment.

Adrenergics

Adrenergics, a group of sympathomimetic drugs, affect alpha and beta receptors in almost all body systems. Some adrenergics affect all three types of alpha and beta receptors, whereas others exert more selective effects. For example, certain adrenergics exert a direct effect on the beta$_2$-receptors in the lungs, causing bronchodilation. Another group of adrenergics stimulates alpha receptors and causes vasoconstriction. They produce a decongestant action when applied topically to the nasal mucosa.

The bronchodilating adrenergics include isoproterenol, isoetharine, and several other drugs. *Isoproterenol* isn't widely used because of its cardiac side effects. It can be given sublingually, by inhalation, or by infusion. *Isoetharine*, which can be given by inhalation, causes fewer side effects than isoproterenol does. Other beta$_2$-selective drugs—*terbutaline, metaproterenol,* and *albuterol*—can be given orally or by inhalation. However, the inhaled form of all bronchodilating adrenergics should be given as soon as possible since a reduced response occurs in prolonged bronchospasm.

The chief side effects of the bronchodilating adrenergics include tachycardia, palpitations, sweating, nervousness, hypertension, and tremors. Typically, the oral form causes more severe tremors than the inhaled form. As a result, oral doses should be started at half strength and gradually increased to full strength.

The adrenergic nasal decongestants include *oxymetazoline, phenylephrine, pseudoephedrine*, and *xylometazoline*. Applied to the nasal mucosa, these drugs provide a rapid decongestant effect. However, rebound congestion may occur after continued use and rapid tolerance may develop.

Epinephrine, with both alpha- and beta-adrenergic action, is no longer widely prescribed as a bronchodilator and decongestant because of its severe side effects. It's contraindicated in patients with coronary artery disease, severe hypertension, acute angle-closure glaucoma, arrhythmias, shock, porphyria, or organic brain damage and for use with general anesthetics.

Purpose and action

Beta$_2$-stimulating adrenergics relax bronchial smooth muscle, resulting in decreased airway resistance and, at times, increased vital capacity. Alpha-stimulating adrenergics cause vasoconstriction, relieving nasal congestion.

Monitoring

Review the patient's drug regimen for possible interactions. For example, concurrent use of an adrenergic and a beta blocker reduces the adrenergic's bronchodilating effect and may lead to bronchospasm. Other sympathomimetics, monoamine oxidase inhibitors, and tricyclic antidepressants can potentiate adrenergic effects.

When administering epinephrine or terbutaline intramuscularly or subcutaneously, pull back on the syringe before injection and check for blood to ensure that the needle isn't in a vein. After injection, massage the site to counteract possible vasoconstriction.

Monitor the patient's respiratory function to assess his response to therapy. An FEV$_1$ (the amount of air exhaled in the first second of a forced expiration after a full inspiration) increase of 15% or more after treatment

suggests that improvement will occur. However, increased airway resistance may indicate an allergic response to the drug or its preservatives.

Monitor the patient for increased blood pressure and heart rate, even if you're giving a beta$_2$-selective drug. Report any such increases to the doctor and reduce the dosage, as ordered.

Tremors, an annoying and common side effect of adrenergics, may reduce patient compliance. If the patient develops a severe hand tremor that interferes with his daily activities, reduce his drug dosage, as ordered.

If the patient's taking an adrenergic nasal decongestant, observe for excessive CNS stimulation and ask about headaches. If these occur, reduce the dosage, as ordered.

Home care instructions

• Explain to the patient that long-term excessive use of adrenergics can reduce their effectiveness. Advise him to report any reduced response. Warn against changing the dosage without guidelines from his doctor.

• If the patient is taking an inhalable bronchodilator, provide him with written directions (see *Using a Metered Dose Inhaler*). Tell him to take his pulse and to assess for side effects according to the amount of drug used. Advise him to notify the doctor if his resting heart rate increases more than 10 beats per minute after starting treatment. Warn him not to use any over-the-counter inhalable drugs without his doctor's permission since these products usually contain epinephrine.

• If the patient will be using a nebulizer, teach him how to clean and troubleshoot any equipment. Explain that the nebulizer can be a source of infection if it is not rinsed and air-dryed between treatments.

• If the patient is taking an adrenergic that doesn't contain a preservative, instruct him to keep it refrigerated. If appropriate, tell him to store the drug in a light-resistant container and not to take it if its color has changed.

USING A METERED DOSE INHALER

Dear Patient:

To use your oral inhaler, just follow these steps:

1

Remove the mouthpiece and cap from the inhaler. Then remove the cap from the mouthpiece. Next, turn the mouthpiece sideways. On one side of the flattened tip you'll see a small hole. Fit the metal stem

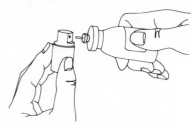

on the inhaler into the hole. After it's assembled, shake the inhaler five times.

2

Open your mouth wide. Then hold the inhaler mouthpiece 1½ to 2 inches in front of your mouth. Exhale fully.

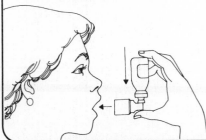

3

Take a slow, deep breath. As you do, firmly press the inhaler against the mouthpiece—one time only—to release one dose of medication. Continue inhaling slowly until your lungs feel full.

4

Take the mouthpiece away from your mouth, and hold your breath for three to five counts of one-1,000, two-1,000, three-1,000. Exhale slowly through pursed lips.

5

If your doctor wants you to take more than one dose, wait a couple of minutes before repeating steps 2 through 4.

6

Rinse your mouth. Gargle and then spit out the fluid.

Remember to clean the inhaler once a day: take it apart and rinse the mouthpiece and cap under warm running water for 1 minute. Shake off the excess water, allow the parts to dry, and then reassemble them.

• If he's taking a nasal decongestant, warn him not to exceed the recommended dosage because headache and CNS stimulation may occur. Explain that habitual use can cause rebound congestion, with mucosal fullness and edema. If he's taking drops, tell him to instill these in the lateral head-down position to reduce the risk of swallowing the drug. If he's using an inhaler, instruct him to close one nostril and inhale through the open one.

Oral Corticosteroids

The oral corticosteroids *prednisone* and *prednisolone* provide symptomatic relief in an asthma attack. They're also prescribed for long-term treatment of chronic obstructive pulmonary disease, aspiration pneumonitis, hypersensitivity pneumonitis, such as farmer's lung, and symptomatic sarcoidosis. Both drugs produce desirable glucocorticoid effects, such as reduced respiratory inflammation. Unfortunately, they also produce undesirable mineralocorticoid effects, such as fluid retention. Worse yet, long-term therapy can cause growth suppression in children, menstrual irregularities, short-term hypokalemia and hyperglycemia, and immunosuppression. An alternate-day regimen may help reduce the number and severity of these effects. Such a regimen can be instituted gradually after a course of daily therapy but, like a daily one, must be tapered slowly to prevent acute adrenal insufficiency.

Oral corticosteroids are contraindicated in patients with systemic fungal infections. They should be used cautiously in patients with GI ulceration, renal or hepatic disease, hypertension, congestive heart failure, osteoporosis, diabetes mellitus, hyperthyroidism or hypothyroidism, uncontrolled viral or bacterial infection, myasthenia gravis, tuberculosis, or acquired immune deficiency syndrome. Because these drugs can precipitate depression or psychotic episodes, especially in high doses, they should be used judiciously in patients with a history of emotional instability or psychotic tendencies.

Purpose and action
Oral corticosteroids suppress respiratory tract inflammation by inhibiting mast cell release of mediators.

Monitoring
Before beginning therapy, weigh the patient to establish a baseline. If the patient's a child, also measure his height. During therapy, assess both height and weight regularly to detect growth retardation or any weight gain caused by corticosteroid-induced appetite stimulation and fluid retention. Notify the doctor if the patient gains weight rapidly or develops edema or hypertension. If the patient's a child, also report failure to grow.

Review the patient's drug regimen for possible interactions. Concurrent use of indomethacin or aspirin, for example, raises the risk of GI distress and bleeding. Barbiturates, phenytoin, and rifampin reduce corticosteroid effects.

In the patient with asthma, monitor FEV_1 and peak flow, especially as dosage changes. Observe the patient's skin for petechiae and bruising, and monitor his serum electrolyte and glucose levels to detect hypokalemia, hypernatremia, and hyperglycemia. If ordered, give potassium supplements and place the patient on a salt-restricted diet.

Periodically assess the patient's mental status, especially if his dosage is high. Report sudden mood swings to the doctor.

When the patient's being withdrawn from therapy or switching from oral to inhaled corticosteroids, watch closely for symptoms of adrenal insufficiency, such as lethargy, weakness, dyspnea, orthostatic hypotension, syncope, fever, rebound inflammation, arthralgia, and anorexia. Report any of these symptoms to the doctor immediately.

Home care instructions

• Emphasize to the patient that he should *never* stop taking his prescribed drug without his doctor's approval because this may precipitate adrenal insufficiency or life-threatening adrenal crisis. Inform him that the dosage must be tapered gradually.

• Provide directions for missed doses. If the patient's on an alternate-day schedule, tell him to take the missed dose if he remembers later that morning; otherwise, he should take the dose the next morning and then skip the following day, resuming an alternate-day schedule. If the patient's on a daily schedule, tell him to make up the missed dose as soon as he remembers, unless it's almost time for his next dose; tell him *not* to double-dose. If he takes the drug several times daily, tell him to take a missed dose as soon as he remembers and to double up if it's time for his next dose.

• Tell the patient to take his prescribed drug with food or milk, to reduce GI upset. Instruct him to avoid alcohol, which can increase the drug's ulcerogenic effects. Warn him not to take any other drug, including aspirin, without his doctor's approval.

• Explain that his prescribed drug impairs resistance to infection. As a result, he must avoid persons with known or suspected infections. He must also avoid vaccinations or immunizations during and directly after therapy.

• Advise him to report minor stress or illness, such as dental extraction or a cold or fever, because the doctor will need to increase his dosage.

• Advise the female patient that prolonged corticosteroid therapy may cause menstrual disturbances.

• If the patient has asthma, explain that proper use of bronchodilators (oral and aerosol) will decrease his need for corticosteroids, thereby minimizing drug side effects.

• Tell him to wear a Medic Alert bracelet, which will advise emergency personnel of his condition and drug regimen.

Inhaled Corticosteroids

Inhaled corticosteroids—primarily *beclomethasone*, *dexamethasone,* and *triamcinolone*—treat chronic asthma that can't be controlled by bronchodilators alone. Like oral corticosteroids, inhaled corticosteroids effectively control symptoms when given prophylactically (twice daily for stable asthma and up to four times daily for unstable or severe asthma). Unlike them, inhaled corticosteroids generally don't cause severe systemic effects, such as growth suppression and cushingoid symptoms, because direct application to the affected site achieves the same result with a lower dose. In mild to moderate asthma, inhaled corticosteroids can sometimes provide the same control achieved by alternate-day doses of 20 mg of oral prednisone.

Inhaled corticosteroids aren't recommended for acute asthma attacks because large doses must reach the lower respiratory tract to be effective. In severe asthma, they may be given along with oral corticosteroids until symptoms improve. Then the oral dose can be tapered gradually.

Chief side effects of inhaled corticosteroids are oral infections and hoarseness. These effects can be prevented by good oral hygiene or by using an extender device with the inhaler.

Purpose and action

Inhaled corticosteroids suppress respiratory tract inflammation, apparently by inhibiting cell-mediated immune reactions and preventing local accumulation of inflammatory cells.

Monitoring

If the patient's temporarily receiving an oral corticosteroid along with an in-

EXTENDERS AND RESERVOIRS:
HANDY INHALER ATTACHMENTS

Metered-dose inhalers work effectively only if the patient has sufficient coordination to inhale slowly while depressing the inhaler's cartridge. For some pediatric and geriatric patients, this proves impossible. To circumvent this problem, an extender or reservoir device can be attached to the inhaler.

Extender: Slow delivery

An extender, or spacer device, attaches to the inhaler at one end and fits into the patient's mouth at the other. This device allows 3 to 5 seconds to elapse between depression of the cartridge and inhalation of the medication. A valve in the extender opens as the patient inhales.

Use of an extender decreases aerosol speed, making the medication droplets smaller as the alcohol solvents evaporate. This greatly reduces the amount of medication deposited in the oropharyngeal and laryngeal areas, which helps to reduce side effects associated with systemic absorption of beta adrenergics and local mucosal irritation or infection associated with inhaled steroids.

Reservoir: A bag of medication

The reservoir, a collapsible bag attached to the inhaler on the side opposite the mouthpiece, provides a closed system in which inhaled air becomes saturated with medication. The patient can slowly inhale the contents of the bag until it collapses.

The reservoir device includes a special detachable mouthpiece containing a reed, which vibrates and makes noise if the patient inhales too quickly. When the patient slows his rate of inspiration, the noise will stop.

INHALER WITH EXTENDER

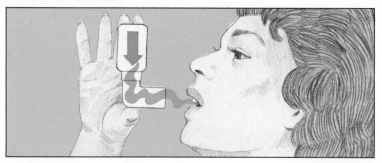

INHALER WITH RESERVOIR

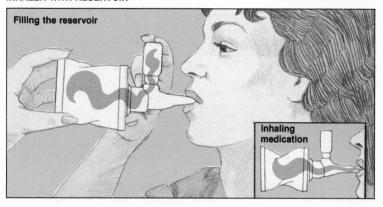

Filling the reservoir

Inhaling medication

haled one, watch for symptoms of adrenal insufficiency as the oral dose is being tapered.

If he's using an inhaled bronchodilator and an inhaled corticosteroid, instruct him to take the bronchodilator at least 15 minutes before the corticosteroid to allow improved airway deposition of the corticosteroid.

Encourage him to rinse out his mouth after each inhalation treatment to reduce the risk of oral fungal infection.

Home care instructions

• Teach the patient to use only the prescribed amount of medication. If he misses a dose, tell him to take it as soon as he remembers, unless it's almost time for his next dose. Instruct him not to double-dose.

• Advise the patient that the medication's full effect may not appear for up to 4 weeks. However, he should check with his doctor if his symptoms worsen or fail to improve, if infection occurs, or if he has an acute asthma attack that's not relieved by bronchodilators.

• Make sure the patient knows how to use his inhaler correctly (see *Using a Metered Dose Inhaler*, page 103). If he has difficulty delivering the medication, you may need to attach an extender or reservoir to the inhaler (see *Extenders and Reservoirs: Handy Inhaler Attachments*).

• Even though systemic absorption of inhaled corticosteroids is low, you'll need to teach the patient the signs of adrenal insufficiency, which may occur during a period of illness or severe stress. Instruct him to notify the doctor immediately if he experiences adrenal insufficiency.

• Tell the patient to wear a Medic Alert bracelet describing his medication and his need for supplemental corticosteroids during an emergency, periods of unusual stress, or an acute asthma attack.

• Advise him to notify any doctor or dentist that he's using inhaled corticosteroids before undergoing any invasive procedure.

Antitussives

These drugs effectively suppress a dry, nonproductive cough, which can tire a patient and interfere with his sleep or everyday activities. They may also be used to suppress coughing in the patient at risk for pneumothorax, tussive syncope, or rib fractures.

Antitussives come in narcotic and nonnarcotic forms. Narcotic antitussives, such as *codeine phosphate* and *codeine sulfate*, effectively suppress coughing. However, their use is limited because of the potential for toxicity and abuse and the range of side effects: from GI upset to CNS depression. Nonnarcotic antitussives, such as *dextromethorphan* and *diphenhydramine*, are common ingredients in over-the-counter cough and cold preparations.

Narcotic antitussives aren't recommended in chronic obstructive pulmonary disease because even slight respiratory depression may have a harmful effect. They must be used cautiously in CNS disorders.

Purpose and action

The centrally acting antitussives suppress the cough reflex by direct action on the medulla oblongata. The locally acting antitussives suppress coughing by anesthetizing the respiratory tract's sensory motor nerve fibers.

Monitoring

When the patient begins therapy, carefully monitor his response to prevent accidents caused by dizziness and drowsiness. Provide assistance with ambulation and raise the side rails of his bed, if necessary. Ask about GI effects, such as nausea.

If the patient's taking a narcotic antitussive, check for diaphoresis and light-headedness. If these symptoms occur along with dizziness and nausea, notify the doctor. He may need to reduce the dosage. Also watch for rash,

EXPECTORANTS: ALTERNATIVE TO ANTITUSSIVES

Not every patient with a cough needs an antitussive. An expectorant, which thins secretions and promotes their expulsion, may be more useful when the patient has pneumonia, bronchitis, cystic fibrosis, or tuberculosis. Thus, make sure you're familiar with these common expectorants.

ACETYLCYSTEINE
This mucolytic agent may be given by direct tracheal instillation or by nebulization through a face mask or mouthpiece. It helps treat acute and chronic bronchopulmonary diseases. It's contraindicated in patients with reactive airways because it may cause bronchospasm.

GUAIFENESIN
A common ingredient in over-the-counter cough preparations, guaifenesin promotes expectoration but can cause drowsiness and GI upset.

TERPIN HYDRATE
This elixir thins secretions and promotes expectoration. The recommended dosage shouldn't be exceeded because of the elixir's high alcohol content.

pruritus, or urticaria, which may signal an allergic reaction. Discontinue the drug and notify the doctor if any of these occur. Encourage fluids and provide a high-fiber diet because codeine may cause constipation.

Check the patient's drug regimen for possible interactions. For example, use of dextromethorphan with a monoamine oxidase (MAO) inhibitor can cause high fever, rigidity, laryngospasm, or bronchospasm. A narcotic antitussive used with narcotic analgesics, tranquilizers, sedatives, hypnotics, tricyclic antidepressants, or MAO inhibitors increases CNS depression and requires close monitoring.

Home care instructions
• Tell the patient to take his medication with food or milk to help prevent GI upset. Instruct him to take a syrup form

undiluted and not to drink liquids afterward.
• Warn the patient that antitussives cause drowsiness. As a result, he should be especially cautious when driving or operating machinery.
• If he experiences a dry mouth, suggest sucking on hard candy or ice chips or chewing sugarless gum.
• Encourage him to drink about 2 quarts (or liters) of fluid daily to thin secretions and ensure hydration. Suggest that he use a vaporizer at night to minimize the drying effects of room air. Recommend hot tea with honey and lemon, other hot beverages, and hard candy or lozenges to relieve his cough.
• If the patient is taking a narcotic antitussive, warn him not to exceed the recommended dosage to prevent oversedation. Caution that long-term use can lead to dependence.

SURGERY

Tracheostomy

Tracheostomy, the surgical creation of an opening into the trachea through the neck, is most commonly performed to provide an airway for the intubated patient who needs prolonged mechanical ventilation. It may also be performed to prevent an unconscious or paralyzed patient from aspirating food or secretions; to bypass upper airway obstruction caused by trauma, burns, epiglottitis, or a tumor; or to help remove lower tracheobronchial secretions in a patient who can't clear them.

Although endotracheal intubation is the treatment of choice in an emergency, tracheostomy may be used if intubation is impossible. For the laryngectomy patient, a permanent tracheostomy in which the skin and the

COMPARING TRACHEOSTOMY TUBES

Tracheostomy tubes, made of plastic or metal, come in cuffed, uncuffed, or fenestrated varieties. Tube selection depends on the patient's condition and the doctor's preference. Make sure you're familiar with the advantages and disadvantages of these commonly used tracheostomy tubes.

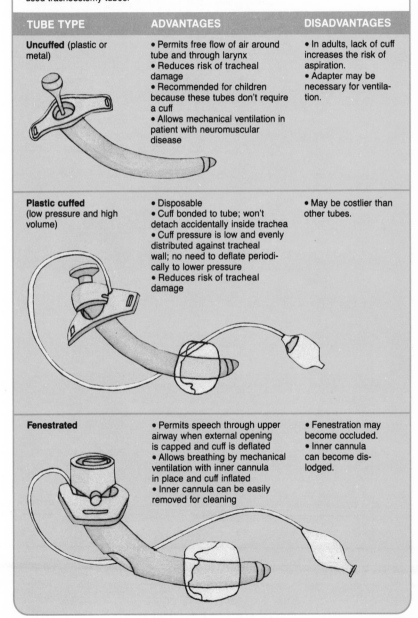

TUBE TYPE	ADVANTAGES	DISADVANTAGES
Uncuffed (plastic or metal)	• Permits free flow of air around tube and through larynx • Reduces risk of tracheal damage • Recommended for children because these tubes don't require a cuff • Allows mechanical ventilation in patient with neuromuscular disease	• In adults, lack of cuff increases the risk of aspiration. • Adapter may be necessary for ventilation.
Plastic cuffed (low pressure and high volume)	• Disposable • Cuff bonded to tube; won't detach accidentally inside trachea • Cuff pressure is low and evenly distributed against tracheal wall; no need to deflate periodically to lower pressure • Reduces risk of tracheal damage	• May be costlier than other tubes.
Fenestrated	• Permits speech through upper airway when external opening is capped and cuff is deflated • Allows breathing by mechanical ventilation with inner cannula in place and cuff inflated • Inner cannula can be easily removed for cleaning	• Fenestration may become occluded. • Inner cannula can become dislodged.

trachea are sutured together provides the necessary stoma.

After creation of the surgical opening, a tracheostomy tube is inserted to permit access to the airway. Selection of a specific tube depends on the patient's condition and the doctor's preference (see *Comparing Tracheostomy Tubes*, page 109).

Tracheostomy can cause serious complications. Within 48 hours after surgery, the patient may develop hemorrhage at the site, bleeding or edema within the tracheal tissue, aspiration of secretions, pneumothorax, or subcutaneous emphysema. After 48 hours, continued attention to sterile suctioning, careful cuff monitoring, and meticulous stoma care can reduce the risk of subsequent complications, such as stoma or pulmonary infection, ischemia and hemorrhage, airway obstruction, hypoxia, and arrhythmias.

Purpose
To provide temporary or permanent access to the lower airway, permitting ventilation and removal of secretions.

Preparation
For an emergency tracheostomy, briefly explain the procedure to the patient, if possible, and quickly obtain supplies or a tracheostomy tray.

For a scheduled tracheostomy, explain the procedure and the need for general anesthesia to the patient and his family. If possible, mention whether the tracheostomy will be temporary or permanent. As needed, discuss a communication system with the patient, such as a letter board, a magic slate, or flash cards, and have him practice using it so he can communicate comfortably while his speech is limited. If the patient will be having a long-term or permanent tracheostomy, introduce him to someone who has undergone a similar procedure and has adjusted well to tube and stoma care.

Ensure that samples for arterial blood gas (ABG) analysis and other diagnostic tests have been collected and that the patient or a responsible family member has signed a consent form.

Procedure
If the patient doesn't have an endotracheal tube in place, the doctor inserts this tube with the patient under general anesthesia. Then the doctor makes a horizontal incision in the skin below the cricoid cartilage and vertical incisions in the trachea. He places a tracheostomy tube between the second and third tracheal rings, and he may also place retraction sutures in the stomal margins to stabilize the opening. Finally, he inflates the tube cuff (if present), provides ventilation, suctions the airways, and provides oxygen by mist.

Monitoring and aftercare
Auscultate breath sounds every 2 hours after tracheostomy, noting crackles, rhonchi, or diminished sounds. Turn the patient every 2 hours to prevent pooling of tracheal secretions. Note the amount, consistency, color, and odor of secretions. As ordered, provide chest physiotherapy to help mobilize secretions. (See *Combating Complications of Tracheostomy* for details on preventing or recognizing complications.)

Provide humidification to reduce the drying effects of oxygen on mucous membranes and to thin secretions. Expect to deliver oxygen through a T-piece connected to a nebulizer or heated cascade humidifier. If your patient's an infant or a young child, be sure to warm the oxygen. Monitor ABG results and compare them with baseline values to help determine if oxygenation and carbon dioxide removal is adequate. As ordered, also monitor the patient's oximetry values.

Using sterile equipment and technique, suction the tracheostomy, as ordered, to remove excess secretions. Use a suction catheter no larger than half the diameter of the tracheostomy tube, and minimize oxygen deprivation and tracheal trauma by keeping the bypass port open while inserting the catheter. Use a gentle, twisting motion on with-

COMBATING COMPLICATIONS OF TRACHEOSTOMY

COMPLI-CATION	PREVENTION	DETECTION	TREATMENT
Aspiration	• Evaluate patient's ability to swallow. • Elevate his head and inflate cuff during feeding and for 30 minutes afterward.	• Assess for dyspnea, tachypnea, rhonchi, crackles, excessive secretions, and fever.	• Obtain chest X-ray, if ordered. • Suction excessive secretions. • Give antibiotics, if necessary.
Bleeding at tracheostomy site	• Don't pull on the tracheostomy tube; don't allow ventilator tubing to do so. • If dressing adheres to wound, wet it with hydrogen peroxide and remove gently.	• Check dressing regularly; slight bleeding is normal, especially if patient has a bleeding disorder.	• Keep cuff inflated to prevent edema and blood aspiration. Give humidified oxygen. • Document rate and amount of bleeding. Check for prolonged clotting time. • As ordered, assist with Gelfoam application or ligation of a small bleeder.
Infection at tracheostomy site	• Always use strict aseptic technique. • Thoroughly clean all tubing. • Change nebulizer or humidifier jar and all tubing daily. • Collect sputum and wound drainage specimens for culture.	• Check for purulent, foul-smelling drainage from stoma. • Be alert for other signs of infection: fever, malaise, increased white blood cell count, and local pain.	• As ordered, obtain culture specimens and administer antibiotics. • Inflate tracheostomy cuff to prevent aspiration. • Suction the patient frequently, maintaining sterile technique; avoid cross-contamination. • Change dressing whenever soiled.
Pneumothorax	• Assess for subcutaneous emphysema, which may indicate pneumothorax. Notify doctor if this occurs.	• Auscultate for decreased or absent breath sounds. • Check for tachypnea, pain, and subcutaneous emphysema.	• If ordered, prepare for chest tube insertion. • Obtain chest X-ray, as ordered, to evaluate pneumothorax or to check placement of chest tube.
Subcutaneous emphysema	• Make sure cuffed tube is patent and properly inflated. • Avoid displacement by securing ties and using lightweight ventilator tubing and swivel valves.	• Most common in mechanically ventilated patients. • Palpate neck for crepitus, listen for escape of air around tube cuff, and check for excessive swelling at wound site.	• Inflate cuff correctly or use a larger tube. • Suction patient and clean tube to remove any blockage. • Document extent of crepitus.
Tracheal malasia	• Avoid excessive cuff pressures. • Avoid suctioning beyond end of tube.	• Dry, hacking cough and blood-streaked sputum when tube is being manipulated.	• Minimize trauma from tube movement. • Keep cuff pressure below 18 mm Hg.

drawal to help minimize tracheal and bronchial mucosal irritation. If secretions are thick and tenacious, instill 3 to 5 ml of sterile normal saline solution during inspiration to help mobilize them. Apply suction for no longer than 10 seconds at a time, and discontinue suctioning if the patient develops respiratory distress. Monitor for arrhythmias, which can occur if suctioning decreases PaO_2 levels below 50 mm Hg. Evaluate the effectiveness of suctioning by auscultating for breath sounds.

A cuffed tube, usually inflated until the patient no longer needs controlled ventilation or is over the risk of aspiration, may cause tracheal stenosis from excessive pressure or incorrect placement. Prevent trauma to the interior tracheal wall by using pressures less than 25 cmH_2O (18 mm Hg) and minimal leak technique when inflating the cuff. Reduce the risk of trauma to the stoma site and internal tracheal wall by using lightweight corrugated tubing for the ventilator or nebulizer and providing a swivel adapter for the ventilator circuit.

Make sure the tracheostomy ties are secure but not overly tight. Refrain from changing the ties unnecessarily until the stoma track is stabler, thereby helping to prevent accidental tube dislodgment or expulsion. Report any tube pulsation to the doctor, since this may indicate its proximity to the innominate artery, predisposing the patient to hemorrhage.

Using aseptic technique, change the tracheostomy dressing when soiled or once per shift, and check the color, odor, amount, and type of any drainage. Also check for swelling, erythema, and bleeding at the site, and report excessive bleeding or unusual drainage immediately.

Keep a sterile tracheostomy tube (with obturator) at the patient's bedside, and be prepared to replace an expelled or contaminated tube. Also keep available a sterile tracheostomy tube (with obturator) that's one size smaller than the tube currently being used, since the trachea begins to close after tube expulsion, making insertion of the same size tube difficult.

Home care instructions
- Tell the patient to notify his doctor if he develops any breathing problems, chest or stoma pain, or any change in the amount or color of his secretions.
- Ensure that the patient can effectively care for his stoma and tracheostomy tube. Instruct him to wash the skin around his stoma with a moist cloth. Emphasize the importance of not getting water in his stoma. He should, of course, avoid swimming. When he showers, he should wear a stoma shield or direct the water below his stoma.
- Tell the patient to place a foam filter over his stoma in winter, thereby warming inspired air, and to wear a bib over the filter.
- Teach the patient to bend at his waist during coughing to help expel secretions. Tell him to keep a tissue handy to catch expelled secretions.

Chest Tube Insertion

Insertion of a tube into the pleural space helps treat pneumothorax, hemothorax, empyema, pleural effusion, or chylothorax. The tube allows drainage of blood, fluid, pus, or air from the pleural space. In pneumothorax, it restores negative pressure to the pleural space by means of an underwater-seal drainage system. The water in the system prevents air from being sucked back into the pleural space during inspiration. (If the leak is through the bronchi and cannot be sealed, suction applied to the underwater-seal system removes air from the pleural space faster than it can collect.) As negative pleural pressure is restored, the lung can reinflate.

Because a collapsed lung is life-threatening, chest tube insertion is often an emergency treatment and has no contraindications. Complications include lung puncture, bleeding, or additional hemothorax at the insertion site. Chest tube obstruction or blockage of the air vent in the underwater-seal drainage system may cause tension pneumothorax, a life-threatening complication.

Purpose
To remove air or fluid from the pleural space, permitting lung reinflation.

Preparation
If time permits, explain the procedure to the patient and tell him that it will allow him to breathe more easily. Take his vital signs to serve as a baseline and obtain a signed consent form. Then administer a sedative, as ordered.

Collect necessary equipment, including a thoracotomy tray and an underwater-seal drainage system. Prepare lidocaine for local anesthesia, as directed. Cleanse the insertion site with povidone-iodine solution. Set up the underwater-seal drainage system according to the manufacturer's instructions, and place it at bedside, below the patient's chest level. Stabilize the unit to avoid knocking it over.

Procedure
Position the patient on his unaffected side. After the doctor injects the local anesthetic at the insertion site, help the patient hold still while the doctor makes a small incision and tunnels the tube through the tissue into the pleural space. Usually, the doctor places the tube anteriorly near the second or third intercostal space if he wants to remove air; laterally and slightly posteriorly at about the eighth intercostal space if he wants to remove fluid.

As soon as the doctor inserts the tube into the pleural space, connect the external end of the tube to the underwater-seal drainage system. The doctor stabilizes the proximal end by suturing the tube into place. Apply petrolatum gauze and a dry sterile dressing. As ordered, tape the tube to the patient's chest wall distal to the insertion site, to help prevent accidental dislodgment. Tape all tube connections and regulate suction, as ordered.

Monitoring and aftercare
Once the patient's chest tube is stabilized, have him take several deep breaths to inflate his lungs fully and help push pleural air out through the tube. Take his vital signs immediately after tube insertion and then every 15 minutes or as ordered. Change the dressing daily to cleanse the site and remove any drainage.

Prepare the patient for a chest X-ray to verify tube placement and to assess the outcome of treatment. As ordered, arrange for daily X-rays to monitor his progress. Palpate the patient's chest above the tube for subcutaneous emphysema and notify the doctor of any increase.

Routinely assess the function of the patient's chest tube. Describe and record the amount of drainage on the intake and output sheet. Once most of the air has been removed, the drainage system should bubble only during forced expiration unless the patient has a bronchopleural fistula. However, constant bubbling in the system when suction is attached may indicate a loose connection, or that the tube has advanced slightly out of the patient's chest. Promptly correct any loose connections to prevent complications.

If the chest tube becomes dislodged, cover the opening immediately with petrolatum gauze and apply pressure to prevent negative inspiratory pressure from sucking air into the patient's chest. Call the doctor and have an assistant obtain the equipment necessary for tube reinsertion while you continue to keep the opening closed. Reassure the patient and monitor him closely for signs of tension pneumothorax (see *Combating Tension Pneumothorax*, page 114).

The doctor will remove the patient's chest tube when the lung has fully reexpanded. As soon as the tube is re-

COMBATING TENSION PNEUMOTHORAX

Fatal if not treated promptly, tension pneumothorax refers to the entrapment of air within the pleural space.

What causes it?
Tension pneumothorax can result from dislodgment or obstruction of the chest tube. In both of these cases, increasing positive pressure within the patient's chest cavity compresses the affected lung and the mediastinum, shifting them toward the opposite lung. The result: markedly impaired venous return and cardiac output and possibly lung collapse.

Telltale signs
Suspect tension pneumothorax if your patient develops any of these untoward signs or symptoms: dyspnea, chest pain, an irritating cough, vertigo, syncope, or anxiety. Is his skin cold, pale, and clammy? Are his respiratory and pulse rates unusually rapid?
   If the patient develops any of these signs or symptoms, palpate his neck, face, and chest wall for subcutaneous emphysema, and palpate his trachea for deviation from midline. Auscultate his lungs for decreased or absent breath sounds on the affected side. Then percuss them for hyperresonance.
   If you suspect tension pneumothorax, notify the doctor at once and help him to identify the cause.

moved, apply an airtight, sterile petrolatum dressing.

Home care instructions
• Typically, the patient will be discharged with a chest tube only if it's being used to drain a loculated empyema, since this doesn't require an underwater-seal drainage system. Teach this patient how to care for his tube, dispose of drainage and soiled dressings properly, and perform wound care and dressing changes.
• Teach the patient with a recently removed chest tube how to cleanse the wound site and change dressings. Tell him to report any signs of infection.

Lung Excision

This treatment, the surgical removal of all or part of a lung, aims to spare healthy lung tissue from disease. Excision may involve pneumonectomy, lobectomy, segmental resection, or wedge resection. (See *Understanding Types of Lung Excision*.)

Pneumonectomy, excision of an entire lung, is usually performed to treat bronchogenic carcinoma but may also be used to treat tuberculosis, bronchiectasis, or lung abscess. It's used only when a less radical approach can't remove all diseased tissue. After pneumonectomy, chest cavity pressures stabilize, and over time fluid fills the cavity where lung tissue was removed, preventing significant mediastinal shift.

Lobectomy, the removal of one of the five lung lobes, can treat bronchogenic carcinoma, tuberculosis, lung abscess, emphysematous blebs or bullae, benign tumors, or localized fungal infections. After this surgery, the remaining lobes expand to fill the entire pleural cavity.

Segmental resection, removal of one or more lung segments, preserves more functional tissue than lobectomy. It's commonly used to treat bronchiectasis. *Wedge resection*, removal of a small portion of the lung without regard to segments, preserves the most functional tissue of all the surgeries but can treat only a small, well-circumscribed lesion. Remaining lung tissue needs to be reexpanded after both resections.

Complications include hemorrhage, infection, and tension pneumothorax. Additional complications include bronchopleural fistula, empyema, and a persistent air space that the remaining lung tissue doesn't expand to fill. Removal of up to three ribs may be necessary to reduce chest cavity size and allow lung tissue to fit the space.

Purpose
To remove diseased lung tissue.

Preparation

Explain the anticipated lung excision to the patient, and inform him that he'll receive a general anesthetic. Prepare him psychologically according to his condition. A patient with lung cancer, for example, faces the fear of dying as well as the fear of surgery and needs ongoing emotional support. In contrast, a patient with a chronic lung disorder, such as tuberculosis or a fungal infection, may view the surgery as a cure for his ailment.

Inform the patient that postoperatively he may have chest tubes in place and may be receiving oxygen. Teach him coughing and deep-breathing techniques, and explain that he'll use these after surgery to facilitate lung reexpansion. Also teach him how to use an incentive spirometer; record the volumes he achieves to provide a baseline.

As ordered, arrange for laboratory studies, such as pulmonary function tests, EKG, chest X-ray, arterial blood gas analysis, bronchoscopy, and possibly cardiac catheterization, to assess cardiac function before pneumonectomy.

Ensure that the patient or a responsible family member has signed a consent form.

UNDERSTANDING TYPES OF LUNG EXCISION

Lung excision may be total (pneumonectomy) or partial (lobectomy, segmental resection, or wedge resection), depending on your patient's condition. The illustrations here show the extent of each of these surgeries for the right lung.

PNEUMONECTOMY

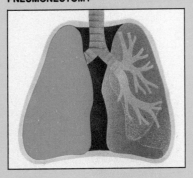

SEGMENTAL RESECTION

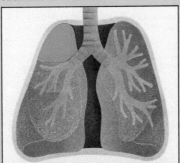

LOBECTOMY

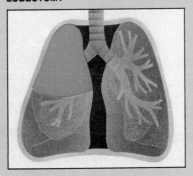

WEDGE RESECTION

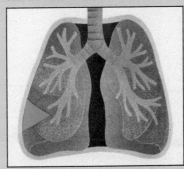

Procedure

After the patient's anesthetized, the surgeon performs a thoracotomy, making a posterolateral incision through the fourth, fifth, sixth, or seventh intercostal space. Then he spreads the ribs and exposes the lung area.

In a pneumonectomy, the surgeon ligates and cuts the pulmonary arteries. Next, he clamps the main stem bronchus leading to the affected lung, divides it, and then closes it with nonabsorbable sutures. Then he removes the lung. To ensure airtight closure, he places a pleural flap over the bronchus and closes it. Then he severs the phrenic nerve on the affected side, allowing it to reduce the size of the pleural cavity. After air pressure in the cavity stabilizes, he closes the chest.

In a lobectomy, the surgeon resects the affected lobe and ligates and cuts the appropriate arteries, veins, and bronchial passages.

In a segmental resection, the surgeon removes the affected segment and ligates and cuts the appropriate artery, vein, and bronchus. In a wedge resection, he clamps and excises the affected area and then sutures it. In both resections, he inserts two chest tubes to aid lung reexpansion.

After completing the excision, the surgeon closes the chest cavity and applies a dressing.

Monitoring and aftercare

If the patient has had a pneumonectomy, make sure he lies only on his operative side or his back until he's stabilized. This prevents fluid from draining into the unaffected lung if the sutured bronchus opens. If he has a chest tube in place, make sure it's functioning and monitor him for signs of tension pneumothorax (see *Combating Tension Pneumothorax*, page 114). Provide analgesics, as ordered.

Have the patient begin coughing and deep-breathing exercises as soon as he's stabilized. Auscultate his lungs, place him in semi-Fowler's position, and have him splint his incision to facilitate coughing and deep breathing. Have him cough every 2 to 4 hours until his breath sounds clear.

Perform passive range-of-motion exercises the evening of surgery and two or three times daily thereafter. Progress to active range-of-motion exercises.

Home care instructions

- Tell the patient to continue his coughing and deep-breathing exercises to prevent complications. Advise him to report any changes in sputum characteristics to his doctor.
- Instruct the patient to continue performing range-of-motion exercises to maintain mobility of his shoulder and chest wall.
- Tell the patient to avoid contact with people who have upper respiratory tract infections and to refrain from smoking.
- Provide him with instructions for wound care and dressing changes, as necessary.

INHALATION THERAPY

Mechanical Ventilation

Mechanical ventilation artificially controls or assists the patient's respirations. Typically requiring an endotracheal or tracheostomy tube, it can deliver room air under positive pressure or oxygen-enriched air in concentrations of up to 100%. It's indicated to correct profoundly impaired gas exchange, as evidenced by hypoxia, hypercapnia, and symptoms of increased work of breathing: nasal flaring, intercostal retraction, decreased blood pressure, and diaphoresis.

Major types of mechanical ventilation systems include positive-pressure, negative-pressure, and high-frequency ventilation (HFV). Positive-pressure systems, the most commonly used, can be volume-cycled or pressure-cycled and may deliver positive end-expiratory pressure or continuous positive airway pressure. Negative-pressure systems provide ventilation for patients unable to generate adequate inspiratory pressures. Still in the experimental stage, HFV systems provide high ventilation rates with low peak airway pressures. (See *Understanding Types of Mechanical Ventilation*, pages 118 and 119, for further information.)

Mechanical ventilators can be used as controllers, assisters, or assister-controllers. In the control mode, a ventilator can deliver a set tidal volume at a prescribed rate, using predetermined inspiratory and expiratory times, to fully regulate ventilation in a patient with paralysis or respiratory arrest. In the assist mode, the patient initiates inspiration and receives a preset tidal volume from the machine, augmenting his respiratory effort while allowing him to determine his own minute ventilation. In the assist-control mode, the patient initiates breathing but a backup control delivers a preset number of breaths at a set volume. In intermittent mandatory ventilation (IMV), the ventilator delivers a set number of specific-volume breaths. The patient may breathe spontaneously between the IMV breaths at volumes that differ from those on the machine. Often used as a weaning tool, IMV may also be used for ventilation.

The patient receiving mechanical ventilation requires ongoing nursing care to provide emotional support, prevent machine failure, and avert such complications as pneumothorax, atelectasis, decreased cardiac output, pulmonary barotrauma, and infection.

Purpose

To deliver room air or oxygen-enriched air according to a preset volume or pressure, thereby decreasing the work of breathing and supporting ventilation in a patient whose respirations are inadequate.

Preparation

Most commonly, the patient will be ventilated using a positive-pressure system. Explain this system to the patient, describing its benefits and the sensations he'll experience. Because the patient will be intubated, set up a communication system with him and provide reassurance that a nurse will be nearby at all times. Keep in mind that the patient's apprehension may make him fight the machine, defeating its purpose.

Place the patient in semi-Fowler's position, if possible, to promote lung expansion. Obtain baseline blood pressure and arterial blood gas (ABG) readings.

If the patient doesn't have an endotracheal or tracheostomy tube in place, he'll be intubated to establish an artificial airway. An oral airway or bite block may be used with an oral endotracheal tube to prevent the patient from biting the tube and interfering with gas flow. Arrange for a chest X-ray following intubation to evaluate tube placement. If necessary, use soft restraints to prevent the patient from extubating himself. Make sure he has a call bell or communication device within reach.

Procedure

As ordered, adjust the positive-pressure ventilator's respiratory rate, tidal volume, flow rate, and oxygen concentration. Keeping the inner lumens sterile, attach the patient's endotracheal or tracheostomy tube to the adapter end of the machine's corrugated tubing.

Reassess ABG levels after the patient has been ventilated for 20 minutes without interruption, which allows enough time for equilibrium to be established at the recommended settings. Then, based on ABG results, readjust the ventilator settings, as ordered.

UNDERSTANDING TYPES OF MECHANICAL VENTILATION

TYPE	DESCRIPTION	NURSING CONSIDERATIONS
Positive-pressure ventilation		
Continuous positive airway pressure	• Applies positive pressure during entire respiratory cycle.	• Useful for patients who are breathing spontaneously but have hypoxemic respiratory failure; also useful during weaning.
Positive end-expiratory pressure	• Applies positive pressure during expiration.	• Useful for treating hypoxemic respiratory failure. • Adults usually receive 5 to 20 cmH$_2$O of pressure, although higher pressures may be used.
Pressure-cycled	• Flow continues until a preset pressure is achieved.	• Useful when excessive inspiratory pressure may damage lungs, as with neonates. • Tidal volume varies with airway resistance and lung compliance. • Alveolar ventilation may not be adequate.
Volume-cycled	• Delivers a preset volume to the patient.	• Effectively treats respiratory failure in adults because it delivers consistent tidal volume despite changes in airway resistance or lung compliance. • Check pressure regularly.
High-frequency ventilation		
High-frequency jet ventilation (HFJV) **High-frequency oscillatory ventilation (HFOV)** **High-frequency positive-pressure ventilation (HFPPV)**	• All three systems deliver gas rapidly under low pressure by means of a special injector cannula. • HFJV delivers 100 to 200 breaths/minute with a tidal volume of 50 to 400 ml. HFOV delivers over 200 breaths/minute, or 900 to 3,000 vibrations, with a tidal volume of 50 to 80 ml. HFPPV delivers 60 to 100 breaths/minute with a tidal volume of 3 to 6 ml/kg (less than the normal 5 to 7 ml/kg).	• High-frequency ventilation is still experimental, but HFJV is used most commonly. • HFJV maintains adequate alveolar ventilation with low airway pressure. Useful for treating tracheal esophageal fistula, bronchopleural fistula, pneumothorax, or pneumomediastinum. May also avert barotrauma in high-risk patients if used early during treatment.

Monitoring and aftercare

Check ABG levels periodically. Overventilation may cause respiratory alkalosis from decreased carbon dioxide. Inadequate alveolar ventilation or atelectasis from an inappropriate tidal volume may cause respiratory acidosis.

Perform the following steps every 1 to 2 hours:

• Check all connections between the ventilator and the patient. Make sure critical alarms are turned on. This includes the low-pressure alarm (not less than 3 cmH$_2$O), which indicates a disconnection in the system, and the high-pressure alarm (set 20 to 30 cmH$_2$O greater than the patient's peak airway pressure) to prevent excessive airway

TYPE	DESCRIPTION	NURSING CONSIDERATIONS
Negative-pressure ventilation		
Chest shell wrap or cuirass	• Creates negative pressure, pulling thorax outward; air flows into lungs for a preset time. • Applies vacuum to the anterior chest and upper abdomen, with minimal pull and some compression of lateral chest wall on inspiration. • Soft plastic type uses Velcro straps at elbow, hip, and neck to confine negative pressure to chest and abdomen; metal or plastic shell under the wrap holds negative pressure away from chest wall, allowing an area for the vacuum to pull on the chest wall.	• Useful for long-term ventilation of select patients unable to generate sufficient inspiratory pressure because of respiratory muscle weakness or inadequate respiratory drive. • Difficult to seal shell tightly; however, patient has greater range of movement than with iron lung.
Pneumobelt	• Applies pressure on the abdomen during expiration, compressing the diaphragm upward. • Releases pressure during inspiration, causing the diaphragm to drop with resulting negative airway pressure and inspiratory airflow.	• Used rarely. • Device requires the patient to be upright or seated.
Tank or iron lung	• Creates negative pressure, pulling thorax outward; air flows into lungs for a preset time. • Negative pressure is felt throughout the body, except for the head. • Device provides controlled ventilation only, which may not synchronize with respirations and may prevent use of respiratory muscles.	• Useful for long-term ventilation of patients unable to generate sufficient inspiratory pressure. • Ventilation may be inadequate because low lung compliance results in decreased tidal volume. • Increased use of chest physiotherapy may be needed to clear airways of mobilized secretions and maintain airway patency. Fluid may also pool in abdomen, leading to decreased cardiac output. • Patient's movement is severely limited.

pressures. Volume alarms, if they are available, should also be used. Make sure that the patient can reach his call bell.

• Verify that ventilator settings are correct and that the ventilator is operating at those settings: compare the patient's respiratory rate with the setting and, for a volume-cycled machine, watch that the spirometer reaches the correct volume. For a pressure-cycled machine, use a respirometer to check exhaled tidal volume.

• Check the humidifier and refill it, if necessary. Check the corrugated tubing for condensation; drain any into another container and discard. (*Do not* drain condensation into the humidifier because the condensation may be contaminated with bacteria.)

• Check the temperature gauges, which should be set between 89.6° F.(32° C.) and 98.6° F. (37° C.). Also check that gas is being delivered at the correct temperature.

• If ordered, give the patient several deep breaths (usually two or three) each hour by setting the sigh mechanism on the ventilator or by using an Ambu bag.

Subsequently, check oxygen concentration every 8 hours and overall ABG values whenever ventilator settings are changed. Assess respiratory status at least every 2 hours in the acutely ill patient and every 4 hours in the stable chronically ill patient to detect the need for suctioning and evaluate the response to treatment. Suction the patient as necessary, noting the amount, color, odor, and consistency of secretions. Auscultate for decreased breath sounds on the left side—an indication of tube slippage into the right main stem bronchus. Arrange for chest X-rays, as ordered.

Monitor the patient's fluid intake and output and his electrolyte balance. Weigh him as ordered. Using aseptic technique, change the humidifier, nebulizer, and ventilator tubing every 48 hours; ventilate the patient manually during this time. Change his position frequently and perform chest physiotherapy, as necessary. Provide emotional support to reduce stress, and give antacids and other medications, as ordered, to reduce gastric acid production and help prevent GI complications. Monitor for decreased bowel sounds and distention, which may indicate paralytic ileus.

If the patient is received high-pressure ventilation, assess for pneumothorax, signaled by absent or diminished breath sounds on the affected side, acute chest pain, and possibly tracheal deviation or subcutaneous or mediastinal emphysema. If he's receiving a high oxygen concentration, watch for signs of toxicity: substernal chest pain,

increased coughing, tachypnea, decreased lung compliance and vital capacity, and decreased PaO_2 levels without a change in oxygen concentration.

If the patient is fighting the ventilator and ineffective ventilation results, give him a sedative or a neuromuscular blocking agent, as ordered, and observe him closely.

Wean the patient, as ordered, based on his respiratory status (see *Weaning the Patient from Mechanical Ventilation*). If he can't be weaned and requires long-term ventilatory support, begin to provide him with instructions on home care.

Home care instructions

• If the patient will need to use a ventilator at home, teach him and a family member to check the device and its settings, the nebulizer, and the oxygen equipment at least once a day. Tell the patient to refill his humidifier, as necessary. Explain that his ABG levels will need to be measured periodically in order to evaluate the effectiveness of therapy.

• Inform the patient that he should call the doctor if he experiences chest pain, fever, dyspnea, or swollen extremities. Teach him to count his pulse rate, and urge him to report any changes in rate or rhythm. If the patient is able to be weighed at home, instruct him to report a weight gain of 5 lb or more within a week.

• Tell the patient to clean his tracheostomy daily, using the technique taught to him by the nurse or respiratory therapist. If he's using nondisposable items, tell him to keep them clean.

• Instruct the patient to try to bring his ventilator with him if he needs to be treated for an acute problem. It may be possible to stabilize him without hospital admission. Provide the patient with emergency numbers, and tell him to call his doctor or respiratory therapist if he has any questions or problems.

WEANING THE PATIENT FROM MECHANICAL VENTILATION

To ensure successful weaning, the patient should have:
- a PaCO$_2$ level less than 50 mm Hg or whatever is normal for the patient
- an FIO$_2$ of 40% or below with a PaO$_2$ of 60 mm Hg or more
- a vital capacity of greater than 10 to 15 ml/kg of body weight
- a negative inspiratory force maneuver greater than −20 cmH$_2$O
- minute ventilation of less than 10 liters/minute with a tidal volume equal to 5 ml/kg of body weight
- an ability to double his spontaneous resting minute ventilation
- a spontaneous respiratory effort
- successful cessation of neuromuscular blocking drugs and absence of infection, acid-base or electrolyte imbalance, hyperglycemia, fever, arrhythmias, renal failure, shock, anemia, or excessive fatigue.

Once the patient meets these criteria, wean him using a conventional T-piece or tracheostomy collar connected to humidified oxygen. Or use continuous positive airway pressure (CPAP), intermittent mandatory ventilation (IMV), synchronized intermittent mandatory ventilation (SIMV), or intermittent demand ventilation (IDV).

Conventional weaning
- Obtain baseline ABG levels, pulse rate, breath sounds, and spontaneous tidal volume, minute ventilation, and negative inspiratory force. Connect a T-piece or tracheostomy collar to a separate humidified oxygen system, and adjust the flow rate or concentration. Deflate the cuff for a T-piece trial unless it's needed to prevent aspiration of saliva or stomach contents.
- If possible, place the patient in semi-Fowler's position. Give a bronchodilator, as ordered, and suction 15 minutes before disconnecting the patient from the ventilator.
- Turn on the oxygen source, detach the patient from the ventilator, and connect his tube to the oxygen source for 5 to 10 minutes/hour at the start and gradually increasing by 5 to 15 minutes/hour.
- Watch closely for signs of hypoxia: restlessness, dyspnea, accessory muscle use, altered skin color and level of consciousness, tachycardia, EKG changes, and altered ABG values. Notify the doctor if the patient's respiratory rate exceeds 30, his pulse rate rises more than 20 beats/minute, his systolic pressure rises or falls more than 15 mm Hg, or his EKG shows a depressed ST segment or more than six extrasystoles per minute. Also notify

him if the patient becomes severely dyspneic or tired. Draw an ABG sample and reconnect the patient to the ventilator.
- Obtain ABG samples, as ordered, while the patient is breathing spontaneously. Compare results to baseline levels and report changes. When the prescribed amount of time for the weaning session has elapsed, return the patient to the ventilator. Increase weaning times as tolerated. (Weaning at night is usually attempted last, to allow the patient rest).

Weaning with CPAP
As ordered, use CPAP to help maintain functional residual capacity and PaO$_2$ when the patient is breathing spontaneously during weaning. Using a T-piece and a high-flow air-oxygen blend, CPAP maintains positive airway pressure throughout the respiratory cycle. Before and during treatment, assess respiratory rate and check for accessory muscle use. Increased rate, reduced volume, and accessory muscle use indicate fatigue.

Weaning with IMV
Generally, the patient will be placed on an IMV mode for periods during the day and then returned to an assist-control mode for sleep or if he's unable to sustain spontaneous efforts. Expect to use IMV if the patient fails to progress satisfactorily with traditional weaning. This method delivers breaths at preset volumes and intervals but also allows the patient to breathe spontaneously in between.

As ordered, gradually decrease the number of machine-delivered breaths/minute until the patient can breathe on his own. Keep in mind that machine weaning doesn't eliminate the risk of hypoxia, so be sure to evaluate the patient's respiratory status and ABG levels. Know the patient's total minute ventilation necessary to maintain stable ABG levels. Monitor spontaneous minute ventilation carefully as IMV is reduced. Acidosis and hypercarbia may stem from inadequate ventilation.

Weaning with IDV and SIMV
Proceed as with IMV, except keep in mind that here the patient triggers the machine-controlled breaths, which are then synchronized with his spontaneous breaths. After you've set one of these ventilators to deliver controlled breaths at regular intervals, notice that the device waits for the patient to initiate the breath and then delivers its full volume as he inspires.

Intermittent Positive-Pressure Breathing

An alternative to deep-breathing exercises and incentive spirometry, intermittent positive-pressure breathing (IPPB) can expand airways, loosen secretions, distend the tracheobronchial tree, and enhance distribution of inspired oxygen. It helps prevent atelectasis in acute exacerbations of chronic obstructive pulmonary diseases, as well as in bronchiectasis, cystic fibrosis, bronchogenic carcinoma, inflammatory lung disease, rib fractures, and pleuritic pain and after upper abdominal surgery. Routine use remains controversial. Many clinicians contend that properly performed deep-breathing exercises and incentive spirometry are equally effective and less costly.

IPPB works by delivering room air or oxygen to the lungs at greater-than-atmospheric pressure. The length of the inspiratory phase is pressure-limited: gas entering the airways gradually meets increasing resistance as the lungs fill or as the patient resists the airflow. Gas delivery ceases when pressure in the mouth or breathing circuit tube equals the machine's preset pressure. Then the patient can exhale passively. Unfortunately, a frightened patient can reduce gas delivery prematurely by blocking the mouthpiece with his tongue or letting the gas fill his cheeks instead of his lungs. In such instances, little gas reaches the lungs before pressure terminates the inspiratory phase. Using low inspiratory flow rates can reduce the problem and make treatment more comfortable. Furthermore, although IPPB easily inflates healthy alveoli, it may have little effect on thickened alveoli or obstructed airways.

IPPB may cause gastric insufflation if air is swallowed during treatment. It may also cause transient dizziness, tachycardia, hypotension, and headache. Spontaneous pneumothorax, although rare, may result from increased intrathoracic pressure, especially in a patient with bullous emphysema. Contraindications for IPPB include untreated pneumothorax, tracheoesophageal fistula, recent gastric surgery, and increased intracranial pressure.

Purpose
To enhance airway and alveolar expansion and loosen secretions.

Preparation
Explain the procedure to the patient, and tell him that his cooperation will help ensure successful treatment. Encourage him to relax.

Auscultate the lungs and take baseline pulse and blood pressure measurements. Place the patient in high Fowler's position or have him sit in a chair, to promote optimal lung expansion. Attach the appropriate tubing to a pressure-cycled positive-pressure ventilator. Don't use a flowmeter, since IPPB requires pressure higher than this device can provide.

Make sure the system's working properly. When giving medication with this treatment, place it in the nebulizer and set delivery only during inspiration, if possible, or use sterile water in the nebulizer to humidify the dry gas when no medication is being given.

Procedure
Tell the patient to breathe deeply and slowly through his mouth, thereby allowing the machine to deliver a breath to him. When the preset pressure is met, the machine cycles off, ending inspiration. Tell him to hold his breath for a few seconds after full inspiration, to allow greater gas distribution and dispersion. Then have him exhale normally. Coach him with each breath and observe the quality of his inspiratory effort.

Work with the patient initially to achieve the best tidal volume possible for each breath while still keeping the pressure limit as low as possible. Use a Wright respirometer attached to the exhalation port to register the volume of each breath, keeping in mind an overall goal of greater than 15 ml/kg of body weight. Set the initial pressure at 5 to 10 cmH_2O; if the machine has a sensitivity control, set it so that the machine cycles on with slight inspiratory effort. Subsequently increase the pressure to the prescribed level, assessing tidal volume with each change. When pressure increases no longer spur volume increases, stop raising the pressure. The risk of gastric distention and pneumothorax increases with pressures over 15 cmH_2O in patients with emphysema and over 25 cmH_2O in patients with restrictive disease.

Monitoring and aftercare

Encourage the patient to pause for several breaths between each IPPB breath because rapid, deep inspirations reduce CO_2 levels quickly and may lead to dizziness and paresthesias. If these symptoms occur despite pauses, stop treatment and notify the doctor.

Take the patient's blood pressure and pulse rate during the initial treatment and compare these with baseline values. Because IPPB raises intrathoracic pressure, it may temporarily decrease cardiac output and venous return, with resulting tachycardia, hypotension, or headache. If the patient's blood pressure changes suddenly or his pulse rate increases by 20 or more beats, stop the treatment and notify the doctor immediately.

If you're giving a bronchodilator along with gas or room air, assess for the patient's response to this. If he tolerates treatment, continue until the medication in the nebulizer is exhausted, usually after 15 to 20 minutes.

Check to see if the patient is swallowing air during the procedure, which may result in gastric distention. If necessary, show him again how to use the machine properly. If the IPPB machine is delivering oxygen, also assess the patient for depressed hypoxic drive.

If the patient reports chest pain, stop the treatment immediately and auscultate his lungs for decreased or absent breath sounds, a possible sign of pneumothorax. The risk of pneumothorax increases at high pressures or if the patient has bullous emphysema.

After treatment, have the patient expectorate into tissues or a specimen cup, or suction him, as necessary. Listen to his breath sounds and compare them with baseline assessments.

Home care instructions

● If the patient will be continuing IPPB treatments at home, have him demonstrate the proper setup, use, and cleaning of the equipment before discharge. Tell him that he shouldn't change the pressure settings without first checking with his doctor.
● Instruct him to discontinue treatment and call his doctor if he experiences dizziness.
● Suggest that the patient avoid using IPPB immediately before or after a meal because of possible nausea and reduced lung expansion.

Continuous Positive Airway Pressure

As its name suggests, continuous positive airway pressure (CPAP) ventilation provides positive pressure in the airways throughout the entire respiratory cycle. First developed to combat respiratory distress in intubated neonates and later used in adults, this treatment was originally delivered with a ventilator. Today CPAP may be used for an intubated or unintubated patient. It may be delivered through an artificial airway, a mask, or nasal prongs by means of a ventilator or a separate high-flow generating system.

CPAP is available as both a demand system and a continuous-flow system.

In the demand system, a valve opens in response to the patient's inspiratory flow. In the continuous-flow system, an air-oxygen blend flows through a humidifier and a reservoir bag into a T-piece. This system requires less work on the part of the patient than the demand system: during inspiration a distended reservoir bag maintains positive pressure.

Besides treating respiratory distress syndrome, CPAP has been used successfully for pulmonary edema, pulmonary emboli, bronchiolitis, fat emboli, pneumonitis, viral pneumonia, and postoperative atelectasis. In mild to moderate cases of these disorders, CPAP provides an alternative to intubation and mechanical ventilation. It increases the functional residual capacity by distending collapsed alveoli. This improves PaO_2 and decreases intrapulmonary shunting and oxygen consumption. It also reduces the work of breathing.

CPAP can also be used to help wean a patient from mechanical ventilation (see "Mechanical Ventilation" in this chapter). Nasal CPAP has proved successful for long-term treatment of obstructive sleep apnea. In this type of CPAP, high-flow compressed air is directed into a mask that covers only the patient's nose. The pressure supplied through the mask serves as a back-pressure splint, preventing the unstable upper airway from collapsing during inspiration.

CPAP may cause gastric distress if the patient swallows air during the treatment (most common when CPAP is delivered without intubation). Because mask CPAP can also cause nausea and vomiting, it shouldn't be used in patients who are unresponsive or at risk for vomiting and aspiration. Rarely, CPAP causes barotrauma or lowers cardiac output.

Purpose
● To improve oxygenation in acute respiratory disorders
● To prevent closure of upper airway

passages in obstructive sleep apnea
● To prevent airway and alveolar collapse in neonates with respiratory distress syndrome
● To assist with weaning from mechanical ventilation.

Preparation
Explain the treatment to the patient or his parents. If the patient is intubated, attach the CPAP device to his tracheostomy or endotracheal tube. Assess his vital signs and lung sounds to provide a baseline.

If CPAP will be delivered through a mask, a respiratory therapist usually sets up the system. After setup, place the mask on the patient. (The mask should be transparent and light-weight and should have a soft, pliable seal. A tight seal isn't required as long as pressure can be maintained.) Obtain arterial blood gas (ABG) determinations and pulmonary function studies, as ordered, to serve as a baseline.

If the patient will be receiving nasal CPAP for sleep apnea, assess for nasal congestion. If needed, have him use a nasal decongestant spray before you start CPAP.

Procedure
For the intubated adult, set the ventilator to CPAP and adjust the setting to the desired cmH_2O; usually the flow required to maintain constant pressure is three to four times the patient's minute ventilation. Attach the T-piece on the CPAP device to the patient's tracheostomy or endotracheal tube.

For mask CPAP, adjust the cmH_2O settings to exceed the patient's maximal inspiratory flow rate.

For nasal mask CPAP, to prevent sleep apnea in an adult, adjust cmH_2O settings, as ordered. Typically, you'll start at 5 cmH_2O and gradually increase pressure until apnea subsides (usually at 10 to 12 cmH_2O). If the patient's routinely hypoxemic when awake, determine his optimal CPAP level without oxygen, and then bleed oxygen into the CPAP circuit with suf-

C.P.A.P. FOR NEONATES

CPAP prevents the collapse of airways and alveoli and elevates PaO_2 levels in neonates with respiratory distress syndrome. It can be delivered through nasal prongs (as shown here) or an endotracheal tube.

To prepare for this treatment, position the neonate on his back with a rolled towel under his neck. This position will help maintain airway patency but avoid hyperextending the neck.

During CPAP, monitor the neonate's arterial blood gas levels, as ordered. Auscultate the lungs for crackles, rhonchi, and bilateral breath sounds.

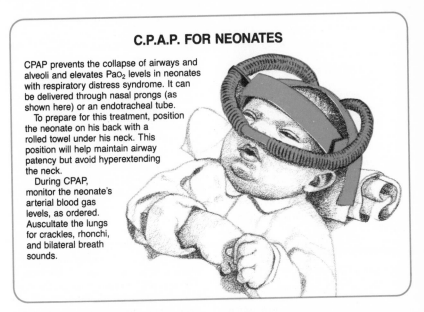

ficient flow to maintain at least 90% oxygen saturation. Adjust the cmH_2O settings based on ABG levels.

Monitoring and aftercare

If the patient is undergoing CPAP for an acute condition, monitor his heart rate, blood pressure, pulmonary capillary wedge pressure, and urine output hourly. Continue to monitor him until he's stable at a CPAP setting necessary to maintain a PaO_2 level greater than 60 with an FIO_2 (fraction of inspired oxygen) of 50% or less. Check for decreased cardiac output, which may result from increased intrathoracic pressure. Watch closely for changes in respiratory rate and pattern. Uncoordinated breathing patterns may indicate severe respiratory muscle fatigue that can't be helped by CPAP. Report this to the doctor; the patient may need mechanical ventilation.

Check the CPAP system for pressure fluctuations. Keep in mind that high airway pressures increase the risk of pneumothorax, so monitor for chest pain and decreased breath sounds. Use oximetry, if possible, to monitor oxygen saturations, especially when you re-

move the CPAP mask to provide routine care. If the patient's stable, remove his mask briefly every 2 to 4 hours to provide mouth and skin care and fluids. Increase the length of time the mask is off as the patient's ability to maintain oxygenation without CPAP improves.

Between treatments, apply benzoin to the skin under the edge of the mask to reduce the risk of breakdown and necrosis. Check closely for air leaks around the mask near the eyes (an area difficult to seal); escaping air can dry the eyes, causing conjunctivitis or other problems. Check air intake ports (present on some CPAP devices) to detect any obstructions.

If the patient is using a nasal CPAP device for sleep apnea, observe him for decreased snoring and mouth breathing while he sleeps, indicating that nasal CPAP is effective. If these symptoms don't subside, notify the doctor; either the system is leaking or the pressure is inadequate.

Home care instructions

CPAP for sleep apnea is the only treatment requiring instructions for home care.

- Ask the patient to demonstrate use of the system to make sure he can prevent excess leakage and maintain the prescribed pressures. Teach him how to clean the mask and change the air filter.
- Explain to the patient that he must use nasal CPAP every night even if he feels well after the initial treatments. Mention that apneic episodes will recur if he doesn't use CPAP as directed. However, he should call his doctor if his symptoms recur despite consistent use of CPAP.
- If the patient's obese, explain that he may be able to reduce the frequency of CPAP treatments if he loses weight.

Oxygen Therapy

Oxygen therapy, delivered by nasal prongs or catheter, mask, or transtracheal catheter, prevents or reverses hypoxemia and reduces the work of breathing. Hypoxemia can result from many causes, including emphysema, pneumonia, Guillain-Barré syndrome, congestive heart failure, and myocardial infarction.

The type of equipment used depends on the patient's condition and on the required concentration of oxygen (FIO_2, the fraction of inspired oxygen). High-flow systems, such as the Venturi mask, deliver a precisely controlled air-oxygen mixture. Low-flow systems, such as nasal prongs or catheter, simple mask, partial rebreather mask, and nonrebreather mask, allow variation in the oxygen percentage delivered, depending on the patient's respiratory pattern. Nasal prongs deliver oxygen at flows from 0.5 to 6 liters/minute. Inexpensive and easy to use, the prongs permit talking, eating, and suctioning without removal and interfere less than any other device with the patient's movement and other functions. However, they may cause nasal drying and can't deliver high oxygen concentrations. In contrast, a nasal catheter can deliver low-flow oxygen at somewhat higher concentrations, but it isn't commonly used because it causes discomfort and dries the mucous membranes. Masks can deliver oxygen concentrations of up to 100%. Transtracheal catheters permit highly efficient oxygen delivery and increased mobility with portable oxygen systems. They also avoid the side effects of nasal delivery systems.

Oxygen therapy, though routinely given, can cause severe complications. For example, high oxygen flows over 24 or more hours can lead to oxygen toxicity, causing cellular damage, which may be permanent. High oxygen concentrations in the patient with chronic hypercapnia can eliminate the patient's stimulus to breathe, thereby increasing carbon dioxide retention, which results in acute respiratory failure.

Purpose
To prevent or treat hypoxemia, thereby decreasing myocardial work load and respiratory effort.

Preparation
Explain the treatment to the patient and gather the necessary equipment. Instruct the patient, his roommate(s), and any visitors not to smoke or use an improperly grounded radio, television, electric razor, or other equipment. Place an "oxygen precautions" sign on the outside of the patient's door.

Perform a cardiopulmonary assessment, and check that baseline arterial blood gas (ABG) values or oximetry values have been obtained. Check the patency of the patient's nostrils (he may need a mask if they're blocked). Consult the doctor if a change in administration route is necessary.

Assemble the equipment, check all the connections, and turn on the oxygen source. Make sure that the humidifier is bubbling and that oxygen is flowing through the prongs, catheter, or mask. Set the flow rate, as ordered. If necessary, have the respiratory therapist check the flowmeter for accuracy.

Procedure

If you're inserting a *nasal cannula*, direct the curved prongs inward, following the nostrils' natural curvature. Hook the tubing behind the patient's ears and under his chin. Set the flow rate, as ordered.

If you're inserting a *nasal catheter*, determine the length to insert by stretching one end of the catheter from the tip of the patient's nose to his earlobe. Mark this spot. Then lubricate the catheter with sterile water or water-soluble lubricant, and gently insert the catheter through the nostril into the nasopharynx to the premeasured length. Use a flashlight and a tongue blade to check that the catheter is positioned correctly: it should be directly behind the uvula but not beyond it (misdirected airflow may cause gastric distention). If the catheter causes the patient to gag or choke, withdraw it slightly. Secure the catheter by taping it at the nose and cheek, and set the flow rate, as ordered.

If you're using a *mask*, make sure the flow rate is at least 5 liters/minute. Lower flow rates won't flush carbon dioxide from any mask but the Venturi model. Now place the mask over the patient's nose, mouth, and chin and press the flexible metal edge so that it fits the bridge of the patient's nose. Use gauze padding, as necessary, to ensure comfort and a proper fit.

The *partial rebreather mask* has an attached reservoir bag that conserves the first portion of the patient's exhalation and also fills with 100% oxygen before the next breath, delivering oxygen concentrations ranging from 40% at a flow rate of 8 liters/minute to 60% at a flow rate of 15 liters/minute, depending on the patient's breathing pattern and rate. The *nonrebreather mask* also has a reservoir bag and can deliver oxygen concentrations ranging from 60% at a flow rate of 8 liters/minute to 90% at a flow rate of 15 liters/minute. Set flow rates for these masks, as ordered, but keep in mind that the reservoir bag should deflate only slightly during inspiration. If it deflates completely or markedly, increase the flow rate as necessary.

The *Venturi mask*, another alternative, delivers the most precise oxygen concentrations: to within 1% of the setting. If you use this mask, make sure its air entrainment ports don't become blocked. Otherwise, the patient's FIO_2 level could rise dangerously.

If a *transtracheal oxygen catheter* will be used to deliver oxygen, the doctor will insert this device into the patient's trachea under local anesthesia.

Monitoring and aftercare

Periodically perform a cardiopulmonary assessment on the patient receiving any form of oxygen therapy. If the patient is on bed rest, change his position frequently to ensure adequate ventilation and circulation. Provide good skin care to prevent irritation and breakdown caused by the tubing, prongs, or mask. Make sure that any oxygen flow exceeding 3 liters/minute is humidified to help prevent drying of mucous membranes.

Assess for signs of hypoxia, including decreased level of consciousness, tachycardia, arrhythmias, diaphoresis, restlessness, altered blood pressure or respiratory rate, clammy skin, and cyanosis. Notify the doctor if any of these occur, and check the oxygen delivery equipment to see if it's malfunctioning. Be especially alert for changes in respiratory status when you change or discontinue oxygen therapy.

If your patient is using a nonrebreather mask, periodically check the valves to see if they are functioning properly. If the valves stick closed, the patient will reinhale carbon dioxide and not get adequate oxygen. Replace the mask, if necessary.

If the patient is receiving high oxygen concentrations (exceeding 50%) for more than 24 hours, ask about symptoms of oxygen toxicity, such as burning, substernal chest pain, dyspnea, and dry cough. Atelectasis and pulmonary edema may also occur. (Encourage coughing and deep breathing to help prevent atelectasis.) Monitor ABGs frequently and reduce oxygen concentrations as soon as ABG results indicate that this is feasible.

If your patient has chronic pulmonary disease, use a low flow rate. However, *don't* use a simple face mask because low flows will not flush carbon dioxide from the mask, resulting in rebreathing of carbon dioxide. Watch for alterations in level of consciousness, heart rate, and respiratory rate, which may signal carbon dioxide narcosis or worsening hypoxemia.

Home care instructions
• If the patient needs oxygen at home, the doctor will order the flow rate of oxygen, the hours per day to be used, and the conditions of use if less than 24 hours. Several types of delivery systems are available, including a tank, a concentrator, and a liquid oxygen system. The choice of system will depend on the patient's needs and on the availability and cost of each system. Make sure the patient can use the prescribed system safely and effectively.
• Tell the patient he'll need regular follow-up care to evaluate his response to therapy.

Humidification and Aerosol Treatments

Humidification refers to the addition of water vapor to inspired gas to prevent loss of airway moisture during inspiration of dry gases. Aerosols, which can be used to deliver medication, refer to fine particles of liquid suspended in a gas.

Humidity may be added directly to the air by a room humidifier or it may be given with oxygen, using an in-line device such as a cold bubble diffuser or cascade humidifier. Some humidification device can be used with every

oxygen delivery device, except for the Venturi mask. (If the patient with a Venturi mask needs humidification, entrained room air, rather than the oxygen, is humidified.)

A large-volume nebulizer supplies cool or heated moisture to the patient whose upper airway has been bypassed by endotracheal intubation or a tracheostomy, or who has recently been extubated. The ultrasonic nebulizer provides intermittent therapy for the patient with thick secretions, helping to mobilize them and promote a productive cough. The small-volume nebulizer is typically used to deliver aerosolized medications, such as bronchodilators, mucolytics, and antibiotics (see *Comparing Humidifiers and Nebulizers*, pages 130 and 131).

Aerosols should be used cautiously in patients susceptible to fluid accumulation and atelectasis, especially those with congestive heart failure, respiratory distress, or a depressed cough reflex. Aerosols should also be given cautiously to asthmatic patients, since they can precipitate bronchospasm.

Purpose
• To reduce moisture loss during oxygen therapy
• To loosen secretions
• To deliver aerosolized medications.

Preparation
Explain the procedure to the patient. Check the doctor's order and make sure the correct equipment has been delivered and set up. (Usually, a respiratory therapist sets up the equipment).

Take the patient's vital signs and assess breath sounds and secretion characteristics to serve as a baseline.

Procedure
For a *room humidifier*, direct the nozzle away from the patient's face and look for visible mist at the nozzle's mouth. Close all doors and windows to maintain humidity in the room. For a *cold bubble humidifier*, set the oxygen flowmeter at the prescribed rate and

check the humidifier for positive pressure release. If this doesn't occur, tighten the connections and check again. Then apply the oxygen delivery device to the patient. The water in the humidifier should bubble as oxygen passes through it. For a *cascade humidifier*, adjust the temperature to 32° to 37° C., as ordered, and arrange the tubing so that condensation flows away from the patient. Check the thermometer, which gives an average reading for inspired air. If the water becomes too hot, lower the temperature, discard all the water in the unit, and replace the water. Have the unit checked if its performance is questionable.

If you're using a *large-volume nebulizer*, attach the nebulizer to the flowmeter and set the flowmeter to at least 10 to 14 liters so the total flow from the nebulizer will be adequate to meet the patient's inspiratory flow needs. If you're administering oxygen, check the percentage delivered. Attach the delivery device to the patient. If you're using an *ultrasonic nebulizer*, turn on the machine and check for misting at the outflow port. Have the patient breathe slowly and deeply to maximize aerosol distribution into his lower tracheobronchial tree.

To deliver medication with the nebulizer, place the patient in a sitting or high-Fowler's position to promote lung expansion and aerosol dispersion. Place any medication in the cup, check that mist is coming from the device, and have the patient take slow, deep, and even breaths. Tell him to hold his breath for up to 10 seconds at the end of inspiration to maximize deposition of medication in the airways. Use the same procedure for a *mininebulizer*; show the patient how to grasp the device and tell him to hold his breath for 2 to 3 seconds with full inspiration.

Monitoring and aftercare

After an aerosol treatment, encourage the patient to cough and deep-breathe to mobilize secretions. Suction him, if necessary. Evaluate the effectiveness of

therapy by comparing current breath sounds with pretreatment findings. Also document the amount, color, and consistency of his sputum. If no improvement occurs or the patient's condition worsens, notify the doctor.

Check the water level in the device frequently and refill or replace it, as needed. Change and clean the equipment regularly, according to your institution's policy. If the patient tires and needs a short rest, stop the treatment and turn off the equipment briefly.

If you're using a cascade humidifier, monitor the temperature closely, and replace the water if it becomes too hot. Make sure the tubing is placed to prevent condensation from flowing toward the patient, where it may be aspirated. When water collects in the tubing, disconnect it from the nebulizer and drain it into a waste container.

If you're using a heated large-volume nebulizer, frequently monitor the temperature, using an in-line thermometer. Tell the patient to report any discomfort, and turn off the heater when the equipment is turned off. Check the patient for signs of overhydration, such as sudden weight gain, crackles, or electrolyte imbalance.

If the patient is receiving ultrasonic nebulizer treatment, watch him for bronchospasm and dyspnea. Stay with him for the duration of treatment (usually 15 to 20 minutes). Be prepared to discontinue treatment promptly.

If you're administering medication by side-stream nebulizer or mininebulizer, take the patient's vital signs before treatment begins and then monitor for drug reactions.

Home care instructions

● Tell the patient using a room humidifier at home that he can fill it with plain tap water or distilled water. Also tell him to run a dilute solution of chlorine bleach and water through the unit every week to prevent the rapid accumulation of mold and bacteria. Instruct him to do this in a well-ventilated room and to rinse the unit well afterward.

COMPARING HUMIDIFIERS AND NEBULIZERS

TYPE	ADVANTAGES	DISADVANTAGES
Humidifiers		
Cold bubble diffuser humidifier	• May be used with all oxygen delivery devices, except Venturi mask	• Delivers 20% to 40% humidity. • Can't be used with endotracheal or tracheostomy tube.
Cascade humidifier	• Delivers 100% humidity at body temperature • Functions as a mainstream humidifier with a ventilator • Most effective of all evaporative humidifiers	• Temperature control can become defective from constant use. • If correct water level isn't maintained, patient's mucosa can become irritated from hot, dry air.
Room humidifier	• Easy to use	• Humidity level difficult to control. • Moisture may damage walls and floors. • High risk of inhaling microorganisms.
Nebulizers		
Large-volume nebulizer (cool or heated)	• Provides both oxygen and aerosol therapy • Provides 100% humidity relative to the temperature of the unit • Useful for long-term therapy	• High risk of bacterial contamination. • If correct water level in reservoir isn't maintained, mucosal irritation can result from hot, dry air. • Infants are at risk for becoming overhydrated.
Mininebulizer	• Compact and disposable; may be used at home • Can be used with any compressed gas system • Allows patient to maximize medication distribution if he inhales correctly	• Distributes medication unevenly if patient inhales inappropriately. • Infection may occur from poor cleaning technique. • Patient may overuse device.
Ultrasonic nebulizer	• Delivers 100% humidity; 90% of particles reach lower airways • Effectively loosens secretions	• May precipitate bronchospasm in asthmatic patient. • Lacks a built-in oxygen system. • May cause pulmonary edema or increased cardiac work load from overhydration.

• Tell the patient to report sudden weight gain, a change in his cough or sputum production, congestion, edema, or dyspnea.

NURSING CONSIDERATIONS

• Watch for irritation caused by drying of mucous membranes and crusting of secretions.
• Replace evaporated water.

• Check temperature every 2 hours; don't let it exceed 37° C. Unplug device if it overheats and attach another cascade to continue humidification.
• Check water level at least every 4 hours. When you add water, empty reservoir completely. Then refill to correct level and attach reservoir tightly.

• Be sure to thoroughly clean unit every 24 hours.
• Empty reservoir completely before refilling.
• Put mat under humidifier and keep device away from walls.
• Not recommended for hospital use.

• Frequently drain condensation and change equipment.
• Check water level and refill, as necessary.
• Watch for sudden weight gain and pulmonary edema, especially in infants.

• Frequently clean and change equipment.
• Teach correct technique and tell patient how often he should use nebulizer treatments.
• Monitor pulse rate before and after treatment. Withhold medication and notify the doctor if rate changes 10 beats/minute at rest.
• Do not power nebulizer with oxygen unless ordered.

• Stay with the patient during treatment.
• Supply another means of oxygen, if necessary.
• Check for signs of overhydration: sudden weight gain, pulmonary edema, crackles, and electrolyte imbalance.

Incentive Spirometry

Primarily used postoperatively to prevent respiratory complications, incentive spirometry measures respiratory flow or volume. A *flow-incentive* spirometer measures the patient's inspiratory effort, or flow rate, in cubic centimeters per second. A *volume-incentive* spirometer does this as well. However, it also calculates the volume of air the patient inhales.

Both types share the same goal: to encourage the patient to produce the deep, sustained inspiratory efforts that normally occur as yawns or sighs. As the patient steadily strives to meet his target flow or volume, he prevents or reverses atelectasis that occurs secondary to shallow respirations.

Purpose
• To prevent or correct atelectasis
• To improve clearance of secretions by increasing the respiratory volume available for coughing.

Preparation
If you plan to use incentive spirometry postoperatively, explain the procedure and familiarize the patient with the device before surgery, when he can practice. Adjust the target respiratory flow or volume, as ordered. Before the patient practices deep breathing, auscultate his lungs to obtain a baseline.

Procedure
Tell the patient his target flow or volume, and instruct him to exhale slowly and completely after each breath. Have him place the mouthpiece between his teeth and close to his lips. Then have

him take a slow, deep breath through his mouth (not through his nose) until he reaches the preset goal. Tell him to remove the mouthpiece, hold his breath for 3 to 5 seconds, and exhale slowly. Have him repeat this procedure 10 times each hour or as ordered, and encourage him to cough after treatment or when he feels the need to clear secretions during treatment.

Monitoring and aftercare
Preoperatively, your patient may understand the need to perform incentive spirometry. But after surgery, when he's weak, sedated, or in pain, you'll need to encourage him. He should show progressive improvement in volume: a daily increase of 20% if he doesn't have underlying lung disease. Document the volume and repetitions he achieves and auscultate his lungs after each treatment. If he doesn't show the expected improvement, notify the doctor and check the patient's temperature, lung sounds, and sputum production. He may be developing a pulmonary infection.

When your patient has met his goal and held it for 2 to 3 days, expect to discontinue incentive spirometry. However, continue to encourage deep breathing, coughing, and ambulation.

Home care instructions
Typically, incentive spirometry doesn't require instructions for home care.

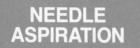

NEEDLE ASPIRATION

Thoracentesis

Thoracentesis refers to the needle aspiration of fluid or air from the pleural space. Although used primarily to determine the cause of pleural fluid ac-

cumulation, this procedure helps treat both transudative and exudative pleural effusions by removing excessive fluid. It improves pulmonary function, relieving such symptoms as dyspnea and tachycardia. However, unless the underlying cause of the fluid accumulation is identified and corrected, pleural effusion will usually recur.

Thoracentesis can cause severe complications. These include pneumothorax, tension pneumothorax, fluid reaccumulation, mediastinal shift, and hypovolemic shock. Thoracentesis should never be performed on a patient with a bleeding disorder.

Purpose
● To help determine the cause of pleural effusion
● To relieve pulmonary compression and respiratory distress
● To instill medication into the pleural space

Preparation
Explain the procedure to the patient. Inform him that he may feel a stinging sensation during injection of the local anesthetic and some pressure during needle insertion and fluid withdrawal. Stress the importance of remaining still during the procedure to reduce the risk of lung injury. Inform him that he'll have a chest X-ray or an ultrasound test to locate the fluid. Assess the patient's respiratory function and take his vital signs as a baseline. If ordered, administer a sedative.

Arrange to have a prepackaged sterile thoracentesis tray at bedside, and a chest tube setup and an oxygen source available. Also have laboratory request slips on hand in case the doctor wants specimens sent to the laboratory for analysis.

Procedure
Position the patient, as ordered. Usually the patient sits on the edge of his bed, with his folded arms resting on an overbed table. Or, if he's unable to sit up, turn him on his side and raise

his arms over his head. Support his arms and head with pillows to make him more comfortable, and expose the affected area. Remind the patient not to move suddenly, cough, or breathe deeply during the procedure.

Open the thoracentesis tray. The doctor disinfects the site and injects the local anesthetic. Then he attaches a three-way stopcock with tubing to the aspiration needle and turns the stopcock to prevent air from entering the pleural space through the needle. Attach the other end of the tubing to the drainage bottle, if instructed.

The doctor inserts the thoracentesis needle into the pleural space and attaches a 50-ml syringe to the stopcock. (He may use a hemostat to hold the needle in place, to prevent pleural tear or lung puncture.) Or he may introduce a Teflon catheter into the needle, remove the needle, and attach a stopcock and syringe or drainage tubing to the catheter. This reduces the risk of pleural puncture by the needle.

Assist the doctor with fluid drainage, specimen collection, or medication administration, as ordered. After the needle is withdrawn, apply a small adhesive bandage to the puncture site. If a specimen was collected, note its color, amount, and character. Arrange for a chest X-ray to check for pneumothorax.

Monitoring and aftercare

During the procedure, take the patient's vital signs frequently. Be alert for apprehension, cyanosis, sudden breathlessness, and tachycardia, which signal pneumothorax. Mediastinal shift may cause the patient to experience labored breathing, arrhythmias, and sudden hypotension.

After the procedure, check his vital signs every 30 minutes for 2 hours and then as ordered. Tell him to call you immediately if he has any difficulty breathing. Watch for a persistent, irritable cough, hemoptysis, and signs of respiratory distress, which may signal pneumothorax or rapid fluid reaccu-

mulation. Check the puncture site for excessive leakage. Finally, be alert for signs of hypovolemic shock if a large amount of fluid was withdrawn. Notify the doctor immediately if these signs occur.

Home care instructions

● Tell the patient to call his doctor if a fever develops. Contamination during thoracentesis can cause infection.
● Instruct the patient to notify his doctor if symptoms recur.

PHYSIOTHERAPY AND BRONCHOSCOPY

Chest Physiotherapy

Chest physiotherapy includes postural drainage, chest percussion and vibration, and coughing and deep-breathing exercises. *Postural drainage* uses gravity to promote drainage of secretions from the lungs and bronchi into the trachea. *Percussion*, which involves cupping the hands and fingers together and clapping them alternately over lung fields, loosens secretions, as does the gentler technique of *vibration*. *Coughing* helps clear the lungs, bronchi, and trachea of secretions and prevents aspiration. And *deep-breathing exercises* help loosen secretions and promote more effective coughing. Especially important for the bedridden patient, these treatments improve secretion clearance and ventilation and help prevent or treat atelectasis and pneumonia, which can hinder recovery.

Indications for chest physiotherapy include the presence of secretions (from such conditions as bronchitis, cystic fibrosis, or pneumonia); chronic obstructive pulmonary disease; diseases that have increased the risk of aspiration (muscular dystrophy, cerebral palsy); postoperative incisional pain that restricts breathing; and prolonged immobility. Often chest physiotherapy is performed with other treatments, such as suctioning, incentive spirometry, and administration of medications, such as expectorants. Improved breath sounds, PaO_2, increased sputum production, and air flow suggest successful treatment.

Contraindications include active or recent pulmonary hemorrhage, untreated pneumothorax, lung contusion, recent myocardial infarction, pulmonary tuberculosis, pulmonary tumor or abscess, osteoporosis, fractured ribs, or an unstable chest wall. It should be performed cautiously in patients with head injuries or with recent eye or cranial surgery because it increases intracranial pressure.

Purpose

To mobilize secretions (especially from peripheral lung areas) and increase clearance of tracheobronchial mucus, promoting maximum ventilation.

Preparation

Explain the procedure to the patient. As ordered, administer pain medication and teach the patient to splint his incision. Auscultate the lungs to determine baseline status, and check the doctor's order to determine which lung areas require treatment.

Obtain pillows and a tilt board, if necessary. Do *not* schedule therapy immediately after a meal; performing chest physiotherapy after a meal increases the risk of nausea and vomiting. Make sure the patient is adequately hydrated before you begin because this liquefies secretions and helps facilitate their removal. If ordered, first administer bronchodilator and mist therapy.

Provide tissues, an emesis basin, and a cup for sputum. If the patient doesn't have an adequate cough to clear secretions, set up suction equipment. If he needs oxygen therapy or is borderline hypoxemic without it, use adequate flows of oxygen during therapy.

Procedure

For *postural drainage*, position the patient as ordered. (The doctor usually determines a position sequence after auscultation and chest X-ray review.) If the patient has a localized condition, such as pneumonia in a specific lobe, expect to start with that area first, to avoid infecting uninvolved areas. If the patient has a diffuse disorder, such as bronchiectasis, expect to start with the lower lobes and work toward the upper ones. Move through the positions in a way that minimizes the patient's repositioning efforts. Tell him to remain in each position for 10 to 15 minutes. During this time, perform percussion and vibration, as ordered.

For *percussion*, place your cupped hands against the patient's chest wall and rapidly flex and extend your wrists, generating a rhythmic, popping sound (a hollow sound helps verify correct performance of the technique). Percuss each segment for a minimum of 3 to 5 minutes. The vibrations you generate pass through the chest wall and help loosen secretions from the airways. Perform percussion throughout both inspiration and expiration, and encourage the patient to take slow deep breaths. *Do not* percuss over the spine, sternum, liver, kidneys, or the female patient's breasts, since you may cause trauma, especially in elderly patients.

For *vibration*, hold your hand flat against the patient's chest wall and, during exhalation, vibrate your hands rapidly by tensing your arm and shoulder muscles. This rapid oscillation aids secretion movement by increasing the velocity and turbulence of exhaled air. Repeat vibration for five exhalations over each chest segment. When the patient says "ah" on exhalation, you should hear a quaver in his voice.

After you complete postural drainage, percussion, or vibration, instruct the patient in *coughing* to remove loosened secretions. Have him take slow deep breaths, and place your hands on his chest wall to help him direct air to the lower and peripheral areas of his

MECHANICAL PERCUSSION AND VIBRATION

Although a mechanical percussion and vibration device may be used in the hospital, this device can also be used by a patient at home to self-administer chest percussion and vibration. Medicare-approved, the device uses directional stroking percussers, which loosen secretions and help move them in the desired direction. A separate pad can be attached to provide chest vibration, and small attachments are available for use with infants.

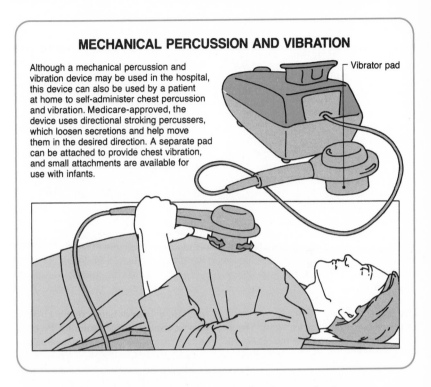

lungs. Tell him to push his abdomen out on inspiration, which will give his diaphragm more room to move downward. Tell him to inhale deeply through his mouth or nose and then exhale in three short huffs or coughs through a slightly open mouth. An effective cough sounds deep and almost hollow; an ineffective cough, shallow and high-pitched. Have the patient repeat the coughing sequence at least two or three times.

For *deep breathing*, place the patient in a sitting position with his feet well supported. Have him inhale slowly and deeply, pushing his abdomen out against his hand to maximize air distribution. Tell him to exhale through pursed lips and to contract his abdomen. Initially, have him do this exercise for 1 minute and then rest for 2 minutes. Gradually increase this to 10 minutes four times each day.

After chest physiotherapy, auscultate the patient's lungs.

Monitoring and aftercare

Evaluate the patient's tolerance for therapy and make adjustments as needed. Watch for fatigue because the patient's ability to cough and breathe deeply diminishes as he tires.

Assess for any difficulty in expectorating secretions, and use suction if the patient has an ineffective cough or a diminished gag reflex. Provide oral hygiene after therapy because secretions may taste foul or have an unpleasant odor.

Home care instructions

The patient with bronchiectasis or cystic fibrosis may need chest physiotherapy at home. Teach him and his family the appropriate techniques and positions, and stress the importance of performing this therapy as ordered. If appropriate, arrange for the patient to obtain a mechanical percussion and vibration device (see *Mechanical Percussion and Vibration*).

Bronchoscopic Removal of Mucus or a Foreign Body

A foreign body or mucus lodged in the tracheobronchial tree can be removed with a rigid metal or a flexible fiberoptic bronchoscope. The rigid bronchoscope allows more room for foreign body removal, but it's normally reserved for use in the operating room. The flexible fiberoptic bronchoscope, a slender tube containing fine glass fibers that transmit light, effectively removes mucous plugs and secretions. This device can be used at bedside, in a minor procedures room, in a radiology suite, or in an operating room.

Bronchoscopic removal of a foreign body or mucus can also be performed for a patient who has an endotracheal or tracheostomy tube in place and is on a ventilator.

Possible complications of bronchoscopy include hypoxemia, hemorrhage (most likely to occur when biopsy is done concurrently), respiratory distress, pneumothorax, bronchospasm, and infection.

Purpose
To visualize and remove a foreign body or mucus from the tracheobronchial tree.

Preparation
Typically, bronchoscopy will be performed using a flexible fiberoptic scope and a local anesthetic. Describe this treatment to the patient and explain that it allows removal of excessive mucus or a foreign body from his airways. Assess his condition and obtain baseline vital signs. If possible, have him fast for 6 to 12 hours before treatment. Tell him who will perform the treatment and where, and that the room will be darkened.

Advise the patient that he may receive a sedative to help him relax. Inform him that a local anesthetic will be sprayed into his nose and mouth to suppress the gag reflex. Warn him that the spray has an unpleasant taste and that he may have a sensation of pharyngeal fullness during treatment. Reassure him that he'll be able to breathe but won't be able to speak.

Make sure the patient or a responsible family member has signed a consent form. Check the patient's history for hypersensitivity to the anesthetic.

Place the patient in a sitting position on an examination table or a bed. If he wears dentures, have him remove them. Tell him to remain relaxed, to hyperextend his neck, to place his arms at his side, and to breathe through his nose. As ordered, give medications such as atropine to decrease secretions and an I.V. barbiturate or narcotic to provide sedation or amnesia and allay anxiety.

Assemble equipment, including intubation equipment and a high-flow oxygen source in case of emergency. Typical equipment consists of a flexible fiberoptic bronchoscope, 2% to 4% lidocaine, sterile gloves, an emesis basin, an Ambu bag with face mask, oral and endotracheal airways, a laryngoscope, suction equipment, and masks and eye protectors for the staff. If the patient requires controlled mechanical ventilation, obtain a bronchoscopy adapter.

Procedure
The doctor sprays a local anesthetic on the patient's throat and nasal cavity, if this approach will be used. Encourage the patient to inspire this anesthetic, and provide tissues and an emesis basin, since excess fluid will cause coughing and gagging. Darken the room to allow easier viewing through the bronchoscope.

While the initial anesthetic takes effect, the doctor lubricates the bronchoscope and introduces it into the upper airway. Once he visualizes the vocal cords, he instills 3 to 4 ml of 2% to 4%

lidocaine to suppress the gag reflex and anesthetize the vocal cords. Remind the patient not to speak from this point on, since the bronchoscope will irritate his vocal cords. Tell him to breathe slowly and to try not to cough. Reassure him and, if necessary, hold his hand to help him relax. Keep oral suction equipment ready.

The doctor advances the broncho-scope through the larynx and into the trachea and bronchi, where he removes mucus, secretions, or a foreign body, as needed; he may also withdraw a specimen for laboratory analysis. If bleeding occurs, he may instill an epi-nephrine solution through the bron-choscope to control it. Place specimens in properly labeled containers and send them to the laboratory immediately.

The doctor withdraws the broncho-scope after removal of the foreign body or mucus.

Monitoring and aftercare

Check the patient's vital signs during the procedure and every 15 minutes afterward until they're stable. Place him in semi-Fowler's position. Keep re-suscitation equipment and a trache-ostomy tray available for 24 hours.

Watch for and immediately report symptoms of respiratory difficulty, such as stridor and dyspnea resulting from laryngeal edema or laryngospasm. Ob-serve for bleeding and listen for wheez-ing, a sign of bronchospasm. Monitor for dyspnea and diminished breath sounds on one side, which may indicate pneumothorax. Report any abnormal findings to the doctor, and prepare for a chest X-ray, if ordered, to confirm pneumothorax.

Provide an emesis basin and instruct the patient to spit out saliva rather than swallow it. Expect to find blood-tinged sputum for up to several hours. How-ever, report prolonged bleeding or per-sisent hemoptysis to the doctor.

Encourage the patient to rest quietly. Restrict all oral intake until after his gag reflex returns. If he experiences hoarseness and a sore throat, provide medicated lozenges when allowed and encourage him not to talk, to rest his vocal cords.

Home care instructions

• If the procedure was performed on an outpatient basis or in the emergency room, tell the patient that he should report any shortness of breath, pain, or prolonged bleeding.
• Advise the patient not to strain his voice, but reassure him that his sore throat and hoarseness are temporary.
• Tell him to report signs of infection, such as fever or thick, yellow sputum.

Selected References

Bayless, et al. *Current Therapy in Internal Medicine, 1984-1985*. St. Louis: C.V. Mosby Co., 1984.

Branson, R., et al. "Mask CPAP: State of the Art," *Respiratory Care* 30(10):846-57, October 1985.

Burton, G., and Hodgkin, J., eds. *Respiratory Care: A Guide to Clinical Practice*, 2nd ed. Philadelphia: J.B. Lippincott Co., 1984.

Donohue, W.J., et al. "Long Term Mechanical Ventilation: Guidelines for Management in the Home and at Alternate Community Sites," *Chest* 90(1), July 1986.

Farzan, S., et al. *A Concise Handbook of Respiratory Diseases*, 2nd ed. East Norwalk, Conn.: Appleton & Lange, 1985.

O'Donohoe, W., ed. *Current Advances in Respiratory Care*. Park Ridge, Ill.: American College of Chest Physicians, 1984.

Stauffer, J., and Silvestri, R. "Complications of Endotracheal Intubation, Tracheostomy and Artificial Airways," *Respiratory Care* 27(4):417-34, April 1982.

Traver, G., ed. *Respiratory Nursing: The Science and Art*. New York: John Wiley & Sons, 1982.

4

Treating Gastrointestinal Dysfunction

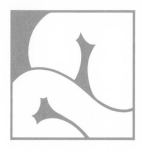

Treating Gastrointestinal Dysfunction

Introduction

Whether used for acute or chronic illnesses, GI treatments will challenge your ability to provide effective patient care before, during, and after them. Before appendectomy, for instance, you'll need to perform an ongoing GI assessment to detect signs of possible rupture. During esophagogastric tamponade, you'll need to carefully monitor the patient for continued variceal bleeding. After surgical insertion of a portal-systemic shunt, you'll need to be on guard for life-threatening pulmonary complications.

Other GI treatments don't entail emergency assessments and interventions. Instead, they require enormous patience and sensitivity to the patient's feelings. Consider the colostomy patient. Not only will you have to teach him about stoma care but you'll also have to help him come to grips with changes in his body image and personal relationships. You'll have to help him deal with pressing personal problems, such as "How will my wife respond to me?" "Will I still have friends?" "How will I be able to hold down my job?"

Now consider a different patient, say, one who requires a bowel training program. Besides extending for weeks or even months, this program can be fraught with disappointment, frustration, and embarrassment for the pa-

tient. To help him overcome these feelings, you'll need to muster your own emotional reserves.

In many other GI treatments, you'll find similarly pressing problems and equally important nursing responsibilities.

Anxiety over treatment and its aftermath

Frequently, GI treatments produce considerable anxiety about their outcome. Consider, for instance, liver transplant. Used as a treatment of last resort for terminally ill patients, this surgery has slim odds of success despite major advances in operative techniques and immunosuppressive therapy. And, if the patient survives the ordeal of surgery, his initial elation may soon subside as complications set in.

You are what you eat

For patients whose self-image rests on their ability to eat or drink whatever they want, dietary restrictions can present a major barrier to compliance with GI treatments. Spicy dishes, for example, may need to be curtailed or even eliminated. Low-fiber foods may need to be replaced by high-fiber ones. To help the patient accept limitations like these, you'll need to clearly demonstrate the link between compliance and health.

DRUG THERAPY

Antacids

Widely used for relieving GI upset, antacids also represent an important adjunctive treatment for peptic ulcers and gastroesophageal reflux. Antacids can be divided into two classes: nonsystemic and systemic. Nonsystemic antacids consist of varying combinations of aluminum, calcium, and magnesium salts; the most commonly used ones include *calcium carbonate, magnesium hydrochloride,* and *aluminum hydroxide.* They work by removing hydrogen ions from the gastric contents. Systemic antacids, such as *sodium bicarbonate,* raise gastric pH by producing some degree of metabolic alkalosis.

Antacids come in powder, tablet, and liquid forms. After ingestion, antacids begin to act almost immediately and exert their effects for 1 to 3 hours, depending on whether they were taken with food or another medication. They're distributed throughout the GI tract and are eliminated primarily in feces.

Common side effects include constipation with calcium- or aluminum-containing antacids and diarrhea with magnesium-containing antacids. What's more, prolonged use of magnesium- or calcium-containing antacids can cause hypermagnesemia or hypercalcemia, whereas overuse of aluminum-containing antacids can cause hypophosphatemia by interfering with phosphorus absorption. All antacids, but most commonly the systemic ones, produce some degree of metabolic alkalosis when taken in large quantities. This effect, negligible in most patients, may lead to milk-alkali

syndrome in patients with acid-base imbalance.

Purpose and action

Antacids help relieve dyspepsia and pyrosis and heal peptic ulcers by neutralizing or removing acid from the gastric lumen to raise gastric pH and inhibit pepsin activity. They also strengthen the gastric mucosal barrier and help increase esophageal sphincter tone.

Monitoring

Assess the patient's bowel function by recording the amount and consistency of stool. Notify the doctor of any constipation or diarrhea; he may change the drug or reduce the dosage.

During long-term therapy with aluminum-containing antacids, regularly monitor the patient's serum phosphorus levels and be alert for signs of hypophosphatemia, such as anorexia, weakness, and malaise.

Monitor the patient taking calcium- or magnesium-containing antacids for signs of hypercalcemia or hypermagnesemia, as appropriate. Be especially aware of these imbalances in patients with impaired renal function.

If the patient's taking a calcium-containing antacid or sodium bicarbonate, check for early symptoms of milk-alkali syndrome: headache, confusion, and anorexia. Monitor blood urea nitrogen and serum calcium and creatinine for elevated levels.

Check the patient's drug regimen for possible interactions with antacids. Aluminum-containing antacids delay gastric emptying and slow the absorption of such drugs as indomethacin, coumadin, isoniazid, and barbiturates. Magnesium-containing antacids decrease the bioavailability of digoxin and tetracycline, and can potentiate the anticoagulant activity of coumadin. All antacids can cause the premature release of enteric-coated drugs in the GI tract; to prevent this, separate doses of antacids and enteric-coated drugs by at least 1 hour.

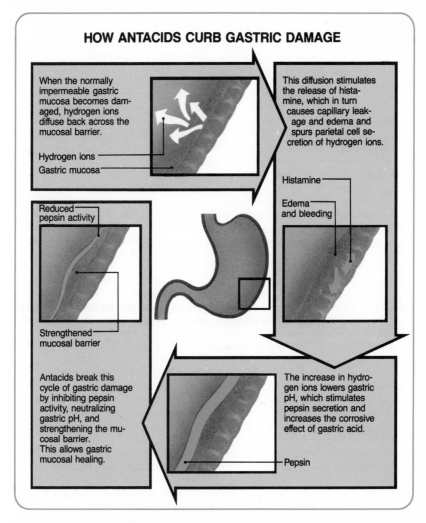

HOW ANTACIDS CURB GASTRIC DAMAGE

When the normally impermeable gastric mucosa becomes damaged, hydrogen ions diffuse back across the mucosal barrier.

Hydrogen ions
Gastric mucosa

This diffusion stimulates the release of histamine, which in turn causes capillary leakage and edema and spurs parietal cell secretion of hydrogen ions.

Histamine
Edema and bleeding

Reduced pepsin activity

Strengthened mucosal barrier

Antacids break this cycle of gastric damage by inhibiting pepsin activity, neutralizing gastric pH, and strengthening the mucosal barrier.
This allows gastric mucosal healing.

The increase in hydrogen ions lowers gastric pH, which stimulates pepsin secretion and increases the corrosive effect of gastric acid.

Pepsin

Home care instructions

• If the patient's taking a liquid antacid, instruct him to shake the suspension thoroughly before pouring. If he's taking antacid tablets, tell him to chew each tablet well before swallowing and to follow the dose with a full glass of water.

• Warn the patient not to take antacids indiscriminately and not to switch brands without his doctor's advice.

• Instruct the patient to keep a record of his bowel movements and to report any changes in his normal pattern.

• Advise him not to take antacids within 2 hours of taking any other medication.

Histamine-Receptor Antagonists

The treatment of choice for ulcer disorders, the histamine (H_2)-receptor antagonists include *cimetidine, ranitidine,* and *famotidine*. They're used for prophylactic and short-term treatment of duodenal and gastric ulcers. They're also used to treat disorders that produce peptic ulcers, such as Zollinger-Ellison syndrome, systemic mastocytosis, and multiple endocrine adenomas. In addition, cimetidine is commonly administered I.V. to prevent GI bleeding in critically ill patients.

The H_2-receptor antagonists, which are usually given orally, are much preferred over surgery. Typically, they help heal ulcers within 6 to 8 weeks. Because these drugs can be effective in a once-a-day dosage form, they provide a good alternative for patients who are noncompliant with prolonged antacid therapy.

Cimetidine, though usually well tolerated, can cause CNS effects, such as dizziness and confusion. These side effects occur most commonly and severely in the elderly and in patients with renal or hepatic dysfunction. Ranitidine and famotidine appear to cause fewer side effects than cimetidine.

Purpose and action
By inhibiting the action of histamine at parietal cell receptor sites, H_2-receptor antagonists reduce gastric secretion of hydrochloric acid. They also reduce the volume of gastric juices and secretion of pepsin and intrinsic factor.

Monitoring
If you're giving cimetidine I.V., rotate injection sites to reduce discomfort. During infusion, carefully monitor the patient's vital signs to prevent adverse cardiac effects. Continue to check vital signs for 2 hours after administration.

Regularly monitor hematologic studies, especially platelet count and prothrombin time, to detect neutropenia, agranulocytosis, or thrombocytopenia. Also watch for signs of hemorrhage: bloody or tarry stools, hematemesis, unusual bleeding or bruising, and signs of shock. Be especially alert for these signs in patients with bleeding ulcers.

Observe for other side effects of H_2-receptor antagonists, such as nausea and vomiting, muscle pain, skin rash, fever, diarrhea or constipation, gynecomastia, jaundice, confusion, and dizziness. If CNS effects occur, notify the doctor. He will probably reduce the dosage or, if severe effects persist, discontinue the drug.

Review the patient's medication regimen for possible interactions, especially if he's taking cimetidine. Cimetidine, for example, decreases the metabolism of theophylline and most benzodiazepines, possibly causing toxic effects. Because antacids interfere with absorption of H_2-receptor antagonists, separate doses of the two drugs by at least 1 hour.

If you're testing gastric juices for blood, keep in mind that the blue dye in cimetidine tablets may cause a false-positive finding. To avoid this spurious result, don't aspirate gastric juices within 15 minutes of administering the tablet.

Home care instructions
• Stress the need to complete the full course of therapy. If the patient has chronic peptic ulcers, explain that abrupt drug discontinuation can cause perforation.
• Instruct the patient to make up a missed dose as soon as he remembers. However, if it's almost time for his next dose, he should skip the missed dose and resume his regular schedule with the next dose. He shouldn't double-dose.
• Tell him to watch for and immediately report any signs of blood dyscrasias, such as easy bruising or bloody stools or bloody vomitus. Also have him report high fever or feelings of confusion, extreme fatigue, and weakness.
• If the patient experiences dizziness or other CNS effects, advise him to avoid driving or other activities that require coordination and alertness.
• If the patient's taking antacids, instruct him not to take them within 1 hour of taking an H_2-receptor antagonist.

• Encourage the patient to refrain from smoking since this interferes with drug action.

• Instruct him to avoid spicy foods, alcohol, hot drinks, caffeine-containing products, and aspirin to prevent GI irritation.

• If the patient's taking cimetidine, tell him to take the drug with or immediately after a meal. Explain that food delays absorption of the drug, thereby prolonging its effects. (Other H_2-receptor antagonists are only slightly affected by food.)

Anticholinergics
[Cholinergic blockers, parasympatholytics]

Typically used as an adjunct to histamine-receptor antagonists and antacids, the anticholinergics inhibit GI motility and prolong gastric emptying, thereby enhancing the effects of these drugs. They're primarily used to help relieve peptic ulcer pain. What's more, they can be used to treat irritable and spastic colon, other functional GI disorders, and neurogenic bowel disorders.

The anticholinergics used for GI dysfunction include the belladonna alkaloids, such as *atropine* and *belladonna elixir*; the quaternary anticholinergics, such as *anisotropine methylbromide, isopropamide iodide, methantheline bromide*, and *propantheline bromide*; and the spasmodics, such as *dicyclomine*. These drugs are usually given orally. However, if the patient requires rapid symptomatic relief, they can be given I.V.

Common side effects of anticholinergics include tachycardia, nausea, vomiting, and visual disturbances, such as blurred or double vision. Because the belladonna alkaloids and antispasmodics are rapidly absorbed and readily cross the blood-brain barrier,

they also cause CNS effects. In contrast, the quaternary anticholinergics don't readily cross the blood-brain barrier and so cause negligible CNS effects.

Anticholinergics are usually contraindicated in patients with narrow-angle glaucoma; tachyarrhythmias or any cardiovascular illness in which an increased heart rate could prove detrimental; any obstructive GI or urologic disorder; severe ulcerative colitis; disorders of GI motility, such as paralytic ileus, intestinal atony, and toxic megacolon; and myasthenia gravis. They shouldn't be used to treat gastric ulcers because the increased gastric emptying time can aggravate the ulcer. They should be used cautiously in infants, the elderly, and patients with autonomic neuropathy, hyperthyroidism, hiatal hernia associated with reflux esophagitis, or hepatic or renal dysfunction.

Purpose and action
Anticholinergics inhibit the effects of the neurotransmitter acetylcholine at the junction between postganglionic nerve endings and effector organs. Specifically, the belladonna alkaloids and quaternary anticholinergics block the action of acetylcholine on the vagus nerve (through a mechanism known as competitive inhibition), which reduces gastric acid secretion and intestinal motility. The antispasmodics directly relax GI smooth muscle.

Monitoring
When administering anticholinergics, check all dosages carefully; even a slight overdosage can lead to toxicity. Generally, you'll administer smaller doses to elderly patients and children, who are most prone to toxic effects.

Observe for drug side effects. Is the patient complaining of a headache? Does he seem dizzy, drowsy, or confused? Restless? Excitable? If you detect any of these CNS effects, notify the doctor; he may need to reduce the dosage. However, if you detect severe CNS effects, such as delirium or paralysis, immediately stop the drug and call the doctor. (Remember that severe CNS effects occur most commonly with belladonna alkaloids or antispasmodics.)

During anticholinergic therapy, carefully monitor the patient's vital signs. In particular, be alert for palpitations and tachycardia. Monitor intake and output and assess for signs of urinary retention, such as bladder enlargement. To help prevent retention, have the patient void before taking the drug.

Ask the patient about visual changes, such as blurred or double vision, mydriasis, and photophobia. If any of these develop, take steps to prevent accidents, such as assisting the patient with ambulation and removing furniture and other objects from his path.

Check the patient's medication regimen for possible interactions. Concurrent use of antacids or antidiarrheals, for example, can interfere with absorption of anticholinergics. These drugs shouldn't be given within 1 hour of an anticholinergic.

Home care instructions

• Instruct the patient to take the drug as prescribed. Generally, he can take it 30 minutes to 1 hour before meals or with meals.
• Tell the patient to immediately report severe side effects: eye pain, blurred vision, rash, significant CNS effects, extreme mucous membrane dryness, fever, and increased or irregular heart rate. Also discuss other possible side effects that, if persistent, warrant notifying the doctor. These include urinary difficulty, constipation, nausea, vomiting, headache, difficulty swallowing, or photophobia.
• Instruct the patient to avoid alcohol and other CNS depressants, which may potentiate side effects.
• Tell him to avoid overexertion in hot or humid weather. Explain that the drug decreases sweating, thereby causing his body temperature to rise and possibly leading to heatstroke. Teach him to watch for and report early signs of heatstroke: fever, confusion, and dry skin and mucous membranes.
• If the patient experiences CNS or visual effects, warn him against driving, operating machinery, or performing other activities that require alertness and clear vision.
• Suggest that he wear sunglasses if he experiences photophobia.
• Advise him to chew sugarless gum or to suck hard candy or ice chips to relieve dry mouth.
• Instruct an elderly patient's caregivers to remove objects that could cause the patient to fall, such as footstools and throw rugs. Explain that the drug may cause dizziness, confusion, and visual problems.

Antiperistaltics
[Antidiarrheals]

By inhibiting peristalsis, these drugs help to control acute or chronic diarrhea resulting from laxative abuse, malabsorption disorders, food or drug reactions, and infectious and inflammatory conditions. The three most commonly prescribed antiperistaltics are *loperamide, diphenoxylate with atropine sulfate,* and *opium derivatives (paregoric).*

These drugs are generally preferred to over-the-counter preparations, such as kaolin and pectin mixtures, because they reduce fluid loss and don't interfere with the absorption of drugs and nutrients. However, because antiperistaltics decrease intestinal motility, they're contraindicated in patients with conditions involving colonic stricture or stenosis (such as ulcerative colitis); in such patients, the drugs could precipitate acute intestinal obstruction or toxic megacolon.

Antiperistaltics are also contraindicated in patients with diarrhea resulting from ingestion of a toxic substance, because they inhibit elimination of toxins from the GI tract. Because of their narcotic effects, these drugs are contraindicated in patients with a history of narcotic dependence. Paregoric's potential for physical dependence is well known. Both loperamide and diphenoxylate, which are chemically related to meperidine, also carry a risk of CNS depression and possibly narcotic dependence.

Purpose and action
Antiperistaltics prolong the transit of intestinal contents by inhibiting motility and propulsion. This, in turn, reduces fluid and electrolyte loss in the stool and increases fecal bulk and viscosity. Certain antiperistaltic preparations may actually stimulate absorption of fluid into the intestine, which further enhances this effect.

Monitoring
Carefully observe the patient for side effects of antiperistaltics. In particular, watch for CNS effects, ranging from dizziness and confusion to stupor and hallucinations. Remember that these effects are especially common and severe in children, the elderly, and patients with impaired renal or hepatic function. If the patient's taking an opium derivative, also watch for nausea and vomiting.

Frequently measure abdominal girth and auscultate for bowel sounds. Abdominal distention and decreased or absent bowel sounds may herald the development of acute intestinal obstruction, such as paralytic ileus or toxic megacolon. Notify the doctor of any abnormal findings.

Home care instructions
● Warn the patient never to exceed the prescribed dosage; doing so could produce sedation, euphoria, and other CNS effects. Explain that prolonged overuse could lead to dependence.
● Instruct the patient to keep an accurate record of the amount and consistency of all stools and to notify the doctor if no improvement occurs within

KAOLIN AND PECTIN MIXTURES

Kaolin and pectin mixtures, such as Kaopectate and Pectokay, are well-known over-the-counter remedies for mild, nonspecific diarrhea. Unlike the antiperistaltics, these preparations don't affect intestinal motility. Instead, they decrease diarrhea by drawing water from the stool.

If your patient is taking one of these preparations, instruct him to use it for no more than 2 or 3 days. If he obtains no relief, tell him to contact his doctor to determine the underlying cause of diarrhea.

Warn the patient that kaolin and pectin mixtures may cause constipation, which, although normally transient, can lead to fecal impaction, particularly in young children or the elderly. Explain that these preparations may affect the absorption of other drugs, especially cardiac glycosides, lincomycin, phenothiazines, and antidyskinetics.

48 hours of starting therapy.
● Tell the patient to maintain adequate fluid intake. Explain that, contrary to popular belief, high fluid ingestion doesn't contribute to diarrhea. Rather, it helps replace the large amounts of fluid lost in diarrhea.
● If diphenoxylate is prescribed for a young child, advise his parents that this drug can mask signs of fluid and electrolyte depletion. Instruct them to make sure the child maintains a high fluid intake and to watch for and report signs of dehydration: lethargy, low-grade fever, poor skin turgor, mucous membrane dryness, decreased urine output, and excessive thirst.
● Tell the patient to immediately report any abdominal pain or discomfort, bloody stools, or constipation.

Laxatives

Laxatives ease the passage of feces through the colon and rectum, thereby relieving or preventing constipation.

COMPARING LAXATIVES

DRUG	CAUTIONS AND CONTRAINDICATIONS	SIDE EFFECTS
Bulk-forming laxatives barley-malt extract calcium polycarbophil methylcellulose psyllium	• Contraindicated in abdominal pain, nausea, vomiting, or other symptoms of appendicitis, intestinal obstruction, or ulceration; disabling adhesions; or swallowing difficulty. • Don't give high-sodium bulk-forming laxatives (Metamucil, Instant Mix) to patients on sodium-restricted diets.	Nausea, vomiting, GI stricture when taken dry, abdominal cramps, laxative dependence with excessive or long-term use
Stool softeners docusate calcium docusate potassium docusate sodium	• Contraindicated in abdominal pain, nausea, vomiting, or other symptoms of appendicitis, intestinal obstruction, or ulceration. • Should be used only occasionally. Don't use for more than 1 week.	Throat irritation, bitter taste, abdominal cramps, diarrhea, dependence with excessive or long-term use
Hyperosmolar laxatives glycerin lactulose magnesium salts sodium salts	• Contraindicated in abdominal pain, nausea, vomiting, or other symptoms of appendicitis, intestinal obstruction, or ulceration; myocardial damage; heart block; imminent delivery; fecal impaction; rectal fissures; and renal disease. Use cautiously in rectal bleeding. • For short-term therapy only; do not use longer than 1 week.	Abdominal cramps, nausea, vomiting, dehydration, electrolyte imbalance (in acute overdose or chronic misuse), acid-base imbalance, dependence with excessive or prolonged use
Stimulant laxatives bisacodyl cascara sagrada castor oil danthron dehydrocholic acid phenolphthalein senna	• Contraindicated in abdominal pain, nausea, vomiting, or other symptoms of appendicitis, intestinal obstruction, or ulceration; anal or rectal fissures; and fecal impactions. Use cautiously in rectal bleeding. • Don't give castor oil to menstruating or pregnant women; it may cause pelvic congestion.	Laxative dependence with excessive or prolonged use; electrolyte and acid-base imbalance with excessive use; nausea, vomiting, abdominal cramps, diarrhea in high doses; breathing difficulty; cardiac arrest; encephalitis; renal irritation; "cathartic colon" (a syndrome resembling ulcerative colitis)
Lubricant laxative mineral oil	• Contraindicated in fecal impaction and in abdominal pain, nausea, vomiting, or other symptoms of appendicitis, intestinal obstruction, or perforation. • Use cautiously in young children; in elderly or debilitated patients because of their susceptibility to lipid pneumonitis; and in rectal bleeding. Enema contraindicated in children under age 2. • To be taken only at bedtime and not for more than 1 week.	Abdominal pain, nausea, vomiting, diarrhea (with excessive use)

SPECIAL CONSIDERATIONS

• Laxative effect usually occurs within 12 to 24 hours but may be delayed up to 3 days.
• Tell the patient to mix the drug well with at least 8 oz (240 ml) of a pleasant-tasting juice and to drink the mixture immediately.
• May reduce appetite if taken before meals.

• Mix liquid form with milk, juice, or infant formula to mask bitter taste.
• The laxative of choice for patients who shouldn't strain during defecation, such as those recovering from myocardial infarction or rectal surgery; in rectoanal disorders that make passage of firm stool difficult; and in postpartum constipation.
• Onset is generally within 24 to 48 hours.
• Store at 59° to 86° F. (15° to 30° C.) and protect from light.
• Discontinue use if severe cramps occur.

• Shake suspension well. Give with large amounts of water.
• Tell the patient to improve flavor of the drug by following dosage with fruit juice or a citrus-flavored carbonated beverage.
• When administering the drug through a nasogastric tube, ensure proper tube placement and patency. After instilling the drug, flush the tube with water to ensure drug delivery and maintain tube patency.
• Don't give oral drugs within 2 hours of administering the laxative.
• Because the laxative produces watery stool within 3 to 6 hours, schedule administration so that it doesn't interfere with activities or sleep.
• Magnesium sulfate is more potent than other saline laxatives.
• Monitor serum electrolytes during prolonged use.

• Don't give oral drugs within 2 hours of administering the laxative.
• Laxative effect usually occurs within 2 to 8 hours. Schedule drug administration to avoid interfering with sleep or activities.
• Monitor serum electrolytes during prolonged use. Some stimulant laxatives may turn alkaline urine reddish pink and acidic urine yellowish brown.

• Don't give drug with meals or immediately after because it delays passage of food from stomach; it's more active on an empty stomach.
• Laxative effect usually occurs in 6 to 8 hours.
• Give with fruit juices or carbonated drinks to disguise taste.
• Warn patient of possible rectal leakage so he can avoid soiling clothing.

Classified according to their mechanism of action, laxatives may be bulk-forming agents, stool softeners, hyperosmolar agents, lubricants, or stimulants.

Bulk-forming laxatives, such as *methylcellulose* and *psyllium*, help treat chronic constipation. Stool softeners, such as *docusate*, prevent constipation and straining during defecation. Hyperosmolar agents, such as *glycerin* and *magnesium salts*, treat constipation and help prepare the bowel for examination or diagnostic or surgical procedures. Lubricants, such as *mineral oil*, and stimulants, such as *castor oil*, have similar indications.

Laxatives vary widely in their speed of action. Typically, bulk-forming laxatives and stool softeners produce elimination in 12 to 48 hours; hyperosmolar laxatives, in 30 minutes to 3 hours.

Purpose and action
• *Bulk-forming laxatives* absorb water and expand, increasing the bulk and fluid content of stool. This, in turn, enhances peristalsis and evacuation.
• *Stool softeners* reduce the surface tension of interfacing liquid bowel contents, thereby increasing the fluid content of stool and softening the fecal mass.
• *Hyperosmolar laxatives* act in different ways. Glycerin draws water into the feces, increasing bulk and promoting peristalsis. Lactulose produces an osmotic effect, which draws water into the colon; the resulting bowel distention stimulates peristalsis. The saline laxatives exert an osmotic effect in the small intestine, producing distention and enhancing peristalsis; they also promote secretion of cholecystokinin by the intestinal mucosa, which stimulates intestinal motility and inhibits fluid and electrolyte absorption in the jejunum and ileum.
• *Lubricant laxatives* create a barrier between the colonic wall and the fecal mass, preventing absorption of fecal water by the colon and promoting its retention in the stool.

• *Stimulant laxatives* are thought to increase peristalsis by exerting a direct effect on intestinal smooth muscle, either by irritating the muscle or by stimulating the colonic intramural plexus. These drugs also promote fluid and electrolyte accumulation in the colon and small intestine.

Monitoring
When administering laxatives, monitor the patient for abdominal cramps, nausea or vomiting, and diarrhea. If you note these or other side effects, notify the doctor. (See *Comparing Laxatives,* pages 146 and 147, for other side effects specific to each class of laxatives.)

Monitor bowel movements and note the amount, consistency, and color. Also note the degree of effort required for defecation.

During long-term therapy, monitor the patient's fluid intake to ensure adequate hydration. (This is especially important if he's taking a bulk-forming laxative.) Regularly assess for signs of dehydration, including fever, tachycardia, hypotension, decreased urine output, poor skin turgor, and extreme thirst. Also monitor serum electrolytes—especially potassium and sodium—and acid-base balance. Watch for signs of electrolyte and acid-base imbalances, such as weakness, diminished reflexes, twitching, vomiting, hypotension, and a rapid, thready pulse.

Home care instructions
• Warn the patient to never take laxatives if he's experiencing abdominal pain, nausea, or vomiting. Explain that these symptoms may herald a more serious condition that a laxative may aggravate.
• Encourage him to drink 6 to 8 glasses of water a day while taking the drug.
• Advise him to notify his doctor if he doesn't have a bowel movement after taking the laxative for the prescribed time and in the prescribed way.
• Reassure the patient that a daily bowel movement isn't essential to good

health; more important is maintaining a consistent elimination pattern. Warn him against overusing laxatives, which can lead to dependence.

• Teach the patient about alternative ways to prevent constipation: regular exercise and adequate fluid and fiber intake. Tell him that good dietary sources of fiber include bran and other cereals, fresh fruits, and vegetables.

Antiemetics

Given to prevent or control nausea and vomiting, antiemetics consist primarily of drugs from four pharmacologic classes: phenothiazines, dopamine antagonists, cannabinoids, and anticholinergics.

The *phenothiazines*, such as chlorpromazine, and the *dopamine antagonists* help control vomiting that results from GI upset, radiation sickness, or cancer chemotherapy. In fact, the dopamine antagonist metoclopramide is the drug of choice for preventing the nausea and vomiting that normally accompany cancer chemotherapy.

The *cannabinoids*, such as nabilone and dronabinol, can control chemotherapy-induced nausea and vomiting when metoclopramide and other antiemetics have failed. Although derived from marijuana, the cannabinoids produce few euphoric effects and have little potential for abuse.

The *anticholinergics*, such as dimenhydrinate and meclizine, help control vomiting that results from vestibular disturbances, such as motion sickness.

Typically, the antiemetics prove most effective when administered prophylactically. Because these drugs produce sedation, they should be used cautiously in patients who are taking other CNS depressants. Dopamine antagonists and phenothiazines can also cause extrapyramidal symptoms, especially if taken for a prolonged period.

Because metoclopramide stimulates GI motility, it's contraindicated in GI ulcers or obstruction. Phenothiazines have the opposite effect on peristalsis, and so should be used cautiously in impaired GI motility. And because phenothiazines may induce transient leukopenia, they're contraindicated in bone marrow depression.

Purpose and action
The phenothiazines and dopamine antagonists prevent or control vomiting by acting on the chemoreceptor trigger zone in the medulla oblongata. The anticholinergics inhibit impulse transmission along the neural pathways from the inner ear. The cannabinoids' mechanism of action isn't known.

Monitoring
During therapy, carefully assess the patient's cardiovascular status; metoclopramide can produce transient hypertension, and phenothiazines and cannabinoids may cause tachycardia and orthostatic hypotension.

If the patient's taking phenothiazines, assess for signs of blood dyscrasias, such as fever, sore throat, and weakness. Similarly, check the results of hematologic studies for evidence of blood dyscrasias. Watch for constipation and urinary retention.

Check the patient's drug regimen for possible interactions. For example, if he's taking phenothiazines, concurrent use of anticholinergics increases anticholinergic activity. Antacids interfere with phenothiazine absorption and shouldn't be given within 2 hours of each other. Barbiturates may decrease the effects of phenothiazines.

If the patient's taking metoclopramide, concurrent use of anticholinergics or narcotic analgesics may antagonize it.

Home care instructions
• Warn the patient to avoid alcohol and over-the-counter preparations that cause CNS depression, such as cough and cold remedies or sleeping pills.
• Instruct him to promptly report chest

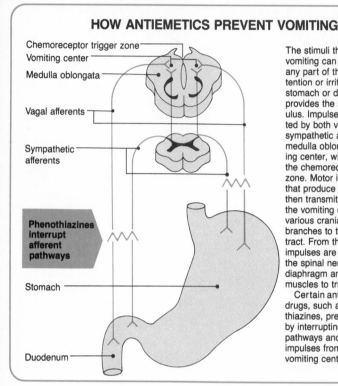

HOW ANTIEMETICS PREVENT VOMITING

Chemoreceptor trigger zone
Vomiting center
Medulla oblongata
Vagal afferents
Sympathetic afferents
Phenothiazines interrupt afferent pathways
Stomach
Duodenum

The stimuli that cause vomiting can originate in any part of the GI tract; distention or irritation of the stomach or duodenum provides the strongest stimulus. Impulses are transmitted by both vagal and sympathetic afferents to the medulla oblongata's vomiting center, which lies in the chemoreceptor trigger zone. Motor impulses that produce vomiting are then transmitted from the vomiting center through various cranial nerve branches to the upper GI tract. From there these impulses are sent through the spinal nerves to the diaphragm and abdominal muscles to trigger vomiting.

Certain antiemetic drugs, such as the phenothiazines, prevent vomiting by interrupting the afferent pathways and preventing impulses from reaching the vomiting center.

pain, palpitations, or persistent headache.
• Because antiemetics usually cause dizziness or drowsiness, tell the patient not to drive or perform any task requiring alertness until his response to the drug has been determined.
• Instruct him to minimize orthostatic hypotension by rising slowly from a sitting or lying position and by avoiding sudden bending or reaching.
• If the patient experiences a dry mouth, tell him to chew sugarless gum, suck hard candy, or rinse with mouthwash.
• If he experiences phenothiazine-induced photosensitivity, advise him to apply a sunscreen and wear protective clothing when outdoors.
• Because antacids inhibit absorption of oral phenothiazines, instruct the patient to separate doses of these by at least 2 hours.

SURGERY

Esophageal Surgeries

In esophageal disorders, surgery may be necessary to manage an emergency, such as acute constriction, or to provide palliative care for an incurable disease, such as advanced esophageal cancer. The primary esophageal surgeries include cardiomyotomy, cricopharyngeal myotomy, esophagectomy, esophagogastrostomy, and esophagomyotomy. (See *Understanding Esophageal Surgeries*, page 152, for details of these surgeries.)

Esophageal surgeries have the potential for serious complications. For example, mediastinitis may result from leakage of esophageal contents into the thorax. Severe inflammation can produce obstruction of the mediastinal structures, such as the superior vena cava, the tracheobronchial tree, and the esophagus. Postoperative reflux, hypersalivation, and impaired clearance of secretions put the patient at risk for aspiration pneumonia. Children who've undergone surgery to repair tracheoesophageal fistula may develop reflex bradycardia, marked by apnea and cyanosis immediately after swallowing.

Purpose
• To restore esophageal patency and motility by correcting a congenital abnormality
• To remove an esophageal obstruction
• To repair traumatic esophageal tissue damage
• To provide comfort in terminal disease.

Preparation
If the patient requires immediate surgery, briefly explain the procedure to him. If he doesn't, focus your preoperative care on evaluating and, if necessary, improving his nutritional status. After all, many patients requiring esophageal surgery have a long history of dysphagia, anorexia, or other eating problems.

Check laboratory results for serum protein, glucose, and electrolyte levels. Also check renal function studies, such as blood urea nitrogen and serum creatinine. If necessary, provide I.V. fluid and electrolyte replacement or protein supplements.

Maintain the patient on a high-protein, high-calorie, soft diet. If he can't tolerate oral feedings, provide gastrostomy tube feedings or I.V. hyperalimentation, as ordered.

Explain the planned surgery to the patient. Inform him that when he awakens from the anesthetic he'll probably have a nasogastric tube inserted to facilitate feeding and provide relief of abdominal distention, and a chest tube inserted to drain fluid from the surgical site. Discuss possible postoperative complications and measures to prevent or minimize them. In particular, discuss the risk of aspiration pneumonia and the importance of good pulmonary hygiene during recovery to prevent it. Demonstrate coughing and deep-breathing exercises, and show him how to splint his incision to protect it and minimize pain.

Ensure that the patient or a responsible family member has signed a consent form.

Procedure
Cardiomyotomy and esophagomyotomy involve either a left thoracotomy or an abdominal incision. After exposing the area of constriction, the surgeon cuts through the muscle fiber but leaves the mucosa intact. This allows the esophageal lumen to expand naturally, relieving constriction.

To perform a cricopharyngeal myotomy, the surgeon makes an incision along the lower anterior border of the left sternonucleomastoid muscle, usually with the patient under local anesthesia. Then the surgeon partially dissects the cricopharyngeal muscle to remove a Zenker's diverticulum, or he severs it to relieve cricopharyngeal spasm. If the patient received a local anesthetic, the surgeon will ask him to swallow periodically.

The surgeon approaches esophagectomy through either a thoracic or an abdominal incision, depending on the abnormality's location. (For example, ligation of a tracheoesophageal fistula requires a right thoracotomy.) He resects diseased tissue or ligates fistulas, as appropriate, and then anastomoses the esophagus to restore patency. If insufficient esophageal tissue remains after massive resection, he may anastomose a segment of the patient's jejunum or colon in place between the esophageal segments.

UNDERSTANDING ESOPHAGEAL SURGERIES

Common esophageal surgeries include cardiomyotomy, esophagomyotomy, cricopharyngeal myotomy, esophagogastrostomy and esophagectomy. Cardiomyotomy, the incision of the muscle wall of the lower esophagus and cardia, relieves achalasia. Esophagomyotomy, the incision of the esophageal muscle wall, relieves diffuse esophageal spasm or intractable esophagitis. The other esophageal surgeries, which have somewhat different indications, are shown below.

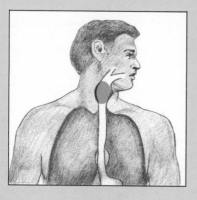

Cricopharyngeal myotomy
Partial or total incision of the cricopharyngeal muscle

Indications
• To allow removal of Zenker's diverticula
• To relieve severe cricopharyngeal spasm

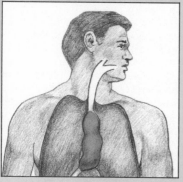

Esophagogastrostomy
Resection of diseased esophageal tissue and anastomosis of the remaining esophageal segment to the stomach

Indications
• To excise lower esophageal malignancy

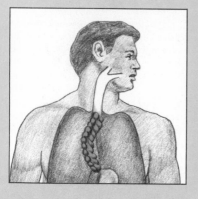

Esophagectomy
Resection of diseased or damaged esophageal tissue, with anastomosis of remaining segments. Extensive resection may require esophagocologastrostomy (anastomosis of a transplanted bowel segment between the esophagus and stomach) to restore esophageal patency.

Indications
• To excise upper or middle esophageal malignancy
• To correct congenital atresia
• To relieve severe esophageal stricture

In esophagogastrostomy, the surgeon performs an extensive right thoracotomy to expose the esophagus and stomach. He resects the diseased portion of the esophagus, then brings the stomach up into the chest cavity and anastomoses it to the remaining esophageal segment.

Emergency repair of esophageal perforation requires a left thoracotomy, with placement of a mediastinal chest tube for postoperative drainage.

Monitoring and aftercare

After surgery, place the patient in semi-Fowler's position to help minimize esophageal reflux. Provide antacids as needed for symptomatic relief.

If surgery involving the upper esophagus produces hypersalivation, the patient may be unable to swallow the excess saliva. Control drooling by using gauze wicks to absorb secretions or by suctioning frequently. If the patient can spit, place an emesis basin within his reach.

To reduce the risk of aspiration pneumonia, keep the head of the patient's bed elevated and encourage him to turn frequently. Carefully monitor his vital signs and auscultate his lungs. Encourage coughing and deep-breathing exercises.

Watch for developing mediastinitis, especially if surgery involved extensive thoracic invasion (as in esophagogastrostomy). Note and report fever, dyspnea, and complaints of substernal pain. If ordered, administer antibiotics to help prevent or correct this complication.

Watch for signs of leakage at the anastomosis site. Check drainage tubes for blood, test for occult blood in stool and drainage, and monitor hemoglobin levels for evidence of slow blood loss.

If the patient has a nasogastric tube in place, avoid manipulating the tube because this may damage the internal sutures or anastomoses. For the same reason, avoid deep suctioning in a patient who has undergone extensive esophageal repair.

Home care instructions

- Advise the patient to sleep with his head elevated, to prevent reflux. He can use three pillows or raise the head of his bed on blocks.
- If the patient smokes, encourage him to stop. Explain that nicotine has a detrimental effect on the lower esophageal sphincter.
- Advise the patient to avoid alcohol, aspirin, and effervescent over-the-counter products (such as Alka-Seltzer) since these may damage the tender esophageal mucosa.
- Also advise him to avoid heavy lifting, straining, and coughing, which could rupture the weakened mucosa.
- Instruct him to report any respiratory symptoms, such as wheezing, coughing, and nocturnal dyspnea.

Hernia Repair

A hernia may be corrected by herniorrhaphy or hernioplasty. Herniorrhaphy, the surgery of choice for inguinal and other abdominal hernias, returns the protruding intestine to the abdominal cavity and repairs the abdominal wall defect. Hernioplasty, a related surgery used to correct more extensive hernias, reinforces the weakened area around the repair with plastic, steel or tantalum mesh, or wire.

Typically, herniorrhaphy and hernioplasty are elective surgeries that can be done quickly and produce few complications. However, emergency herniorrhaphy may be necessary to reduce a strangulated hernia and prevent ischemia and gangrene.

Purpose

To return herniated tissue to its original position and to repair the underlying muscle wall defect.

Preparation

Explain the surgery to the patient, gearing your discussion to his age and level of comprehension. Tell him that the surgery will relieve the discomfort of hernia. If the patient is having elective surgery, assure him that recovery is usually rapid; if no complications occur, he may return home the day of surgery and usually can resume normal activities within 4 to 6 weeks. If the patient is having emergency surgery for a strangulated or incarcerated hernia, explain that he may be hospitalized from 1 to 2 weeks and may have a nasogastric tube in place for several days before he's allowed to eat or get out of bed.

Ensure that the patient or a responsible family member has signed a consent form.

Prepare the patient for surgery by shaving the surgical site and administering a cleansing enema and a sedative, as ordered.

Procedure

With the patient under general or spinal anesthesia, the surgeon makes an incision over the area of herniation. He manipulates the herniated tissue back to its proper position and then repairs the defect in the muscle or fascia. If necessary, he reinforces the area of the defect with wire, mesh, or another material. Then he closes the incision and applies a dressing.

Monitoring and aftercare

Take steps to reduce pressure on the incision site. For example, teach the patient how to get up from a lying or sitting position without straining his abdomen. Also teach him how to splint his incision when he coughs or sneezes, and reassure him that coughing or sneezing won't cause the hernia to recur. As ordered, administer a stool softener to prevent straining during defecation. Encourage early ambulation but warn against bending, lifting, or other strenuous activities.

Make sure the patient voids within 12 hours after surgery. If swelling interferes with normal urination, insert an indwelling (Foley) catheter.

Provide comfort measures. Administer analgesics, as ordered. After inguinal hernia repair, apply an ice bag to the patient's scrotum to reduce swelling and pain. If appropriate, apply a scrotal bridge or truss; for best results, apply it in the morning before the patient gets out of bed.

Regularly check the dressing for drainage and the incision site for inflammation or swelling. Assess the patient for other symptoms of infection. Report possible infection to the doctor, and expect to administer antibiotics, as ordered.

Home care instructions

● Instruct the patient to avoid lifting, bending, and pushing or pulling movements for 8 weeks after surgery or until his doctor allows them.
● Tell him to watch for and report signs of infection, including fever, chills, diaphoresis, malaise, lethargy, and pain, inflammation, swelling, and drainage at the incision site. Instruct him to keep the incision clean and covered until the sutures are removed.
● Stress the importance of regular follow-up examinations to evaluate wound healing and the success of hernia repair.
● If the patient's job involves heavy lifting or other strenuous activity, discuss the possible need for a job change.

Gastric Surgeries

If chronic ulcer disease doesn't respond to medication, dietary therapy, and rest, gastric surgery may be necessary to remove diseased tissue and prevent recurrence of ulcers. This surgery may also be used to excise a malignancy or relieve an obstruction. In an emergency, it may be performed to control severe GI hemorrhage resulting from a perforated ulcer.

Gastric surgery can take various forms, depending on the location and extent of the disorder. For example, a partial gastrectomy may be performed to reduce the amount of acid-secreting mucosa. A bilateral vagotomy may be performed to relieve ulcer symptoms and to eliminate vagal nerve stimulation of gastric secretions. A pyloroplasty may be performed to improve drainage and prevent obstruction. Most commonly, though, two gastric surgeries are combined, such as vagotomy with gastroenterostomy or vagotomy with antrectomy. (See *Understanding Common Gastric Surgeries*, pages 156 and 157, for descriptions of these and other gastric surgeries.)

Gastric surgery carries the risk of serious complications, including hemorrhage, obstruction, dumping syndrome, paralytic ileus, vitamin B_{12} deficiency, and atelectasis. Your nursing care needs to focus on measures to prevent these complications and on early detection and prompt intervention if they do develop. Careful postoperative monitoring, including maintaining nutritional status and fluid and electrolyte balance, is essential.

Purpose
• To excise areas of gastric ulceration or malignancy
• To reduce acid secretion by removing portions of the gastric mucosa
• To relieve gastric obstruction.

Preparation
The extent of preoperative preparation obviously depends on the nature of surgery. If emergency surgery is necessary, preparation may be limited to immunohematologic studies and measures to control acute hemorrhage, such as iced gastric lavage and administration of vasopressors. Planned surgery allows more extensive preparation.

Before planned surgery, evaluate and take steps to stabilize the patient's fluid and electrolyte balance and nutritional status—all of which may be severely compromised by chronic ulcer disease or other GI disorders. Monitor the patient's intake and output, and draw serum samples for hematologic studies. As ordered, begin I.V. fluid replacement and parenteral nutrition. Also as ordered, prepare the patient for abdominal X-rays. On the night before surgery, administer cleansing laxatives and enemas, as necessary. On the morning of surgery, insert a nasogastric (NG) tube.

As time permits, discuss postoperative care measures with the patient. Explain that the NG tube will remain in place for 2 to 3 days to remove fluid, blood, and air from the abdominal cavity and to prevent distention; he'll also have abdominal drains inserted at the surgical site and an I.V. line in place for several days.

Remember that the patient will have fears about the surgery and concerns about its effect on his life-style even if he doesn't express them. Take the time to reassure him. Point out that other, more conservative treatments haven't worked and that surgery is now necessary to relieve his symptoms and prevent more serious, possibly even life-threatening, complications. Explain that with successful surgery, he should be able to lead a near-normal life with few restrictions on his activity.

Discuss how surgery will affect his diet. Explain that he'll be fed through a gastrostomy tube for several days after surgery and then gradually resume oral feeding with clear liquids and eventually solid foods. If gastric surgery is extensive, he may receive I.V. hyperalimentation for a week or longer.

Explain the need for postoperative deep-breathing exercises and coughing to prevent pulmonary complications. Stress the importance of performing these measures even though incisional pain may make him reluctant to do so.

Ensure that the patient or a responsible family member has signed a consent form.

Procedure
Surgery begins with an upper abdominal incision, such as an upper paramedial incision, to expose the stomach

UNDERSTANDING COMMON GASTRIC SURGERIES

Besides treating chronic ulcers, gastric surgeries help remove obstructions and malignancy. Be sure you're familiar with these commonly performed gastric surgeries.

VAGOTOMY WITH GASTROENTEROSTOMY

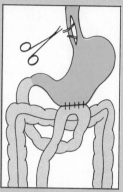

In this procedure, the surgeon resects the vagus nerves and creates a stoma for gastric drainage. He'll perform selective, truncal, or parietal cell vagotomy, depending on the degree of decreased gastric acid secretion required.

VAGOTOMY WITH ANTRECTOMY

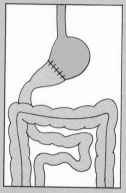

After resecting the vagus nerves, the surgeon removes the antrum. Then he anastomoses the remaining stomach segment to the jejunum and closes the duodenal stump.

and part of the intestine. Total gastrectomy, the removal of the entire stomach, requires a more extensive incision.

The rest of the procedure varies, depending on the type of surgery. (See *Understanding Common Gastric Surgeries*.) To complete the operation, the surgeon inserts abdominal drains and closes the incision. Then he applies a dressing.

Monitoring and aftercare

When the patient awakens from surgery, place him in a low or semi-Fowler's position—whichever he finds more comfortable. Either position will ease breathing and prevent aspiration if he vomits.

Check the patient's vital signs every 2 hours until his condition stabilizes. Watch especially for hypotension, bradycardia, and respiratory changes, which may signal hemorrhage and shock. Periodically check the wound site, NG tube, and abdominal drainage tubes for bleeding.

Maintain tube feedings or I.V. hyperalimentation, and I.V. fluid and electrolyte replacement therapy, as ordered. Monitor blood studies daily. Watch for signs of dehydration, hyponatremia, and metabolic alkalosis, which may result from gastric suctioning. Weigh the patient daily and monitor and record intake and output, including NG tube drainage.

Auscultate the patient's abdomen daily for the return of bowel sounds. When they return, notify the doctor, who'll order clamping or removal of the NG tube and gradual resumption of oral feeding. During NG tube clamping, watch for nausea and vomiting; if they occur, unclamp the tube immediately and reattach it to suction.

VAGOTOMY WITH PYLOROPLASTY

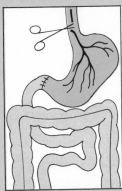

In this procedure, the surgeon resects the vagus nerves and refashions the pylorus to widen the lumen and aid gastric emptying.

BILLROTH I

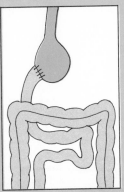

In this partial gastrectomy with a gastroduodenoscopy, the surgeon excises the distal third to half of the stomach and anastomoses the remaining stomach to the duodenum.

BILLROTH II

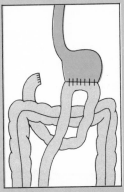

In this partial gastrectomy with a gastrojejunostomy, the surgeon removes the distal segment of the stomach and antrum. Then he anastomoses the remaining stomach and the jejunum, and closes the duodenal stump.

Throughout recovery, have the patient cough, deep-breathe, and change position frequently. Provide incentive spirometry, as necessary. Teach him to splint his incision while coughing to help reduce pain. Assess his breath sounds frequently to detect atelectasis.

Assess for other complications, including vitamin B_{12} deficiency, anemia (especially common in patients who've undergone total gastrectomy), and dumping syndrome, a potentially serious digestive complication marked by weakness, nausea, flatulence, and palpitations within 30 minutes after a meal.

Home care instructions

● Instruct the patient to notify the doctor immediately if he develops any signs of life-threatening complications, such as hemorrhage, obstruction, or perforation.

● Explain dumping syndrome and ways to avoid it. Advise the patient to eat small, frequent meals evenly spaced throughout the day. He should chew his food thoroughly and drink fluids between meals rather than with them. In his diet, he should decrease intake of carbohydrates and salt while increasing fat and protein. After a meal, he should lie down for 20 to 30 minutes.

● Advise the patient to avoid or limit foods high in fiber, such as fresh fruits and vegetables and whole-grain breads.

● If the doctor has prescribed a GI anticholinergic to decrease motility and acid secretion, instruct the patient to take the drug 30 minutes to 1 hour before meals.

● If the patient is being discharged on tube feedings, make sure that he and his family understand how to give the feeding.

• Encourage the patient and his family to help speed healing and lessen the risk of recurrence by identifying and eliminating sources of emotional stress at home and in the workplace. Instruct the patient to balance activity and rest and to schedule a realistic pattern of work and sleep. Suggest that he learn and apply stress management techniques, such as progressive relaxation and meditation. If the patient finds self-management difficult, encourage him to seek professional counseling.

• Advise the patient to avoid smoking because it alters pancreatic secretions that neutralize gastric acid in the duodenum.

Abdominoperineal or Bowel Surgery with Ostomy

An ostomy involves the resection of diseased colonic and rectal segments and the creation of a stoma on the outer abdominal wall to allow elimination of feces. This surgery is performed for such intestinal maladies as inflammatory bowel disease, familial polyposis, diverticulitis, and especially advanced colorectal cancer if conservative surgery and other treatments aren't successful or if the patient develops acute complications, such as obstruction, abscess, or fistula.

Depending on the nature and location of the problem, the surgeon chooses among several types of surgery. For instance, intractable obstruction of the ascending, transverse, descending, or sigmoid colon requires permanent colostomy, with removal of the affected bowel segments. Cancer of the rectum and lower sigmoid colon often mandates abdominoperineal resection, which involves creation of a permanent colostomy and removal of the remaining colon, rectum, and anus.

Perforated sigmoid diverticulitis, Hirschsprung's disease, rectovaginal fistula, and penetrating trauma often call for temporary colostomy to interrupt the intestinal flow and allow healing of inflamed or injured bowel segments. After healing occurs (usually within 6 to 8 weeks), anastomosis of the divided segments restores bowel integrity and function. In a double-barrel colostomy, the transverse colon is divided and both ends are brought out through the abdominal wall to create a proximal stoma for fecal drainage and a distal stoma leading to the nonfunctioning bowel. Loop colostomy, done as an emergency procedure to relieve acute obstruction, involves creating proximal and distal stomas from a loop of intestine that has been pulled through an abdominal incision and supported with a plastic or glass rod.

Severe, widespread colonic obstruction may require total or near-total removal of the colon and rectum and creation of an ileostomy from the proximal ileum. A permanent ileostomy requires that the patient wear a drainage pouch or bag over the stoma to receive the constant fecal drainage. In contrast, a continent, or Kock, ileostomy doesn't require an external pouch. (See *Continent Ileostomy: Guidelines for Patient Care*, page 161.)

Common complications of ostomies include hemorrhage, sepsis, ileus, and fluid and electrolyte imbalance from excessive drainage through the stoma. Skin excoriation may occur around the stoma from contact with acidic digestive enzymes in the drainage, and irritation may occur from pressure of the ostomy pouch. Excoriation occurs more commonly with an ileostomy than with a colostomy because of the greater acidity of fecal drainage.

Ostomates commonly exhibit some degree of emotional and psychological problems, such as depression and anxiety, related to altered body image and worries about life-style changes associated with the stoma and ostomy pouch.

REVIEWING TYPES OF OSTOMIES

The type of ostomy depends on the patient's condition. Temporary ones, such as a double-barrel or loop colostomy, help treat perforated sigmoid diverticulitis, penetrating trauma, and other conditions in which intestinal healing is expected. They're also used to bypass an inoperable intestinal tumor.

Permanent colostomy or ileostomy typically accompanies extensive abdominal surgery, often for removal of a malignant tumor.

PERMANENT COLOSTOMY

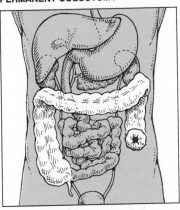

DOUBLE-BARREL COLOSTOMY

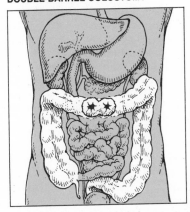

LOOP COLOSTOMY

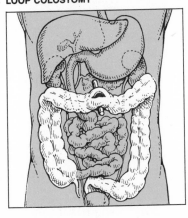

ILEOSTOMY

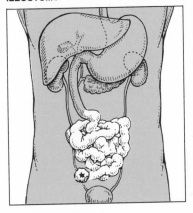

Effective nursing care for an ostomy patient means anticipating and taking steps to help prevent or minimize these complications. Such care includes careful monitoring of fluid and electrolyte balance and nutritional status before and after surgery. It also involves teaching proper stoma care and drainage techniques, dietary modifications, and other long-term treatment measures.

Purpose

To remove diseased colonic and rectal tissue and create a surgical opening, or stoma, through the abdominal wall for elimination of feces.

Preparation

If emergency surgery is necessary, briefly explain that the diseased or injured portion of the bowel will be repaired, if possible, and isolated to allow healing. Mention that a small portion of the unaffected bowel will be temporarily brought to an opening in the skin to allow elimination.

If immediate surgery isn't required, supplement the doctor's explanation of the surgery, as necessary, and answer all questions in clear, simple terms. Include family members or caregivers in your discussion, if appropriate. Prepare the patient for postoperative pain, especially if he's scheduled for an abdominoperineal resection, and mention that analgesics will be provided.

Describe the type of ostomy the patient will have and explain how fecal matter drains through it. Try using simple illustrations to facilitate your explanation. Discuss selection and use of ostomy appliances; if possible, show him the actual appliances. Prepare him for the foul smell and consistency of fecal drainage. This consistency varies, depending on the stoma's location: a constant watery stool with an ileostomy to a soft, semisolid stool with a colostomy in the descending colon.

Inform the colostomy patient that he'll initially wear a pouch to collect fecal drainage. Point out that he may learn to control bowel movements by irrigating the colostomy. If he does learn bowel control, he may no longer need to use a pouch.

Reassure the patient that once he becomes comfortable with the ostomy management routine, he should be able to resume his normal level of activity with few restrictions.

Before surgery, try to arrange for a visit with an enterostomal therapist, who can provide more detailed information. The therapist can also help the patient select the best location for the stoma. If possible, arrange for the patient to meet with former ostomy patients (from groups such as the United Ostomy Association) before surgery; these ostomates can share their personal insights into the realities of living with and caring for a stoma.

If chronic bowel disease has seriously compromised the patient's condition, evaluate his nutritional and fluid status for 3 to 4 days before surgery (if time permits). Typically, the patient will be receiving I.V. hyperalimentation to prepare him for the physiological stress of surgery. Record the patient's fluid intake and output and weight daily, and watch for early signs of dehydration. Expect to draw periodic blood samples for hematocrit and hemoglobin determinations. Be prepared to transfuse blood, if ordered.

If the patient is on long-term, low-dose steroid therapy, continue to administer the drug to prevent rebound adrenocortical insufficiency. Explain that the drug will be withdrawn gradually after surgery. Also administer antibiotics, as ordered, to reduce intestinal flora.

Ensure that the patient or a responsible family member has signed a consent form.

Procedure

In an *abdominoperineal resection*, the surgeon makes a low abdominal incision and divides the sigmoid colon. He brings the proximal end of the colon out through another, smaller abdominal incision to create a permanent colostomy. He then makes a wide perineal incision and resects the anus, rectum, and distal portion of the sigmoid colon. He closes the abdominal wound and places one or more abdominal sump drains; he usually leaves the perineal wound open and packs it with gauze, but he may close it and place several Penrose drains.

To create a stoma for a colostomy or ileostomy, the surgeon sutures a loop of the remaining intestinal segment to the peritoneal wall to stabilize it and prevent prolapse or volvulus, then pulls the end of the segment through the outer abdominal wall, everts it, and sutures it to the skin.

CONTINENT ILEOSTOMY: GUIDELINES FOR PATIENT CARE

For some patients, a *continent ileostomy* provides a desirable alternative to a conventional ileostomy. In a conventional ileostomy, fecal drainage flows continuously into a pouch. In a continent ileostomy, though, drainage is automatically controlled by a stoma valve.

To perform a continent ileostomy, the surgeon creates an intraabdominal pouch from the terminal ileum and intussuscepts the end of the ileum to form a nipple valve (which shuts against pressure from the filled pouch). He then sutures the pouch to the inner abdominal wall and sutures the nipple valve flush with the abdomen to create a stoma.

Providing care after surgery

The patient returns from surgery with a catheter inserted in the stoma to drain fecal matter from the reservoir and prevent it from filling and placing pressure on the sutures. Be sure the catheter is connected to low intermittent suction. Check the patency of the catheter regularly, and irrigate it with 20 to 30 ml of normal saline solution every 2 to 4 hours to prevent obstruction.

If no complications develop, the color of pouch drainage will change 2 to 4 days after surgery from blood-tinged to greenish brown, indicating the return of peristalsis. When this occurs, give the patient clear liquids and gradually introduce low-residue solids.

Provide instructions for clamping and unclamping the pouch to increase its capacity.

Teaching pouch care

Typically, the catheter remains in place for 2 to 6 weeks after surgery. After it's removed, teach the patient how to empty the pouch by inserting a lubricated #28 French Silastic catheter through the stoma. He can empty the pouch while sitting or standing, though the latter position usually gives better results. He can also quicken drainage by contracting his abdominal muscles.

Provide guidelines for draining the pouch. Right after surgery, the pouch usually holds 70 to 100 ml. One month later, it will hold about 200 ml. After 6 months, it will hold about 600 ml and will need to be emptied three or four times daily.

Be sure the patient knows to carry a catheter with him at all times. Between intubations, he should cover his stoma with gauze to prevent mucus from soiling his clothes. Before applying the gauze, he should wash the stomal area with warm water and dry it.

Demonstrate how to irrigate the pouch. Suggest irrigation weekly or whenever undigested food obstructs drainage.

For a *loop colostomy*, the surgeon brings a portion of intestine out through an abdominal incision. He slips an ostomy bridge (a short plastic or glass rod) under the intestinal loop to support it on the outer abdominal wall, incises the intestine to create a temporary stoma, then closes the wound around the exposed intestinal loop. For a *double-barrel colostomy*, the surgeon divides the colon and brings both ends through an abdominal incision to create a proximal stoma for fecal drainage and a distal stoma leading to the inactive bowel. He inserts abdominal sump drains and closes the incision around the stomas. Later, when the intestinal injury has healed or the inflammation subsided, the loop or double-barrel temporary colostomy is discontinued, and the divided ends of the colon are anastomosed to restore bowel integrity.

For an *ileostomy*, the surgeon resects all or part of the colon and rectum (proctocolectomy). He creates a permanent ileostomy by bringing a loop of the proximal ileum out through a small abdominal incision, typically located in the right lower quadrant between the midline and the right anterior ileum, then fashioning a stoma.

Monitoring and aftercare

In the immediate postoperative period, carefully monitor intake and output and weigh the patient daily. Maintain fluid and electrolyte balance, and watch for signs of dehydration (decreased urinary output, poor skin turgor) and electrolyte imbalance. Provide analgesics, as ordered. Be especially alert for pain in the patient with an abdominoperineal resection because of the extent and location of the incisions.

Note and record the color, consistency, and odor of fecal drainage from the stoma. If the patient has a double-barrel colostomy, check for mucous drainage from the inactive (distal) stoma. The nature of fecal drainage is determined by the type of ostomy surgery; generally, the more colon tissue that is preserved, the more closely drainage will resemble normal stool. For the first few days after surgery, fecal drainage probably will be mucoid (and possibly slightly blood-tinged) and mostly odorless. Report excessive blood or mucous content, which could indicate hemorrhage or infection.

Observe the patient for signs of peritonitis or sepsis, caused by leakage of bowel contents into the abdominal cavity. Remember that patients receiving antibiotics or I.V. hyperalimentation are at an increased risk for sepsis.

Provide meticulous wound care, changing dressings often. Check dressings and drainage sites frequently for signs of infection (purulent drainage, foul odor) or fecal drainage. If the patient has had an abdominoperineal resection, irrigate the perineal area, as ordered.

Regularly check the stoma and the surrounding skin for irritation and excoriation, which may develop from contact with fecal drainage or from pressure caused by an overfilled or improperly fitted drainage pouch. Take measures to correct any such problems. Also observe the stoma's appearance. The stoma should look smooth, cherry-red, and slightly edematous; immediately report any discoloration or excessive swelling, which may indicate circulatory problems that could lead to ischemia.

During the recovery period, don't neglect the patient's emotional needs. En-

courage him to express his feelings and concerns; if he's anxious and depressed, reassure him that these common postoperative reactions should fade as he adjusts to the ostomy. Continue to arrange for visits by an enterostomal therapist, if possible.

Home care instructions

• If the patient has a colostomy, teach him or a caregiver how to apply, remove, and empty the pouch. And when appropriate, teach him how to irrigate the colostomy with warm tap water to gain some control over elimination. Emphasize that continence can be achieved with dietary control and bowel retraining.

• Instruct the colostomy patient to change the stoma appliance as needed, to wash the stoma site with warm water and mild soap every 3 days, and to change the adhesive layer. These measures help prevent skin irritation and excoriation.

• If the patient has an ileostomy, instruct him to change the drainage pouch only when leakage occurs. Also emphasize meticulous skin care and use of a protective skin barrier around the stoma site.

• Discuss dietary restrictions and suggestions to prevent stoma blockage, diarrhea, flatus, and odor. (See *Dietary Modifications for Ostomates* for details.)

• Explain the need for maintaining a high fluid intake to help ensure fluid and electrolyte balance. This is especially important in times of increased fluid loss, such as during periods of hot weather or bouts of diarrhea.

• Warn the patient to avoid alcohol, laxatives, and diuretics, which will increase fluid loss and may contribute to an imbalance.

• Tell the patient to report persistent diarrhea through the stoma, which can quickly lead to fluid and electrolyte imbalance.

• If the patient had an abdominoperineal resection, suggest sitz baths to help relieve perineal discomfort. Rec-

DIETARY MODIFICATIONS FOR OSTOMATES

Dear Patient:

As an ostomate, you need to restrict your diet initially to allow your ostomy time to heal completely and your digestive tract time to adjust gradually. Eventually, however, you'll be able to enjoy a near-normal diet. Just remember to keep in mind these instructions.

• Chew your food well. Food that isn't well chewed may not be completely digested. When eliminated, it may block your stoma.

• If the doctor has prescribed a low-fiber diet, you should stay on it for 6 to 8 weeks after surgery. This diet limits foods high in indigestible cellulose, such as vegetables, seeds, fruits, and grains. The reason? These foods may block your stoma.

• Gradually add foods to your diet. This way you'll be able to tell which foods are causing indigestion, gas, or a foul odor from your stoma.

Typically, foods that cause odor include corn, dried beans, onions, cabbage, fish, and spicy foods. Some vitamin and mineral supplements and antibiotics may also cause odor. You may want to use an ostomy deodorant or an odorproof pouch if you include odor-producing foods in your diet.

Trial and error will help you determine which foods cause gas. Vegetables that cause foul stoma odor, such as beans, cabbage, and corn, may also cause gas. Gas-producing fruits include apples, melons, avocados, and cantaloupe.

• Because you have an ostomy, you're especially susceptible to fluid and electrolyte losses. So be sure to drink plenty of fluids, especially in hot weather or when you have diarrhea. Fruit juice and bouillon, which contain potassium, are particularly helpful.

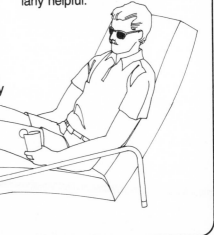

ommend refraining from intercourse until the perineum heals.

• Encourage the patient to discuss his feelings about resuming sexual intercourse. Mention that the drainage pouch won't dislodge if the device is empty and fitted properly. Suggest avoiding food and fluids for several hours before intercourse.

• Remind the patient and his family that depression commonly occurs after ostomy surgery. However, recommend counseling if depression persists.

Bowel Resection and Anastomosis

Surgical resection of diseased intestinal tissue (colectomy) and anastomosis of the remaining segments helps treat localized obstructive disorders, including diverticulosis (with an area of acute diverticulitis or abscess formation), intestinal polyps, adhesions that cause bowel dysfunction, and malignant or benign intestinal lesions. It's the preferred surgical technique for localized bowel cancer, but not for widespread carcinoma, which usually requires massive resection with creation of a temporary or permanent colostomy or an ileostomy.

Unlike the patient who undergoes total colectomy or more extensive surgery, the patient who undergoes simple resection and anastomosis usually retains normal bowel function. He is, however, at risk for many of the same postoperative complications, including bleeding from the anastomosis site, peritonitis and resultant sepsis, and problems common to all patients undergoing abdominal surgery, such as wound infection and atelectasis.

Purpose

To remove diseased portions of the bowel and join the remaining segments to restore bowel integrity and function.

Preparation

Explain that the surgery will remove a diseased portion of the patient's bowel and will connect the remaining healthy segments. Keep in mind that the patient and his family will probably have many questions about the surgery and its effect on the patient's life-style. Take the time to listen to their concerns and to answer their questions.

Discuss anticipated postoperative care measures. Tell the patient that he'll awaken from surgery with a nasogastric (NG) tube in place to drain air and fluid from the intestinal tract and prevent distention. Explain that when peristalsis returns, usually within 2 to 3 days, the tube will be removed. Tell him to anticipate ambulation on the first day after surgery, to promote return of peristalsis. Also prepare him for the presence of an I.V. line, which will provide fluid replacement, and abdominal drains.

To reduce the risk of postoperative atelectasis and pneumonia, teach the patient how to cough and deep-breathe properly and emphasize the need to do so regularly throughout the recovery period. Demonstrate incisional splinting to protect the sutures and reduce discomfort.

Before surgery, as ordered, administer antibiotics to reduce intestinal flora, and laxatives or enemas to remove fecal contents.

Ensure that the patient or a responsible family member has signed a consent form.

Procedure

The incision site varies, depending on the pathology's location. If the surgeon's performing a right colectomy, he makes an incision in the lower right abdominal quadrant through the rectus muscle. He then resects the right colonic structures, including the ascending colon, hepatic flexure, proximal portion of the transverse colon, cecum, and appendix. Next, he anastomoses the ileum and transverse colon to create an ileotransverse colostomy.

In the "no touch" technique, he performs as much of the operation as possible (such as ligation of vessels and removal of lymph nodes) before manipulating the malignancy; theoretically, this helps prevent metastasis.

In a radical left colectomy, the surgeon resects the splenic flexure, descending colon, and proximal portion of the sigmoid. Depending on the extent of carcinoma, he also may excise the attached mesentery, the spleen, and the tail of the pancreas.

In a conservative colectomy, the surgeon limits the resection to the diseased area and a wide margin of surrounding normal tissue. One such segmental resection is an anterior resection of the rectosigmoid, which preserves the anus and sphincters and allows the patient to retain some degree of normal bowel control. This procedure can be performed only if enough undiseased rectal tissue remains to allow anastomosis to the sigmoid.

After excising the diseased colonic tissue, the surgeon then anastomoses the remaining bowel segments to restore patency. End-to-end anastomosis provides the most physiologically sound junction and is the quickest to perform, but it requires that the approximated bowel segments be large enough to prevent postoperative obstruction at the anastomosis site. Side-to-side anastomosis minimizes the danger of obstruction, but this lengthy procedure may be contraindicated in an emergency.

Monitoring and aftercare

For the first few days after surgery, carefully monitor intake and output and weigh the patient daily. Maintain fluid and electrolyte balance through I.V. replacement therapy, and check the patient regularly for signs of dehydration, such as decreased urinary output and poor skin turgor.

Keep the NG tube patent. Warn the patient that, if the tube becomes dislodged, he should never attempt to reposition it himself; doing so could damage the anastomosis.

To detect possible complications, carefully monitor the patient's vital signs and closely assess his overall condition. Remember that anastomotic leakage may produce only vague symptoms at first; watch for low-grade fever, malaise, slight leukocytosis, and abdominal distention and tenderness. Also be alert for more extensive hemorrhage from acute leakage; watch for signs of hypovolemic shock (precipitous drop in blood pressure and pulse rate, respiratory difficulty, decreased level of consciousness) and bloody stool or wound drainage.

Observe the patient for signs of peritonitis or sepsis, caused by leakage of bowel contents into the abdominal cavity. Remember that a patient receiving antibiotics or I.V. hyperalimentation is at increased risk for sepsis. Sepsis also may result from "wicking" of colonic bacteria up the NG tube to the oral cavity; to prevent this problem, provide frequent mouth and tube care.

Provide meticulous wound care, changing dressings often. Check dressings and drainage sites frequently for signs of infection (purulent drainage, foul odor) or fecal drainage. Also watch for sudden fever, especially when accompanied by abdominal pain and tenderness.

Regularly assess the patient for signs of postresection obstruction. Examine the abdomen for distention and rigidity, auscultate for bowel sounds, and note passage of any flatus or feces.

Once the patient regains peristalsis and bowel function, take steps to prevent constipation and straining during defecation, both of which can damage the anastomosis. Encourage him to drink plenty of fluids, and administer a stool softener or other laxatives, as ordered. Note and record the frequency and amount of all bowel movements, as well as characteristics of the stool.

Encourage regular coughing and deep breathing to prevent atelectasis; remind him to splint the incision site, as necessary.

Home care instructions

• Instruct the patient to record the frequency and character of bowel movements and to notify the doctor of any changes in his normal pattern. Warn against using laxatives without consulting his doctor.

• Caution the patient to avoid abdominal straining and heavy lifting until the sutures are completely healed and the doctor grants permission to do so.

• Instruct the patient to maintain the prescribed semibland diet until his bowel has healed completely (usually 4 to 8 weeks after surgery). In particular, urge him to avoid carbonated beverages and gas-producing foods.

• Because extensive bowel resection may interfere with the patient's ability to absorb nutrients from food, emphasize the importance of taking prescribed vitamin supplements.

Hemorrhoidectomy

Hemorrhoidectomy refers to the surgical removal of hemorrhoidal varicosities through cauterization or excision. The most effective treatment for intolerable hemorrhoidal pain, excessive bleeding, or large prolapse, it's used when diet, drugs, sitz baths, and compresses fail to provide symptomatic relief.

A relatively quick and simple surgery, hemorrhoidectomy carries only one potentially serious complication: hemorrhage due to the rich vascularity of the region. This risk is greatest during the first 24 hours after surgery and then again after 7 to 10 days when the sutures slough off. Because of this risk, hemorrhoidectomy is contraindicated in patients with blood dyscrasias or certain GI cancers, or during the first trimester of pregnancy.

Although the patient usually is discharged on the same day as surgery, postoperative healing of delicate rectoanal tissues can be slow and painful.

For this reason, nursing care focuses on measures to promote postoperative comfort and speed healing. Such measures include administration of analgesics, frequent dressing changes and wound cleansing, and maintenance of a regular elimination schedule.

Purpose

To remove hemorrhoidal varicosities from the anus and rectum.

Preparation

Tell the patient that this operation will remove his hemorrhoids and relieve pain and bleeding. Explain the details of postoperative care, including frequent dressing changes and regular perianal cleansing. Reassure him that the nursing staff will respect his need for privacy as much as possible during these procedures. Prepare the patient for surgery by administering an enema (usually 2 to 4 hours before surgery), and by shaving and cleansing the perianal area.

Ensure that the patient or a responsible family member has signed a consent form.

Procedure

After administering a local anesthetic, the surgeon digitally dilates the rectal sphincter. He then removes the hemorrhoidal varicosities, either by clamping and cauterization or by ligation and excision. (See *Ligating Hemorrhoidal Tissue.*) He may place a small, lubricated tube in the patient's anus to drain air, fluid, blood, and flatus, or he may elect to pack the area with petrolatum gauze.

Monitoring and aftercare

After surgery, position the patient comfortably in bed; support his buttocks with pillows, if necessary. Encourage him to shift position regularly and to assume the prone position for 15 minutes every few hours to reduce edema at the surgical site.

Keep alert for acute hemorrhage and hypovolemic shock. Monitor vital signs every 2 to 4 hours, check and record intake and output, and assess for signs of fluid volume deficit, such as poor skin turgor, dry mucous membranes, and feelings of faintness, weakness, and confusion.

Check the dressing regularly, and immediately report any excessive bleeding or drainage. If bleeding is excessive, you may be asked to insert a balloon-tipped catheter into the rectum and inflate it to exert pressure on the hemorrhagic area and reduce blood loss.

Ensure that the patient voids within the first 24 hours after surgery. If necessary, help stimulate voiding with measures such as massages and warm sitz baths; catheterize him only if other measures fail to induce urination.

Using warm water and a mild soap, cleanse the perianal area to prevent infection and irritation. Gently pat the area dry. After spreading petrolatum on the wound site to prevent skin irritation, apply a wet dressing (a 1:1 solution of cold water and witch hazel) to the perianal area.

As needed, provide analgesics and sitz baths or hot compresses to reduce local pain, swelling, and inflammation and to prevent rectoanal spasms.

As soon as the patient can resume oral feeding, administer a bulk-forming or stool-softening laxative, as ordered, to ease defecation. Explain that he needs to pass stools shortly after surgery to dilate the anus and prevent the formation of strictures from scar tissue during wound healing. If he experiences pain during defecation, administer analgesics, as ordered.

Home care instructions
• Before discharge, teach the patient proper perianal hygiene: wiping gently with soft, white toilet paper (the dyes used in colored paper may cause irritation), cleansing with mild soap and warm water, and applying a sanitary pad.
• Encourage him to take sitz baths three to four times daily and after each

LIGATING HEMORRHOIDAL TISSUE

Removal of large internal hemorrhoids often requires ligation. In this surgical technique, the doctor inserts an anoscope to dilate the rectal sphincter, then uses grasping forceps to pull the hemorrhoid into position. He then inserts a ligator through the anoscope and slips a small rubber band over the pedicle of the hemorrhoid to bind it and cut off blood flow. He then excises the hemorrhoid or allows it to slough off naturally, which usually occurs within 5 to 7 days.

GRASPING THE HEMORRHOID

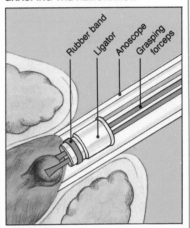

LIGATING THE HEMORRHOID

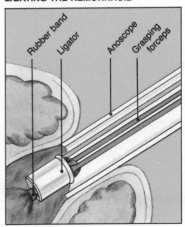

bowel movement to reduce swelling and discomfort.

- Instruct him to report increased rectal bleeding, purulent drainage, fever, constipation, or rectal spasm.
- Stress the importance of regular bowel habits. Provide tips on avoiding constipation, including regular exercise and adequate intake of dietary fiber and fluids (8 to 10 glasses of water a day).
- Warn against overusing stool-softening laxatives. Explain that a firm stool is necessary to dilate the anal canal and prevent stricture formation.

Appendectomy

With rare exceptions, the only effective treatment for acute appendicitis is appendectomy, the surgical removal of an inflamed vermiform appendix. Commonly performed in an emergency, this surgery aims to prevent imminent rupture or perforation of the appendix. When completed before these complications can occur, appendectomy is generally effective and uneventful. If the appendix ruptures or perforates before surgery, its infected contents spill into the peritoneal cavity, possibly causing peritonitis—the most common and deadly complication of appendicitis, with a mortality of 10%.

Purpose
To remove an inflamed appendix.

Preparation
Typically, you'll have little time to prepare the patient for appendectomy. Begin by reassuring him that the surgery will relieve his pain and won't interfere with normal GI functioning.

Briefly explain the surgery and answer any questions the patient and his family might have. Explain that before surgery he'll receive prophylactic antibiotics to prevent infection and I.V. fluids to maintain blood pressure during surgery. He'll have a nasogastric (NG) tube inserted to decompress the stomach and reduce postoperative nausea and vomiting, and he'll be given a sedative and general anesthetic. Tell him that he'll awaken from the general anesthetic with a dressing over the surgical site and possibly several drains in the incision; the drains will remain in place for 3 to 5 days.

Assure the patient that recovery is usually rapid; if no complications occur, he should be walking and gradually resuming oral feeding the day after surgery. He can expect to be discharged after 3 days and return to his normal activity level in 2 to 4 weeks.

While awaiting surgery, place the patient in Fowler's position to reduce pain. Avoid giving analgesics, which can mask the pain that heralds rupture. Also never apply heat to the abdomen or give cathartics or enemas; these measures could trigger rupture.

Ensure that the patient or a responsible family member has signed a consent form.

Procedure
With the patient under general anesthesia, the surgeon makes an incision in the right lower abdominal quadrant (using either a muscle-splitting, or "gridiron," incision or a McBurney's point incision) to expose the appendix. After dividing and ligating the appendicular blood vessels, he divides the appendix from the cecum and removes it. He ligates the base of the appendix and places a purse-string suture in the cecum. Then he removes any excess fluid or tissue debris from the abdominal cavity and closes the incision.

If perforation complicates appendicitis, the surgeon may insert one or more Penrose drains or abdominal sump tubes (or both) before closing the incision, to drain the abdominal cavity.

Monitoring and aftercare
After the patient awakens from the anesthetic, place him in Fowler's position to decrease the risk of any contami-

nated peritoneal fluid infecting the upper abdomen. Carefully monitor his vital signs and record intake and output for 2 days after surgery. Auscultate the abdomen for bowel sounds, indicating the return of peristalsis.

Regularly check the dressing for drainage, and change it as necessary. If abdominal drains are in place, check and record the amount and nature of drainage, and maintain drain patency. Also check drainage from the NG tube, and suction, as necessary.

Encourage ambulation within 12 hours after surgery, if possible. Assist the patient, as necessary. Also encourage coughing, deep breathing, and frequent position changes to prevent pulmonary complications. On the day after surgery, remove the NG tube and gradually resume oral foods and fluids, as ordered.

Throughout the recovery period, assess the patient closely for signs of peritonitis. Watch for and report continuing pain and fever, excessive wound drainage, hypotension, tachycardia, pallor, weakness, and other signs of infection and fluid and electrolyte loss. If peritonitis develops, expect to assist with emergency treatment, including GI intubation, parenteral fluid and electrolyte replacement, and antibiotic therapy.

Home care instructions
• Instruct the patient to watch for and immediately report fever, chills, diaphoresis, nausea, vomiting, or abdominal pain and tenderness.
• Encourage him to keep his scheduled follow-up appointments to monitor healing and detect any developing complications.

Gallbladder Surgery

When drug therapy, dietary changes, and supportive treatments fail to control gallbladder or biliary duct disease, surgery may be necessary to restore biliary flow from the liver to the small intestine.

Gallbladder removal, or *cholecystectomy*, restores biliary flow in gallstone disease (cholecystitis or cholelithiasis) and widespread carcinoma. The third most commonly performed surgery in the United States, cholecystectomy relieves symptoms in roughly 95% of patients with gallstone disease. In the remaining 5% of patients and in those who aren't considered good candidates for cholecystectomy, *cholecystostomy* or *choledochostomy* is often performed with this surgery.

After gallbladder resection, *choledochoduodenostomy* or *choledochojejunostomy* may be necessary to restore biliary flow. Similarly, biliary obstruction may require duct resection and either *cholecystoduodenostomy* or *cholecystojejunostomy*: the anastomosis of the gallbladder to the duodenum or jejunum, respectively.

Complications of gallbladder surgery, though relatively rare, can be grave. Peritonitis, for instance, may occur from obstructed biliary drainage and resultant leakage of bile into the peritoneum. Postcholecystectomy syndrome, marked by fever, jaundice, and pain, may occur. And, as in all abdominal surgeries, postoperative atelectasis may result from hampered respiratory excursion.

Purpose
To correct biliary tract obstruction and restore biliary flow from the liver to the small intestine.

Preparation
Explain the planned surgery to the patient, using clear, simple terms and diagrams. Reassure him that the surgery will relieve his symptoms and that his recovery should be rapid and uneventful. Explain that he probably will be ambulatory the day after surgery, discharged within 1 to 2 weeks, and allowed to resume his full range of activities within 4 to 6 weeks.

UNDERSTANDING GALLBLADDER SURGERIES

Gallbladder surgeries include cholecystectomy and a number of less commonly performed procedures.

CHOLECYSTECTOMY

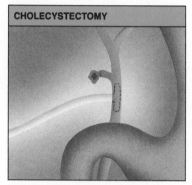

Performed under general anesthesia, this surgery begins with a right subcostal or paramedial incision. The surgeon then surveys the abdomen and uses laparotomy packs to isolate the gallbladder from the surrounding organs. After identifying biliary tract structures, he may use cholangiography or ultrasonography to help identify gallstones. Using a choledoscope, he directly visualizes the bile ducts and inserts a Fogarty balloon-tipped catheter to clear the ducts of stones.

The surgeon ligates and divides the cystic duct and artery and removes the entire gallbladder. Typically, he performs a choledochostomy: the insertion of a T tube into the common bile duct to decompress the biliary tree and prevent bile peritonitis during healing. He may also insert a Penrose drain into the ducts.

CHOLEDOCHODUODENOSTOMY OR CHOLEDOCHOJEJUNOSTOMY

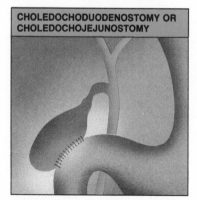

In these procedures, performed under

general anesthesia, the surgeon makes a right subcostal incision and anastomoses the common bile duct to the duodenum or jejunum. These bypass procedures avoid further jaundice from an obstruction in the distal end of the common duct.

CHOLECYSTOSTOMY

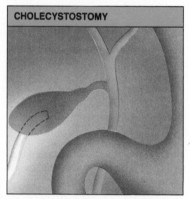

After administering a local anesthetic, the surgeon inserts a trocar with suction through a small incision in the fundus of the gallbladder to decompress and aspirate the gallbladder. Using forceps, he removes any retained gallstones or inflammatory debris. Then he inserts a drain.

CHOLEDOCHOSTOMY

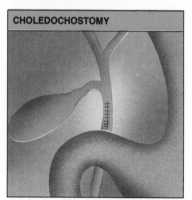

This surgery involves an incision into the common bile duct for exploration and removal of stones or other obstructions. T-tube implantation isn't usually required in this surgery. Instead, the duct is irrigated and closed.

Inform him that after surgery he'll have a nasogastric tube (NG) in place for 1 or 2 days and an abdominal drain at the incision site for 3 to 5 days. If appropriate, tell him that a T tube will be inserted in the common bile duct during surgery to drain excess bile and allow removal of retained stones. Explain that the T tube may remain in place for up to 2 weeks, depending on the surgery, and that he may be discharged with it.

Teach the patient how to perform coughing and deep-breathing exercises to prevent postoperative atelectasis, which can lead to pneumonia. Tell him that an analgesic can be administered before these exercises to relieve discomfort. Ensure that the patient or a responsible family member has signed a consent form.

Monitor and, if necessary, help stabilize the patient's nutritional status and fluid balance. Such measures may include administering vitamin K, blood transfusions, or glucose and protein supplements. For 24 hours before surgery, give the patient clear liquids only. As ordered, administer preoperative medications and assist with insertion of an NG tube.

Procedure

See *Understanding Gallbladder Surgeries* for details on the different procedures.

After completion of the surgery and, if necessary, implantation of the T tube, the surgeon removes blood and debris from the abdomen, closes the incision, and applies a dressing.

Monitoring and aftercare

When the patient returns from surgery, place him in low Fowler's position. As ordered, attach the NG tube to low intermittent suction. Monitor the amount and characteristics of drainage from the NG tube, as well as from any abdominal drains. Check the dressing frequently and change it as necessary.

If the patient has a T tube in place, frequently assess the position and patency of the tube and drainage bag. The drainage bag should be level with the abdomen to prevent excessive drainage. Also note the amount and characteristics of drainage; bloody or blood-tinged bile normally occurs for only the first few hours after surgery. Provide meticulous skin care around the tube insertion site to prevent irritation.

After a few days, expect to remove the NG tube and begin to introduce foods: first liquids, then gradually soft solids. As ordered, clamp the T tube for an hour before and an hour after each meal to allow bile to travel to the intestine to aid digestion.

Be alert for signs of postcholecystectomy syndrome (such as fever, abdominal pain, and jaundice) and other complications involving obstructed bile drainage. For several days after surgery, monitor vital signs and record intake and output every 8 hours. If any untoward signs occur, report them to the doctor and collect urine and stool samples for laboratory analysis of bile content.

Assist the patient with ambulation on the first postoperative day, unless contraindicated. Have him cough, deep-breathe, and perform incentive spirometry every 4 hours; as ordered, provide analgesics to ease discomfort during these exercises. Assess his respiratory status every 3 hours to detect hypoventilation and signs of atelectasis.

Home care instructions

• If the patient's being discharged with a T tube in place, stress the need for meticulous tube care.
• Tell the patient to immediately report any signs of biliary obstruction: fever, jaundice, pruritus, pain, dark urine, and clay-colored stools.
• Instruct the patient to maintain a diet that's low in fats and high in carbohydrates and protein. Explain that as bile flow to the intestine increases, so will his ability to digest fats; as this happens, usually within 6 weeks, he may gradually add fats to his diet.

Liver Transplant

For the patient with a life-threatening liver disorder that doesn't respond to any other medical or surgical treatments, a liver transplant may represent the only means of survival. But the many problems and risks inherent in this complex and costly surgery make it a rarely used option. It's typically reserved for the terminally ill who stand a realistic chance of surviving the surgery and withstanding postoperative complications. Candidates include patients with congenital biliary abnormalities, inborn errors of metabolism, or end-stage liver disease (with the exception of liver cancer or alcohol-induced cirrhosis).

Many qualified transplant candidates are awaiting suitable donor organs. Often the wait proves fatal. And even if a compatible healthy liver is located and transplantation performed, the patient faces many obstacles to recovery. Besides the characteristic complications associated with extensive abdominal and vascular surgeries, liver transplant carries a high risk of tissue rejection, owing to antigenic differences between the donor and recipient. Successful transplantation depends on overcoming rejection. But despite recent advances in immunosuppressive therapy and improved surgical techniques and postoperative care, the long-term survival rate for the transplant patient remains low.

Purpose
To remove a diseased liver from a terminally ill patient and replace it with a healthy donor organ.

Preparation
By the time the patient's in the hospital awaiting a liver transplant, he'll have received a thorough physical examination and undergone such tests as the barium swallow and enema, hepatic arteriography, and ultrasonography to determine his suitability as a transplant candidate. Any potentially dangerous sequelae of liver disease—portal hypertension, hepatic encephalopathy, hepatorenal syndrome, or coagulopathy—may disqualify him.

In addition, the patient will have undergone an extensive battery of tests designed to match him with a donor, including ABO compatibility, histocompatibility studies, and lymphocyte cross matching.

In the period before transplantation, work with other members of the health care team to prepare the patient for surgery. As necessary, take steps to help improve his nutritional and fluid status and to stabilize his metabolic state in preparation for the extreme demands of transplantation.

Reinforce the doctor's explanation of the transplant procedure to the patient and, if the patient's a child, to his parents. Honestly discuss the prospects of success and of postoperative complications. Point out that transplantation, even if successful, doesn't guarantee a life free from medical problems. Stress the need for lifetime follow-up care to minimize these problems.

Discuss anticipated postoperative care measures. Inform the patient that he probably will remain in the intensive care unit (ICU) for 2 to 4 weeks, in modified reverse isolation, and subsequently will be transferred to another area to continue his recovery. If possible, arrange for the patient and his family to visit the ICU and meet staff members. Prepare him for the array of equipment he'll have in place or at bedside: an endotracheal tube and mechanical ventilator, a nasogastric tube, hemodynamic monitoring lines and an EKG machine, I.V. lines, and abdominal drains. Inform him of expected fluid and food restrictions.

As ordered, begin immunosuppressive therapy to decrease the risk of tissue rejection, using such drugs as cyclosporine and corticosteroids. While doing so, explain the need for lifelong therapy to prevent rejection.

Before transplant surgery, also take time to address the patient's (and his family's) emotional needs. Discuss the typical stages of emotional adjustment to a liver transplant: overwhelming relief and elation at surviving the operation, followed—as complications set in—by anxiety, frustration, and depression. Assure him that you and other members of the health care team will be there to support him through the difficult times. Offer to refer him to a staff psychologist or psychiatric clinical nurse specialist for further support both before and after the surgery.

Ensure that the patient or a responsible family member has signed a consent form.

Procedure

The donor liver is excised from the cadaver and then preserved by inducing hypothermia and injecting an electrolyte solution into the portal vein. These methods can preserve the liver for up to 10 hours. The organ is then transported in an ice-slush solution to the transplant center.

To prepare the recipient for transplantation, the surgeon opens the abdomen, clamps and frees the vena cava and portal and hepatic vessels, and excises the diseased liver. During this critical stage, he decompresses venous return from the lower half of the body with a Partex pump connected between the iliac and axillary arteries.

Working as quickly as possible, he then positions the donor organ in place and anastomoses the upper and lower vena cava, portal vein, and hepatic artery to restore circulation. After controlling all bleeding, he reconstructs the common bile duct. The surgical assistant then evacuates the abdominal cavity of blood and debris, inserts abdominal drains, and closes and dresses the incision.

Monitoring and aftercare

Focus your aftercare on four areas: maintaining immunosuppressive ther-apy to combat tissue rejection; monitoring for early signs of rejection and other complications; preventing opportunistic infections, which can lead to rejection; and providing reassurance and emotional support to the patient throughout the prolonged recovery period. (See *Managing Complications of Liver Transplant*, page 174, for detailed instructions.)

Home care instructions

● Make sure the patient and his family understand the early indicators of tissue rejection: pain and tenderness in the right upper quadrant, right flank, or center of the back; fever; tachycardia; jaundice; and changes in the color of urine or stool. Stress the need to call the doctor immediately if any of these signs or symptoms develop.

● Instruct them to watch for and report any signs of liver failure, such as abdominal distention, bloody stool or vomitus, decreased urine output, abdominal pain and tenderness, anorexia, or altered level of consciousness.

● To reduce the risk of tissue rejection, advise the patient to avoid contact with any person who has or may have a contagious illness. Emphasize the importance of reporting any early signs of infection, including fever, weakness, lethargy, and tachycardia.

● Stress the importance of strict compliance with the prescribed immunosuppressive drug regimen. Explain that noncompliance can trigger rejection, even of a liver that has been functioning well for years. Also warn the patient of the potential side effects of immunosuppressive therapy, such as infection, fluid retention, acne, glaucoma, diabetes, or cancer.

● Emphasize the importance of regular follow-up examinations to evaluate the integrity of the surgical site and continued tissue compatibility.

● If appropriate, suggest that the patient and his family seek psychological counseling to help them cope with the effects on their lives of the patient's long-term and perilous recovery.

MANAGING COMPLICATIONS OF LIVER TRANSPLANT

COMPLICATION	ASSESSMENT AND INTERVENTION
Hemorrhage and hypovolemic shock	• Assess vital signs and other indicators of fluid volume hourly, and note trends indicating hypovolemia: hypotension; narrowed pulse pressure; rapid, weak, and occasionally irregular pulse; oliguria; decreased level of consciousness; and signs of peripheral vasoconstriction. • Monitor hematocrit and hemoglobin levels daily. • Maintain the patency of all I.V. lines, and reserve two units of blood for possible transfusion.
Vascular obstruction	• Be alert for symptoms of acute vascular obstruction in the right upper quadrant: cramping pain or tenderness, nausea, and vomiting. Notify the doctor immediately of any such symptoms. • As ordered, prepare for emergency thrombectomy. Maintain I.V. infusions, check and document vital signs, and maintain airway patency.
Wound infection or abscess	• Assess the incision site daily and report any inflammation, tenderness, drainage, or other signs of infection. • Change the dressing daily. • Note and report any symptoms of peritonitis or abscess: fever, chills, leukocytosis (or leukopenia with bands), and abdominal pain, tenderness, and rigidity. • Take the patient's rectal temperature every 4 hours. • Collect abdominal drainage for culture and sensitivity studies. Document the color, amount, odor, and consistency of drainage. • Assess for signs of infection in other areas, such as the urinary tract, respiratory system, and skin. Document and report any signs of infection.
Pulmonary insufficiency or failure	• Maintain ventilation at prescribed levels. • Monitor arterial blood gases daily, and change ventilator settings according to results and the patient's clinical status. • Auscultate for abnormal lung sounds every 8 hours. • Suction the patient frequently.
Effects of immunosuppressive therapy	• Note any signs of opportunistic infection: fever, tachycardia, chills, leukocytosis or leukopenia, and diaphoresis. • Maintain reverse isolation. • Report drug side effects, such as fluid retention, diabetes, and acne. • Check the patient's weight daily.
Hepatic failure	• Monitor nasogastric tube drainage for upper GI bleeding. • Frequently check the patient's orientation, level of consciousness, limb movement, and deep tendon reflexes. • Note development of ascites and peripheral edema. • Carefully monitor renal function by checking urine output, blood urea nitrogen levels, and serum creatinine and potassium levels. Monitor serum amylase values daily.

Liver Resection or Repair

Resection or repair of diseased or damaged liver tissue may be indicated for various hepatic disorders, including cysts, abscesses, tumors, and lacerations or crush injuries from blunt or penetrating trauma. Usually surgery is performed only after conservative measures prove ineffective. For instance, if aspiration fails to correct a liver abscess, resection may be necessary.

Liver resection procedures include a partial or subtotal hepatectomy (excision of a portion of the liver) and lobectomy (excision of an entire lobe). Lobectomy is the surgery of choice for primary liver tumors, but partial hepatectomy may be effective for small tumors. However, because liver cancer is often advanced at diagnosis, few tumors are resectable. In fact, only single tumors confined to one lobe are usually considered resectable, and then only if the patient is free of complicating cirrhosis, jaundice, or ascites.

Owing to the liver's anatomic location, surgery usually is performed through a thoracoabdominal incision. As a result, it carries many of the risks associated with both thoracic and abdominal surgery, such as atelectasis, ascites, and renal failure. What's more, impaired liver function due to surgery can result in such diverse complications as hypoglycemia from decreased hepatic gluconeogenesis, hypovolemia from a reduction in the liver's blood-storing capacity, and hepatic encephalopathy from interference with hepatic conversion of ammonia to urea. And because of the liver's friability, acute hemorrhage remains a threat during and after surgery.

Purpose
- To resect diseased hepatic tissue
- To repair hepatic injury.

Preparation
If emergency surgery is necessary, briefly explain the procedure to the patient. If surgery is elective, you'll have ample time to prepare the patient. In fact, the preparation period may extend up to 6 weeks. During this time, explain the purpose of coagulation studies; blood chemistry tests, including serum ammonia and creatinine, SGOT, SGPT, blood urea nitrogen (BUN), blood glucose, and serum electrolyte levels; arterial blood gas analysis; and blood typing and cross matching. Depending on the results of these tests, give fluid and electrolyte replacements, transfuse blood or blood components, or provide protein supplements, as ordered. Encourage rest and good nutrition and provide vitamin supplements, as ordered, to help improve liver function.

Prepare the patient for additional diagnostic tests that help locate and identify lesions. Such tests may include a liver scan, ultrasonography and a computed tomography scan, percutaneous needle biopsy, hepatic angiography, and cholangiography.

Next, explain postoperative care measures. Tell the patient that he'll awaken from surgery with a nasogastric tube, chest tube, and hemodynamic lines in place. Tell him to expect frequent checks of vital signs, fluid and electrolyte balance, and neurologic status, as well as I.V. fluid replacement and possibly blood transfusions and hyperalimentation. If possible, arrange for him to visit the intensive care unit before surgery to familiarize himself with the setting.

Because of the liver's anatomic position, surgery often interferes with normal respiratory excursion, increasing the risk of postoperative atelectasis. To reduce this risk, encourage the patient to practice coughing and deep-breathing exercises as preparation for postoperative use.

Ensure that the patient or a responsible family member has signed a consent form.

Procedure

To repair a liver laceration or crush injury, the surgeon usually makes a vertical incision in the right upper quadrant. This allows him to quickly extend the incision if he finds more damage than suspected. He resects damaged liver tissue and sutures any lacerations, then carefully explores surrounding tissue and organs for additional injury. When he has repaired all the damage and controlled bleeding, he places a chest tube or abdominal drains and closes the incision.

In elective surgery, the technique depends on the location and extent of liver disease. For a right lobectomy, the surgeon makes a thoracoabdominal incision or a right subcostal incision extending to the seventh or eighth intercostal space; for a left lobectomy, he makes a large paramedial incision.

After exposing the targeted lobe, the surgeon divides the appropriate ligamentous attachments and ligates involved hepatic vessels, rotates the liver forward, and resects the diseased tissue. Because hepatic tissue is highly friable, he handles and resects the liver cautiously and uses large, blunt, noncutting needles for suturing.

In a right lobectomy, he inserts a chest tube in the right lateral chest wall and connects it to suction to remove accumulated blood, fluid, and air. Because a left lobectomy usually doesn't involve the pleural space, no chest tube is needed. Instead, the surgeon may place one or more abdominal drains to remove fluid, blood, and air from the abdominal cavity.

Monitoring and aftercare

After surgery, frequently assess for complications, such as hemorrhage and infection. Monitor the patient's vital signs and evaluate his fluid status every 1 to 2 hours. Report any signs of volume deficit, which could indicate intraperitoneal bleeding. Be sure to maintain I.V. line patency for possible emergency fluid replacement or blood transfusion. Provide analgesics, as ordered.

At least daily, check laboratory test results for hypoglycemia, increased prothrombin time, increased ammonia levels, azotemia (increased BUN and creatinine levels), and electrolyte imbalances (especially potassium, sodium, and calcium imbalances). Promptly report any such findings and take corrective actions, as ordered. For example, give vitamin K intramuscularly to decrease prothrombin time or infuse hypertonic glucose solution to correct hypoglycemia.

Check dressings often and change them as needed. Note and report excessive bloody drainage on the dressings or in the drainage tube. Also note the amount and characteristics of nasogastric tube drainage; keep in mind that excessive drainage could trigger metabolic alkalosis. If the patient has a chest tube in place, maintain tube patency by milking it, as necessary, and make sure the suction equipment's operating properly.

Encourage the patient to cough, deep-breathe, and change position frequently to prevent pulmonary complications. Periodically auscultate his lungs and report any adventitious breath sounds.

Watch for symptoms of hepatic encephalopathy: behavioral or personality changes, such as confusion, forgetfulness, lethargy or stupor, and hallucinations. Also observe for asterixis, apraxia, and hyperactive reflexes.

Throughout the recovery period, take measures to enhance patient comfort. Promote rest and relaxation, and provide a quiet atmosphere. Assist with ambulation, as ordered.

Home care instructions

• Inform the patient that adequate rest and good nutrition will conserve his energy and reduce metabolic demands on the liver, thereby speeding healing. For the first 6 to 8 months after surgery, he should gradually resume normal activities, balance periods of activity and rest, and avoid overexertion.
• As ordered, instruct him to maintain

a high-calorie, high-carbohydrate, and high-protein diet during this period to help restore the liver mass. However, if the patient had hepatic encephalopathy, advise him to follow a low-protein diet, with carbohydrates making up the balance of caloric intake.
• Emphasize the importance of follow-up examinations to evaluate liver function.

Insertion of a LeVeen Shunt

Drainage of ascitic fluid from the abdominal cavity into the superior vena cava, using the LeVeen peritovenous shunt, helps control intractable ascites resulting from chronic liver disease.

Often used with diuretic therapy, the LeVeen shunt represents an effective alternative to traditional treatments for ascites. For example, paracentesis—the aspiration of ascitic fluid from the peritoneal cavity—was once performed routinely but is now done less commonly because ascites tends to recur rapidly and protein depletion follows each aspiration.

Despite its advantages, the LeVeen shunt can cause potentially serious complications, including ascitic fluid leakage from incisions, wound infection, subcutaneous bleeding, disseminated intravascular coagulation (DIC), and congestive heart failure (CHF). These complications, serious in any patient, pose an even greater threat to a patient with chronic liver disease.

Purpose
To drain excess fluid from the abdominal cavity into the venous system, thereby relieving chronic ascites.

Preparation
Explain to the patient that the LeVeen shunt redirects excess fluid from his abdomen into a large vein. Point out,

though, that the shunt doesn't correct the underlying cause of fluid buildup. As a result, he still needs to comply with other treatments for chronic liver disease, such as diuretic therapy.

Show the shunt to the patient and describe how it works. (See *How the LeVeen Shunt Works*, page 178.) Tell him that he'll receive a local anesthetic to prevent discomfort during shunt insertion. Also take the opportunity to teach him how to use a blow bottle; explain that breathing against resistance will promote ascitic fluid drainage once the shunt's in place.

Before surgery, measure and record the patient's weight and abdominal girth to serve as a baseline. Monitor and record his intake and output, send 24-hour urine specimens to the laboratory for electrolyte analysis, and administer prophylactic antibiotic therapy, as ordered. For 2 days before surgery, draw serum samples, as ordered, for a complete blood count (CBC). If the patient has a low hematocrit level, transfuse blood, as ordered.

Ensure that the patient or a responsible family member has signed a consent form.

Procedure
After injecting a local anesthetic at the insertion site, the surgeon makes a small incision through the abdominal wall and peritoneum. He inserts the shunt's peritoneal tube into the abdominal cavity and sutures the one-way valve in place under the skin to prevent shifting and leakage. Then he tunnels the venous tube through the subcutaneous tissue, implants it in the superior vena cava, and closes the incision.

Monitoring and aftercare
After the patient returns from surgery, take steps to enhance his comfort. Place him in low- or semi-Fowler's position, whichever he prefers. Administer analgesics, as ordered.

Monitor the patient's vital signs frequently, watching for hypervolemia or

HOW THE LeVEEN SHUNT WORKS

The LeVeen shunt consists of a peritoneal tube, a venous tube, and a one-way pressure-sensitive valve that controls fluid flow.

How does the shunt work? As the patient inhales, pressure within his abdomen increases while pressure in his superior vena cava decreases. This pressure differential causes the shunt's valve to open, allowing ascitic fluid to drain from the abdominal cavity into the superior vena cava. When the patient exhales, superior vena cava pressure rises and intraabdominal pressure falls; this pressure differential forces the valve shut, stopping fluid flow.

The valve's one-way design prevents backflow of blood into the tubing, reducing the risk of clotting and shunt occlusion. It also prevents the valve from opening if superior vena cava pressure remains higher than intraabdominal pressure, as often occurs in congestive heart failure. This reduces the risk of fluid overload in the vascular system.

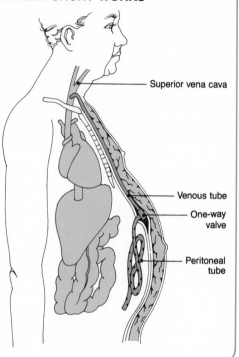

Superior vena cava

Venous tube

One-way valve

Peritoneal tube

hypovolemia. As ordered, administer an I.V. or I.M. diuretic, such as furosemide, to reduce fluid retention. Check and record intake and output hourly for the first 24 hours after surgery, then daily until discharge. Measure abdominal girth and weight daily; compare the findings with baseline data to assess fluid drainage.

As ordered, draw serum samples for CBC; serum electrolyte, blood urea nitrogen, creatinine, and albumin levels; and other studies. Monitor the results of these tests and notify the doctor of any abnormalities.

Instruct the patient to use the blow bottle for at least 15 minutes four times daily. As ordered, apply an abdominal binder for the first 24 hours after surgery. Explain that both blow bottle and binder raise intraabdominal pressure and enhance ascitic fluid drainage.

Regularly check the incision site for bleeding, swelling, inflammation, drainage, and hematoma formation. Change dressings as needed. Also be alert for signs of CHF, DIC, and GI bleeding.

Home care instructions
• Instruct the patient to continue using the blow bottle four times a day, 15 minutes at a time, for as long as the shunt is in place.
• Tell him to avoid putting pressure on the shunt to prevent clot formation and shunt occlusion.
• Advise him to watch for and immediately report bleeding or drainage from the incision site, fever, chills, diaphoresis, or other signs of infection.
• Stress the importance of regular follow-up examinations to assess shunt patency and control of ascites.

Insertion of a Portal-Systemic Shunt

In patients with intractable portal hypertension, a portal-systemic shunt reduces portal pressure and prevents or controls bleeding from esophageal varices. Typically, this surgery is performed only after more conservative measures—diet and drug therapy, electrocoagulation, and injection sclerotherapy—prove ineffective. If possible, it's performed after esophageal bleeding is controlled and the patient's condition stabilized. However, emergency surgery may be necessary if esophagogastric tamponade or vasopressor drugs can't control hemorrhage from ruptured varices.

Three types of portal-systemic shunting are performed. *Portacaval shunting*, the most common, diverts blood from the portal vein to the inferior vena cava, thereby reducing portal pressure. *Splenorenal shunting*, used in portal vein obstruction and when hypersplenism accompanies portal hypertension, diverts blood from the splenic vein to the left renal vein. *Mesocaval shunting*, indicated in portal vein thrombosis, previous splenectomy, or uncontrollable ascites, routes blood from the superior mesenteric vein to the inferior vena cava.

A delicate and complicated surgery, portal-systemic shunting possesses grave risks. For example, diversion of large amounts of blood into the inferior vena cava may cause pulmonary edema and ventricular overload. And shunting of blood away from the liver inhibits the conversion of ammonia to urea, possibly causing hepatic encephalopathy, which can progress rapidly to hepatic coma and death. Other possible complications include hemorrhage from a leaking anastomosis, which can cause peritonitis, and respiratory complications.

Because of these complications, portal-systemic shunting has a mortality of 25% to 50%. In fact, research suggests that the surgery does little to prolong survival, with patients succumbing to hepatic complications more commonly than to uncontrolled esophageal bleeding.

Purpose

To reduce portal pressure and control bleeding esophageal varices by shunting blood away from the portal venous system.

Preparation

If emergency surgery is necessary, you won't have time to provide the patient with a detailed explanation of the procedure. Instead, you'll need to focus on stabilizing the patient's condition, including assisting with measures to control bleeding.

If surgery is planned, however, explain the procedure and why it's needed. Also discuss what the patient can expect after surgery and during the recovery period. Inform him that he'll return from surgery with a nasogastric tube and a chest tube in place. He'll also be connected to a cardiac monitor and will have pulmonary artery, arterial, and central venous pressure catheters in place to monitor hemodynamic status. Tell him to expect frequent vital sign checks and neurologic assessments to detect any complications in their early stages.

While dealing with the patient's physical concerns, don't neglect his emotional needs. For example, if the patient's esophageal varices and portal hypertension are related to alcoholism (a common sequela), explain the need to stop drinking. As appropriate, offer to refer the patient to a local chapter of Alcoholics Anonymous or another self-help group for more support.

Portal-systemic shunting can only prevent or control life-threatening bleeding; it can't correct any underlying liver disease. If the patient suffers from terminal liver disease, help pre-

COMPLICATIONS

HAZARDS OF PORTAL-SYSTEMIC SHUNTING

Careful postoperative assessment can help you detect complications from portal-systemic shunting and perhaps even prevent death. For 48 to 72 hours after surgery, closely monitor the patient's fluid balance. At least hourly, check his vital signs and record intake and output. Monitor cardiac output and other hemodynamic measurements. Auscultate the patient's lungs at least every 4 hours to detect signs of pulmonary edema, such as crackles.

Watch closely for neurologic changes, such as lethargy, disorientation, apraxia, or hyperreflexia, which may point to hepatic encephalopathy and developing hepatic coma. As ordered, draw a serum sample for determination of ammonia levels. (Blood decomposition in the intestinal tract raises serum ammonia levels; a damaged liver may be unable to metabolize the ammonia, resulting in neurotoxic effects.) Also as ordered, draw blood for liver function and electrolyte studies.

Take steps to prevent respiratory complications. Encourage the patient to cough, deep-breathe, and change position at least once every hour. Provide an incentive spirometer and show him how to use it.

pare him and his family for impending death. If possible, refer them for psychological counseling.

Procedure

After the patient receives a general anesthetic, the surgeon makes an abdominal incision. In a portacaval shunt, he joins the portal vein and the inferior vena cava. The end-to-side anastomosis reduces portal pressure most effectively, but the side-to-side anastomosis allows some portal blood flow through the liver.

In a splenorenal shunt, the surgeon joins the splenic vein and the left renal vein. The end-to-side anastomosis involves splenectomy, unlike the side-to-side anastomosis, which may be used in the absence of hypersplenism.

In a mesocaval shunt, the surgeon

joins the superior mesenteric vein to the inferior vena cava. However, neither the side-to-side nor the Dacron graft anastomosis performs as well as the other shunts, and both carry the risk of thrombosis.

Monitoring and aftercare

After surgery, be sure to monitor the patient carefully for signs of developing complications. (See *Hazards of Portal-Systemic Shunting.*) Provide analgesics, as ordered.

Home care instructions

●Explain to the patient that although surgery has stopped the bleeding and will reduce the risk of future rupture, it has not corrected the underlying liver disease. Emphasize the importance of complying with his prescribed dietary and drug regimens, including strict abstention from alcohol. Also stress the need for adequate rest to reduce the risk of bleeding and infection.

● Tell the patient and his family to watch for and immediately report disorientation, lethargy, amnesia, slurred speech, asterixis, apraxia, and hyperreflexia. Explain that these signs and symptoms may herald hepatic encephalopathy, a potentially fatal complication.

● Stress the importance of regular follow-up examinations to evaluate shunt patency and liver function.

INTUBATION

Nasoenteric Decompression

In this treatment, a doctor or a specially trained nurse inserts a long, weighted nasoenteric tube through the patient's stomach and into the intestinal tract. The tube is then propelled by peristalsis through the intestine to, and possibly through, the obstruction, thereby relieving it.

Along with fluid and electrolyte replacement, nasoenteric decompression normally represents the initial treatment for acute intestinal obstruction resulting from polyps, adhesions, fecal impaction, volvulus, or localized carcinoma. It usually relieves the obstruction, especially in the small intestine. However, if the patient fails to show signs of improvement, or if his condition deteriorates, bowel resection may be necessary.

Nasoenteric decompression may also be performed to aspirate gastric contents or to prevent GI upset after abdominal surgery. It can, however, cause complications. The most common include reflex esophagitis, nasal or oral inflammation, and nasal or laryngeal ulcers. Rarely, atelectasis and pneumonia may result from the presence of the tube in the esophagus and its interference with normal coughing. And excessive intestinal drainage can produce acid-base imbalance or malposition of the tube within the intestine. Fortunately, these complications can be prevented by scrupulous postoperative care.

Purpose
• To relieve acute intestinal obstruction
• To aspirate gastric contents for examination
• To prevent nausea, vomiting, and abdominal distention after GI surgery.

Preparation
Briefly explain the procedure to the patient. Tell him that he'll experience mild discomfort as the doctor inserts and advances the tube. Reassure him that he'll be given a sedative if intubation proves difficult or painful.

Next, gather and prepare the equipment. If you're using a Cantor tube, inject the proper amount of mercury

into the balloon. If you're using a Miller-Abbott tube, inflate the balloon and check for leaks. Be sure to deflate the balloon completely before insertion; it will be filled with mercury or water only after it passes through the pylorus and into the duodenum.

After preparing the equipment, place the patient in semi-Fowler's position and help him to relax.

Procedure
After determining how far the tube must be advanced to reach the pylorus, the doctor applies a water-soluble lubricant to the first few centimeters of the tube to reduce friction and ease insertion. He then inserts the tube into the selected nostril, telling the patient to breathe through his mouth. When the tube reaches the nasopharynx, he instructs the patient to lower his chin to his chest and swallow repeatedly to help advance the tube. After the tube passes the trachea, the doctor may allow the patient to sip water to facilitate swallowing. If intubation proves difficult, administer a sedative, as ordered.

The doctor advances the tube slowly and carefully until it reaches the stomach. After confirming correct placement of the tube, he orders the patient positioned to help gravity and normal peristaltic action advance the tube further. Usually the patient is positioned on his right side until the tube passes through the pylorus, and then he's placed on his back in Fowler's position as it advances through the duodenum. To confirm the tube's passage into the duodenum, the doctor tests the pH of an intestinal aspirate; normal intestinal pH is less than 7.0.

If a Miller-Abbott tube is being used, the doctor injects mercury into the balloon lumen when the tube enters the duodenum.

Once the tube is inserted the premeasured distance (or if tube advancement is halted by the obstruction), the doctor orders abdominal X-rays to confirm its location. If these confirm proper tube placement, secure the tube to prevent further advancement and to keep it from being pulled out. (Never tape the tube directly to the patient's skin; rather, wrap it with gauze, then tape the gauze to the cheek.) As ordered, connect the tube to intermittent suction.

Monitoring and aftercare

The patient with a nasoenteric tube in place needs to receive special care and continuous monitoring. Frequently check the tube's patency and the effectiveness of intestinal suction and decompression. Note and record the amount and nature of drainage. As ordered, irrigate the tube with normal saline solution.

Regularly check the patient's vital signs and assess his fluid and electrolyte status. Record his intake and output and be sure to watch for signs of fluid imbalance, such as decreased urine output, poor skin turgor, skin and mucous membrane dryness, lethargy, and fever.

Monitor for acid-base imbalance. Watch for signs of metabolic alkalosis (altered level of consciousness, slow and shallow respirations, hypertonic muscles, and tetany) or acidosis (dyspnea, disorientation and, later, weakness, malaise, and deep, rapid respirations). Also watch for signs of secondary infection, such as fever and chills.

Provide mouth care and apply petrolatum to the nostril openings at least every 4 hours. Check for signs that indicate the return of peristalsis. These include the presence of bowel sounds, decreased abdominal distention, passage of flatus, or a spontaneous bowel movement. If these signs occur, notify the doctor and assist with tube removal.

Home care instructions

The nasoenteric tube is removed before discharge. As a result, the patient doesn't require treatment-related directions for home care.

Iced Gastric Lavage

Using ice water or an iced saline solution, gastric lavage represents an emergency treatment for GI hemorrhage caused by peptic ulcer disease or ruptured esophageal or gastric varices. It involves intubation with a large-bore single- or double-lumen tube, instillation of irrigating fluid, and aspiration of gastric contents. The iced fluid causes vasoconstriction of GI vessels, thereby controlling hemorrhage. In some cases, a vasoconstrictor such as norepinephrine may be added to the irrigating fluid to enhance this action.

Complications of iced gastric lavage, although rare, may become serious if untreated. The most common one is vomiting with subsequent aspiration. Fluid overload may develop, especially in elderly or debilitated patients, as may electrolyte imbalance or metabolic alkalosis. Bradyarrhythmias may occur as a result of vagal stimulation and lowered body temperature.

Iced saline solution may be contraindicated for patients on sodium-restricted diets. For such patients, ice-water lavage is preferred.

Purpose

To control upper GI hemorrhage.

Preparation

Tell the patient (or his family, if the patient's uncommunicative) that this treatment rinses the stomach with cold fluid to stop internal bleeding. Tell him that he may experience some discomfort during intubation, but reassure him that the procedure isn't usually painful. Stress the importance of his relaxation and cooperation during treatment.

Assemble the necessary equipment at the patient's bedside: a bulb syringe with solution container, a basin filled with ice, 2 to 3 liters of irrigating fluid (normal saline solution or water, as ordered), an empty basin for return fluid, a measuring cup, an emesis basin, towels and a bed-saver pad, tissues, a water-soluble lubricant, and a large-lumen gastric tube, as ordered. (See *Comparing Nasogastric Tubes*, page 184.) Make sure a suction machine with catheter is readily available.

Position the patient in high Fowler's position and help him relax. Cover his gown with a bed-saver pad and put a blanket over him to keep him warm. If he's wearing dentures, remove them.

If time permits, draw blood samples for a complete blood count, typing, and cross matching.

Procedure

Chill the irrigating solution in a basin of ice and pour the solution into the container. Cover the end of the tube with a water-soluble lubricant; then insert it into the patient's mouth or nostril, as ordered. Advance the tube through the pharynx and trachea and into the stomach. If you've intubated the patient nasally, have him sip water or suck ice chips to aid tube passage; however, don't give the patient water or ice if you've intubated orally.

Once you think the tube is in the patient's stomach, check tube placement. First, attach a bulb or piston syringe to the tube and try to aspirate gastric fluid. (Caution: Never aspirate gastric fluid forcefully; you may injure the gastric mucosa.) If you cannot, reposition the tube and try again. Even if you can aspirate fluid, you can't assume the tube is properly placed. To confirm placement, attach a bulb syringe to the tube and inject about 30 ml of air. Using a stethoscope, auscultate for air entering the stomach (marked by swooshing or gurgling sounds). If you can't hear these sounds, the tube may be in the bronchus or esophagus.

When the tube is in place, lower the head of the bed to 15 degrees and reposition the patient on his left side, if possible. (If this position is contraindicated, keep him in high Fowler's po-

---

GASTRIC LAVAGE: SOME GIVE IT TEPID

Although an iced solution is normally used for lavage, some hospitals now recommend instilling a room-temperature solution.

Why? This recommendation is based on the premise that the vagal stimulation produced as the iced solution moves down the esophagus stimulates gastric secretion of hydrochloric acid. This increased secretion stimulates GI motility and can aggravate bleeding.

---

sition to prevent aspiration of vomitus.) Next, fill the syringe with 30 to 50 ml of irrigating solution and begin instillation. Instill a total of about 250 ml of fluid, wait 30 seconds, and then begin to withdraw the fluid into the syringe. If you're unable to withdraw any fluid, allow the tube to drain into the emesis basin.

If the doctor has ordered a vasoconstrictor added to the irrigating fluid, wait for a prescribed period of time before withdrawing fluid, to allow the drug to be absorbed into the gastric mucosa.

Carefully measure and record fluid return and document the character of the aspirate. Abdominal distention and vomiting will occur if the volume of return doesn't at least equal the amount of fluid instilled. If it doesn't, reposition the tube. If this doesn't increase return, stop lavage and notify the doctor.

Continue lavage until the return fluid is clear, or as ordered. After completing lavage, aspirate any remaining fluid from the patient's stomach. Then remove the tube or secure it, as ordered.

Monitoring and aftercare

Never leave the patient alone during gastric lavage. Watch him continuously for developing complications, such as vomiting and aspiration. Monitor his vital signs every 30 minutes until his condition stabilizes. Stay alert for bradyarrhythmias, hypothermia, and signs of hypovolemia, such as hypoten-

COMPARING NASOGASTRIC TUBES

Five types of gastric tubes are commonly used: the Argyle Salem sump, Bard-Parker, Edlich, Ewald, and Levacuator.

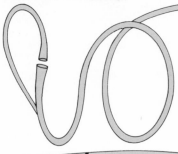

Argyle Salem sump
This 48" (122 cm) long, double-lumen, clear plastic tube has holes at the tips and along the sides, a blue sump port (which helps prevent mucosal damage during suctioning), and markings at 18", 22", 26", and 30". It also has a radiopaque Sentinel Line for X-ray confirmation of placement. The tube is used for gastric lavage, aspiration of gastric contents, and tube feedings.

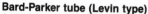

Bard-Parker tube (Levin type)
A 50" (127 cm) long, single-lumen, clear plastic tube with holes at the tip and along the sides, this tube has the same clinical uses as the Argyle Salem sump.

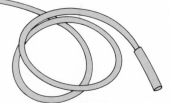

Edlich tube
This wide-bore, single-lumen, clear plastic tube has four openings near the closed distal tip. It's used for gastric lavage and aspiration of gastric contents. The wide-bore design allows rapid evacuation of gastric contents, making the tube especially useful in emergency situations.

Ewald tube
This wide-bore, single-lumen, clear plastic tube has several openings at the distal end. It's used for gastric lavage and aspiration of gastric contents. Like the Edlich tube, the Ewald tube's wide bore allows rapid aspiration of gastric contents.

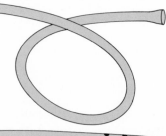

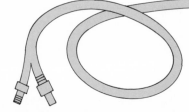

Levacuator tube
This wide-bore, clear plastic tube has a large lumen for aspirating gastric contents and a small one for instilling irrigating fluid. It's used for gastric lavage and aspiration of gastric contents. Like the Edlich and Ewald tubes, the Levacuator tube allows rapid evacuation of gastric contents.

sion and an increased respiratory rate. Also watch for other indicators of fluid volume deficit: decreased level of consciousness, dry skin and mucous membranes, and poor skin turgor. As ordered, provide I.V. fluid replacements or blood transfusions to correct any volume deficit.

Suction the patient's mouth, as necessary, to prevent aspiration and airway obstruction. Make sure emergency equipment is readily available in case obstruction occurs.

Home care instructions

Because the patient who undergoes iced gastric lavage is discharged only after he's stabilized, he doesn't require treatment-related instructions for home care.

Esophagogastric Tamponade

In this emergency treatment, insertion of a multilumen esophageal tube helps to control esophageal or gastric hemorrhage resulting from ruptured varices. The most commonly used esophageal tubes include the Minnesota, the Linton, and the Sengstaken-Blakemore tubes. (See *Comparing Esophageal Tubes*, page 186.)

The tube is inserted through a nostril, or sometimes through the mouth, and then passed through the esophagus into the stomach. Inflation of the tube's esophageal and gastric balloons exerts pressure on the varices and stops bleeding, while a suction lumen allows esophageal and gastric contents to be aspirated. A nasogastric (NG) tube may also be used to aspirate oral secretions and to check for bleeding above the esophageal balloon.

Typically, the balloons are deflated within 48 hours, after measures have been taken to identify and control the source of the bleeding. Balloon infla-

tion for more than 48 hours may cause pressure necrosis, which can produce further hemorrhage. Other potential complications include airway obstruction from tube migration or balloon rupture and tissue necrosis at the insertion site.

Purpose

To provide temporary control of esophageal or gastric hemorrhage and prevent excessive blood loss.

Preparation

Explain to the patient (or to his family, if the patient's unable to communicate) that this treatment aims to stop bleeding from the esophagus and stomach. Provide reassurance and emotional support. Stress the importance of relaxing and cooperating during intubation. Administer a sedative, as ordered, to help the patient relax.

Place the patient in semi-Fowler's position to aid gastric emptying and prevent aspiration of vomitus. However, if the patient's unconscious, position him on his left side with the head of the bed raised about 15 degrees.

As ordered, draw blood samples to determine serum electrolyte levels, complete blood count, Rh type, and cross matching. Also draw arterial samples for blood gas measurements.

Next, gather and prepare the equipment: an esophageal tube (as ordered), an NG tube, an irrigation set, a piston syringe, a bulb syringe, a large basin with ice, a water-soluble lubricant, four hemostats, a small sponge block or a football helmet with face mask, a Hoffman clamp, and adhesive tape. Make sure a suction machine is on hand and in good working order. Keep emergency resuscitation equipment readily available. Tape a pair of scissors to the head of the bed to cut the tube in case of acute respiratory distress.

Determine the length of NG tube needed by measuring the distance between the esophageal balloon and the suction lumen on the esophageal tube; mark the NG tube at the appropriate

COMPARING ESOPHAGEAL TUBES

Three commonly used esophageal tubes include the Sengstaken-Blakemore tube, the Linton tube, and the Minnesota esophagogastric tamponade tube.

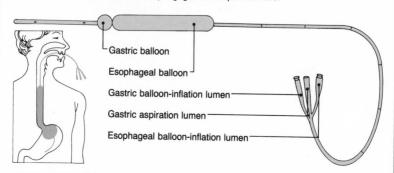

Gastric balloon

Esophageal balloon

Gastric balloon-inflation lumen

Gastric aspiration lumen

Esophageal balloon-inflation lumen

The Sengstaken-Blakemore tube, a three-lumen device with esophageal and gastric balloons, has a gastric aspiration port that allows drainage from below the gastric balloon and enables instillation of medication.

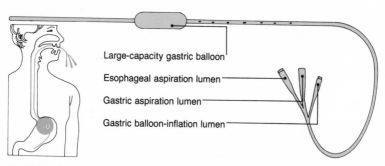

Large-capacity gastric balloon

Esophageal aspiration lumen

Gastric aspiration lumen

Gastric balloon-inflation lumen

The Linton tube, a three-lumen, single-balloon device, has ports for esophageal and gastric aspiration. Because the tube doesn't have an esophageal balloon, it isn't used to control bleeding from esophageal varices. When used to treat gastric bleeding, the tube carries a decreased risk of esophageal necrosis.

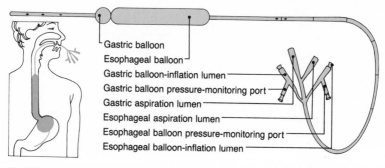

Gastric balloon

Esophageal balloon

Gastric balloon-inflation lumen

Gastric balloon pressure-monitoring port

Gastric aspiration lumen

Esophageal aspiration lumen

Esophageal balloon pressure-monitoring port

Esophageal balloon-inflation lumen

The Minnesota esophagogastric tamponade tube has four lumens and two balloons. It has pressure monitoring ports for both balloons, thus eliminating the need for Y connectors.

spot. Open the disposable irrigation set, and fill the container with normal saline solution. Then, check the balloons for air leaks by inflating them and holding them under water. If you don't detect any leaks, deflate the balloons and clamp their lumens so that they remain deflated during intubation. Run water through the esophageal and NG tubes to test patency. Also check the patency of all aspiration lumens, and make sure they're labeled properly.

Finally, chill the distal ends of the esophageal and NG tubes in ice to stiffen them and aid insertion.

Procedure
First, the doctor checks the patency of the patient's nostrils to determine the best nostril for tube insertion. However, if nasal intubation is contraindicated, he'll insert the tube orally. He then sprays the posterior pharynx and nostril (as appropriate) with an anesthetic to minimize discomfort and prevent gagging during intubation.

After applying a water-soluble lubricant to the tip of the esophageal tube, the doctor twists both balloons around the tube and inserts it. As he does so, he encourages the patient to breathe through his mouth.

To aid passage of the tube into the esophagus, the doctor asks the patient to tilt his chin downward toward his chest and swallow. He may allow the patient to sip water or suck ice chips to prevent gagging.

Once the tube reaches the stomach, the doctor aspirates gastric contents with a bulb syringe attached to the tube's suction port. Document the amount, color, and consistency of the aspirate.

Next, the doctor inserts the NG tube through the other nostril and advances it the premeasured distance into the lower esophagus. Connect the tube to low-continuous suction and tape it in place on the patient's cheek.

After confirming proper esophageal tube placement by X-rays, the doctor inflates the gastric balloon with 250 to 500 ml of air. He then double-clamps the gastric port with hemostats. As ordered, apply gentle traction to the tube by placing a small sponge block around the tube and under the patient's nose, then taping the tube to the sponge. Or you can slide a football helmet over the patient's head and tape the tube to the lower bar of the face mask. Once the tube is securely in place, the doctor inflates the esophageal balloon to the desired pressure (usually 30 to 40 mm Hg) and double-clamps the tube.

Connect intermittent gastric suction to the large suction port to empty the stomach, help prevent nausea and vomiting, and allow continuous observation of gastric contents for bleeding.

Monitoring and aftercare
Never leave the patient unattended during esophagogastric tamponade. Closely monitor his condition and the tube's lumen pressure. Check vital signs every 30 to 60 minutes; a change may indicate recurrence of bleeding or other complications.

As ordered, maintain drainage and suction on the esophageal and gastric aspiration ports to prevent fluid accumulation. Irrigate the gastric aspiration port with normal saline solution to prevent clogging.

Watch for signs of respiratory distress while the esophageal tube's in place. If it develops, have someone else notify the doctor. Then quickly pinch the tube at the patient's nose and cut it with scissors. Next, remove the tube.

Be alert for esophageal rupture, heralded by signs of shock, increased respiratory difficulty, and increased bleeding. Rupture can occur at any time but is most common during intubation or esophageal balloon inflation. Be prepared to transfuse blood, if needed.

Keep the patient warm and comfortable. Instruct him to remain as still and quiet as possible; if ordered, administer a sedative to help him relax. Provide frequent mouth and nose care, applying a water-soluble ointment to the nostrils to prevent tissue irritation and pressure sores.

When bleeding has been controlled, assist with tube removal.

Home care instructions

Because the patient who undergoes esophagogastric tamponade is discharged only after he's stabilized, he doesn't require treatment-related instructions for home care.

ENDOSCOPY

Endoscopic Retrograde Sphincterotomy

Originally developed to remove retained gallstones from the common bile duct after cholecystectomy, endoscopic retrograde sphincterotomy (ERS) is now also used to treat high-risk patients with biliary dyskinesia and to insert biliary stents for drainage of malignant or benign strictures in the common bile duct.

In ERS, the doctor advances a fiberoptic endoscope through the stomach and duodenum to the ampulla of Vater. He then passes a cutting wire, known as a sphincterotome or papillotome, through the endoscope and makes a small incision to widen the biliary sphincter. The stone may drop out into the duodenum on its own, or the doctor may need to introduce a Dormier basket, a balloon, or a lithotriptor through the endoscope to remove or crush the stone. Alternatively, the doctor may introduce an endobiliary prosthesis, or stent, through the endoscope to bypass a bile duct obstruction and restore normal biliary drainage.

ERS allows treatment without general anesthesia or a surgical incision, assuring a quicker and safer recovery. And it may be performed on an outpatient basis for some patients, making it a cost-effective alternative to surgery. Complications of ERS include hemorrhage, transient pancreatitis, cholangitis, and sepsis.

Purpose

To relieve obstruction of biliary drainage.

Preparation

Explain the treatment to the patient, and answer any questions he may have. Tell him that he'll have an anesthetic sprayed in his throat to eliminate any discomfort during insertion of the endoscope and that he may also receive a sedative to help him relax and to reduce secretions. Reassure him that the sphincterotomy should cause little or no discomfort.

Position the patient on the fluoroscopy table in a left side-lying position, with his left arm behind him. Encourage him to relax and, if ordered, administer a sedative.

Procedure

After anesthetizing the patient's throat, the doctor inserts the fiberoptic endoscope. He passes it through the stomach, into the duodenum, and to the ampulla of Vater. Then he injects a radiopaque dye to allow fluoroscopic visualization of the obstruction. After dye injection, he asks the patient to shift to the prone position, which helps the dye flow to the ampulla and bile duct.

Once the doctor locates the obstruction, he passes the sphincterotome through the endoscope and, under fluoroscopic guidance, into the ampulla of Vater. He then sends an electric current through the sphincterotome to incise the papillary sphincter and widen the duct.

Depending on the size and position of the stones, the doctor either allows them to pass naturally through the

TRANSHEPATIC BILIARY CATHETERIZATION

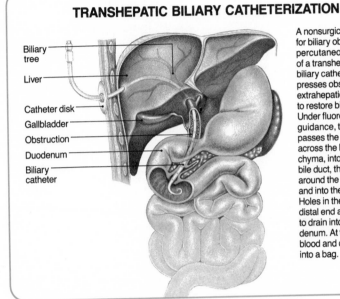

Biliary tree

Liver

Catheter disk

Gallbladder

Obstruction

Duodenum

Biliary catheter

A nonsurgical treatment for biliary obstruction, percutaneous insertion of a transhepatic biliary catheter decompresses obstructed extrahepatic bile ducts to restore bile flow. Under fluoroscopic guidance, the doctor passes the catheter across the liver parenchyma, into the common bile duct, through or around the obstruction, and into the duodenum. Holes in the catheter's distal end allow bile to drain into the duodenum. At the other end, blood and debris drain into a bag.

widened duct and into the duodenum or removes them with a balloon catheter or Dormier basket. If the doctor detects an extremely large stone, he may crush it using a lithotriptor. Cholangiography confirms stone passage or removal.

After sphincterotomy, the doctor may choose to insert a nasobiliary catheter to drain bile and temporarily decompress the biliary tree. To do so, he inserts a large-bore (#10 or #12 French) catheter into the common bile duct, then attaches the proximal end to a collection device.

To insert an endobiliary prosthesis, the doctor passes a stent through the endoscope and through the sphincterotomy opening. He positions it with the distal tip above the obstruction and the proximal end in the duodenum to reestablish duct continuity and allow free flow of bile.

Monitoring and aftercare

After treatment, help the patient maintain good pulmonary hygiene. To prevent aspiration of secretions, instruct him to cough, deep-breathe, and expectorate regularly. Keep in mind that the anesthetic's effects may hinder expectoration and swallowing. Withhold food and fluids until the anesthetic wears off and the patient's gag reflex returns.

Check the patient's vital signs frequently and monitor carefully for signs of hemorrhage: hematemesis, melena, tachycardia, and hypotension. If any of these signs develop, notify the doctor immediately.

Also observe for other complications. Cholangitis, for instance, produces hyperbilirubinemia, high fever and chills, abdominal pain, jaundice, and hypotension. Pancreatitis may be marked by abdominal pain and rigidity, vomiting, low-grade fever, tachycardia, diaphoresis, and elevated serum amylase levels (although elevated serum amylase by itself doesn't confirm pancreatitis). If you note any complications, call the doctor and prepare to draw serum samples for culture and sensitivity studies and to administer antibiotics, as ordered.

Home care instructions
• Instruct the patient to immediately report any signs of hemorrhage, sepsis, cholangitis, or pancreatitis.
• Advise him to report any recurrence of the characteristic jaundice and pain of biliary obstruction. He may need repeat ERS to remove new stones or replace a malfunctioning biliary stent.

BOWEL MANAGEMENT

Bowel Training

Establishing a bowel training routine can help correct constipation and, in some patients, incontinence. Bowel training attempts to reestablish a regular pattern of elimination through changes in diet and life-style, supplemented by limited use of laxatives, enemas, or suppositories, as necessary.

The success of a bowel training program depends on the patient's ability to perform self-care measures, his willingness to do so, and the presence of a strong support system of family or friends. What's more, this program requires considerable time and patience to be effective. On your part, it requires sensitivity to the patient's feelings of discomfort and embarrassment.

Purpose
To help the patient establish a normal elimination pattern.

Preparation
Assess the patient's overall condition to ensure that he's well enough—and sufficiently stable—to withstand the lengthy and sometimes frustrating bowel training program. Next, take a complete bowel history. Remember that many patients, especially elderly ones, may be reluctant to discuss elimina-

tion. To help the patient overcome such reluctance, provide privacy and use a supportive tone of voice.

Begin by asking the patient how often he defecates. Does he usually have a bowel movement after meals? Immediately upon arising in the morning?

Explore his use of medications. Does he take laxatives to stimulate evacuation or kaolin-pectin preparations to suppress incontinence? If so, how long has he used them? Does he have any particular dietary preferences or restrictions?

Begin bowel training by discussing the overall goals of the program. Be sure to tell the patient that, contrary to popular wisdom, a daily bowel movement isn't necessary for good health. In fact, for an elderly person, a bowel movement every 2 or 3 days may be sufficient. Emphasize that a regular pattern of elimination, based on his individual needs and abilities, is the goal of training.

Procedure
Essential components of a bowel training program include:
• Adequate fluid intake—usually between 2,000 and 4,000 ml/day, unless contraindicated. Fluids promote softer stool and help stimulate peristalsis.
• Increased dietary fiber to contribute bulk to the stool and stimulate peristalsis. Good sources of dietary fiber include whole-grain and bran cereals, fresh fruits, and raw vegetables.
• A regular schedule for defecation. Toileting should follow each meal so that attempts at defecation are made at about the same time each day. Approximately 30 minutes after a meal (when the gastrocolic reflex reaches its peak effect), place the patient on a toilet (or commode or bedpan, as appropriate). Have him remain there for a minimum of 10 to 15 minutes. Raising his feet and having him lean forward may help him to defecate. If the patient must use a bedpan, he should assume a sitting position, if possible.

• Increased level of activity, as appropriate, to stimulate and maintain intestinal motility and tonicity. If the patient's able, encourage regular ambulation and teach him how to perform abdominal and perineal exercises to strengthen and retrain the anal musculature.

• If necessary, a laxative, enemas, or glycerin suppositories to stimulate defecation. If you must use these measures, you should gradually phase them out during the duration of the training program (usually 6 to 8 weeks), until the patient can defecate consistently without them.

• Digital stimulation to relax the anal sphincter and promote elimination. For a patient with spinal cord injury or other neurologic damage, it may be a necessary part of the training program. To perform this procedure, insert a lubricated finger of a gloved hand about 1 to 2 cm into the patient's rectum. Then gently rotate the finger for 30 to 60 seconds.

• Operative conditioning to improve sphincter muscle tone in a patient who is incontinent. To accomplish this, you'll insert a balloon attached to a monitor into the rectum and inflate it. Instruct the patient to contract his sphincter against the pressure from the balloon and to check his progress on the monitor.

Monitoring and aftercare

Because consistency is crucial to successful bowel training, be sure that all caregivers follow the program strictly. Careful, detailed documentation of each step of the program, along with the patient's response, is also essential.

Consult with other health care providers, as necessary, to eliminate any impediments to successful training. For example, dental work may be required if bad teeth or poorly fitting dentures interfere with maintaining the prescribed diet.

Home care instructions

• Tell the patient never to ignore the urge to defecate.

• Make sure he has convenient access to clean, private toilet facilities. Consult with family or caregivers to ensure such access.

• Instruct the patient or his caregivers about dietary measures necessary to his bowel management program.

• Warn the patient against overingestion of bran, which can impair iron absorption.

Selected References

Barrett, N. "Ileal Loop and Body Image," *AORN Journal* 36:712, October 1982.

Broadwell, D., and Jackson, B. *Principles of Ostomy Care.* St. Louis: C.V. Mosby Co., 1981.

Cohen, S., ed. *Clinical Gastroenterology: A Problem-Oriented Approach.* New York: John Wiley & Sons, 1983.

Daly, J., and DeCosse, J. "Complications in Surgery of the Colon and Rectum," *Surgical Clinics of North America* 63(6):1215-31, December 1983.

Duranceau, A.C. "Symposium on Esophageal Surgery," *Surgical Clinics of North America* 63:4, 1984.

Fazio, V.W. "Regional Enteritis: Indications for Surgery and Operative Strategy," *Surgical Clinics of North America* 63(1):27-48, February 1983.

Gebhart, E. M. "Perioperative Care of the Ostomy Patient," *AORN Journal* 36:296, August 1982.

Groah, L. *Operating Room Nursing.* East Norwalk, Conn.: Appleton & Lange, 1982.

Nyhus, L., and Watell, C. *Surgery of the Stomach and Duodenum,* 3rd ed. Boston: Little, Brown & Co., 1977.

5

Treating Nutritional and Metabolic Dysfunction

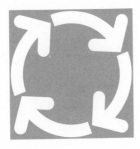

Treating Nutritional and Metabolic Dysfunction

Introduction

Of all the treatments in which you play a role, perhaps the most unique are those for metabolic and nutritional disorders. Where other therapies typically involve drugs or surgery, these are characteristically centered around specialized diets.

A sound solution
The premise of all these diets is straightforward and sound: to reduce symptoms of disease by altering intake of substances that the patient's body can't properly digest, metabolize, or excrete. But though they're deceptively simple, these diets can work wonders. In infants born with phenylketonuria, for instance, they sidestep the disease's grim—and, at one time, inevitable—prognosis of neurologic damage and mental retardation. For patients with elevated cholesterol levels or celiac disease, they can permit a long and virtually normal life.

Drawbacks and obstacles
These therapies also have some drawbacks, the most important of which can be summarized in a single word: compliance. When you ask a patient to change his eating habits, you're challenging some of his most basic and deeply ingrained behavior patterns. Indeed, you're not simply up against *his* behavior; you're often faced with an entire cultural heritage that places strong emotional values on how one eats, when one eats, and most important of all, *what* one eats.

That's why you have to do a lot of groundwork to help patients make positive changes in their lives. The dietary history, for example, is vital; so is thorough patient teaching and follow-up care to help the patient identify and overcome obstacles. And because of the cultural aspects, it's important to remember that your nursing care can't be limited to the patient; to be successful, it must include the family—especially the person who does most of the cooking for the patient.

An important reminder
One last thing to keep in mind: tread carefully. For example, to you, the dangers of red meat for a patient with high cholesterol levels may be a simple fact of chemistry; to the elderly patient who struggled through the Depression to feed her family, your recommendations may seem to border on heresy, and she may be insulted if you seem to imply that her cooking is responsible for her husband's heart problems. It's these sorts of unexpected (and often unexpressed) reactions that can sabotage your best efforts, so remember: whenever possible, season your suggestions tastefully and tactfully.

DRUG THERAPY

Bile Acid–Sequestering Resins

Bile acid–sequestering resins—which include the drugs *cholestyramine* and *colestipol*—are sometimes used to treat hyperlipoproteinemia. They're prescribed for patients in whom diet, exercise, and diabetic control haven't reduced serum lipid levels and for patients with familial hypercholesterolemia, who have high levels of low-density lipoproteins (LDLs) and normal levels of very low-density lipoproteins (VLDLs). They're also used to treat combined hyperlipoproteinemia, a condition in which both LDL and VLDL levels are elevated.

Bile acid–sequestering resins have a number of drawbacks, however. For one, these drugs can only be used prophylactically; they can't remove fatty deposits that are already present in the patient's arteries. And even their prophylactic value isn't clearly established; although they reduce the incidence of nonfatal myocardial infarction (MI), they haven't been shown to lessen the risk of other cardiovascular disorders or of death.

In addition, patient compliance is often difficult to achieve; the drugs must be taken two to four times a day and may cause constipation and GI upset. They must be used cautiously in patients with coronary artery disease, since straining because of constipation can trigger angina or MI. What's more, the drugs can worsen peptic ulcers and malabsorption states—especially steatorrhea. In patients with impaired renal function, they increase the risk of hyperchloremic acidosis. And they must be used cautiously in patients with biliary obstruction or atresia, since bile acids are diminished or absent in such patients.

For all of the reasons just given, bile acid–sequestering agents aren't widely used.

Purpose and action
Cholestyramine and colestipol bind with bile acids in the intestine, preventing reabsorption of cholesterol and thereby increasing the rate at which the liver converts cholesterol into bile acids. In addition, cholestyramine speeds LDL removal by stimulating LDL receptors.

Monitoring
Monitor serum cholesterol and triglyceride levels to evaluate drug effects. Watch for adverse reactions, especially in a patient with peptic ulcers, malabsorption, or impaired renal function.

Encourage fluids to help prevent constipation. However, if constipation occurs, notify the doctor and administer stool softeners, as ordered.

If the patient's taking other oral medications, give them an hour before or 4 hours after he takes cholestyramine or colestipol. Because both drugs can inhibit the absorption of vitamins A and D (which are fat-soluble) and calcium, administer supplements, as ordered.

Home care instructions
● To prevent esophageal irritation or blockage, instruct the patient to take the drug with large amounts of water, fruit juice, soup, or pulpy fruit.
● Give the patient dietary guidelines (see "Low-Cholesterol Diet," page 208), and urge him to eat high-fiber foods to help combat constipation. Tell him that if he experiences constipation, he should call his doctor, who may reduce the drug dosage or prescribe a stool softener.
● Explain that other side effects, such as heartburn, nausea, indigestion, and

abdominal pain, usually diminish with time.
• Tell the patient that if he misses a dose, he should take it as soon as possible; however, he shouldn't double-dose.

Antihyperlipidemics

The antihyperlipidemic drugs *gemfibrozil* and *clofibrate* provide adjunctive treatment for severe Type III or IV primary hyperlipidemia that doesn't respond to dietary restrictions, weight loss, exercise, or good diabetic control.

The use of antihyperlipidemics is controversial. Although these drugs lower serum triglyceride levels, some studies suggest that this reduction doesn't diminish the risk of cardiovascular disease and mortality. In addition, the antihyperlipidemics have numerous drawbacks: they can cause cholelithiasis and cholecystitis and shouldn't be given to patients with primary biliary cirrhosis, since they could further elevate cholesterol levels. What's more, clofibrate may reactivate peptic ulcers and increase the risk of peripheral vascular disease, pulmonary embolism, thrombophlebitis, angina pectoris, arrhythmias, and intermittent claudication.

Purpose and action
Clofibrate and gemfibrozil reduce serum levels of very low–density lipoprotein by inhibiting their hepatic production or release.

Monitoring
Watch for biliary complications in patients with gallstones. Monitor kidney and liver function, since antihyperlipidemics are cleared through these organs.

Be alert for nausea, vomiting, diarrhea, or flatulence, especially in a patient with a peptic ulcer. If any of these signs occur, notify the doctor; he may

reduce the dosage or discontinue the drug altogether.

Monitor hepatic enzyme levels and complete blood counts monthly to detect liver dysfunction, anemia, or leukopenia. If any of these occur, notify the doctor; he'll probably discontinue the drug.

Home care instructions
• Emphasize to the patient that the prescribed drug can help control his condition but can't cure it. Urge him to follow a low-fat diet (see "Low-Fat Diet," page 211).
• Tell the patient to take the drug with food to minimize GI distress.
• If the patient has renal disease, instruct him to call his doctor if he experiences flulike symptoms or muscle pain or soreness.
• Tell the patient to take a missed dose as soon as possible but not to double-dose.
• Emphasize the importance of frequent checkups. Tell the patient that the doctor may discontinue therapy if triglyceride levels do not drop within 3 months.

Vitamin Supplements

Prescribed when dietary sources fail to provide adequate vitamins, these organic compounds are most commonly needed by pregnant and lactating women, infants, strict vegetarians, the elderly, and people who are on a calorie-restricted diet. In addition, supplements are often indicated for postsurgical patients and those undergoing treatment for cancer, alcoholism, GI disturbances, anorexia, or hyperthyroidism.

Vitamin supplements are widely promoted as a treatment for conditions ranging from cancer to the common cold. However, controlled clinical studies haven't substantiated these claims, pointing out instead that vita-

UNDERSTANDING VITAMIN SUPPLEMENTS

Most people know that vitamins are essential for growth and development. But how they're stored and given can greatly influence their intended effects. And how they act can depend on the patient's condition, his use of prescription or over-the-counter drugs, and other factors. When you're administering a vitamin supplement, review the appropriate section below for important nursing concerns.

Vitamin C
• Don't give to infants by I.M. injection since tissue necrosis can occur.
• Give I.V. doses of vitamin C slowly; rapid injection can cause dizziness and syncope. Administer cautiously in renal insufficiency since excess amounts are excreted in urine.

• Protect parenteral solution from light.
• Avoid giving sodium-containing preparations of vitamin C to patients on a sodium-restricted diet. Similarly, avoid giving preparations containing calcium to patients who are receiving digitalis since cardiac disturbances may result.

Thiamine (vitamin B₁)
• Perform sensitivity tests before giving large I.V. doses. During administration, keep epinephrine readily available to treat anaphylaxis.
• Keep in mind that B vitamins act together; an excess amount of one can cause an increased need for the others.

• In a patient with Wernicke's syndrome, give thiamine before I.V. glucose to prevent worsening of symptoms.
• Don't add thiamine to alkaline I.V. solutions; it will decompose.
• Rotate I.M. injection sites to reduce discomfort.

Riboflavin (vitamin B₂)
• Before riboflavin is absorbed, it must be combined with phosphorus. Give with dairy products.
• Because riboflavin supplements are

sensitive to light, keep them in an opaque container.
• Don't give riboflavin with alkaline substances.

Niacin (vitamin B₃)
• Don't give niacin to patients with an active peptic ulcer, hepatic dysfunction, severe hypotension, hemorrhage, or arterial bleeding. Use cautiously in patients with gallbladder disease, diabetes mellitus, or gout.
• Give I.V. only for severe niacin deficiency. Use slow injection.
• Begin therapy with small doses to minimize side effects; increase dosage gradually. Initial therapeutic response usually occurs within 48 hours.
• Administer niacin supplements with meals to reduce GI upset. Tell the patient to avoid taking niacin with hot beverages because of increased vasodilation.

• Inform the patient that tingling, itching, headache, or a sensation of warmth—especially around the head, neck, and ears—can occur shortly after administration but that these effects usually subside with continued therapy. Niacinamide or timed-release niacin may be given to minimize them.
• Monitor hepatic function and blood glucose levels frequently.
• Caution the patient against prolonged exposure to bright sunlight. Also warn him against engaging in hazardous activities because he may experience dizziness or weakness—particularly early in the course of therapy.

Pyridoxine (vitamin B₆)
• Keep in mind that pyridoxine requirements may be increased in patients taking isoniazid, cycloserine, oral contraceptives,

hydralazine, or penicillin.
• Give the vitamin cautiously during lactation since it blocks prolactin.

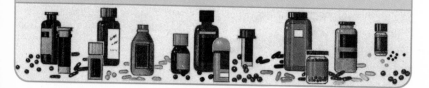

UNDERSTANDING VITAMIN SUPPLEMENTS *(continued)*

Cyanocobalamin (vitamin B₁₂)
- To prevent impaired vitamin absorption, don't give neomycin, colchicine, para-aminosalicylic acid, or chloramphenicol with cyanocobalamin. Don't administer parenterally to a patient with a hypersensitivity to cobalt. Don't mix with other parenteral medications.
- Because I.V. administration may cause an anaphylactic reaction, give by this route only when other routes are ruled out.
- Protect it from light and heat.
- Closely monitor serum potassium levels for first 48 hours. Give potassium, if necessary.

Vitamin A
- Oral administration contraindicated in malabsorption syndrome. However, if malabsorption results from inadequate bile secretion, oral route may be used with concurrent administration of bile salts. Also contraindicated in hypervitaminosis A.
- I.V. administration contraindicated except for special water-miscible forms intended for infusion with large parenteral volumes. Never give any form of vitamin A by I.V. push since *death may occur.*
- Don't give vitamin A or carotene (its precursor) with mineral oil, cholestyramine resin, or colestipol. These drugs can impair vitamin absorption.
- Because of the potential for additive toxicity, vitamin A should be used cautiously with isotretinoin.
- In severe hepatic dysfunction, diabetes, or hypothyroidism, use vitamin A rather than carotene. However, if carotene is prescribed, dosage should be doubled.
- Adequate vitamin A absorption requires suitable protein intake, bile, concurrent recommended-daily-allowance doses of vitamin E, and zinc.
- Absorption is fastest and most complete with water-miscible preparations, intermediate with emulsions, and slowest with oil suspensions.
- Watch for symptoms of hypervitaminosis, such as bone pain and irritability. Closely monitor for skin disorders, since high doses may induce chronic toxicity.
- Carefully evaluate vitamin A intake from fortified foods, dietary supplements, and drugs to help avoid toxicity. Discourage self-administration of megadoses.
- In pregnant women, avoid doses exceeding recommended daily allowance.
- Liquid preparations are available if nasogastric administration is necessary. This vitamin may be mixed with cereal or fruit juice.
- Record eating and bowel habits. Report abnormalities to the doctor.
- Protect from light and heat.

Vitamin D
- Contraindicated in hypercalcemia, hypervitaminosis A, and renal osteodystrophy with hyperphosphatemia because of the risk of metastatic calcification. Use cautiously in renal impairment.
- If I.V. route is necessary, use only water-miscible solutions intended for dilution in large-volume parenterals. Use cautiously in cardiac patients, especially if they're receiving cardiotonic glycosides.
- Monitor eating and bowel habits; dry mouth, nausea, vomiting, metallic taste, and constipation can herald toxicity.
- If the patient has hyperphosphatemia, enforce dietary phosphate restrictions and give binding agents to avoid metastatic calcification and renal calculi.
- When high doses are used, monitor serum and urine calcium, potassium, and urea levels. Doses of 60,000 units/day can cause hypercalcemia.
- Malabsorption due to inadequate bile or to hepatic dysfunction may require addition of exogenous bile salts to oral vitamin D. Space doses. Use together cautiously.
- I.M. injection of vitamin D dispersed in oil is preferable in patients who are unable to absorb oral form.
- This vitamin is fat-soluble. Warn patient against increasing dosage on his own.
- Tell the patient to restrict his intake of magnesium-containing antacids.

(continued)

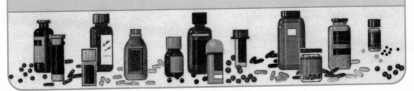

UNDERSTANDING VITAMIN SUPPLEMENTS *(continued)*

Vitamin E

• Use cautiously with aluminum-containing antacids since large amounts of aluminum hydroxide may precipitate bile acids in the upper small intestine, thereby decreasing absorption of fat-soluble vitamins. Also use cautiously with antihyperlipidemics, iron supplements, and vitamin A.

• Water-miscible forms are more completely absorbed in GI tract than other forms.
• Adequate bile is essential for absorption.
• Requirements increase with rise in dietary polyunsaturated acids.
• Vitamin E may protect other vitamins against oxidation.

Folic acid

• Folic acid is contraindicated in normocytic and aplastic anemias; in the treatment of overdose of methotrexate, pyrimethamine, or trimethoprim; and in undiagnosed anemia (since it may mask pernicious anemia) or refractory anemia. It's also contraindicated as the sole agent in treating

pernicious anemia since it may mask neurologic effects.
• If the patient has a sore mouth and tongue, provide soft bland foods or liquids.
• Don't mix folic acid with other medications when administering intramuscularly.
• Protect it from light and heat.

Vitamin K

• Use cautiously, if at all, during last weeks of pregnancy to avoid toxic reactions in newborns, and in glucose-6-phosphate dehydrogenase deficiency to avoid hemolysis. Use large doses cautiously in severe hepatic disease since they could further impair function.
• Use cautiously with other drugs. Concurrent use of antihyperlipidemics, for instance, may decrease vitamin K absorption.
• Administer I.V. over 2 to 3 hours. Mix in normal saline solution, dextrose 5% in water, or dextrose 5% in normal saline solution. Observe patient closely for flushing,

weakness, tachycardia, and hypotension.
• Failure to respond to vitamin K may indicate coagulation defects.
• In severe bleeding, don't delay other measures, such as transfusion.
• Protect parenteral products from light. Wrap infusion container with aluminum foil.
• Effects of I.V. injections are more rapid but shorter-lived than S.C. or I.M. injections.
• Monitor prothrombin time to determine dosage effectiveness.
• Phytonadione (vitamin K_1) therapy in infants causes fewer adverse reactions than do other vitamin K analogues.

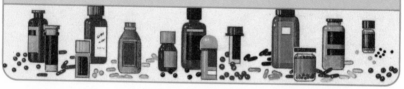

min supplements aren't necessary for well-nourished, healthy individuals. In fact, they may cause a variety of ill effects, such as anorexia, headache, nausea, and vomiting.

Purpose
• To help correct vitamin deficiency
• To supplement dietary intake in patients with high vitamin requirements.

Monitoring
Vitamins vary greatly in their route of administration, their side effects, and their interactions. (See *Understanding*

Vitamin Supplements, pages 196 to 198, for a summary of nursing considerations.)

Home care instructions
• Warn the patient about the dangers of taking megadoses of vitamins without his doctor's approval. Encourage him to eat a well-balanced diet instead.
• To preserve water-soluble vitamins, instruct the patient to steam vegetables and not to overcook them.
• Explain that synthetic vitamins are no less effective than natural vitamins despite their lower cost.

Mineral Supplements

Supplements correct mineral deficiency caused by dietary deficiency, increased metabolic demands, or disease. They're most commonly prescribed for children, pregnant women, the elderly, and patients with burns or other injuries. Mineral supplements are also given to patients receiving intravenous hyperalimentation.

Purpose
- To correct mineral deficiencies or to help meet increased metabolic demands

- To offset poor mineral absorption.

Monitoring
Minerals vary considerably in their route of administration, their side effects, and their interactions. (See *Understanding Mineral Supplements* for a summary of important nursing considerations.)

Home care instructions
Inform the patient that many mineral supplements are sold in combination with vitamin preparations. Point out, though, that these preparations are appropriate for patients requiring a general supplement. However, he should be sure to take only his prescribed supplement.

UNDERSTANDING MINERAL SUPPLEMENTS

Minerals help build bone and soft tissue and form hair, nails, and skin. They serve other purposes, too. Iron and copper, for instance, promote synthesis of hemoglobin and red blood cells. Other minerals help regulate muscle contraction and relaxation, blood clotting, and acid-base balance.
  When administering a mineral supplement, keep in mind these important considerations.

Calcium
- Give cautiously if the patient has a history of renal calculi since calcium can precipitate into the urine.
- If the patient's taking a cardiac glycoside, monitor serum drug levels. Increased calcium levels can heighten the risk of drug toxicity.
- Don't give calcium with dairy products, bran cereal, spinach, rhubarb, or corticosteroids to prevent impaired absorption.
- If the patient's receiving a calcium supplement, tell him to take it 1 hour after meals to reduce GI upset.
- Monitor serum and urine calcium levels. Report excessive increases, which could indicate hypercalcemia.

Potassium
- Keep in mind that the parenteral form must be diluted in large amounts of fluid and given slowly. *Direct injection of undiluted potassium can cause death.*
- Don't give to patients with severe renal impairment or heart block, acute dehydration, or excessive tissue damage or to those receiving captopril or cardiac glycoside therapy. Hyperkalemia could occur.
- Use cautiously with potassium-sparing diuretics, salt substitutes, low-salt milk, or other potassium-containing drugs.
- Use oral potassium supplements cautiously if the patient's taking atropine or related compounds since GI lesions can occur.
- Monitor intake and output to check kidney function. Check EKG for possible arrhythmias; if they occur, notify the doctor.
- Tell the patient to take potassium supplements immediately after meals to help prevent GI upset.
- Don't give postoperatively until urine flow is established.

(continued)

Ca Cu Fe K Mg Na Zn

UNDERSTANDING MINERAL SUPPLEMENTS (continued)

Phosphorus
• Dilute phosphorus in a large amount of fluid and infuse slowly to prevent vessel irritation. Monitor sodium or potassium levels, depending on which salt is used. Report elevations.

• Be alert for symptoms of tetany (muscle spasms, paresthesias around the mouth and in the extremities, abdominal pain, hair loss, and arrhythmias) from insufficient calcium or excessive phosphorus.

Sodium
• Use cautiously in patients with congestive heart failure, impaired renal function, or edema.
• Monitor serum electrolyte levels frequently since imbalances can occur during therapy.
• Check intake and output daily since excessive sodium can cause fluid retention.
• Weigh the patient daily.

Oral iron
• Contraindicated in hemosiderosis and hemochromatosis. Use cautiously in peptic ulcer, regional enteritis, and ulcerative colitis. Also use cautiously in long-term therapy.
• Tell the patient that GI upset is related to dose. Instruct him to take iron between meals since food may decrease absorption; however, if he experiences nausea, he may take the supplements with food. (Enteric-coated products reduce GI upset, but they also reduce iron absorption.)
• Advise him not to take iron supplements for at least 2 hours after eating dairy products, eggs, coffee, tea, or whole grain bread or cereals since these foods interfere with absorption.
• If he's taking a liquid iron preparation, instruct him to dilute it in juice (preferably orange juice) or water, but not in milk or antacids. If he's taking tablets, tell him to take them with orange juice to promote absorption.
• Warn the patient that iron is toxic and that such symptoms as vomiting, upper abdominal pain, pallor, cyanosis, diarrhea, and drowsiness indicate toxicity. Provide the phone number of the local poison control center, and suggest keeping ipecac syrup available.
• To prevent iron toxicity, tell the patient to continue with the regular dosage schedule if he misses a dose; he shouldn't double-dose.
• Let the patient know that his stools may turn black because of unabsorbed iron. Reassure him that this effect is harmless.
• Check for constipation and record the color and amount of stool. Teach dietary measures for preventing constipation.
• To avoid staining teeth, give iron elixir with a glass straw.
• Monitor hemoglobin and reticulocyte counts during therapy.

Parenteral iron
• Contraindicated in hemosiderosis, hemochromatosis, and all anemias other than iron deficiency anemia. Use with extreme caution in impaired hepatic function and rheumatoid arthritis.
• Check policy before giving I.V. iron dextran. Some hospitals don't permit infusion because of its questionable safety.
• Inject deeply in upper outer quadrant of buttock—never into an arm or other exposed area—with a 2" to 3", 19G or 20G needle. Use Z-track technique to avoid leakage into subcutaneous tissue and tatooing of skin. However, use I.V. route when muscle mass is insufficient for deep I.M. injection; when absorption from muscle is impaired; when massive and prolonged parenteral therapy may be necessary; and when I.M. injection may cause severe bleeding.
• Minimize skin staining by using a separate needle to withdraw drug from container.
• Monitor the patient's vital signs during I.V. administration. Reactions are varied, ranging from pain, inflammation, and myalgia to hypotension, shock, and even death.
• Monitor hemoglobin and hematocrit levels, and reticulocyte count.
• Upon completion of I.V. iron dextran infusion, flush the vein with 10 ml of 0.9% sodium chloride injection. Tell the patient to rest for 15 to 30 minutes.

Ca Cu Fe K Mg Na Zn

UNDERSTANDING MINERAL SUPPLEMENTS (continued)

Magnesium
• Contraindicated in impaired renal function, myocardial damage, heart block, and active labor.
• Use parenteral magnesium with extreme caution in patients receiving cardiac glycosides. Treating magnesium toxicity with calcium in such patients could cause serious alterations in cardiac conduction; heart block may result.
• I.V. bolus dose must be injected slowly to avoid respiratory or cardiac arrest.
• If available, use an infusion pump for I.V. administration. The maximum flow rate is 150 ml/minute. Rapid drip causes a feeling of heat.
• Monitor vital signs every 15 minutes when giving I.V. for severe hypomagnesemia. Watch for respiratory depression and signs of heart block. Respirations should exceed 16/minute before dose is given since magnesium can cause respiratory depression.
• Monitor intake and output. Output should be 100 ml or more during 4-hour period before dose.
• Test knee jerk and patellar reflexes before each additional dose. If absent, give no more magnesium until reflexes return. Otherwise, the patient may develop temporary respiratory failure and need CPR or I.V. calcium.
• Check magnesium levels after repeated doses. Keep I.V. calcium available to reverse magnesium intoxication.
• After giving to toxemic mothers within 24 hours before delivery, watch the neonate for signs of magnesium toxicity, including neuromuscular and respiratory depression.

Copper and zinc
• Monitor serum levels during therapy.
• Tell the patient to take zinc with meals.
However, warn him not to take it with dairy products, which can decrease absorption.

Ca Cu Fe K Mg Na Zn

Appetite Suppressants

Chemically related to amphetamines, the appetite suppressants include *benzphetamine, diethylpropion, fenfluramine, mazindol, phenmetrazine,* and *phentermine.* They're used with dietary restrictions, behavior modification, and exercise to treat obesity. They can be taken only for 6 to 12 weeks, since tolerance and dependence develop with longer use. Typically, they're reserved for patients who lose weight with great difficulty or who've reached a plateau in their weight-loss program.

Because appetite suppressants act like amphetamines in stimulating the CNS, they're contraindicated for patients who are known drug abusers. They must be used cautiously in patients with cardiovascular disease, hyperthyroidism, and hyperexcitability states. Chronic overuse can cause severe dermatoses, insomnia, hyperactivity, irritability, and personality alterations—including psychosis. Diethylpropion may cause increased seizure activity.

Purpose and action
Appetite suppressants exert their effects on the appetite control center in the hypothalamus. Most of them work by affecting dopamine and norepinephrine metabolism. Fenfluramine, by contrast, appears to influence serotonin metabolism.

Monitoring
Review the patient's drug regimen for possible interactions. Appetite sup-

pressants, for instance, shouldn't be used for at least 2 weeks after a patient has discontinued a monoamine oxidase inhibitor; otherwise, hypertensive crisis could occur.

During therapy, observe the patient for signs of excessive stimulation—for example, hypertension, restlessness, or dizziness. Assess for cardiac effects, such as palpitations, an irregular pulse, and tachycardia. If the patient's diabetic, also monitor blood and urine glucose levels since these drugs can alter glucose metabolism. If any adverse effects occur, notify the doctor; he'll probably reduce the dosage or discontinue the drug.

Home care instructions
• Emphasize to the patient that drug therapy is an adjunct to dietary restrictions and exercise.
• Tell him not to consume excessive amounts of meat, dried fish, beer, or Chianti wine. These high-tyramine foods and beverages could increase blood pressure when combined with appetite suppressants.
• Caution the patient to avoid caffeine-containing products because of the additive stimulant effect.
• Tell the patient to take the drug 30 to 60 minutes before meals and to take the last dose of the day 4 to 6 hours before bedtime to reduce insomnia. However, if the drug causes GI irritation, instruct him to take it at mealtime. Or, if he's taking an extended-release or long-acting drug, tell him to take it when he awakens in the morning.
• Instruct the patient to swallow extended-release capsules whole. If he were to chew or crush them, a large quantity of the drug could be released quickly, causing severe side effects.
• Tell the patient not to increase the drug dosage on his own. Explain that when tolerance begins to develop, the doctor will discontinue the drug gradually to prevent withdrawal symptoms.
• Warn him to avoid activities requiring alertness or good psychomotor coordination until his response to the drug has been determined.
• If the patient's taking fenfluramine, explain that the drug can cause drowsiness.
• Suggest ice chips or sugarless candy or gum to relieve dry mouth.

DIETARY THERAPY

Calorie-Modified Diet

Say the word "diet" to most patients and they'll think of a calorie-modified diet—specifically, a low-calorie diet. These diets are among the most popular—and most abused—forms of self-treatment, and a large part of your job with obese patients will be to counter the misinformation they've been exposed to. You'll need to emphasize that dieting is just one part of an overall treatment plan that may also include exercise, behavior modification, psychotherapy, drugs, or even surgery. In addition, you'll need to stress the dangers of unbalanced fad diets, "quick" diets, and fasting, explaining that a balanced low-calorie diet that results in a weight loss of a pound or so a week is the most effective means of long-term weight loss.

For some patients, a calorie-modified diet means *increased* caloric intake. Patients may be underweight because of poor eating patterns; excessive activity (for example, athletic training); improper food absorption; wasting diseases, such as cancer or hyperthyroidism; or anorexia nervosa. For these patients, the goal of therapy is to add 500 to 1,000 calories/day through a diet that's high in protein and carbohydrates, with moderate amounts of fat.

Compliance, of course, is the major obstacle for patients on a calorie-modified diet. That's obvious with patients requiring a low-calorie diet, but keep in mind that those on a high-calorie diet may also find it difficult to adhere to their dietary regimen. In fact, such patients can pose the more difficult challenge, at least in the hospital; for while food can simply be withheld from an obese patient, it's much more difficult to persuade an underweight patient to eat if he doesn't want to.

With both types of patients, you'll need to use a great deal of ingenuity to help them maintain their diets over the long term. Be flexible—creative, even—in your approach. For example, if the patient doesn't like to count calories, help him develop a food-exchange plan similar to the one diabetic patients use. Encourage the obese patient to learn low-calorie cooking techniques. Suggest that he record his daily intake in a food diary to help him understand his eating patterns. Tell him that he can eat several small meals throughout the day instead of three regular ones (but tell him not to eat too heavily in the evening hours, since these calories will tend to be converted into fat as he sleeps). Warn the patient to expect setbacks, and explore ways of overcoming them.

Above all, be positive; tell the patient that although change may come slowly and painfully, the benefits are well worth the struggle.

Purpose
To help correct weight imbalances.

Preparation
Before beginning a calorie-modified diet, all patients—underweight as well as overweight—should receive a thorough medical examination.

After you've reviewed the results of this examination, take a dietary history. Ask the patient what kinds of foods he likes and dislikes and how they're prepared. Talk about eating habits; find out if the patient eats regular meals, skips some meals, or snacks between meals.

Also explore food-related behavior. For example, ask the patient whether he sits down at a table to eat or eats while standing, driving, or watching television. Ask him if he smokes and whether he's trying to quit; a patient trying to stop smoking will often have difficulty following a diet.

With an obese patient, also discuss the benefits of exercise and the role of behavior modification, psychotherapy, and prescribed drugs in weight loss. Encourage him to join a weight-loss support group. In addition, help him set reasonable weight-loss goals, and stress that gradual reduction helps keep weight from returning.

With an underweight patient, set a realistic goal for weight gain—for most patients, about 1 lb/week. Recommend a hearty breakfast and regular meals, and explore ways of adding more calories to the diet—for example, by eating extra snacks or by using a concentrated liquid supplement. Depending on the patient's underlying condition, you may wish to use a behavior modification plan.

Procedure
Depending on the *obese patient's* sex, weight, and activity level, the doctor may prescribe a diet providing 1,000 to 1,800 calories/day, with about 20% of them coming from protein. For the patient whose obesity presents an immediate threat to life, the doctor will probably recommend an extremely low-calorie diet—about 300 to 700 calories/day—that includes high-quality protein and few carbohydrates.

A weight-reduction diet includes foods from all four groups. Besides limiting carbohydrates, it restricts fats and alcohol and includes fiber to reduce caloric density and slow digestion.

The *underweight patient* requires a high-protein and high-calorie diet providing 500 to 1,000 additional calories/day. To prevent anorexia and nausea, fat intake remains normal.

UNMASKING THE FAD DIET

"Take off 16 pounds in 2 weeks!" "Melt away ugly bulges forever!" "Lose weight on watercress!" The claims of fad diets are everywhere, it seems—emblazoned in bold type in magazine ads, capturing headlines in disreputable papers at supermarket checkout stands, prominently featured in window displays of book stores and health-food stores. A large part of your role as a health educator is to counter these pie-in-the-sky claims and help your patients develop a realistic weight-loss plan.

But it may take some salesmanship of your own to convince patients that gradual, moderate weight loss is not only the most healthy, but also the most effective, method of dieting. You'll need to explain, for example, that although pounds may be shed rapidly with a fad diet, they usually come right back. The reasons? Much of the initial weight that's lost is simply fluid, and it'll start to return the first time the dieter drinks a glass of water. And even when the diet actually reduces fat tissue, it doesn't affect the "set point"—a sort of natural thermostat in the hypothalamus that governs the body's metabolic rate. Thus, the pounds quickly return as soon as the diet's over. What's more, studies show that when a person loses and regains weight, he'll have much more difficulty losing it a second time.

Fad facts

Admittedly, a gimmick can sometimes help motivate a person to stick with a diet. And not all popular diets are bad; just be sure the one your patient chooses is sound. Here are some telltale signs that can help you spot a fad diet:
- They promise rapid success.
- They're promoted as "easy" or "painless."
- They involve some "new," "exclusive," or "patented" nutritional theory or system—which, upon close inspection, is almost always unproven.
- They cost money—for a book, videotape, program, formula, or pills.
- They're often based on repetition; for example, they may call for the dieter to eat grapefruit or ice cream every day.
- They're nutritionally deficient, usually in one of the calorie-containing food groups (protein, fat, or carbohydrates).

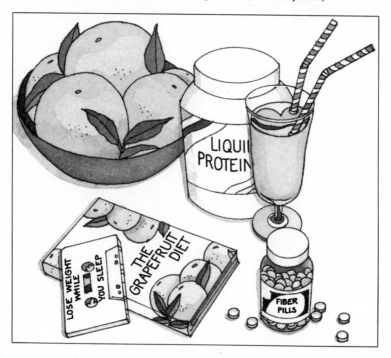

For the patient on a high-calorie diet, gradually increase caloric intake over time so that he can adjust to the added amounts. Use extra helpings, snacks, and concentrated supplements to increase caloric intake.

Monitoring

Weigh the patient weekly to chart his progress. Since he will ideally be gaining or losing only 1 lb/week, explain to him that more frequent weighings aren't necessary. In fact, daily fluctuations primarily result from fluid retention and are likely to be misleading.

Have both overweight and underweight patients bring in food diaries when they're weighed, and review the choices and amounts of foods that they've eaten. Be sure that the patient is drinking sufficient fluids to prevent orthostatic hypotension.

Monitor urine nitrogen levels in an overweight patient. The reason? Nitrogen imbalance and loss of lean tissue mass are especially prevalent in a patient on an extremely low-calorie diet.

Home care instructions

• Enlist the support of the patient's family. Their encouragement and cooperation are vital to help the patient maintain his diet.
• Suggest that the overweight patient plan menus and shopping lists for the week to prevent impulse buying and eating. Encourage him to have fish and poultry instead of red meat, to substitute polyunsaturated fats for saturated ones, and to eat vegetables and fruits instead of sweets.
• Suggest to the underweight patient that he eat dried fruits and nuts for between-meal snacks, since they're high in calories and nutritious. Recommend that he eat bananas with breakfast and that he have potatoes, pasta, noodles, or rice at least twice a day.
• Arrange a consultation with a dietitian for the patient with a severe weight imbalance. A team effort—with doctor, nurse, dietitian, and therapist partic-

ipating—may be necessary to help the patient.
• Encourage the patient not to abandon his diet simply because he sometimes "cheats"; explain that occasional noncompliance matters little to long-term success. Help him use behavior modification techniques to reduce noncompliance; for example, set a goal of slowly reducing the number of "cheating" episodes per week.
• Tell the patient on a reducing diet to avoid alcohol since it can cause a hypoglycemic response.
• Tell the female patient who's losing weight to watch for menstrual disorders and to report them to her doctor. Prolonged dieting can cause amenorrhea.
• Be sure that the patient regulates his energy expenditure. The underweight patient may need to cut down on his activities; the overweight person should develop an exercise program.

Fiber-Modified Diet

Fiber makes up a crucial part of the diet—and yet, paradoxically, it's completely indigestible. Its benefits are primarily mechanical in nature: it promotes peristalsis, reduces intestinal transit time, and increases stool volume and weight.

A high-fiber diet can help prevent diverticulitis by distending the colon and relieving pressure on the intestinal wall. It can help treat obesity by decreasing caloric density and promoting a feeling of fullness. Water-soluble fibers, such as pectin, can lower serum cholesterol levels and help prevent coronary artery disease. A high-fiber, low-cholesterol diet can help diabetic patients reduce—and in some cases, eliminate—their need for insulin and oral hypoglycemic drugs, apparently by promoting a moderate blood glucose response to ingested food and enhancing tissue sensitivity to insulin. Some researchers even believe that a high-fiber diet can prevent bowel cancer by reducing the concentration of carcinogens in fecal matter.

Although dietary fiber is usually beneficial, its use may need to be restricted in patients who are suffering from indigestion, gastric reflux, or diarrhea. In addition, a low-fiber diet is normally ordered both before and after GI surgery. In all of these instances, the diet aims to eliminate mechanical stimulation of an inflamed or irritated GI tract.

Because low-fiber diets lack sufficient vitamins and minerals, they can be used for only a limited time.

Purpose

- *For a high-fiber diet:* to prevent constipation and to treat diverticulitis, obesity, hypercholesterolemia, or diabetes mellitus.
- *For a low-fiber diet:* to reduce mechanical stimulation of the bowel and limit gastric secretions.

Preparation

For a high-fiber diet, review the patient's dietary intake and explain the benefits that the diet offers. You may find the patient with diverticulitis apprehensive about eating high-fiber foods in the mistaken belief that they're difficult to digest. If so, explain how dietary fiber can relieve his symptoms by helping to stretch the colon and prevent pouching of the intestinal wall from excess pressure. Tell the patient that side effects, such as a bloated feeling and diarrhea, can be minimized by adding fiber to his diet gradually.

With the dietitian, help the patient and his family identify foods that are high and low in fiber. Explain that mineral and vitamin deficiencies may occur with either a high-fiber diet (because of reduced absorption) or a low-fiber diet (because of the foods that are eaten). Mention that the patient needs to eat a variety of foods and may have to take vitamin and mineral supplements.

Procedure

Diabetic patients on a high-fiber diet should consume 30 to 50 g of fiber a day; for other patients, the diet is more flexible and should simply include as much fiber as practical.

A high-fiber diet should include breads and baked goods made from 100% whole wheat or whole rye flour instead of white flour. Other sources of high fiber include granola, oatmeal, unpeeled apples and other fruits, and raw and leafy vegetables, such as carrots and lettuce. Coarsely ground bran can be added to cereals, muffins, or bread as a further fiber supplement. Fiber supplements made from guar gums or methylcellulose may also be added.

A low-fiber diet consists of soft, mild food. It excludes raw vegetables and fruits, nuts, seeds, coarse breads, and strong seasonings. Fried foods and fats are limited, since they can increase gastric reflux. The patient may eat milk and dairy products and should cook meats and vegetables until they're quite tender.

Monitoring

The patient on a high-fiber diet may initially experience cramping or diarrhea; if he does, he should eliminate some high-fiber foods and reintroduce them gradually. Suggest that he substitute whole grain bread and cereals first. After he's able to tolerate them, he may add fibrous cooked fruits and vegetables, and then finally switch to raw fruits and vegetables.

If the patient on a high-fiber diet doesn't have at least one soft stool per day, tell him to add a bran supplement to his diet.

If the patient's on a low-fiber diet, ask him about the type and frequency of GI distress to determine his response to the diet.

Home care instructions

- Tell the female patient on a high-fiber diet to increase her calcium intake to prevent osteoporosis. Tell her to drink at least two glasses of milk a day and to eat cheese and yogurt. If she's trying to lose weight or suffers from diabetes, recommend skim milk and low-fat cheese.

• Tell the patient on a high-fiber diet to eat plenty of iron-rich foods, such as liver. To increase his zinc intake, recommend meat, nuts, beans, wheat germ, and cheese.

• Instruct him to take a list of high-fiber foods with him when he grocery shops. The list will remind him of which foods to buy.

• Remind all patients on a fiber-modified diet to schedule follow-up appointments to evaluate their progress and assess their nutritional status.

Protein-Modified Diet

Protein—the raw material for building cells and regulating bodily functions—is normally supplied in abundance by a well-balanced diet. But a high-protein diet may be necessary for those with increased body-building needs, such as growing children, athletes, and pregnant women. In addition, a high-protein diet can benefit patients with increased tissue breakdown or with nitrogen depletion caused by stress or increased secretions of thyroid or glucocorticoid hormones. And it's often used in patients who've suffered protein loss because of immobilization, dietary deficiency, advanced age, infection, alcoholism, drug addiction, or chronic disease.

The beneficial effects of a high-protein diet can be striking. In just a few weeks the patient's general health and well-being begin to improve. He gains weight and feels stronger; his resistance to infection increases and wounds heal more quickly.

In contrast to these patients, others suffer from an *excess* of protein and must adhere to a low-protein regimen. Typically, these patients have illnesses that impair the body's ability to eliminate the products of protein catabolism—for example, end-stage renal disease or severe hepatic disease.

Purpose
To meet the body's increased or decreased requirements for protein.

Preparation
Begin by discussing the patient's dietary history with him and providing information about sources of complete and incomplete protein. If the patient requires a high-protein diet, explain that he also needs to eat plenty of carbohydrates; otherwise, the body simply burns protein as fuel.

If the patient requires a low-protein diet, work with the dietitian to develop an individualized plan. Emphasize to the patient that he'll need to limit the size of portions as well as the types of foods that he eats; using the food on his hospital tray or plastic models, show him the correct portion size for various foods. In addition, show him how to use a food scale, and have him give you a return demonstration. Include the patient's family—especially the primary food preparer—in these discussions. Also, be especially sensitive to ethnic and cultural influences; most Americans consume large amounts of protein.

Procedure
The goal of a *high-protein diet* is to provide approximately 125 g of protein and 2,500 calories each day. Tell the patient to select one half to two thirds of the day's protein allowance from complete-protein foods and to divide his protein allowance as evenly as possible among the meals of the day. Suggest that he add nonfat dry milk to regular milk and to casseroles to increase their protein content.

A *low-protein diet* should provide 75% of the dietary protein allowance in the form of high-value protein, such as that found in eggs. As with high-protein regimens, the protein allowance should be distributed as evenly as possible among meals. To minimize protein catabolism, be sure the diet includes enough calories to meet the patient's energy requirements. The prescribed diet may also include supplements to prevent amino acid deficiencies.

Monitoring

If the patient on a high-protein diet is hospitalized, weigh him daily; if he's an outpatient, weigh him weekly. Expect to see a weight gain of 1 to 2 lb/week. Monitor him for signs of protein deficiency, such as weakness, decreased resistance to infection, and low hemoglobin levels. In severe protein deficiency, monitor serum albumin levels. Also check for edema, a sign of albumin deficiency.

If the patient on a low-protein diet has end-stage renal disease, monitor his blood urea nitrogen and serum creatinine levels; these levels reflect the clearance of the end products of protein metabolism. Also monitor the glomerular filtration rate (GFR); it can serve as a guide for the degree to which proteins need to be restricted. For example, a patient with a GFR of 10 to 15 ml/minute should restrict protein intake to 40 to 55 g/day. Similarly, monitor urine flow to determine how much fluid the patient should be consuming; daily fluid intake should be 500 to 600 ml more than urine output.

If the patient's receiving a low-protein diet because of liver disease, monitor his serum ammonia levels daily and watch for signs of ammonia intoxication, such as flapping hand motions or tremors. Elevated levels will require further dietary restrictions.

Home care instructions

• Reinforce the dietary guidelines, and if necessary, arrange a referral to a nutritionist or dietitian.
• Encourage the patient to return for frequent checkups.

• If the patient's on a high-protein diet, remind him to increase his protein and calorie consumption gradually.
• If the patient's on a low-protein diet, recommend a vegetarian cookbook.

Low-Cholesterol Diet

Dietary therapy represents the first line of defense in the fight against high serum cholesterol levels and their cardiovascular complications. It's one important part of an overall campaign against risk factors for heart disease; the patient must also be encouraged, if necessary, to stop smoking, lose weight, and exercise more. If he suffers from hereditary hypercholesterolemia, he may also require drug therapy.

A low-cholesterol diet isn't curative, so most patients must remain on it permanently. Typically, results don't become apparent for at least 3 months.

Because serum cholesterol levels reflect overall fat intake, a low-cholesterol diet has much in common with a low-fat diet. But there are some differences because of the role that certain foods play in hypercholesterolemia. For example, research has shown that serum cholesterol levels can be significantly reduced by substituting monounsaturated and polyunsaturated fats (such as olive oil, safflower oil, and corn oil) for saturated fats. Dietary fiber also lowers serum cholesterol levels, and some research suggests that leafy and root vegetables do so as well.

Purpose

To lower serum cholesterol levels by decreasing saturated fats and increasing dietary fiber.

Preparation

If possible, arrange a referral with a dietitian to help the patient plan a low-cholesterol diet. Before he meets with the dietitian, take a careful dietary history. Ask him whether he cooks with animal fats, whether he uses margarine or butter, and whether he usually bakes, broils, or fries his food. How many eggs does he eat each week? Does he eat processed foods or frozen prepared dinners? Does he eat out often? If so, what kinds of foods does he eat?

After taking the patient's history, explain to him how high cholesterol levels increase his risk of cardiovascular disease and how dietary control can reduce this risk. Explain that not all fats are the same; saturated fats (which are often solid, such as butter or animal fat) tend to be converted to cholesterol. Tell him to strive toward a diet in which the ratio of polyunsaturated to saturated fats is about 1:1 (in the typical American diet, it's about 1:3).

Also explain the role of low-density lipoprotein (LDL) in cardiovascular disease. Tell the patient that LDL carries cholesterol to the cells and that high LDL levels can therefore promote the accumulation of cholesterol in arterial walls. Explain that high-density lipoprotein (HDL), by contrast, is desirable, since it helps remove cholesterol from the blood and transport it to the liver for elimination.

Stress that new, tasty foods can be exchanged for foods that are high in saturated fats. For example, suggest beans as an alternate source of protein, and whole grain cereal and bread, fruits, and raw vegetables to increase fiber content. Oat cereals and apples help to reduce cholesterol levels.

Procedure
Usually, the patient is advised to follow one of three diets recommended by the American Heart Association (see *Three Ways to Combat Cholesterol*). All of these diets provide adequate nutrition. If necessary, caloric intake can be reduced to help the patient lose weight, and salt may be restricted to curb hypertension. Phase in the low-cholesterol diet gradually, both to improve compliance and to permit assessment of the patient's response, which can vary greatly.

Monitoring
Schedule a visit with a dietitian, who will provide support and reinforcement of dietary measures. The dietitian can

---

THREE WAYS TO COMBAT CHOLESTEROL

The American Heart Association recommends three diets for combating elevated cholesterol levels. These diets range from a slightly restrictive one, which aims to prevent excessive cholesterol intake, to a severely restrictive one.

Accent on prevention
In the preventive diet, suitable for most people, about a third of the calories are evenly divided among saturated, monounsaturated, and polyunsaturated fats. Carbohydrates—ideally, complex ones—make up half of the calories, with protein making up the remainder. Total cholesterol intake doesn't exceed 300 mg/day.

This diet limits egg yolks to two weekly. Most organ meats are omitted. Soft margarine, vegetable oils and shortening, skim milk, and egg whites replace butter, lard, whole milk, and whole eggs. Beef can be eaten three times weekly.

Strictly lean
The AHA's "phase 2" diet aims to correct mild hypercholesterolemia. It contains the same distribution of fats, carbohydrates, and protein as the preventive diet but restricts cholesterol to 200 mg/day. It also limits intake of meat, poultry, and seafood to 6 oz a day, while emphasizing legumes, grains, fruits, and vegetables. Only extremely lean cuts of meats and skim milk cheeses are permitted.

Lean and mean
The most restrictive diet is used for severe hypercholesterolemia. Fats amount to no more than 25% of the calories consumed (again, equally distributed among saturated, monounsaturated, and polyunsaturated fats). Between 55% and 60% of calories come from carbohydrates. Meat, shellfish, and poultry servings are limited to 3 oz daily.

COMPARING FATS AND OILS

For a patient on a low-cholesterol diet, you'll need to emphasize the importance of curbing intake of saturated fats, replacing them with polyunsaturated or monounsaturated ones. The graph shows the ratio of polyunsaturated fats to saturated ones for a select group of fats and oil. Tell your patient to use fats with a high ratio. Or suggest substituting olive oil, a highly monounsaturated fat, for saturated ones. Keep in mind, though, that all fats are calorie-rich and may need to be restricted if the patient must also lose weight.

Ratio of polyunsaturated to saturated fats

Ratio	Fats and oils
8:1	Safflower oil
6:1	Sunflower oil
5:1	Canola oil Corn oil
4:1	Soybean oil Mayonnaise
3:1	Safflower oil margarine (tub) Sesame oil Salad dressing
2:1	Corn oil margarine (tub) Safflower oil margarine (stick) Cottonseed oil
1:1	Corn oil margarine (stick) Peanut oil Vegetable oil margarine (tub)
0.6:1	Vegetable oil margarine (stick) Vegetable shortening
0.3:1	Lard
0.05:1	Butter Coconut oil, palm kernel oil

suggest ways to make meal preparation easier for the whole family.

The low-cholesterol diet doesn't usually produce side effects. However, if the patient's dietary cholesterol level is very low, he may require vitamin A supplements. He may also require mineral supplements, since large amounts of dietary fiber may interfere with absorption of calcium, iron, and zinc.

Monitor serum cholesterol level and HDL, LDL, and VLDL fractions to evaluate treatment. Have the patient keep a chart of these values to provide positive reinforcement of the diet.

Home care instructions

• Review low-cholesterol food choices with the patient (see *Nurse's Guide to Food Values*, pages 229 to 235).
• Explain that he may need several months to adapt to new eating patterns. To promote compliance, encourage him to master one part of the diet at a time. For example, he may choose to limit his consumption of red meat before reducing the number of eggs that he eats.
• When the patient eats out, recommend that he select salads and vegetables, that he choose poultry over red meat, and that he have simply prepared dishes (but not fried food) rather than those that come with rich sauces or dressings. Pasta and Chinese dishes—especially vegetarian ones—are often good choices; however, tell the patient to avoid pasta dishes that contain large amounts of whole milk cheeses.
• Be sure the patient ingests enough dairy products to make up for impaired calcium absorption. He should eat beans and leafy vegetables to obtain iron and zinc, which may be poorly absorbed with high amounts of fiber.
• Recommend a cooking spray for frying and baking.
• Tell the patient to use tub margarines rather than the stick form and to select a type that's high in polyunsaturated or monounsaturated fat. Tell him to buy a brand that shows vegetable oils first in the list of ingredients.
• Suggest that he make soups or stews

a day ahead of time and refrigerate them; he can then skim off the hardened fat before reheating it.
• Recommend to the patient that he use egg substitutes or egg whites in recipes calling for eggs. Advise him that low-cholesterol substitutes are available for mayonnaise, salad dressings, hot dogs, egg noodles, ice cream, and many other foods.

Low-Fat Diet

Although fat supplies energy and fat-soluble vitamins, most Americans eat too much of it—about 160 g/day, on average, accounting for some 40% of their caloric intake. In fact, excessive dietary fat has been linked not only to obesity but also to cardiovascular disease and colon, prostate, and breast cancer.

Authorities on nutrition recommend that fat be limited to no more than 30% of total caloric intake—that is, about 120 g/day. Patients with certain disorders may require a diet that's even lower in fat: either one containing only 50 g of fat per day or an extremely low-fat diet containing only 25 to 30 g of fat per day.

A low-fat diet benefits a variety of patients. For instance, in patients with malabsorption disorders secondary to hepatic or pancreatic disease, it reduces problems caused by impaired fat digestion and absorption. In those with gallbladder disease, it can diminish fat-induced contractions of the gallbladder; and while it can't dissolve gallstones or prevent attacks, it can provide symptomatic relief. In patients with gout, the diet can help prevent uric acid retention. Many researchers believe that it can also help patients with multiple sclerosis, slowing the progression of disease and reducing the incidence of new attacks. And in patients with hyperlipoproteinemia, a low-fat diet can sometimes reduce serum levels of lipoproteins and, if it's started early in life, can help prevent atherosclerosis in patients with hereditary hyperlipoproteinemia.

Compliance is the major problem with these diets. Simply reducing fat intake to 30% of ingested calories, for example, limits the patient to three eggs a week and requires substitution of skim milk, margarine, and vegetable oils for whole milk, butter, and lard. The more stringent diets, of course, are even more limiting.

Purpose

To prevent or reduce elevated lipid levels in the blood, lymph system, gallbladder, and other tissues by reducing dietary fat.

Preparation

Discuss the low-fat diet with the patient and members of his family—especially the food preparer. Explain why a low-fat diet is necessary and the role that fat plays in the patient's condition. Emphasize that the diet won't cure the underlying condition but that it can relieve symptoms and prevent complications.

Take a dietary history, focusing on the patient's likes and dislikes and the ways his food is prepared. Ask him how often he eats out in restaurants, especially fast-food establishments.

Help the patient to identify dietary sources of fat. Point out that fat is often invisible—for example, when it's a component in cream, milk, eggs, or some meat.

Discuss methods of food preparation. Explain that the patient should remove visible fat and skin from meat and should broil or bake foods rather than fry them.

If the patient suffers from hyperlipoproteinemia, explain the difference between saturated and polyunsaturated fats (see "Low-Cholesterol Diet," page 208). You needn't go into this distinction with patients who aren't at risk for hyperlipoproteinemia, however; they should simply reduce their total intake of fat.

Procedure

A diet of 30 to 40 g of fat per day excludes whole milk and its products. However, the patient may use skim milk and products made from it and have 1 tbsp of oil, lard, butter, or mayonnaise and 4 oz of lean meat daily. Eggs are limited to three a week. The patient should avoid such high-fat snacks as chocolate, nuts, cheese crackers, and chips. Substitutes include vegetables, fruits, bread, cereals, rice, and pasta.

If necessary, this basic diet can be modified further, for example, by eliminating eggs and reducing intake of other high-fat foods.

Monitoring

Make sure the patient receives a vitamin supplement since intake of fat-soluble vitamins will be reduced. In addition, watch for signs that he's deficient in these vitamins.

Monitor the patient's protein intake since a low-fat diet tends to restrict high-protein foods. Also keep an eye on his weight, since a low-fat diet also tends to be low in calories. For many patients, weight loss may be beneficial, but caloric intake may need to be increased if weight loss is excessive.

Home care instructions

• Teach the patient how to shop for low-fat foods. For example, tell him to look for dairy products made with skim milk and for pasta that doesn't contain eggs. Suggest that the patient explore ethnic foods, such as Italian, Japanese, and Chinese dishes; they're often low in fat and offer some variety to his diet. However, tell him to watch the amount of cheese in Italian dishes.
• Explain that foods must be properly prepared to reduce dietary fat. For example, tell him to put baked meats or poultry on a rack away from the drippings and to remove skin and fat from foods before cooking them.
• Recommend that he use egg substitutes or egg whites for cooking.
• Counsel the patient about eating out. Suggest that he order juice for an ap-

petizer and use lemon juice or vinegar on salads. Remind him that he must limit portions of meat, and should order foods that are broiled, baked, or poached. Tell him to omit sauces and gravies and to select ices, fruit, or a liqueur for dessert.

• Check with the doctor to see if the patient's diet can include medium-chain triglycerides. These synthetic substances, which are absorbed directly into the portal vein, may be used in place of cooking oil. Although they're expensive, they can improve the patient's compliance with fat restrictions and increase his caloric intake.

Low-Sodium Diet

Among the most difficult diets for a patient to accept, the low-sodium diet is often described as tasteless and bland. Most Americans typically consume 3,000 to 5,000 mg of sodium daily. A low-sodium diet may restrict this amount to as little as 200 mg daily.

Why is a low-sodium diet necessary for some patients? The answer first requires an understanding of sodium's role in maintaining homeostasis. By osmotic pressure, it regulates the volume of intracellular and extracellular fluids. Most of the body's sodium is found in extracellular fluid. This fluid has a constant composition of 3.3 g of sodium per liter of fluid. The body retains sodium only in solution, excreting any excess primarily through the skin and also through the kidneys and bowels. However, if excess sodium is retained, excess water will also be retained, resulting in an abnormal accumulation of extracellular fluid. Restricting dietary sodium can help correct this imbalance and may be prescribed for congestive heart failure, hypertension, chronic renal failure with edema, and cirrhosis with ascites.

When counseling a patient about sodium restriction, remember that he may equate sodium with table salt (which is 46% sodium). So, you'll need to do more than simply advise him to cut down on table salt. Also teach him about the sodium content of specific foods. Avoiding sodium entirely is almost impossible because sodium is naturally found in most foods. Examples of some high-sodium foods are milk, eggs, cheese, meat, poultry, fish, celery, carrots, and spinach. Although most dietary sodium comes from table salt, there are also sodium compounds present as additives. For example, monosodium glutamate (MSG) is used to enhance flavor in many prepared foods, and sodium alginate is added to chocolate milk to keep the chocolate in suspension and to ice cream for smoother texture. What's more, many prescription and over-the-counter drugs contain sodium as does the water in some areas. Softened water has an especially high sodium content.

Purpose
To restrict dietary sodium, thereby preventing or correcting water retention associated with increased cardiac work load and edema or ascites.

Preparation
Take a dietary history to estimate the sodium content of the patient's usual food choices as well as the amount of salt he adds to food at the table. Note any specific cultural or ethnic influences on his diet. Also, determine how often the patient eats in restaurants or away from home. This will help you plan a realistic sodium-restricted diet and give you an idea of how easily the patient will adjust to such a diet.

To encourage compliance, explain to the patient sodium's role in water retention within the body. Note how water retention contributes to edema, ascites, and hypertension.

Next, help him identify all dietary sources of sodium. Typically, the patient can easily recognize salt (sodium chloride) because of its distinctive taste. Make sure he realizes, though, that sodium is a natural constituent of all foodstuffs. Generally, meat, fish, milk, and eggs contain more sodium than do whole grain cereals, fruits, and vegetables. (See *Nurse's Guide to Food Values*, pages 229 to 235, for the sodium content of hundreds of foods.) What's more, food additives, such as MSG and baking soda (sodium bicarbonate), can significantly increase the sodium content of his diet. Point out that many of these additives don't give food a salty taste.

Procedure
Typically, the doctor restricts sodium in the patient's diet to one of five levels: 2,000 to 3,000 mg; 1,000 mg; 800 mg; 500 mg; or 200 mg. (See *Meal Planning for a Low-Sodium Diet*.)

On a 200-mg sodium diet, distilled water must be used for drinking and for making beverages, such as coffee and tea. All other diets contain an allowance of 100 mg of sodium for 1 qt of tap water.

Monitoring
Usually, the patient on a sharply restricted sodium diet (500 mg or less of sodium) is hospitalized. You'll need to monitor him carefully—especially when sodium restriction is prolonged—to avoid hyponatremia, hypochloremia, and, eventually, sodium-depletion azotemia. Watch for complaints of weakness, lassitude, anorexia and vomiting, confusion, abdominal cramps, and aching skeletal muscles. To detect fluid retention, weigh the patient daily and report any sudden increase to the doctor. Also watch for diminished fluid output, which may signal renal failure.

And, finally, check the patient's food tray before he eats, to be sure that salt hasn't been added accidentally.

Home care instructions
• Teach the patient how to read food labels when grocery shopping to determine an item's sodium content. The sodium content is noted on the label

(200 mg of salt equals 80 mg of sodium). Also, inform him that additives are listed in order of greatest quantity. Tell him to avoid a product if one of these additives is among the first five listed: salt, sodium benzoate, sodium nitrate, or MSG.
• Warn him that many over-the-counter medications contain sodium. Some examples include Alka-Seltzer, Di-Gel, Maalox Plus, Metamucil, Rolaids, and Vicks Formula 44 Cough Mixture. Have him consult his doctor or pharmacist about the sodium content of any unprescribed medicine that he wishes to take.
• To help make the sodium-restricted diet more palatable, suggest seasoning foods with herbs and spices instead of salt. (See *"Nothing Tastes Good Anymore,"* page 216.) Tell the patient to avoid salt substitutes, unless his doctor approves. Explain that some products advertised as low-sodium salt substitutes contain another salt and sodium chloride, giving them only half as much sodium as regular table salt. What's more, they may contain potassium or ammonium salt, which could be harmful if the patient has kidney or liver disease. Other products classified as vegetized salts use powdered dehydrated vegetables as a base and may contain considerable sodium.
• At restaurants, advise the patient to order baked, broiled, or roasted foods and to skip gravies, juices, soups, and cheesy dressings.
• Teach the patient how to modify ethnic food practices, as necessary. For example, advise the patient who likes Southern cuisine or "soul food" not to cook with bacon or salt pork.

Help the Jewish patient who wishes to follow orthodox dietary laws regarding meat and poultry. To be kosher, freshly slaughtered meat and poultry must be salted for 1 hour to remove the blood. Although the meat or poultry is thoroughly washed before cooking, some sodium is retained, increasing its sodium content by as much as 400%. Suggest using ammonium

MEAL PLANNING FOR A LOW-SODIUM DIET

When the patient's on a low-sodium diet, he'll need your guidance to plan his meals appropriately.

MODEST RESTRICTIONS

If the patient's sodium intake is restricted to 2,000 to 3,000 mg, instruct him to:

- cook food with a minimum of salt and not to use salt at the table
- stay away from obviously salty foods, such as potato chips, pretzels, and snack crackers, and other high-sodium foods, such as canned soups and vegetables, prepared foods (such as TV dinners and frozen entrees), luncheon meats, cheeses, or pickles and any other foods preserved in brine
- refrain from using canned tomatoes and tomato products
- avoid salted sauces or seasonings, such as chili sauce, mustard, catsup, and relish
- include unsalted meat, broth, soups, and butter in his diet.

STRICTER GUIDELINES

Have the patient follow these same guidelines for all other levels of sodium restriction, except tell him to cook his food without salt. Then suggest the daily meal plan below, as appropriate.

Sodium restricted to 1,000 mg:
- Regular milk, 1 pt
- Unsalted egg, one
- Unsalted meat, 6 oz, cooked
- Unsalted vegetables, three servings
- Citrus fruit, as desired
- Unsalted bread and its exchanges, as desired
- Regular bread, two slices
- Unsalted fats, sugars, and jellies that are free from sodium preservatives

Sodium restricted to 800 mg:
- Regular milk, 1 pt
- Unsalted egg, one
- Unsalted meat, 6 oz, cooked
- Unsalted vegetables, three servings
- Citrus fruit, as desired
- Unsalted bread and its exchanges, as desired
- Regular bread, one slice
- Unsalted fats, sugar, and jelly that's free from sodium preservatives

Sodium restricted to 500 mg:
- Regular milk, 1 cup
- Low-sodium milk, 1 cup
- Unsalted egg, one
- Unsalted meat, 6 oz, cooked
- Unsalted vegetables, three servings
- Citrus fruit, one serving
- Unsalted bread and its exchanges, as desired
- Unsalted fats, sugar, and jelly that's free from sodium preservatives

Sodium restricted to 200 mg:
- Low-sodium milk, 1 pt
- Unsalted meat, 5 oz, cooked (one unsalted egg can be substituted for 3 oz meat)
- Unsalted vegetables, three servings
- Citrus fruit, three servings
- Unsalted bread and its exchanges, six servings
- Unsalted fats, sugar, and jelly that's free from sodium preservatives

"NOTHING TASTES GOOD ANYMORE"

That's the most common complaint you'll hear about a low-sodium diet. But just because food lacks salt, it doesn't have to be bland.

Common herbs and spices can enhance the flavor of food without adding salt. Basil and fresh garlic, for instance, can liven up tomato sauces, stews, and Italian dishes. Curry, cayenne pepper, or dry mustard can add zest to beef, poultry, and seafood. Rosemary, sage, and other spices can give taste to gravies.

Of course, these aren't the only taste-enhancing herbs and spices. Consider tarragon, paprika, bay leaf, thyme, dill, and fennel. The list goes on.

However, warn the patient that not all spices, herbs, and condiments are salt-free. Some are notoriously high in sodium, such as catsup, mustard, monosodium glutamate, soy or Worcestershire sauce, meat sauces or tenderizers, relish, horseradish, and pickles. Some dehydrated products, such as celery or parsley flakes, also contain large amounts of sodium.

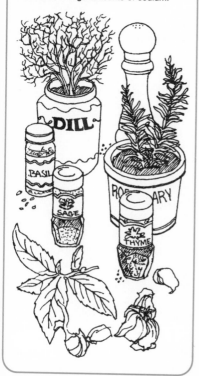

chloride instead of sodium chloride for drawing out the blood. Or have the patient boil the meat and discard the broth before serving.

Advise the Italian patient to use fresh tomatoes whenever possible for soups and sauces or to use unsalted canned tomatoes, tomato paste, or tomato juice. Have him avoid or restrict his intake of olives, Italian cheese, and Italian bread.

Caution the Japanese or Chinese patient not to season his food with MSG or soy sauce. A low-salt soy sauce is available.

• Inform the patient about the availability of specially prepared low-sodium products, such as low-sodium milk, unsalted canned vegetables, unsalted butter and margarine, low-sodium soups, and low-sodium baking powder.

• Collaborate with the dietitian to help the patient plan low-sodium menus and methods of preparing foods at home. Dietitians use a system similar to counting calories for counting the milligrams of sodium eaten. The patient can eat small portions of sodium-containing food as part of the daily sodium allotment. Suggest where he might locate low-sodium recipes to keep his diet varied and enjoyable.

• Explain that bottled soft drinks may be high in sodium, depending on the sodium content of the water in the area where they're manufactured. In low-caloric beverages, substituting sodium saccharin for sugar increases the sodium content even more.

• Eliminating salt from his diet may place the patient at risk for iodine deficiency if his iodine intake depends mainly on the use of iodized salt. Teach him about other dietary sources of iodine, such as seafood and vegetables grown in iodine-rich soil. Explain that he can have the iodine content of his garden soil analyzed. Advise him to take supplemental iodine tablets, as ordered, if the iodine content of his diet and local drinking water is inadequate. Tell him to contact his water authority or have his well water tested for its iodine content.

● Refer the patient to the American Heart Association for additional information about sodium-restricted diets.

Gluten-Free Diet

A gluten-free diet prevents the bloating, projectile vomiting, and poor growth patterns that are the hallmarks of celiac disease. In this disorder, which is usually first diagnosed in infancy or early childhood, the intestinal lining is damaged by the glutamine-bound fraction of protein found in many grain products. Researchers aren't sure why celiac disease occurs; it may be the result of an abnormal enzyme in the mucosal cell that doesn't digest a toxic peptide in gluten, or it may involve an immune reaction within the mucosal cell membrane.

A gluten-free diet can't reverse the intestinal damage of celiac disease. However, it can prevent further damage, improve symptoms, and correct malabsorption of nutrients. Children who are placed on a gluten-free diet may improve within 2 weeks; in adults, results take a little longer—typically, a month or two.

Initially, the patient's diet not only excludes sources of gluten but also is high in protein, calories, vitamins, and minerals to correct previous dietary deficiencies. Once these deficiencies are corrected, the patient adheres to a diet that's normal except for the gluten content. He must follow this diet scrupulously for the rest of his life; those who go on and off the diet repeatedly may eventually fail to respond to it.

Purpose
To prevent complications of celiac disease.

Preparation
Begin by taking a dietary history. Ask the child's parents about symptoms, including the frequency and characteristics of stool.

Coordinate the patient's therapy. Schedule a visit by the dietitian, who will outline the specific restrictions of the diet. Reinforce the dietitian's instructions, emphasizing the need to plan menus carefully to prevent dietary deficiencies. Tell parents to read labels carefully, since many ready-to-eat foods use gluten for processing.

Procedure
A gluten-free diet eliminates all products containing wheat, rye, oats, barley, malt, and buckwheat. In their place, the patient may eat cereals and breads made from rice, corn, soy, and potatoes. Initially, milk and milk products are also withheld, since intestinal damage often causes an intolerance to lactose. As symptoms improve, these dairy products can be gradually reintroduced.

Monitoring
The patient may initially require hospitalization to stabilize his condition and provide nutritional supplementation. While he's in the hospital, monitor hemoglobin and hematocrit values for signs of anemia, and administer iron, folate, or vitamin B_{12}, as ordered. Bleeding may result from vitamin K deficiency; monitor prothrombin time. Osteomalacia may develop because of vitamin D and calcium deficiencies; watch for rheumatic-type pain in the pelvis and limbs. In addition, monitor intake and output carefully.

Home care instructions
● Explain that the gluten-free diet is difficult to follow. Gluten is hidden in many foods—for example, in chocolate syrup (where it's used as a stabilizing and thickening agent); in sausages, hot dogs, and turkey injected with hydrolyzed vegetable protein; and in distilled white vinegar and whiskeys.
● Tell the parents that some foods are specially made for the patient with ce-

liac disease; the dietitian can recommend brands. Suggest that they look for them in health-food stores or gourmet shops.
• Suggest that they visit an Asian food store, where many of the products are made entirely from rice and rice flour.
• Explain that foods made with special gluten-free flours may be less grainy if the flour is mixed with the liquid in a recipe. Tell the parents to boil the flour with the liquid and cool this mixture before adding it to other ingredients.
• For older children and adults, discuss foods that can be eaten in restaurants. Suggest broiled or baked meat or fish; tell the patient to avoid sauces, gravies, and breaded foods.
• Emphasize the need for frequent checkups.

Low-Purine Diet

This diet restricts foods with preformed purines—for example, liver, eggs, and sardines—which the body breaks down into uric acids. It's primarily used to control gout and prevent renal calculi, two conditions caused by high uric acid levels. In addition, a low-purine diet can be used for patients with increased uric acid levels secondary to obesity, hypertension, hypertriglyceridemia, fasting, alcoholism, lead toxicity, toxemia of pregnancy, leukemia, polycythemia, psoriasis, or diuretic therapy.

Since the body synthesizes purines, dietary measures alone won't always control these conditions. For that reason, the diet's usually supplemented with drugs, such as allopurinol and probenecid, that reduce uric acid levels, as well as an exercise and weight-control program.

Purpose
To lower uric acid levels, thereby controlling gout and preventing formation of renal calculi.

Preparation
Review the patient's dietary history. Specifically ask about alcohol consumption, which can aggravate gout. In addition, review the patient's drug history, since hydrochlorothiazide, pyrazinamide, and other drugs can cause a buildup of uric acid in body tissues.

Emphasize that the low-purine diet is only part of a comprehensive regimen.

Procedure
The low-purine diet contains limited amounts of fats, moderate amounts of protein, and plentiful amounts of complex carbohydrates. In addition, it includes about 2 qt of fluid a day to help promote uric acid excretion, as well as vegetables and fruit to increase the alkalinity of the urine and thereby increase the solubility of uric acid.

The diet limits the patient's weekly intake of animal protein to about 15 oz of lean beef, veal, lamb, poultry, or fish—in other words, about five servings of no more than 3 oz. Dairy products are limited to 4 cups of skim milk and 2 oz of cheese daily.

The patient must avoid all high-purine foods, such as organ meats (kidney, liver, brain), meat extracts, bouillon, gravies, fish eggs, shrimp, mackerel, herring, anchovies, mussels, and sardines. In addition, he should avoid alcohol or at least limit it to one drink daily, preferably diluted with water.

The patient can have three to four daily servings of vegetables, including potatoes and most kinds of green, leafy vegetables. (However, dried beans, peas, spinach, and lentils have moderate amounts of purine and should be restricted to one serving a day.) He can also eat two to three servings of fruit a day, one serving of enriched cereal, and four to six slices of enriched bread with 2 tbs of margarine or butter. Moderate amounts of coffee and tea are permitted; the purines that they contain break down to methyl uric acid, which isn't deposited in body tissues.

If the patient's on an exceedingly strict diet—for example, during an acute attack of gout—he may need to eliminate animal protein, eggs, and cheese altogether. He should drink skim milk and eat cottage cheese to get enough protein and should avoid alcohol entirely.

Monitoring

If the patient's hospitalized, closely monitor his serum uric acid levels. Notify the doctor if levels begin to rise sharply.

Assess the patient regularly for diffuse swelling in the joints and for nodular deposits of sodium urate crystals. In addition, closely monitor his intake and output, and encourage fluids.

Check urine pH. If ordered, administer sodium bicarbonate or potassium carbonate to increase urine alkalinity.

Antigout drugs can decrease absorption of sodium, potassium, carotene, riboflavin, and vitamin B_{12}, so watch for deficiencies. If ordered, administer vitamin and mineral supplements.

Home care instructions

• Emphasize the need for follow-up visits to monitor his progress and detect dietary deficiencies.

• Suggest that the patient keep a food diary, and review it with him when he comes in for follow-up visits.

• Tell the patient not to diet during an acute gout attack since the breakdown of adipose tissue decreases uric acid excretion. If he wishes to lose weight, tell him to do so gradually and to avoid fasting, which can precipitate a gout attack.

• Suggest ways that the patient can add fluids to his diet—for example, by eating soup or drinking a glass of water before each meal and at bedtime.

• Help the patient develop an exercise and weight-control program.

• Tell him to avoid taking aspirin or other salicylates; they can interact with some antigout drugs to prevent uric acid excretion.

Low-Phenylalanine Diet

For a child born with phenylketonuria, a congenital deficiency of the liver enzyme phenylalanine hydroxylase, the low-phenylalanine diet is a blessing. If it's begun shortly after birth and followed scrupulously until adolescence, it can prevent the mental retardation and neurologic damage that are otherwise inevitable in this disease.

But it's a mixed blessing. Not only is the diet difficult to follow but it also must be adhered to scrupulously. The child must begin to take responsibility for the diet early on and may not understand the consequences of noncompliance. As he leaves the sheltered home environment, he often finds that the diet sets him apart from his friends.

Some controversy exists over how long the diet must be followed. Although children have been taken off it at age 7 or 8, reports of learning and behavior problems have prompted researchers to recommend that the diet be observed into adolescence. At that time the patient requires no special dietary restrictions—with one important exception: female patients who want to become pregnant must return to the diet before and for the duration of the pregnancy, since excess phenylalanine can be transmitted to the fetus and cause congenital defects.

Purpose

To reduce phenylalanine intake while providing sufficient amino acids and nutrients for normal growth and development.

Preparation

Explain to parents the effects of excess phenylalanine on the developing nervous system and how this diet can help prevent them. Stress that the child will be physically and psychologically normal *only if he carefully adheres to the diet.* Provide suggestions early in treat-

INQUIRY

QUESTIONS PARENTS ASK ABOUT DIETARY RESTRICTIONS

Why can't I nurse my baby?

Even though breast milk is an excellent source of protein, your baby can't digest the phenylalanine that it contains. Nursing would cause him to have too much phenylalanine in his bloodstream. This, in turn, would damage his brain. In place of breast milk or regular formula, you can feed your baby a substitute milk called Lofenalac, from which 95% of the phenylalanine has been removed.

When can we discontinue this special diet and start giving our child regular food?

You'll need to continue the diet for a long time, probably until your child becomes an adolescent. For the first few years of your child's life, his brain is rapidly maturing and the diet can prevent mental retardation. Even when your child starts school, he should continue the diet. School-age children who have stopped following their diet have experienced learning and behavior difficulties.

Are there any other restrictions that we should know about?

If you have a boy, there are no other restrictions. However, if you have a girl, there may be some dietary restrictions later in her life if she decides to marry and become pregnant. That's because phenylketonuria (PKU) is carried as an autosomal recessive gene. If your daughter and her husband both possessed the gene, they would have a one in four chance that their child would have PKU. If her husband didn't carry the gene, the child wouldn't have PKU. However, your daughter would have to follow a low-phenylalanine diet before and during her pregnancy. Otherwise, her increased phenylalanine levels could endanger the fetus.

---

ment to limit psychosocial problems. For example, warn the parents against overemphasizing food intake or over-protecting their child; tell them to treat him as normally as possible. Suggest that they seek family counseling to help them adjust to the dietary regimen.

Procedure

The infant is given a special formula made of enzymatic hydrolysate of casein, which contains exceedingly low levels of phenylalanine, normal amounts of other amino acids, and added amounts of carbohydrate and fat. Since he requires some phenylalanine for normal development, he also receives small supplements of evaporated milk or regular infant formula.

As the child grows older, the diet restricts foods to those with a low or moderate phenylalanine content. Since most natural proteins contain phenylalanine, the diet is similar to the low-protein diet (see "Protein-Modified Diet," page 207).

Monitoring

Check serum phenylalanine levels weekly in early infancy and monthly as the child matures to determine his response to therapy. Serum levels should be kept between 2 and 10 mg/dl.

Assess the child's height, weight, and head circumference regularly to ensure that the diet provides adequate nutrition. In addition, monitor hemoglobin levels, since the diet is low in protein and in magnesium and zinc levels. If deficiencies develop, the doctor will order vitamin and mineral supplements.

Overzealous adherence to the diet may result in excessively low phenylalanine levels. In addition to monitoring blood values, watch for signs of phenylalanine deficiency: listlessness, anorexia, or stunted growth.

Home care instructions

● Instruct the parents to keep a daily food diary. When they come in for follow-up visits, review the diary with them to assess both phenylalanine intake and overall nutrition.

• Tell them that supplemental milk should be mixed with the low-phenylalanine formula so that the infant doesn't develop a taste for regular milk.

• Explain that during illness, tissue breakdown can cause an accumulation of phenylalanine in the blood; during this time, the child may be restricted to clear liquids. Tell parents to reintroduce the formula or diet as soon as possible after the child recovers.

• Parents need additional support and guidance as they introduce new foods to an infant. Have them demonstrate their ability to weigh and measure food properly and to make appropriate choices from the exchange lists.

• Stress to parents that as the child matures, he must become responsible for his own diet. Help them develop this responsibility early; for example, explain that by age 3 or 4, children can learn that some foods are "no" foods and others are "yes" foods, and they can be taught to count out the number of crackers that they're allowed to eat.

• Help the parents find sources of low-protein foods, such as specialty shops and mail-order firms, and suggest that they use cookbooks designed for a low-phenylalanine diet and vegetarian cookbooks that include dairy products.

Lactose-Reduced Diet

A lactose-reduced diet is the only treatment for lactose intolerance, a common disorder in which patients have difficulty digesting dairy products.

Some degree of lactose intolerance develops in most people after the age of 5. But for reasons that aren't entirely understood, it's usually more pronounced among blacks, Asians, Orientals, and South Americans. And in a few cases, complete lactose intolerance is present from birth. Secondary lactose intolerance may occur in patients with celiac disease, sprue, colitis, enteritis,

cystic fibrosis, or malnutrition and in patients who've undergone a gastrectomy or small-bowel resection.

Few patients require a diet that's totally free of lactose; most can tolerate some milk as long as it's carefully spaced throughout the day. In addition, many patients are able to consume cheese or yogurt, in which the lactose is broken down by the active cultures, as well as sweet acidophilus milk, which contains an enzyme that hydrolyzes lactose.

Because the diet has some flexibility, it's one of the easiest to follow. And unlike many other diets, a reduced-lactose diet need not be permanent; many patients can gradually add dairy products without suffering ill effects.

Purpose
To reduce dietary lactose, thereby alleviating GI symptoms.

Preparation
Before prescribing a lactose-reduced diet, the doctor will measure the patient's ability to digest lactose. He may perform either of two tests: the lactose tolerance test or the lactose malabsorption test. The tolerance test involves serial blood samples taken after oral administration of lactose; patients with lactose intolerance usually won't achieve the normal 20% rise in blood glucose over the fasting level. The diagnosis is confirmed by diarrhea, gas, or cramps during the test and a drop in stool pH from 7 or 8 to 5.5. In the lactose malabsorption test, an increase in exhaled hydrogen after lactose ingestion shows that bacteria are acting on undigested lactose.

If these tests confirm lactose intolerance, work with the patient to reduce his intake of lactose. Take a dietary history, focusing on the kinds and amounts of dairy products that he eats.

Explain to the patient why he has trouble digesting these products. Tell him that undigested lactose is fermented by intestinal bacteria and that it draws water into the intestine; the

WHAT HAPPENS IN LACTOSE INTOLERANCE

The classic signs of lactose intolerance—bloating, flatulence, diarrhea, and malabsorption—result from undigested lactose making its way into the small intestine. Once there, it's attacked by bacteria, giving off hydrogen as it's broken down. The lactose also draws water into the intestine by osmosis. The gas and increased fluid load trigger hyperperistalsis—which, in turn, inhibits absorption of other nutrients.

NORMAL DIGESTION

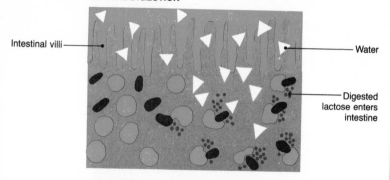

Intestinal villi

Water

Digested lactose enters intestine

DIGESTION IN LACTOSE INTOLERANCE

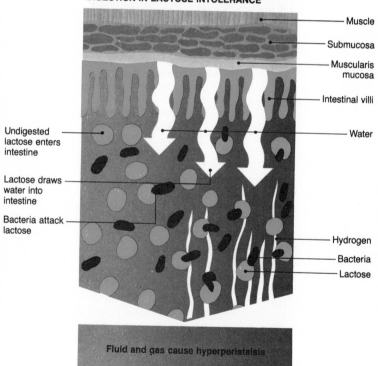

Muscle

Submucosa

Muscularis mucosa

Intestinal villi

Undigested lactose enters intestine

Water

Lactose draws water into intestine

Bacteria attack lactose

Hydrogen

Bacteria

Lactose

Fluid and gas cause hyperperistalsis

acids and gases formed by fermentation combine with the excess water to cause bloating, cramping, and diarrhea. Explain that milk and milk products are the only sources of lactose and that limiting them can prevent GI distress.

Procedure
The patient should limit or eliminate his consumption of ordinary milk and milk products. As a guideline, suggest that he drink no more than half a cup of ordinary milk per day; recommend that he substitute sweet acidophilus milk. If he wishes, he can try eating small quantities of cheese or drinking small amounts of buttermilk or yogurt, since they contain bacteria that break down lactose. He should avoid baked goods made with milk, sausages that contain milk solids, creamy sauces and gravies, and processed foods that contain lactose. He should also avoid other, less obvious sources of lactose, such as chocolate; caramel; cocoa mixes; certain nondairy creamers, vitamins, and medications; instant potatoes; and frozen french fries.

Monitoring
Monitor the patient's intake of calcium and riboflavin; both are usually supplied by milk. Provide dietary supplements, if ordered. Also assess his diet to be sure he's taking in sufficient protein and calories.

Home care instructions
• Tell the patient to carefully read food labels to detect the presence of milk, milk solids, whey, lactose, or casein.
• Suggest that he substitute water or fruit juices for milk in recipes.
• Explain that if he eats out, he should avoid foods prepared with sauces, gravies, or breading.
• Tell the patient that if his symptoms improve, he can try adding small amounts of dairy products at one meal; if he tolerates them well, he may gradually increase his intake of them. Inform him that sometimes chocolate milk is tolerated better than regular

milk. If he wants to try adding cottage cheese to his diet, tell him to experiment with different brands; the amount of lactose they contain varies widely.

ENTERAL AND PARENTERAL NUTRITION

Enteral Nutrition

Enteral nutrition bypasses the upper GI tract, introducing pureed food or a special liquid enteral formula directly into the stomach or small intestine via a feeding tube. It's indicated for patients whose GI tract is functional but who can't take adequate food by mouth—for example, those suffering from Crohn's disease, ulcerative colitis, short-bowel syndrome, head and neck injuries, neurologic disease, or psychiatric disorders. In such cases, enteral nutrition offers a number of advantages over intravenous hyperalimentation: it maintains the integrity of the intestinal mucosa, causes fewer metabolic complications, provides better nutrition and greater weight gain, and costs less.

Complications of enteral nutrition may be mechanical, gastrointestinal, or metabolic. Fortunately, most can often be managed without removing the feeding tube (see *Correcting Complications of Tube Feedings*, page 225).

Purpose
To provide necessary nutrition in patients who can't take food by mouth.

Preparation
Before inserting the tube, explain to the patient why enteral nutrition is necessary and how it will be performed. In addition, give him the opportunity to ask questions and express any fears or concerns.

If the patient will be having a feeding

tube surgically placed, provide routine preoperative care. If you're inserting a nasogastric, nasoduodenal, or nasojejunal tube, explain to the patient that the initial discomfort he feels will resolve as he becomes accustomed to the presence of the tube. Before inserting the tube, assess both nostrils for pathology, patency, and ease of air exchange. Ask the patient if he has ever suffered nasal trauma or undergone nasal surgery. Then have him breathe through his nose as you occlude each nostril in turn. Note which nostril is more patent.

Next, place the patient in the semi-Fowler or high Fowler position. Make sure he doesn't lean forward. Drape the front of his gown with a linen-saver pad and give him an emesis basin.

Measure the tube length. To estimate the distance needed to reach the pylorus, extend the distal end of the tube from the tip of the patient's nose to his earlobe; coil this portion of the tube around your finger so that it will remain curved until you insert it. Then extend the uncoiled portion from the earlobe to the xiphoid process. Use a small piece of nonallergenic tape to mark the total length on the tube.

Lubricate the curved tip of the tube with a small amount of water-soluble lubricant. Then insert the tip into the more patent nostril and advance it along the nasal passage toward the ear on the same side. When it passes the nasopharyngeal junction, turn it 180 degrees to aim it into the esophagus; then continue to pass it until the tape reaches the patient's nose.

To insert an oral tube, first have the patient lower his chin to close the trachea. Then place the tube at the back of his tongue and give him a cup of water with a straw. Have him sip the water, and tell him to swallow frequently and not to bite down on the tube. Advance the tube as he swallows.

To place a tube in the duodenum, position the patient on his right side (so that gravity will help the tube pass through the pylorus) and advance it 2″ to 3″ every hour until its placement is confirmed.

For all types of tubes, correct placement can be verified by X-ray. In addition, placement of stomach tubes can be verified by aspirating gastric secretions through the tube. If necessary, manipulate the tubing or place the patient on his left side to pool the gastric contents in the greater curvature and facilitate aspiration. Don't check tube placement by injecting air into the tube and auscultating the abdomen; it's an unreliable method.

Procedure

To give enteral nutrition, first warm the formula to room temperature. Then position the patient: if he has a gastric tube, put him in a high semi-Fowler's position. For a duodenal or jejunal tube, you don't need to elevate the bed; since the formula is infused beyond the cardioesophageal and pyloric sphincters, gastric reflux is unlikely.

Next, unclamp the tube. Assess the abdomen and auscultate for bowel sounds. If ordered, check the placement of the feeding tube.

To prevent vomiting, aspirate the stomach contents through the tube before you administer the feeding. Measure the volume of these contents to assess gastric retention. Then irrigate the tube with 50 ml of water.

The feeding is administered by one of several methods. For a continuous feeding—the most common method—set up an infusion pump or controller, add enteral formula, set the rate (which shouldn't exceed 150 ml/hour), and push the start button. For a bolus feeding, use a 50- or 60-ml syringe to administer the ordered amount of formula every 3 or 4 hours. For intermittent continuous feeding, use a feeding bag; regulate the flow rate so that the feeding takes place over a 20- to 30-minute period every 3 to 4 hours (the rate shouldn't exceed 50 to 60 ml/minute).

Unless the doctor has ordered fluid restriction, the patient may receive additional water (up to an amount equal-

CORRECTING COMPLICATIONS OF TUBE FEEDINGS

COMPLICATION	INTERVENTIONS
Aspiration of gastric secretions	• Discontinue feeding immediately. • Perform tracheal suction of aspirated contents, if possible. • Notify the doctor. Prophylactic antibiotics and chest physiotherapy may be ordered. • Check tube placement before feeding to prevent complication.
Tube obstruction	• Flush tube with warm water or cranberry juice. If necessary, replace tube. • Flush tube with 50 ml of water after each feeding to remove excess sticky formula, which could occlude the tube.
Nasal or pharyngeal irritation or necrosis	• Provide frequent oral hygiene, using mouthwash or lemon and glycerin swabs. Use petrolatum on cracked lips. • Change position of tube. If necessary, replace tube.
Vomiting, bloating, diarrhea, or cramps	• Reduce flow rate. • Administer metoclopromide to increase GI motility. • Warm formula. • For 30 minutes after feeding, position the patient on his right side with his head elevated to facilitate gastric emptying. • Notify doctor. He may want to reduce the amount of formula being given during each feeding.
Constipation	• Provide additional fluids, if the patient can tolerate them. • Administer bulk laxative. • Fruit, vegetable, or sugar content of feeding may be increased.
Electrolyte imbalance	• Monitor serum electrolyte levels. • Notify doctor. He may want to adjust formula content, to correct deficiency.
Hyperglycemia	• Monitor blood glucose levels. • Notify doctor of elevated levels. • Administer insulin, if ordered. • Doctor may change formula, to correct sugar content.
Congestive heart failure	• Monitor the patient's intake, output, and respiratory status. • Reduce flow rate. • Notify doctor. • Administer diuretics and digoxin, as ordered. • Decrease the patient's fluid intake and enforce bed rest.

ing 25% of his total feeding volume), either mixed with the formula or given afterward.

After the feeding is complete, again irrigate the feeding tube with 50 ml of water and clamp the tube.

Monitoring and aftercare

Record the amount of ingested formula. Increase the volume or concentration of the feeding over 2 days; be sure to note the patient's tolerance of these increases, as evidenced by such signs as nausea, vomiting, diarrhea, and abdominal distention. If the patient vomits, promptly discontinue the feeding and notify the doctor; also report excessive diarrhea.

Weigh the patient daily at the same time, in the same type of clothing, and using the same scale to assess the results of therapy. Monitor laboratory studies, including blood urea nitrogen, hematocrit, hemoglobin, and serum protein levels. Provide meticulous care for the patient's mouth and nares, and change the anchoring tapes and dressings daily to prevent skin breakdown and infection.

Home care instructions

• Intermittent and continuous feedings can be performed at home by family members. Explain that the procedure is generally done the same way as in the hospital, with a few modifications. For example, if the patient doesn't have a hospital bed at home, he may need to be propped up with pillows.

Have family members and the patient observe you as you administer tube feedings. Coach them a step at a time until they can perform the feedings independently under your supervision.

• If the patient will have an enteral feeding pump, show family members how to operate it and how to detect and correct problems.

• Tell family members that prepared feeding solutions should be stored in the refrigerator and that food given through a gastrostomy tube should be fully cooked and pureed in a food processor or blender.

• Tell them to weigh the patient three times a week at the same time of day and in the same type of clothing. To detect distention, they should measure the patient's abdominal girth before and after feedings.

• If indicated, show the patient how to test his urine for glucose and acetone.

• Before discharge, refer the patient to a social worker to make arrangements for home feeding and follow-up care by a visiting nurse.

Intravenous Hyperalimentation
[Total parenteral nutrition]

Intravenous hyperalimentation (IVH) refers to the parenteral administration of a solution containing dextrose, proteins, electrolytes, vitamins, and trace elements in amounts that exceed the patient's energy expenditures. IVH can be used for patients in whom GI feeding is contraindicated or ineffective, such as those suffering from severe Crohn's disease, short-bowel syndrome, intestinal fistulas, or ulcerative colitis. It's also used to provide supplemental nutrition in patients who are malnourished, comatose, or suffering from burns, trauma, or malignancy.

Parenteral nutrition may be administered through a central catheter or a peripheral vein. Direct central lines carry the risk of pneumothorax, but they offer several advantages: they're easily dressed and don't restrict activity; they permit the administration of any type of solution, regardless of its osmolarity; and they eliminate the need for repeated venipuncture. Peripheral administration, by contrast, can be used only for solutions that are isotonic or slightly hypertonic.

IVH can cause potentially severe

DEALING WITH HAZARDS OF I.V. HYPERALIMENTATION

I.V. hyperalimentation (IVH) can cause potentially severe complications. These may be related to the IVH equipment or to a metabolic or nutritional problem caused by prolonged or overly rapid feedings.

Equipment-related complications
Air embolism and infection are perhaps the most serious complications caused by the IVH equipment. Suspect *air embolism* if the patient reports chest pain and you detect cyanosis, dyspnea, and coughing. Treat this problem by clamping the catheter, placing the patient in the left Trendelenburg position, and having him perform Valsalva's maneuver. Then notify the doctor.

Suspect *infection* if the patient develops a fever or if redness, swelling, or drainage appears at the catheter insertion site. If he is lethargic, sweating profusely, or shivering, stop the IVH solution and replace it with dextrose 10% in water. Change the I.V. tubing and dressing, and notify the doctor, who'll order cultures of the tubing, solution, and the patient's blood. If fever subsides within 6 hours of stopping IVH, suspect contamination of the solution or the delivery apparatus. If it persists, suspect catheter-related sepsis and again notify the doctor, who will then order blood and urine cultures. If necessary, he'll remove the catheter.

Be alert for other complications, such as pneumothorax, hydrothorax, extravasation, and injury to the brachial plexus.

Metabolic and nutritional complications
A whole array of disturbances in glucose metabolism, fluid and electrolyte balance, and nutrition can result from I.V. hyperalimentation. *Hyperglycemia*, for instance, can develop from overly rapid delivery of the solution, decreased glucose tolerance, or excessive total glucose load. If it develops, you'll need to add insulin to the solution. *Hypoglycemia*, in contrast, can develop from excessive endogenous production of insulin after abrupt termination of feeding. It can also result from excessive addition of insulin to the IVH solution. To correct hypoglycemia, give carbohydrates orally, if possible. Or you can infuse dextrose 10% in water or give a bolus of dextrose 50% in water.

Fluid deficit or excess can stem from inadequate or excessive replacement, electrolyte imbalance, or other problems. To correct fluid imbalance, adjust the patient's fluid intake as ordered.

Electrolyte imbalances, such as *hypokalemia* and *hypocalcemia*, require addition of the deficient electrolyte to the solution. *Essential fatty acid deficiency*, which can result from absent or inadequate fat intake for a prolonged period, requires infusion of two or three bottles of 10% to 20% fat emulsion daily. Deficiency of trace elements, such as *copper* and *zinc*, requires addition of these elements to the solution.

complications, such as infection, hyperglycemia, and hypokalemia (see *Dealing with Hazards of I.V. Hyperalimentation*). Fortunately, though, most complications can be prevented by careful monitoring of the catheter site, infusion rate, and laboratory studies.

Purpose
• To provide essential nutrients for patients who can't take food via the GI tract
• To provide supplemental nutrients for patients suffering from protein-wasting conditions.

Preparation
Explain the procedure to the patient and give him an opportunity to express his concerns. Be alert for signs of depression or resistance to IVH, especially in a patient who requires long-term therapy; the loss of the ability to eat may be devastating to the patient's self-image.

Next, gather the infusion pump and a prepackaged sterile kit containing the necessary equipment. If ordered, establish a peripheral line or assist with insertion of a central venous line.

Remove the hyperalimentation solution from the refrigerator and allow it to stand for at least 30 minutes to reach room temperature. Before hanging it, check the label against the doctor's orders. And inspect the solution for cloudiness, turbidity, and particles and the container for cracks.

Procedure

Begin by placing the patient in the Trendelenburg position, setting up the I.V. fluid and tubing, and dressing the catheter insertion site. Review the patient's chart to be sure that placement of the venous access device has been confirmed by X-ray.

Using sterile technique, connect the solution to the I.V. line. If you're using an Infuse-a-Port device or a Hickman catheter, flush it with heparin and saline solution. Then infuse the solution as ordered, using an infusion pump.

To minimize side effects, begin the infusion slowly, gradually increasing the flow rate. Similarly, if you need to discontinue the infusion, taper it slowly.

Monitoring and aftercare

Check the infusion rate, catheter integrity, and dressings hourly. Carefully record the patient's intake and output, and collect urine specimens every 6 hours for laboratory analysis. Monitor laboratory studies daily.

Weigh the patient every day at the same time, on the same scale, and in the same type of clothing. Watch for edema and, if it occurs, notify the doctor.

Change the I.V. tubing and dressings every 48 hours. When you change the dressing, inspect the catheter insertion site and report any redness, swelling, discharge, or drainage.

To prevent oral lesions and parotitis, have the patient brush his teeth and tongue frequently and use mouthwash and lip balm as necessary.

Home care instructions

• If the patient will be receiving parenteral nutrition at home, have his family practice the procedures in the hospital under your supervision.

• For these patients, also review instructions for storing the solution. For most patients, it will be delivered daily or will need to be picked up from a local pharmacy. Explain that the solution must be refrigerated and that each bag has an expiration date. Tell the patient or a family member to check the solution's date, composition, and appearance. Then, if the solution is suitable for use, allow it to warm to room temperature before using it.

• Tell family members to change the patient's dressing whenever it becomes soiled or loose, or at least once a week (for transparent polyurethane dressings) or every other day (for gauze dressings). Teach them to use aseptic technique when changing the dressing.

• Instruct them to regularly inspect the catheter insertion site for swelling, redness, or drainage. Suggest using a mirror if the patient must inspect his own dressing.

• Demonstrate how to irrigate the catheter. Long-term venous access devices need to be heparinized to remain patent; silicone silastic atrial catheters require daily irrigation with 3 ml of a heparin/saline solution. Implanted infusion ports must be flushed with 3 to 5 ml of a heparin/saline solution every 4 weeks. In addition, the catheter should be irrigated with saline solution after every infusion to clear the lumen of residual solution.

• Explain that the patient should be weighed daily at the same time, on the same scale, and while wearing similar clothing. Show the patient and his family how to check urine glucose levels and how to monitor intake and output. Caution them to watch for swelling—which indicates electrolyte imbalances—and to be on guard for signs of infection.

• Review the potential complications of IVH. Advise the patient to keep the telephone numbers of his local police and fire department, ambulance company, hospital, and doctor within easy reach.

NURSE'S GUIDE TO FOOD VALUES

Use this chart as a handy reference to help your patient select foods that meet his special dietary requirements. If the patient's on a low-cholesterol diet, for example, you can select foods from the four major groups that provide necessary nutrients while containing low levels of cholesterol.

FOOD AND AMOUNT	CALORIES	PROTEIN (g)	CHOLESTEROL (mg)	CARBOHYDRATE (g/100 g)	CALCIUM (mg)	SODIUM (mg)	POTASSIUM (mg)	PHOSPHORUS (mg)	PHENYLALANINE (mg)
Bread Barley, uncooked, 1 c, 200 g	700	16	0	158	32	6	320	378	1,322
Italian, 1 slice, 30 g	85	3	0	17	5	151	22	23	149
Pumpernickel, 1 slice, 32 g	80	3	0	17	27	161	145	73	136
Rye, 1 slice, 25 g	60	2	0	13	19	139	36	37	106
White, 1 slice, 25 g	70	2	0	13	21	127	26	24	116
Whole wheat, 1 slice, 28 g	65	3	0	14	24	148	72	71	143
Flour All-purpose, 1 c, 125 g	455	13	1	95	20	3	119	109	721
Whole wheat, 1 c, 120 g	400	16	0	85	49	3	444	446	788
Breakfast cereal Cornflakes, plain, 25 g	95	2	0	21	4	251	30	9	89
Farina, quick-cooking, 1 c, 240 g	105	3	0	22	147	1656	25	113	1,419
Oatmeal or rolled oats, 1 c, 240 g	130	5	0	23	22	523	146	137	1,819
Wheat germ, 1 tbsp, 6 g	25	2	0	3	3	0	57	70	54
Crackers and grains Graham, 2 crackers, 14 g	55	1	0	10	6	94	55	21	52
Macaroni, cooked firm, 1 c, 130 g	190	7	0	39	14	30	103	85	870
Noodles, egg, 1 c, 160 g	200	7	150	37	16	3	70	94	976
Popcorn, plain, 1 c, 6 g	25	1	0	5	1	5	23	17	93
Rice, long grain, 1 c, 205 g	225	4	0	50	21	767	57	57	783
Saltines, 4 crackers, 11 g	50	1	0	8	2	121	13	10	58
Spaghetti, 1 c, 130 g	190	7	0	39	14	30	103	85	870

KEY: c = cup, **g** = gram, **mg** = milligram, **t** = trace, **tbsp** = tablespoon, **tsp** = teaspoon

(continued)

NURSE'S GUIDE TO FOOD VALUES *(continued)*

FOOD AND AMOUNT	CALORIES	PROTEIN (g)	CHOLESTEROL (mg)	CARBOHYDRATE (g/100 g)	CALCIUM (mg)	SODIUM (mg)	POTASSIUM (mg)	PHOSPHORUS (mg)	PHENYLALANINE (mg)
Dairy products Butter, 1 tbsp	100	t	36	t	3	152	4	3	2
Cheese, cheddar, 1 oz, 28 g	115	7	25	t	204	207	28	145	348
Cheese, cottage, 1 c, 225 g	235	28	28	6	135	515	190	297	2,063
Cheese, parmesan, 1 oz, 28 g	110	11	27	1	312	206	42	218	540
Ice cream, 1 c	270	5	49	32	176	115	257	134	120
Milk, evaporated, ½ c, 100 g	137	7	31	10	252	118	303	205	340
Milk, whole, 1 c	150	8	32	11	291	120	370	228	450
Milk, 2%, 1 c	120	8	14	12	297	120	377	232	450
Milk, 1%, 1 c	100	8	7	12	300	120	381	235	450
Milk, skim, 1 c	85	8	4	12	302	120	406	247	450
Yogurt, whole milk, 8 oz	140	8	30	11	274	115	351	215	430
Eggs Egg, 1 whole, 50 g	80	6	252	1	27	57	65	90	349
Egg white, 1, 33 g	15	3	0	t	3	48	50	4	227
Egg yolk, 1, 17 g	65	3	252	t	24	9	15	86	122
Fats and dressings Corn oil, 1 tbsp	120	0	0	0	0	0	0	0	0
French dressing, 1 tbsp	65	t	0	3	2	206	13	2	5
Italian dressing, 1 tbsp	85	t	0	1	2	314	2	1	1
Lard, 1 tbsp	115	0	13	0	0	0	0	0	0
Margarine, 1 pat	100	t	0	t	3	152	4	3	5
Mayonnaise, 1 tbsp	100	t	11	t	3	90	5	4	5
Olive oil, 1 tbsp	120	0	0	0	0	0	0	0	0
Peanut oil, 1 tbsp	120	0	0	0	0	0	0	0	0
Thousand Island dressing, 1 tbsp	80	t	3	2	2	130	18	3	4

KEY: c = cup, **g** = gram, **mg** = milligram, **t** = trace, **tbsp** = tablespoon, **tsp** = teaspoon

NURSE'S GUIDE TO FOOD VALUES *(continued)*

FOOD AND AMOUNT	CALORIES	PROTEIN (g)	CHOLESTEROL (mg)	CARBOHYDRATE (g/100 g)	CALCIUM (mg)	SODIUM (mg)	POTASSIUM (mg)	PHOSPHORUS (mg)	PHENYLALANINE (mg)
Fruits and juices Apple (medium), 138 g	80	t	0	20	10	1	152	14	14
Apple juice, 1 c, 248 g	120	t	0	30	15	2	250	22	8
Applesauce, sweetened, 1 c, 255 g	230	1	0	61	10	5	166	13	12
Apricot, canned, ½ c, 100 g	38	1	0	10	12	1	246	16	20
Apricot, dried, 1 c, 130 g	340	7	0	86	87	34	1273	140	16
Avocado, 216 g	370	5	0	13	22	9	1303	91	97
Banana, 119 g	100	1	0	26	10	1	440	31	52
Blueberries, 1 c, 145 g	90	1	0	22	22	1	117	19	21
Cantaloupe, half, 477 g	80	2	0	20	38	57	682	44	102
Cherries, sweet, 10, 68 g	45	1	0	12	15	1	129	13	9
Cranberry juice, 1 c, 253 g	165	t	0	42	13	3	25	8	10
Dates, whole, 10, 80 g	220	2	0	58	47	1	518	50	50
Grapefruit, pink/red, half, 241 g	50	1	0	13	20	1	166	20	0
Grapefruit, white, half, 241 g	45	1	0	12	19	1	159	19	
Grapes, Thompson seedless, 10, 50 g	35	t	0	9	6	2	87	10	5
Lemon, raw, 74 g	20	1	0	6	19	1	102	12	0
Lime juice, canned, unsweetened, 1 c, 246 g	65	1	0	22	22	3	256	27	0
Orange, 131 g	65	1	0	16	54	1	263	26	15
Orange juice, diluted, frozen, 1 c, 249 g	120	2	0	29	25	2	503	42	21
Peach, raw, 100 g	40	1	0	10	9	1	202	19	18
Peaches, canned in water, 244 g	75	1	0	20	10	5	334	32	22

KEY: c = cup, **g** = gram, **mg** = milligram, **t** = trace, **tbsp** = tablespoon, **tsp** = teaspoon

(continued)

NURSE'S GUIDE TO FOOD VALUES *(continued)*

FOOD AND AMOUNT	CALORIES	PROTEIN (g)	CHOLESTEROL (mg)	CARBOHYDRATE (g/100 g)	CALCIUM (mg)	SODIUM (mg)	POTASSIUM (mg)	PHOSPHORUS (mg)	PHENYLALANINE (mg)
Pear, Bartlett, raw, 164 g	100	1	0	25	13	2	213	18	14
Pineapple juice, unsweetened, 1 c, 250 g	140	1	0	34	38	3	373	23	21
Plum, 66 g	30	t	0	8	8	1	112	12	24
Prune juice, 1 c, 256 g	195	1	0	49	36	0	602	51	32
Raisins, seedless, 1 c, 145 g	420	4	0	112	90	1	1106	146	203
Raspberries, 1 c, 123 g	70	1	0	17	27	1	207	27	32
Strawberries, 1 c, 149 g	55	1	0	13	31	1	244	31	36
Tangerine, 86 g	40	1	0	10	34	1	108	15	10
Watermelon, 4" × 8" wedge, 926 g	110	2	0	27	30	9	426	43	100
Legumes and nuts Almonds, slivered, 1 c 115 g	690	21	0	22	269	5	889	580	1318
Beans, canned, lima, 1 c, 190 g	260	16	0	49	55	44	1163	293	2321
Beans, dried, great northern, 1 c, 180 g	210	14	0	38	90	10	749	266	2126
Cashew nuts, roasted, 1 c, 140 g	785	24	0	41	53	21	650	522	1324
Coconuts, shredded, 1 c, 80 g	275	3	0	8	10	0	205	76	139
Lentils, whole, cooked, 1 c, 200 g	210	16	0	39	50	10	498	238	2208
Peanut butter, 1 tbsp, 16 g	95	4	0	3	9	97	100	61	242
Peanuts, roasted, 1 c, 144 g	840	37	0	27	107	7	971	577	2242
Walnuts, black, chopped, 1 c, 125 g	785	26	0	19	t	2	575	713	959
Meat Bacon, 2 slices, 15 g	85	4	6	t	2	153	184	114	65

KEY: c = cup, **g** = gram, **mg** = milligram, **t** = trace, **tbsp** = tablespoon, **tsp** = teaspoon

NURSE'S GUIDE TO FOOD VALUES *(continued)*

FOOD AND AMOUNT	CALORIES	PROTEIN (g)	CHOLESTEROL (mg)	CARBOHYDRATE (g/100 g)	CALCIUM (mg)	SODIUM (mg)	POTASSIUM (mg)	PHOSPHORUS (mg)	PHENYLALANINE (mg)
Beef, pot roasted, 3 oz, 85 g	245	23	78	0	10	65	189	159	566
Beef, ground, 10% fat, 3 oz, 85 g	185	23	75	0	10	65	261	196	559
Beef, ground, 21% fat, 2.9 oz, 82 g	235	20	78	0	9	63	221	159	540
Beef, rib roast, 3 oz, 85 g	375	17	78	0	8	65	189	159	608
Beef, steak, sirloin, 3 oz, 85 g	330	20	78	0	9	65	220	162	604
Lamb chop, broiled, 3.1 oz, 89 g	360	18	84	0	8	62	200	139	539
Lamb leg, roasted, 3 oz, 85 g	235	22	81	0	9	60	241	177	622
Liver, beef, fried, 3 oz, 85 g	195	22	366	5	9	156	323	405	814
Pork, fresh, loin chop, broiled, 2.7 oz, 78 g	305	19	68	0	9	51	216	209	504
Pork, ham, cured, 3 oz, 85 g	245	18	75	0	8	791	199	46	549
Pork, roast, 3 oz, 85 g	310	21	75	0	9	55	233	218	398
Pork, sausage, 1 link, 13 g	60	2	75	t	1	125	35	21	51
Veal, cutlet, 3 oz, 85 g	185	23	84	0	9	68	258	196	673
Poultry Chicken, dark meat, skinned, roasted, 3½ oz, 100 g	220	30	88	2	14	86	321	225	811
Chicken, light meat, skinned, roasted, 3½ oz, 100 g	197	32	77	1	12	64	441	280	811
Turkey, skinned, roasted, 3½ oz, 100 g	176	33	77	0	8	130	410	251	960
Seafood Bluefish, broiled, 3½ oz, 100 g	159	26	63	0	29	76	325	287	761

KEY: c = cup, **g** = gram, **mg** = milligram, **t** = trace, **tbsp** = tablespoon, **tsp** = teaspoon

(continued)

NURSE'S GUIDE TO FOOD VALUES (continued)

FOOD AND AMOUNT	CALORIES	PROTEIN (g)	CHOLESTEROL (mg)	CARBOHYDRATE (g/100 g)	CALCIUM (mg)	SODIUM (mg)	POTASSIUM (mg)	PHOSPHORUS (mg)	PHENYLALANINE (mg)
Cod, broiled, 3½ oz, 100 g	170	29	63	0	31	110	407	274	612
Crabmeat, canned, 1 c, 135 g	135	24	117	1	61	1350	65	90	1128
Flounder, baked, 3½ oz, 100 g	202	30	63	0	23	76	325	344	553
Haddock, 3½ oz, 100 g	165	20	63	6	40	177	348	247	676
Halibut, 3½ oz, 100 g	171	25	63	0	16	134	525	248	690
Salmon, fresh, broiled or baked, 3½ oz, 100 g	182	27	60	0	*	116	443	414	646
Sardines, canned in oil, 3 oz, 85 g	175	20	51	0	372	700	502	224	666
Shrimp, canned, 3 oz, 85 g	100	21	119	1	98	158	194	199	590
Tuna, canned in water, 3½ oz, 100 g	127	28	60	0	16	41	279	190	1000
Vegetables Asparagus, raw, 1 c	30	3	0	5	30	18	265	73	81
Beans, green, frozen, 1 c	35	2	0	8	54	18	205	43	11
Beans, yellow, frozen, 1 c	35	2	0	8	47	18	221	42	11
Beets, 1 c	55	2	0	12	24	37	354	39	28
Broccoli, 1 c, 155 g	50	5	0	9	100	28	392	104	184
Brussels sprouts, 1 c, 155 g	50	5	0	10	33	18	457	95	229
Cabbage, white, raw, 1 c	20	1	0	5	44	33	210	26	48
Carrot, raw, 1, 72 g	30	1	0	7	27	46	246	26	22
Carrots, cooked, 1 c, 155 g	50	1	0	11	51	50	344	48	28
Cauliflower, cooked, 1 c, 125 g	30	3	0	5	26	12	258	53	90
Celery, raw, 1 c, 120 g	20	1	0	5	47	149	409	34	0

KEY: c = cup, g = gram, mg = milligram, t = trace, tbsp = tablespoon, tsp = teaspoon
* Varies according to presence or absence of bone.

NURSE'S GUIDE TO FOOD VALUES *(continued)*

FOOD AND AMOUNT	CALORIES	PROTEIN (g)	CHOLESTEROL (mg)	CARBOHYDRATE (g/100 g)	CALCIUM (mg)	SODIUM (mg)	POTASSIUM (mg)	PHOSPHORUS (mg)	PHENYLALANINE (mg)
Corn, canned, 1 c	175	5	0	43	6	30	204	153	196
Cucumber, peeled, 6½ large pieces	5	t	0	1	5	2	45	5	7
Lettuce, iceberg, ¼ head	20	1	0	4	27	12	236	30	92
Mushrooms, raw, 1 c, 70 g	20	2	0	3	4	11	290	81	0
Onion, raw, sliced, 1 c, 115 g	45	2	0	10	31	16	181	41	49
Peas, whole, canned, 1 c, 170 g	150	8	0	29	44	39	163	129	223
Pepper, sweet, raw, 74 g	15	1	0	4	7	8	157	16	41
Potato, baked, peeled, 156 g	145	4	0	33	14	18	782	101	117
Potato, boiled, peeled, 137 g	105	3	0	23	10	16	556	72	102
Spinach, cooked, 1 c, 80 g	40	5	0	6	167	91	583	68	79
Sweet potato, baked, 114 g	160	2	0	37	46	21	342	66	114
Tomato, raw, 135 g	25	1	0	6	16	25	300	33	38
Turnip, cooked, ⅔ c	23	1	0	5	35	34	188	24	32

KEY: c = cup, g = gram, mg = milligram, t = trace, tbsp = tablespoon, tsp = teaspoon

Selected References

Dickerson, J., and Booth, E. *Clinical Nutrition for Nurses, Dieticians and Other Health Care Professionals.* Winchester, Mass.: Faber & Faber, 1985.

Green, M., and Harry, J. *Nutrition in Contemporary Nursing Practice.* New York: John Wiley & Sons, 1981.

Guthrie, H. *Introductory Nutrition,* 6th ed. St. Louis: C.V. Mosby Co., 1986.

Hui, Y. *Essentials of Nutrition and Diet Therapy.* Boston: Jones & Bartlett, 1985.

Krause, M., and Mahan, K. *Food, Nutrition and Diet Therapy,* 6th ed. Philadelphia: W.B. Saunders Co., 1979.

Patrick, M., et al. *Medical-Surgical Nursing: Pathophysiological Concepts.* Philadelphia: J.B. Lippincott Co., 1986.

6

Treating Neurologic Dysfunction

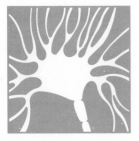

Treating Neurologic Dysfunction

Introduction

With ongoing advances in treating neurologic dysfunction, you need an in-depth understanding of current drug therapy, surgery, and related treatments to provide effective nursing care.

Drug therapy
Drug therapy forms the backbone of treatment for many neurologic disorders. Anticonvulsants, for instance, help control seizures. Beta-adrenergic blockers prevent migraine headache, whereas ergot alkaloids can relieve it. Steroids help lower intracranial pressure.

When caring for a patient undergoing drug therapy, you'll need to be alert for severe side effects and for interactions with other drugs. Some drugs, such as the barbiturates, also carry a high risk of toxicity and dependence.

Keep in mind that therapy's success hinges on the patient's strict adherence to his medication schedule. Compliance is especially critical for drugs that require steady-state blood levels for therapeutic effectiveness, such as anticonvulsants, or for drugs used prophylactically, such as beta-adrenergic blockers.

Surgery
Life-threatening neurologic disorders usually call for emergency surgery. For example, an epidural hematoma typi-cally requires immediate aspiration. A cerebral aneurysm requires correction through clipping or another technique. These and other surgeries often involve a craniotomy, a procedure that opens the skull and exposes the brain.

As a nurse, you assume a multifaceted role when caring for a patient undergoing neurologic surgery. For example, you're responsible for the patient's preoperative assessment and postoperative care. You're also responsible for answering questions raised by the patient and his family and for providing appropriate teaching—whether it involves ventricular shunt care or cosmetic care after craniotomy. And because the prospect of surgery usually provokes fear and anxiety, you'll need to provide ongoing emotional support.

Related treatments
Other treatments, such as barbiturate coma and implantation of intracranial electrodes to control uncoordinated neuromuscular activity, may require you to take on an even larger role. Even if you don't participate in these treatments, you'll be responsible for patient preparation as well as for assessment and monitoring before, during, and after them. What's more, you may need to help the patient and his family face an uncertain and perhaps unfavorable prognosis.

DRUG THERAPY

Barbiturate Anticonvulsants

Typically, these long-acting CNS depressants provide a useful adjunct to other anticonvulsant drugs, such as the benzodiazepines. They're not in the forefront of seizure treatment because their dosage must be carefully regulated to provide control without causing oversedation.

The barbiturate anticonvulsants include phenobarbital, mephobarbital, metharbital, and primidone. *Phenobarbital,* the barbiturate of choice for most patients, can be given orally for long-term treatment of generalized tonic-clonic and focal seizures. The parenteral form can be used for emergency treatment of status epilepticus and seizures caused by eclampsia, meningitis, or tetanus. *Mephobarbital,* administered orally, provides an alternative to phenobarbital for patients who can't tolerate phenobarbital's sedative effects. *Metharbital,* also given orally, is seldom used because it causes excessive sedation. Although not a true barbiturate, *primidone* is structurally similar to phenobarbital. It's used as primary or adjunctive treatment for generalized tonic-clonic, psychomotor, and focal seizures.

Barbiturate anticonvulsants are contraindicated in patients with a hypersensitivity to at least one of the drugs; in patients with porphyria, cardiac or hepatic dysfunction, respiratory disease with dyspnea or obstruction, or nephritis; and in pregnant or lactating women. They should be used cautiously in elderly or debilitated patients and in those with severe anemia, diabetes mellitus, hyperthyroidism, or hypoadrenalism. Prolonged use of these drugs can lead to blood dyscrasias, physiologic and psychological dependence, and tolerance. And, when taken with alcohol or other CNS depressants, barbiturates can cause excessive CNS depression and death.

Intravenous doses of barbiturates should be administered slowly into a large vein to reduce the risk of venous irritation, thrombosis, and hypotension. For I.M. injection, no more than 3 ml should be given at any one site to prevent tissue irritation.

Purpose and action
To reduce seizure activity by depressing monosynaptic and polysynaptic transmission in the CNS and increasing the threshold for electrical stimulation of the motor cortex.

Monitoring
When administering I.V. barbiturates, carefully monitor the patient's vital signs, especially respirations. Watch for signs of toxicity: respiratory depression, bradycardia or tachycardia, oliguria, hypotension, lowered body temperature, and decreased level of consciousness. Because overdose can be fatal, keep emergency equipment readily available in the event of respiratory or cardiac arrest.

While the patient's adjusting to therapy, he may experience lethargy, drowsiness, confusion, decreased attention span, and slurred speech. In addition, an elderly or young patient may develop paradoxical hyperexcitability. Typically, these effects occur in the early stages of therapy, when dosage is being gradually increased to achieve optimum seizure control, and subside after the patient develops tolerance, usually within 3 weeks. To prevent injury, assist him with ambulation and raise the side rails of his bed.

During early therapy, also watch for systemic or local dermatologic reactions, such as facial edema, purpura, urticaria, and skin rash or blisters.

Such reactions may dictate discontinuing the drug or reducing its dosage.

Be alert for other common side effects, such as anorexia or nausea. Encourage the patient to maintain a well-balanced diet, even if he doesn't feel like eating. Because fluid loss from vomiting can affect serum barbiturate concentrations, monitor intake and output and ensure adequate hydration.

Check the patient's drug history for medications that may potentiate barbiturate effects: monoamine oxidase inhibitors, valproic acid, and diazepam. Also check for rifampin, which may lower barbiturate levels.

During long-term barbiturate therapy, monitor hematologic status carefully to detect blood dyscrasias.

Home care instructions

• Warn the patient to avoid activities requiring alertness and good coordination until he has adjusted to therapy.

• Warn him that loss of consciousness and even death can result from using alcohol or other CNS depressants with barbiturates.

• Discuss side effects that the patient should report immediately: breathing difficulty, chest pain, eye pain or redness, eye discharge or decreased tearing, skin redness or peeling, hair loss, and facial edema. The doctor may adjust the dose or discontinue the drug.

• Also explain the need to report any increased bruising or bleeding, which may indicate a blood dyscrasia.

• Instruct the patient to follow his medication schedule closely. If he misses a dose, he should take it right away if he remembers within an hour or so of the missed dose. If he doesn't remember until later, he should skip the missed dose and return to the regular dosing schedule. He should never double-dose.

• Tell him never to break, crush, or chew extended-release capsules. He should swallow them whole.

• Warn him not to stop taking the drug abruptly without his doctor's approval; seizures and delirium may result.

Benzodiazepine Anticonvulsants

Used alone or with other anticonvulsant drugs, the benzodiazepines clonazepam, clorazepate, and diazepam prevent seizures or reduce their frequency or severity. *Clonazepam* proves useful in treating absence, akinetic, and myoclonic seizures, whereas *clorazepate* provides adjunctive therapy for simple partial seizures. In the parenteral form, *diazepam* helps treat status epilepticus. In the oral form, it's used adjunctively for seizures.

Typically, the benzodiazepines are preferred over the barbiturate anticonvulsants because they're more predictable and produce fewer side effects at therapeutic doses. What's more, they have less potential for dependence, abuse, and interaction with other drugs. In overdoses, they're less toxic. Nonetheless, prolonged use of benzodiazepines can produce psychological and physiologic dependence. And when they're taken with alcohol or other CNS depressants, the benzodiazepines can cause increased CNS depression and death.

Because benzodiazepine dependence occurs most commonly in patients with a history of alcohol and drug abuse, these drugs should be avoided in such patients, if possible. They should be used cautiously in patients with suicidal tendencies or in those whose history suggests potential abuse. They're contraindicated in patients with a known hypersensitivity to any benzodiazepine and in patients with hepatic disease or acute angle-closure glaucoma. They should be administered judiciously to patients with renal impairment, chronic respiratory disease, or chronic open-angle glaucoma. Intravenous administration should be avoided in shock or coma or with respiratory depression.

COMPARING SERUM LEVELS
OF ANTICONVULSANTS

To evaluate the safety and effectiveness of anticonvulsant drugs, you need to monitor the patient's serum drug levels. This table, which presents therapeutic ranges, toxic levels, and information on the onset and duration of action for some common anticonvulsants, will help you assess your patient's response to his drug regimen.

DRUG	THERAPEUTIC RANGE (mcg/ml)	TOXIC LEVEL (mcg/ml)	SERUM HALF-LIFE	TIME TO REACH STEADY STATE
Carbamazepine	4 to 10	≥12	10 to 25 hr	4 to 6 days
Clonazepam	0.03 to 0.06	≥0.08	19 to 48 hr	4 to 6 days
Ethosuximide	40 to 100	≥150	30 to 60 hr	4 to 8 days
Phenobarbital	15 to 25	≥35	50 to 120 hr	14 to 21 days
Phenytoin	10 to 20	>20	18 to 22 hr	5 to 7 days
Primidone	6 to 12	≥15	6 to 8 hr	2 to 3 days
Valproic acid	50 to 100	>100	8 to 15 hr	2 to 3 days

Purpose and action

Benzodiazepines produce an anticonvulsant effect by interfering with electrical transmission through the limbic structure, thalamus, and cortex and suppressing the spread of seizure activity produced in these areas. The precise sites and mechanisms of action are unclear. Apparently, the drugs facilitate the action of gamma-aminobutyric acid, an inhibitory neurotransmitter, after interacting with a specific neuronal membrane receptor.

Monitoring

Keep in mind that I.V. administration can cause apnea, hypotension, bradycardia, or cardiac arrest, particularly in elderly or severely ill patients and in those with limited pulmonary reserve or unstable cardiovascular status. For this reason, always keep resuscitation equipment on hand when using this administration route. After I.V. administration, check for redness, pain, or swelling at the injection site.

Watch for common side effects of benzodiazepines: drowsiness, dizziness, light-headedness, feelings of clumsiness or unsteadiness, and confusion. Be especially alert for these effects in elderly or debilitated patients, children and infants, and patients with hepatic disease or low serum albumin levels. Even if the patient takes the drug at bedtime, he may feel less alert on rising. Typically, these effects occur during the early stages of therapy and subside within a few days. During this period, take steps to protect the patient from injury, such as raising side rails and assisting him with ambulation.

Also watch for GI effects, such as anorexia, nausea, excessive thirst, and constipation or diarrhea. Try reducing or eliminating some of these effects by giving the drug with food.

During long-term therapy, regularly monitor hepatic and renal function tests and blood counts, especially for the patient with liver or kidney impairment. Check his drug regimen for cimetidine, which may slow clearance of clorazepate and diazepam.

Because abrupt withdrawal from benzodiazepines may precipitate status epilepticus, make sure the patient takes all of his scheduled medication.

Home care instructions
• To prevent dependence, warn the patient not to exceed the dosage, even if he feels the drug isn't working.
• Tell him to report confusion, depression, blurred vision, ataxia, or unusual fatigue.
• Instruct the patient to avoid activities that require alertness or coordination, such as driving, until his response to the drug has been determined.
• To reduce GI distress, advise taking the drug with food.
• Warn him that concurrent use of alcohol and benzodiazepines can cause severe CNS depression and even death.
• Instruct him to avoid smoking. Although the mechanism of interaction is unclear, tobacco apparently speeds metabolism of benzodiazepines, thereby reducing their effectiveness.
• Tell the patient to make up a missed dose as soon as he remembers, as long as it's within an hour of the scheduled administration. Otherwise, he should resume his regular schedule with the next dose. He shouldn't double-dose.
• If the patient is taking an extended-release capsule, instruct him to swallow it whole. He should never crush, break, or chew it.
• If the patient is on prolonged therapy, explain that his doctor will evaluate the effectiveness of therapy about every 4 months. Warn against stopping the drug without his doctor's approval.
• Explain to the patient that after he stops taking the drug, his body may take some time to adjust to withdrawal—from a few days up to 3 weeks, depending on the dosage and the duration of therapy. Tell him to notify his doctor if he experiences withdrawal symptoms, such as extreme irritability, nervousness, incoordination, or weakness.

Hydantoin Anticonvulsants

The hydantoin derivatives—phenytoin, ethotoin, mephenytoin, and phenacemide—treat generalized tonic-clonic and complex partial seizures. Because of their effectiveness and minimal side effects, these drugs are considered the first-line treatment for these seizures.

Phenytoin is typically the hydantoin of choice. Unlike the other hydantoins, which are administered only orally, phenytoin may be given orally or intravenously. It can also be used in status epilepticus and nonepileptic seizures, but it must be used cautiously in patients with cardiac disease.

Ethotoin, less toxic but also less effective than phenytoin, is most com-

COMPARING DRUGS

COMPARING SIDE EFFECTS OF HYDANTOINS

Although all hydantoin derivatives produce some similar side effects, several significant differences may influence the selection of one drug over the others.

Blood dyscrasias, although possible from any of the hydantoins, most commonly occur with mephenytoin.

CNS effects, such as ataxia, confusion, and slurred speech, also may occur with all the hydantoins. However, they're most common and severe with phenytoin. In contrast, mephenytoin's CNS effects usually are limited to drowsiness.

Because *gingival hyperplasia* occurs most commonly with phenytoin but rarely with ethotoin, the latter hydantoin is prescribed for patients predisposed to this problem, such as children and the elderly. Likewise, *hypertrichosis* develops commonly with phenytoin but rarely with ethotoin, making ethotoin the preferred hydantoin if this side effect occurs.

Life-threatening *ventricular fibrillation* has occurred with phenytoin but not with mephenytoin or ethotoin.

UNDERSTANDING OTHER KEY ANTICONVULSANTS

Besides the barbiturates, benzodiazepines, and hydantoin derivatives, several other drugs help treat seizure disorders, as described below.

DRUG AND INDICATIONS	MECHANISM OF ACTION	MONITORING
Carbamazepine Treatment of generalized tonic-clonic, complex partial, and mixed seizures and trigeminal neuralgia	Exact mechanism of action is unknown. Drug is thought to stabilize neuronal membranes and limit seizure activity by increasing efflux or decreasing influx of sodium ions across cell membranes in the motor cortex during generation of nerve impulses.	• Check for signs of hyponatremia. • Observe for signs of latent psychosis, confusion, or agitation. • If the patient complains of blurred or double vision, notify doctor. • Monitor CBC, liver function tests, blood urea nitrogen (BUN) levels, and urinalysis.
Suximide derivatives (ethosuximide, methsuximide, phensuximide) Treatment of absence seizures	Increase seizure threshold and reduce the paroxysmal spike-and-wave pattern of absence seizures by depressing impulse transmission in the motor cortex.	• Monitor CBC for blood dyscrasias; liver function tests for impaired hepatic function; and BUN level and urinalysis for impaired renal function.
Valproic acid Treatment of absence seizures and mixed seizures; used investigationally for generalized tonic-clonic seizures	Increases levels of gamma-aminobutyric acid, which transmits inhibitory nerve impulses in the CNS.	• Every 6 months during therapy, monitor CBC and platelet count for signs of thrombocytopenia; liver and kidney function tests for signs of dysfunction; and serum ammonia for elevated levels.

monly prescribed for children, who are especially prone to the gingival hyperplasia caused by phenytoin. Because of potentially life-threatening blood dyscrasias, *mephenytoin* is used infrequently. *Phenacemide*, the most toxic hydantoin anticonvulsant, is usually reserved for patients who fail to respond to other anticonvulsants.

Because hydantoin derivatives are metabolized in the liver and excreted by the kidneys, they're usually contraindicated in hepatic and renal disorders. They're also contraindicated in patients with hematologic disorders or hydantoin hypersensitivity. Phenacemide, meanwhile, shouldn't be used for patients with personality disorders because it can cause severe psychotic episodes. All the hydantoins should be used cautiously in elderly or debilitated patients and in those with hypotension, myocardial insufficiency, or respiratory depression.

Purpose and action

Hydantoin derivatives provide anticonvulsant action by stabilizing neuronal membranes in the motor cortex during generation of nerve impulses. They do so either by increasing efflux or decreasing influx of sodium ions across the cell membranes.

Monitoring

While the patient builds therapeutic levels of the prescribed hydantoin, watch for common side effects: drowsiness, dizziness, rash, urticaria, ataxia, nausea or vomiting, insomnia, visual disturbances, hirsutism, and blood dyscrasias. Motor disturbances, drowsiness, and dizziness typically subside after the first few days of therapy. Until they do, take measures to protect the patient from falls, such as assisting him with ambulation and raising side rails. Reducing hydantoin dosage may diminish some of the per-

HOME CARE INSTRUCTIONS

• Emphasize the importance of complying with the dosing schedule to maintain consistent blood levels. Warn the patient not to stop taking the drug without first consulting his doctor.
• Because this drug causes drowsiness, warn the patient not to drive or operate machinery until his response to the drug has been determined.

• Tell the patient to notify his doctor immediately if fever, sore throat, mouth ulcers, or easy bruising occurs.
• Tell him to take the drug with meals to prevent GI irritation.
• Remind the patient to continue regular medical visits to monitor the safety and effectiveness of therapy.

• Warn the patient not to discontinue the medication without first consulting his doctor.
• Tell him not to drive or operate machinery until he has adjusted to the drug's CNS effects.
• Instruct him to never take damaged tablets; the drug's effectiveness will be reduced.

• Explain that phensuximide may turn his urine red, pink, or reddish brown but that the effect is harmless.
• Instruct him to take the prescribed drug with food or milk to reduce GI irritation.

• Emphasize the importance of complying with treatment to ensure steady-state drug levels. Explain that noncompliance may bring on seizures.
• Tell the patient to report any malaise, fever, or lethargy, which may be early symptoms of serious or even fatal hepatotoxicity.

• Tell the patient to swallow the capsules whole with water. He shouldn't chew or break capsules or take them with milk.
• Warn the patient not to drive a car or operate machinery until he has adjusted to the drug's CNS effects.

sistent side effects. Or, if the patient experiences nausea and vomiting, give the drug with or after meals.

Carefully monitor the patient's serum drug levels and physical status (including level of seizure activity) to determine the safety and effectiveness of therapy. Pay special attention to toxic effects in an elderly patient, who will tend to metabolize hydantoins slowly. Such a patient may receive therapeutic benefit from lower doses.

Check the patient's drug and dietary regimen for possible interactions with the prescribed hydantoin. Folic acid, dexamethasone, and tube feedings of Osmolite or Isocal may decrease hydantoin activity. In contrast, anticoagulants, cimetidine, antihistamines, diazepam, salicylates, and sulfonamides increase it.

If you're giving I.V. phenytoin, infuse the drug at a rate of less than 5 mg/ minute to prevent hypotension, ar-

rhythmias, or even cardiac arrest. If you're giving phenacemide, monitor for personality changes, especially depression and suicidal tendencies.

Home care instructions

• Advise the patient to immediately report blurred or double vision, uncontrollable eye movements, confusion, severe drowsiness, dizziness, hallucinations, slurred speech, or nausea.
• Instruct him to avoid alcohol, which interferes with drug metabolism.
• Explain to the patient that he should avoid activities requiring alertness and good psychomotor coordination while he's adjusting to the prescribed drug.
• Stress the importance of regular physical examinations and blood tests to evaluate the safety and effectiveness of hydantoin therapy.
• Explain how good oral hygiene and regular dental checkups can help combat gingival hyperplasia (occurs most

commonly in children receiving prolonged phenytoin therapy).

• Instruct the patient to strictly comply with his medication schedule. If he misses a dose, he should take it right away if he remembers within an hour or so of the missed dose. If he doesn't remember until later, he should skip the missed dose and return to his regular dosing schedule. He should never double-dose.

• If the patient is taking liquid phenytoin, show him how to mix it correctly.

• Tell the patient to learn the trade or generic name of the hydantoin he's taking and to take *only that specific drug.* Warn him not to switch from a trade to a generic form or vice versa. Doing so could alter drug blood levels and bring on seizures.

• Advise wearing an identification bracelet or carrying a card that specifies the name and dosage of his prescribed drug.

Ergot Alkaloids

This group of adrenergic blocking agents, which includes *dihydroergotamine mesylate* and *ergotamine tartrate*, provides relief from vascular (migraine and cluster) headaches. When given in the prodromal phase of such a headache, these drugs effectively constrict dilated cerebral vessels and relieve pain.

Ergotamine tartrate, considered the more effective of the two ergot alkaloids, is available in oral, inhalant, and sublingual forms; the latter two forms provide more rapid action in treating acute episodes. Ergotamine also serves as an ingredient in products containing varying mixtures of the belladonna alkaloids, phenobarbital, and caffeine.

Dihydroergotamine mesylate, administered intramuscularly or intravenously, produces fewer and less serious GI side effects than ergotamine

and may be indicated for patients prone to GI reactions.

Because the ergot alkaloids cause vasoconstriction, they're contraindicated in severe hypertension, peripheral or occlusive vascular disease, coronary artery disease, phlebitis, impaired renal or hepatic function, and other debilitating diseases. Patients over age 40 should undergo a complete cardiovascular evaluation, including an electrocardiogram, before starting ergot therapy.

Purpose and action
These drugs inhibit the effects of epinephrine, norepinephrine, and other sympathomimetic amines. This causes cerebral vasoconstriction, counteracting the pain-producing vasodilation of a vascular headache.

Monitoring
During ergot therapy, carefully monitor the results of cardiac and renal function tests, complete blood count, and erythrocyte sedimentation rate. Check for signs of drug intolerance, such as insomnia or drowsiness, malaise, abdominal pain, nasal congestion, rash, and dermatitis. Report any abnormal test findings or adverse effects to the doctor, who may need to alter the patient's drug regimen.

Because of these drugs' vasoconstrictive effects, be alert for signs of reduced peripheral circulation: coldness, numbness, tingling, muscle pain and weakness, and localized edema in the extremities. Severe vasoconstriction can result in tissue damage.

Review the patient's drug regimen for possible interactions. For example, propranolol or other beta blockers and vasopressors can dangerously intensify the vasoconstrictive effects of ergot alkaloids. If the patient's taking these drugs concurrently, carefully monitor his pulse rate, blood pressure, and respirations. Immediately report bradycardia or tachycardia, hypertension or hypotension, chest pain, or shortness of breath.

Home care instructions

• Tell the patient to take the drug during the prodromal stage of a headache or as soon as possible after onset. To help him relax, which will enhance the drug's effectiveness, advise him to lie down in a quiet, darkened room, if possible.

• Teach the patient how to use the sublingual or inhalant forms of ergotamine, if appropriate.

• Warn him not to increase drug dosage without first consulting his doctor.

• To reduce the frequency and severity of vascular headaches, help the patient identify possible precipitating factors, such as stress or the ingestion of caffeine, chocolate, or alcohol.

• Instruct the patient on long-term therapy to report any coldness, numbness, tingling, or pain in his hands and feet; leg cramps; or chest or flank pain. Show him how to assess for peripheral edema, and tell him to report this effect as well.

• Tell the patient to avoid overexposure to cold temperatures, which may increase drug side effects.

• If he experiences nausea, vomiting, or other GI effects, tell him to take the drug with food or milk.

• Explain to the patient that ergotamine rebound—increased severity and frequency of headaches—may occur after discontinuing therapy.

Beta-Adrenergic Blockers

[Beta blockers]

Besides their well-known cardiovascular applications, the beta-adrenergic blockers—*atenolol, metoprolol, nadolol, pindolol, propranolol,* and *timolol*—can be used prophylactically for patients with frequent or disabling migraine headaches. They're not indicated for acute or infrequent attacks.

Because the beta blockers lower blood pressure, they're contraindicated in patients with cardiogenic shock, second- or third-degree atrioventricular block, sinus bradycardia, or hypotension. Because they can reduce peripheral circulation, they should be used cautiously in peripheral vascular disease. Beta blockers can also produce bronchospasm, especially at high doses. As a result, they should be given cautiously to patients with respiratory problems. Because beta blockers are metabolized by the liver and excreted by the kidneys, they should be used judiciously in patients with hepatic or renal impairment.

Patients with hyperthyroidism may experience severe exacerbation of symptoms from abrupt withdrawal of beta blockers. In these patients, therapy must be discontinued gradually.

Purpose and action

These drugs block response to beta stimulation and depress renin secretion, producing an antihypertensive effect. Their mechanism of action in preventing migraine headaches is unclear. Apparently, they prevent cerebral vasodilation—the physiologic action that produces migraines.

Monitoring

Before administering a beta blocker, check the patient's apical pulse rate. If you note bradycardia, tachycardia, or arrhythmias, withhold the drug and notify the doctor.

When first giving a beta blocker, be alert for signs of drug toxicity, such as bradycardia or tachycardia, pulse irregularities, dyspnea, bluish-tinged fingernails and palms, severe dizziness or syncope, and possibly seizures. These signs typically develop within 1 to 2 hours after drug ingestion.

During therapy, regularly check the patient's vital signs, especially blood pressure and pulse rate. Closely monitor his complete blood count to detect possible thrombocytopenia and leukopenia.

Review the patient's medication regimen for possible interactions. Concurrent use of cardiac glycosides, for example, can cause excessive bradycardia and myocardial depression. Antihypertensives and diuretics may produce severe hypotension. Paradoxically, the antihypertensive clonidine can cause hypertension.

Check for use of monoamine oxidase inhibitors, phenothiazines, I.V. phenytoin, adrenergics, and xanthines. All of these drugs must be used cautiously with beta blockers.

Home care instructions

• Teach the patient how to take his pulse rate and stress the importance of notifying the doctor if he detects bradycardia, tachycardia, or irregular beats.

• Also emphasize the importance of immediately reporting breathing difficulty, cyanosis, cold or swollen hands or feet, and chest, back, or joint pain. He should report fever, sore throat, rash, unusual bleeding or easy bruising, and any CNS effects (such as confusion, depression, hallucinations, dizziness, and fainting).

• Instruct the patient to take the drug at the same time each day for most effective prophylaxis. If he misses a dose, he should take it as soon as he remembers, unless he doesn't remember until within 4 hours of his next scheduled dose of metoprolol or timolol or within 8 hours of his next scheduled dose of atenolol, nadolol, or extended-release propranolol. In such cases, he shouldn't take the drug, resuming his schedule with the next dose.

• To help evaluate therapy's effectiveness, ask the patient to record the frequency and severity of migraine attacks.

• To possibly reduce the patient's need for migraine prophylaxis, help him identify and avoid aggravating factors. These may include smoking, alcohol, fatigue, stress, chocolate, and tyramine-containing foods, such as cheddar cheese.

Antimyasthenics
[Cholinesterase inhibitors]

The treatment of choice for relieving myasthenic symptoms, the antimyasthenic drugs include neostigmine, ambenonium, and pyridostigmine. *Neostigmine*, which has the shortest duration of action of the antimyasthenics, is sometimes used in the Tensilon test to help diagnose myasthenia gravis. Slower-acting *pyridostigmine* may produce fewer and less serious side effects than neostigmine. Even slower-acting *ambenonium* provides an alternative for patients with a hypersensitivity to the bromide ion contained in neostigmine and pyridostigmine. However, this drug possesses the greatest potential for toxicity.

The choice of a specific antimyasthenic drug and its dosage depend on clinical experience, the patient's response, and the route of administration. No matter what the drug or dosage, the oral form is preferred to treat recurrent myasthenic symptoms. The I.V. route may be used to treat myasthenic crisis or to circumvent swallowing difficulty.

Because the antimyasthenics can constrict the bronchi and cause breathing problems, they should be administered cautiously in patients with asthma, pneumonia, or atelectasis and in all postoperative patients. Typically, the antimyasthenics are contraindicated in patients with arrhythmias, intestinal or urinary tract obstruction, or urinary tract infection.

Purpose and action

• To treat myasthenic symptoms by inhibiting the disease-induced destruction of acetylcholine. Accumulating acetylcholine promotes increased stimulation of nerve receptors and, ultimately, improved muscle innervation and increased muscle strength.

HOW ANTIMYASTHENICS WORK

Acetylcholine, a powerful neurotransmitter, is synthesized in the presynaptic terminal endings of cholinergic nerve fibers. These terminals contain vesicles that, when stimulated, release acetylcholine into the synaptic cleft to mediate impulse transmission between the presynaptic terminal and the target receptor neuron, or postsynaptic receptor. Most secreted acetylcholine is quickly split into acetate ions and choline by the enzyme anticholinesterase, which appears both on the presynaptic terminal and on the surface of the receptor neuron. Antimyasthenic drugs work by inhibiting anticholinesterase, resulting in a higher concentration of acetylcholine in the synaptic cleft and improved impulse transmission.

NORMAL ACETYLCHOLINE ACTION

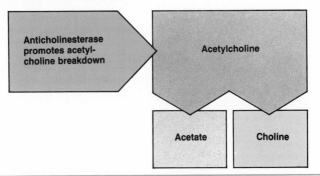

EFFECT OF ANTIMYASTHENICS ON ACETYLCHOLINE

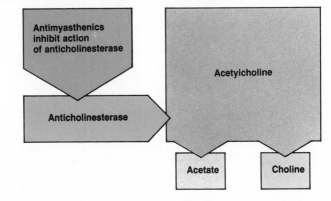

● *For neostigmine and pyridostigmine:* To serve as an antidote for nondepolarizing neuromuscular blocking agents used in surgery, such as tubocurarine.

● *For neostigmine:* To prevent and treat postoperative nonobstructive urinary retention and ileus.

Monitoring

During administration, carefully monitor the patient's vital signs, especially respirations. Keep atropine injection and emergency equipment readily available in the event of respiratory arrest. To help determine the most effective dose, document the patient's muscle strength, ease of swallowing, and respiratory effort after each dose.

Throughout therapy, watch for signs of drug toxicity or underdosage, which can cause myasthenic crisis. Signs of toxicity include headaches, weakness, diaphoresis, abdominal pain, nausea and vomiting, diarrhea, excessive salivation, and bronchospasm. Myasthenic crisis is marked by bradycardia, difficulty breathing or swallowing, blurred vision, diarrhea, nausea or vomiting, excessive salivation, and weakness. Inform the doctor of any untoward symptoms, since he'll need to distinguish between drug toxicity and myasthenic crisis.

Check the patient's drug regimen for possible interactions. For example, concurrent use of aminoglycosides, anesthetics, lidocaine, capreomycin, polymyxin, lincomycin, quinidine, or procainamide may antagonize the effects of antimyasthenics. The antihypertensives guanadrel, guanethidine, mecamylamine, and trimethaphan may worsen myasthenic symptoms. Atropine and related compounds may reduce or prevent some side effects of antimyasthenics and may mask initial signs of toxicity. Concurrent use of other cholinesterase inhibitors, particularly edrophonium, can cause rapid toxicity.

Home care instructions
• Tell the patient and his family the signs of drug toxicity and myasthenic crisis. Instruct them to report any such signs immediately.
• Allow the patient some freedom in determining his medication dose and schedule. To maximize the drug's effectiveness, encourage him to schedule his largest doses before usual periods of fatigue, such as in the afternoon and before meals. Also encourage him to schedule rest times for such periods.
• Teach him how to evaluate and record variations in muscle strength. Instruct him to keep a daily record of these variations, correlated to the time of day and his medication schedule, to help his doctor evaluate therapy.

• While the patient's adjusting to therapy, have him take the drug with food or milk to minimize GI distress. Explain that scheduling a dose for 30 minutes before meals may help alleviate dysphagia.
• Because even a minor respiratory infection can aggravate myasthenic symptoms, instruct the patient to avoid contact with all persons with infections.
• Advise him to wear an identification bracelet or necklace indicating his condition and current drug regimen.

Antidyskinetics
[Cholinergic blockers, parasympatholytics]

These synthetic anticholinergics have supplanted the belladonna alkaloids as the drugs of choice in treating Parkinson's disease. Commonly used with levodopa, the antidyskinetics can be used alone in mild cases of the disease. They also prove effective in treating drug-induced extrapyramidal symptoms, such as tremors and akinesia. However, they're not indicated for relief of tardive dyskinesia.

Four drugs constitute the antidyskinetic family: *benztropine, biperiden, procyclidine,* and *trihexyphenidyl.* The choice of a specific antidyskinetic depends on the patient's response and the drug's pharmacokinetic profile. For example, because both procyclidine and trihexyphenidyl have a direct antispasmodic effect on smooth muscle, they may be especially useful for the patient with muscle rigidity.

Typically, the antidyskinetics are contraindicated in acute angle-closure glaucoma. They should be used cautiously in hypertension or hypotension, arrhythmias, prostatic hypertrophy, hepatic or renal disease, obstructive disease of the genitourinary or GI tract, urinary retention, tardive dyskinesia,

COMPARING LEVODOPA AND LEVODOPA-CARBIDOPA

Often, levodopa or the combination drug levodopa-carbidopa is used with an antidyskinetic drug to relieve symptoms of Parkinson's disease. Which of these two drugs is the better choice for this application?

The answer hinges on several factors. Because levodopa quickly metabolizes in the GI tract and the liver, less than 1% of the dose reaches the CNS for conversion to dopamine—a process known as decarboxylation. But in the combination drug, carbidopa inhibits GI metabolism of levodopa without affecting levodopa's metabolism within the CNS, thus making more levodopa available for decarboxylation in the brain. As a result, less levodopa is needed to achieve therapeutic results. In fact, the combination drug can reduce the amount of levodopa needed by up to three quarters.

But levodopa-carbidopa has its drawbacks. Because it enhances the action of levodopa, it produces not only therapeutic effects but also adverse reactions more rapidly and at lower doses than does levodopa alone.

Whichever drug the doctor chooses, you'll need to monitor the patient carefully. In particular, watch for CNS effects, such as dyskinesias and altered mental status. Report them promptly; the doctor may need to change the drug or adjust the dosage.

---

or myasthenia gravis, and in alcoholic, elderly, or debilitated patients. Because these drugs can produce or worsen psychotic symptoms, they should be used carefully in patients with personality disorders.

Purpose and action

To relieve parkinsonian and extrapyramidal symptoms by partially blocking central cholinergic receptors, which helps balance cholinergic and dopaminergic activity in the basal ganglia.

Monitoring

Throughout antidyskinetic therapy, monitor the patient for common side effects. In children and in alcoholic, elderly, or debilitated patients, watch especially for antimuscarinic effects, such as skin and mucous membrane dryness, skin warmth and flushing, and tachycardia; these effects usually disappear after the early stages of therapy or with a reduction in drug dosage. Also observe for signs of anhidrosis and hyperthermia; to decrease the likelihood of these effects, keep the patient's room cool. Carefully check for GI effects, including nausea, diarrhea or constipation, and abdominal pain and distention; such effects may indicate paralytic ileus. In addition, watch older male patients for difficult or painful urination. Monitor intake and output for signs of urinary retention.

Because long-term antidyskinetic therapy can lead to glaucoma, have the patient report any eye pain, blurred vision, or photosensitivity. Check for mydriasis or increased intraocular pressure. Report any such effects immediately so that the patient can receive an ophthalmologic evaluation. Also watch for and report any changes in mental status, such as confusion, agitation, delirium, hallucinations, depression, and memory loss. Such changes may indicate drug toxicity.

Because the ocular and CNS effects of these drugs can lead to falls, take precautionary measures, such as raising side rails and assisting the patient with ambulation.

Review the patient's medication regimen for possible interactions. Concurrent use of antidyskinetics with antihistamines, magnesium sulfate, or CNS depressants may cause excessive sedation. Cyclobenzaprine, haloperidol, monoamine oxidase inhibitors, phenothiazines, procainamide, and tricyclic antidepressants may intensify antimuscarinic effects and lead to paralytic ileus. Chlorpromazine may increase anticholinergic activity and actually aggravate parkinsonian symptoms.

Because antacids and absorbent antidiarrheals may reduce the therapeutic effects of antidyskinetics, give these drugs at least 1 hour before or after an antidyskinetic.

Home care instructions

• Warn the patient never to stop taking the drug without his doctor's approval. Explain that abrupt withdrawal may cause sudden exacerbation of parkinsonian symptoms.
• Instruct him to adhere strictly to the prescribed dosage schedule—even if he feels the drug isn't working. Explain that therapeutic effects may not be apparent for up to several weeks.
• Emphasize the need to immediately report any abdominal pain, distention, diarrhea, or constipation, which may signal paralytic ileus.
• Explain to the patient that he should avoid activities that require alertness and coordination, such as driving and operating machinery, until his CNS response to the drug has been determined.
• Warn him to avoid alcohol and other CNS depressants, which increase the sedative effects of antidyskinetics.
• To help minimize gastric irritation, tell the patient to take his medication with or immediately after meals.
• Explain that he can alleviate dry mouth with frequent sips of water, ice chips, or sugarless gum or hard candy.
• If the patient experiences anhidrosis, warn him to avoid overexertion. His inability to perspire could lead to hyperthermia, especially in hot weather.
• Discuss the importance of regular ophthalmologic examinations to help identify any eye problems caused by long-term therapy.

Benzodiazepine Sedative-Hypnotics

The benzodiazepines *flurazepam*, *temazepam*, and *triazolam* produce hypnosis and skeletal muscle relaxation. As a result, they're useful in treating insomnia associated with difficulty falling asleep, frequent nocturnal awakenings, and early morning awakening. In fact, they're preferred over barbiturates for these sleep problems. That's because they're more predictable and produce fewer side effects at therapeutic doses. What's more, they have less potential for dependence, abuse, and interaction with other drugs. In overdoses, they're less toxic.

Although benzodiazepines have proven effective and safe for both short- and long-term therapy, prolonged use can result in psychological and physiologic dependence. And when taken with alcohol or other CNS depressants, the benzodiazepines can produce increased CNS depression and death.

Because benzodiazepine dependence occurs most commonly in patients with a history of alcohol or drug abuse, these drugs should be avoided in such patients, if possible. They also should be used cautiously in patients with suicidal tendencies or in those whose history indicates that they may increase drug dosage on their own initiative. Benzodiazepines are contraindicated in patients with a known hypersensitivity to any drug in the benzodiazepine family and in patients with hepatic disease or acute angle-closure glaucoma. They should be administered judiciously to patients with renal impairment, chronic respiratory disease, or chronic open-angle glaucoma.

Purpose and action

These drugs produce a hypnotic effect by interfering with electrical transmission through the limbic structures, thalamus, and hypothalamus. Although the benzodiazepines' mechanism of action isn't fully understood, they apparently facilitate the action of gamma-aminobutyric acid, an inhibitory neurotransmitter, after interacting with a specific neuronal membrane receptor in the ascending reticular activating system.

Monitoring

During benzodiazepine therapy, watch for common side effects: drowsiness, dizziness, light-headedness, unsteadiness, and confusion. Be especially alert for these effects in elderly or debilitated patients and in those with hepatic disease or low serum albumin levels. Typically, these effects occur during the early stages of therapy and subside within a few days. During this period, take steps to protect the patient from injury, such as raising side rails and assisting him with ambulation.

Watch for GI effects, such as loss of appetite, nausea, excessive thirst, and constipation or diarrhea. Try reducing or eliminating some of these effects by giving the drug with food.

Check the patient's drug regimen for use of other sedatives and hypnotics, narcotic and opioid analgesics, antihypertensives, monoamine oxidase inhibitors, or cimetidine, which may enhance the CNS-depressant and hypotensive effects of benzodiazepines.

During long-term therapy, regularly monitor hepatic and renal function tests and blood counts, especially for the patient with liver or kidney impairment.

Home care instructions

● Warn the patient never to increase benzodiazepine dosage on his own, even if he feels the drug isn't working effectively. Doing so will increase his risk of drug overdose or dependence. Explain that drug effects may not be apparent for a day or two.
● Discuss common, reportable side effects: dizziness, drowsiness, lethargy,

---

BENZODIAZEPINES: A SAFER ALTERNATIVE

Until recently, doctors regularly prescribed barbiturates, such as amobarbital and phenobarbital, for treating sleep disorders and anxiety. Or they may have ordered nonbarbiturate sedative-hypnotics, such as chloral hydrate and glutethimide, for the same reasons. Some of these drugs possess the potential for dependence, toxicity, and life-threatening interactions. However, even though they can be used successfully, the safer and equally effective benzodiazepines are used more commonly.

---

impaired coordination, and confusion.
● Instruct the patient to avoid activities that require alertness and coordination, such as driving, until his response to the drug has been determined.
● To prevent GI distress, advise taking the drug with meals.
● Explain that benzodiazepines accentuate the effects of alcohol and other CNS depressants—possibly causing severe CNS depression and even death. As a result, he should avoid these substances during therapy.
● Also tell him not to use tobacco. Although the mechanism of interaction is unclear, tobacco apparently speeds metabolism of benzodiazepines, thereby reducing their effectiveness.
● Explain to the patient that after he stops taking the drug, his body may take some time to adjust to withdrawal—anywhere from a few days to 3 weeks, depending on the dosage and the duration of therapy. Tell him to notify his doctor if he experiences extreme irritability, nervousness, incoordination, or weakness. Alert him to the possibility of rebound insomnia, which should persist for no more than 2 or 3 nights.
● Encourage the patient to seek alternative therapy to deal with the underlying cause of his insomnia and to explore nonchemical sleep aids, such as biofeedback and progressive relaxation therapy.

Corticosteroids

[Adrenocorticosteroids, glucocorticoids]

Besides their many other uses, the corticosteroids *cortisone, prednisolone, methylprednisolone, dexamethasone,* and *hydrocortisone* can relieve cerebral edema resulting from head injury, neurosurgical procedures, or tumors. At therapeutic levels, they exert an anti-inflammatory effect that stabilizes cell membranes and helps prevent secondary CNS damage.

Usually, the corticosteroids are initially administered intravenously or by deep I.M. injection for cerebral edema. As treatment progresses, the oral form may be introduced gradually.

Prolonged corticosteroid therapy requires careful monitoring of the patient's vital signs, fluid and electrolyte balance, mental status, and overall condition. That's because these drugs have been linked to hypokalemia, hyperglycemia, growth suppression in children, menstrual irregularities in women, and other untoward effects. By increasing protein catabolism, they can interfere with normal wound healing and immune response.

Because of their immunosuppressant effects, the corticosteroids are contraindicated in patients with systemic fungal infections. They should be given cautiously in patients with GI ulcers, renal or hepatic disease, hypertension, congestive heart failure, osteoporosis, diabetes mellitus, hyperthyroidism or hypothyroidism, uncontrolled viral or bacterial infections, myasthenia gravis, tuberculosis, or acquired immune deficiency syndrome. Because these drugs can precipitate depression or psychotic episodes, especially in high doses, they should be given judiciously in patients with a history of emotional instability or psychotic tendencies.

Abrupt withdrawal of corticosteroids can precipitate potentially fatal adrenal crisis. For this reason, the drug dosage should always be tapered gradually under close supervision.

Purpose and action

Glucocorticoids stabilize cell membranes and inhibit the release of proteolytic enzymes, preventing the cerebral tissue's normal inflammatory response and reducing edema.

Monitoring

Check the patient's drug regimen for possible interactions with corticosteroids. Barbiturates, phenytoin, rifampin, and ephedrine may decrease glucocorticoid effects, possibly requiring a dosage increase. Antacids can impair absorption of the drugs. Amphotericin B and diuretics can potentiate hypokalemia.

During therapy, regularly check the patient's body weight, blood pressure, intake and output, and blood glucose and serum potassium levels. Compare them to baseline levels. Similarly, check the patient's skin for delayed wound healing or skin compromise.

Observe the patient for increased thirst and frequent urination, which may indicate hyperglycemia. Be alert for signs of hypokalemia, such as muscle cramps, arrhythmias, hypotension, confusion, lethargy, and hypoactive reflexes. If weight gain, edema, and hypertension occur, suspect sodium and fluid retention. If the patient reports visual disturbances, inform the ophthalmologist. The patient may have glaucoma, cataracts, or optic nerve damage.

If the patient's receiving prolonged therapy, watch for cushingoid signs, such as moon face and purple striae on the limbs, trunk, or face. Also observe for insomnia, emotional lability, and psychotic behavior—especially in a patient with a history of instability.

During withdrawal of corticosteroids, monitor the patient for symptoms of possible adrenal insufficiency: lethargy, weakness, dyspnea, orthostatic hypotension, syncope, fever, arthralgia, and anorexia. Report any of these effects to the doctor immediately.

Home care instructions
• Warn the patient never to stop taking the drug without his doctor's consent. Sudden withdrawal can be fatal.
• Instruct him to take a missed dose as soon as he remembers and to then return to his normal schedule. He shouldn't take a double dose unless he's taking the drug several times a day.
• To reduce GI upset, tell him to take the prescribed drug with food or milk. He should also avoid alcohol, which can increase the ulcerogenic effects of corticosteroids.
• Explain that corticosteroids impair resistance to infection. As a result, the patient must avoid exposure to any person with a known or suspected infection. He must also avoid any vaccinations or immunizations during therapy and the withdrawal period.
• Instruct the patient to carry an identification card specifying the name and dosage of his prescribed drug.

SURGERY

Craniotomy

This procedure involves creation of a surgical incision into the skull, thereby exposing the brain for any number of treatments. These treatments may include ventricular shunting, excision of a tumor or abscess, hematoma aspiration, and aneurysm clipping. Craniotomy has many potential complications, including infection, hemorrhage, respiratory compromise, and increased intracranial pressure (ICP); the degree of risk depends largely on the patient's condition and the surgery's complexity.

Your role in a craniotomy is largely supportive. Your clear explanation of the surgery and thorough answers to questions can help allay some of the patient's and family's concerns. After surgery, your close monitoring for complications can improve the chances of recovery.

Purpose
To expose the brain for surgical intervention.

Preparation
Help the patient and family cope with the surgery by clarifying the doctor's explanation and by encouraging them to ask questions. When answering their questions, be informative and honest. While you can't guarantee a complete and uncomplicated recovery, you can help instill a sense of confidence in the surgeon and in a successful outcome.

Explain preoperative procedures. Tell the patient that his hair will be washed with an antimicrobial shampoo on the night before surgery. In the operating room, his head will be shaved, and he'll receive steroids to reduce postoperative inflammation. His legs may also be wrapped with elastic bandages to improve venous return and reduce the risk of thrombophlebitis. And because craniotomy is a lengthy procedure, he may also have a urinary catheter inserted.

Also prepare the patient for postoperative recovery. Explain that he'll awaken from surgery with a large dressing on his head to protect the incision. He also may have a surgical drain implanted in his skull for a few days and will be receiving prophylactic antibiotics. Warn him to expect a headache and facial swelling for 2 to 3 days after surgery, and reassure him that he'll receive medication to reduce the pain. Explain that, if all goes well, he should be ambulatory within 2 to 3 days after surgery. The doctor will usually remove the sutures within 7 to 10 days.

Before surgery, perform a complete neurologic assessment. Carefully record your assessment data to use as a baseline for postoperative evaluation.

Because the patient will go to the intensive care unit (ICU) after surgery, arrange a preoperative visit for him and his family. Explain the equipment and introduce them to the staff.

Procedure

After the patient receives a general anesthetic, the surgeon marks an incision line and cuts through the scalp to the cranium, forming a scalp flap that he turns to one side. He then bores two or more holes through the skull in the corners of the cranial incision, using an air-driven or electric drill, and cuts out a bone flap with a small saw. After pulling aside or removing the bone flap, he incises and retracts the dura, exposing the brain. (See *Craniotomy: A Window into the Brain* for a more detailed explanation.)

The surgeon then proceeds with the surgery (see other surgeries in this chapter for details). Afterward, he reverses the incision procedure and covers the site with a sterile dressing. Then the patient is taken to the ICU for recovery.

Monitoring and aftercare

After surgery, carefully monitor the patient's vital signs and neurologic status. Check him every 15 minutes for the first 4 hours, then once every 30 to 60 minutes for the next 24 to 48 hours.

To help prevent increased ICP, position the patient on his side. Elevate his head 15 to 30 degrees to increase venous return and help him breathe more easily. With another nurse's help, turn him carefully every 2 hours.

Throughout the course of postoperative care, observe the patient closely for signs of increased ICP. Immediately notify the doctor if you note worsening mental status, pupillary changes, or focal signs, such as increasing weakness in an extremity.

Closely observe the patient's respi-

ratory status, noting rate and pattern. Immediately report any abnormalities. Encourage him to deep-breathe and cough, but warn him not to do this too strenuously. Suction gently, as ordered.

Carefully monitor fluid and electrolyte balance. The doctor will probably restrict fluid intake severely to minimize cerebral edema and prevent increased ICP. Monitor and record intake and output, check urine specific gravity every 2 hours, and weigh the patient, as ordered. Check serum electrolyte levels every 24 hours and watch the patient for signs of imbalance. Remember, low potassium levels may cause confusion and stupor; reduced sodium and chloride levels may produce weakness, lethargy, and even coma. Because fluid and electrolyte imbalance can precipitate seizures, report any of these signs immediately.

Provide good wound care. Make sure the dressing stays dry and in place, and that it's not too tight. Excessive dressing tightness may indicate swelling—a sign of increased ICP. If the patient has a closed drainage system, periodically check drain patency and note and document the amount and characteristics of any discharge. Notify the doctor of excessive bloody drainage, possibly indicating cerebral hemorrhage, or of clear or yellow drainage, which may indicate a cerebrospinal fluid leak. Also monitor the patient for signs of wound infection, such as fever and purulent drainage.

Finally, provide supportive care. Ensure a quiet, calm environment to minimize anxiety and agitation and help lower ICP. Administer anticonvulsants, as ordered, and maintain seizure precautions. Provide other ordered medications, such as steroids to prevent or reduce cerebral edema, stool softeners to prevent increased ICP from straining, and analgesics to relieve pain.

Home care instructions

● Before discharge, teach the patient proper wound care techniques. Tell him to keep the suture line dry and to

CRANIOTOMY: A WINDOW INTO THE BRAIN

To perform a craniotomy, the surgeon incises the skin, clamps the aponeurotic layer, and retracts the skin flap. He then incises and retracts the muscle layer and scrapes the periosteum off the skull.

Next, using an air-driven or electric drill, he drills a series of burr holes in the corners of the skull incision. During drilling, warm saline solution is dripped into the burr holes and the holes are suctioned to remove bone dust. Once drilling is com-

plete, the surgeon uses a dural elevator to separate the dura from the bone around the margin of each burr hole. He then saws between the burr holes to create a bone flap. He either leaves this flap attached to the muscle and retracts it, or detaches the flap completely and removes it. In either case, the flap is wrapped to keep it moist and protected.

Finally, the surgeon incises and retracts the dura, exposing the brain.

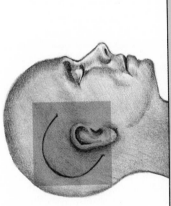

1   Initial incision

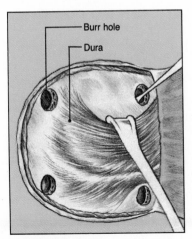

2   Retraction of skin flap

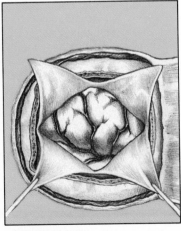

Burr hole
Dura

3   Burr holes drilled

4   Brain exposed

regularly cleanse the incision with hydrogen peroxide and saline solution. Instruct him to evaluate the incision regularly for redness, warmth, or tenderness and to report any of these findings to the doctor.

• If the patient is self-conscious about his appearance, suggest that he wear a wig, hat, or scarf until his hair grows back. As his hair begins to grow back, tell him to apply a lanolin-based lotion to keep his scalp supple and decrease itching. Remind him not to apply lotion to the suture line, however.

• Remind the patient to continue taking prescribed anticonvulsant medications to minimize the risk of seizures. Depending on the type of surgery performed, he may need to continue anticonvulsant therapy for up to 12 months after surgery. Also remind him to report any drug side effects, such as excessive drowsiness or confusion.

Cerebral Aneurysm Repair

For a patient with a cerebral aneurysm, surgical treatment represents the only sure method to prevent initial rupture or rebleeding. The surgeon can choose among several techniques, depending on the shape and location of the aneurysm. These techniques include clamping the affected artery, wrapping the aneurysm wall with a biological or synthetic material, or clipping or ligating the aneurysm. If the aneurysm isn't readily accessible for ligation, the treatment of choice, most often he'll choose clipping. In this procedure, the surgeon performs a craniotomy and then applies a metal spring clip around the neck of a berry aneurysm, thereby excluding the defective area from circulation. (See *Techniques for Repairing Aneurysms.*) Later, the arterial wall repairs itself, and the necrotic tissue detaches and is reabsorbed.

Preoperative nursing care for a patient undergoing aneurysm repair involves careful monitoring of neurologic status, maintenance of a stress-free environment, and other measures to prevent rupture or rebleeding and their complications, such as increased intracranial pressure (ICP) and pulmonary emboli. It also includes patient teaching and ongoing emotional support to prepare him for surgery. Postoperative care seeks to promote healing of the craniotomy site and gradual resumption of the patient's normal activities.

Purpose
To repair a cerebral aneurysm, thereby preventing possible rupture or rebleeding and stabilizing cerebral blood flow.

Preparation
If the patient's aneurysm will be clipped, explain to him that this surgical technique seals off the aneurysm from the cerebral circulation, preventing vessel rupture. If his aneurysm will be wrapped, explain that this technique supports the arterial wall. Tell him he'll receive a general anesthetic and then undergo a craniotomy to open the skull and expose the aneurysm. (See "Craniotomy," pages 253 to 256, for detailed patient preparation information for this procedure.)

Before the operation, frequently monitor the patient's neurologic status, checking his pupillary response, level of consciousness, and motor function. Record your assessment data to use as a baseline for your postoperative evaluation.

Because stress and activity elevate arterial pressure, which in turn can cause the aneurysm to rupture or rebleed, enforce bed rest and encourage the patient to rest and sleep as much as possible. Provide him with a darkened, quiet environment and try to anticipate all of his physiologic needs. Restrict his activities and limit visitors. Explain the reasons for these precautions and restrictions to the patient and his family, and enlist the family's help in enforcing them.

Despite these restrictions, the patient needs some activity to prevent skin breakdown and reduce the risk of pulmonary complications. Encourage him to deep-breathe, but warn him that coughing and sneezing may cause problems. If you need to suction the patient, do so gently. Carefully turn the patient every 2 hours. As appropriate, encourage him to perform range-of-motion exercises every 2 hours. (If the patient can't perform active exercises, provide passive exercise for his legs more often than every 2 hours to help prevent thrombus formation.) To also help prevent thrombus formation, apply antiembolism stockings, elastic bandages, or automatic compression boots.

Administer medications, as ordered. These may include anticonvulsants to prevent seizures, corticosteroids to prevent cerebral edema, stool softeners to prevent increased ICP from straining, and analgesics to relieve headache. If the patient's receiving I.V. fluids, carefully monitor and record his intake and output.

The aneurysm can rupture at any time, so watch for and immediately report early signs of it: a new or worsening headache, renewed or increased nuchal rigidity, or decreasing level of consciousness. Also notify the doctor of signs of increased ICP, including pupillary changes and focal neurologic deficits (such as increasing weakness in an extremity).

If the patient is awaiting surgery for an already-ruptured aneurysm, observe him for signs of rebleeding and elevated ICP.

Procedure

After cerebral arteriography has ruled out vasospasm, the surgeon performs a craniotomy to expose the aneurysm. Because cerebral aneurysms usually occur in the internal carotid or middle cerebral artery, craniotomy is usually done in the suboccipital or subfrontal

TECHNIQUES FOR REPAIRING ANEURYSMS

Using a metal spring clip, a berry aneurysm (named after its shape) can be isolated from the cerebral circulation. With other kinds of aneurysms, such as a fusiform aneurysm, the arterial wall can be supported by wrapping it with biological or synthetic material.

CLIPPING A BERRY ANEURYSM

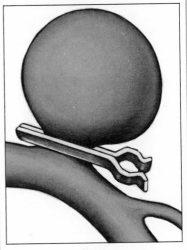

WRAPPING A FUSIFORM ANEURYSM

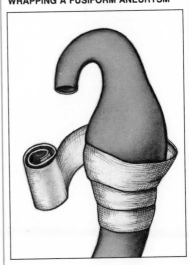

areas. Once the surgeon visualizes the aneurysm, with the aid of a microscope, he then carefully frees the aneurysm from the arachnoid tissue.

The surgeon then wraps the aneurysm with a biological or synthetic material. Or, if he plans to clip the aneurysm, he opens a small, spring-loaded clip and slips it over the neck of the aneurysm or over its feeder vessel. (A large aneurysm may require more than one clip.) Once the clip is in position, he releases it, letting it close to block blood flow to the aneurysm. The surgeon may leave the clip as is or he may elect to secure it with methyl methacrylate or a similar liquid agent, which quickly solidifies around the clip and the aneurysm. He then ligates and removes the sac of the aneurysm.

Next, the surgeon reverses the craniotomy procedure to close the incision.

Monitoring and aftercare

Monitor the patient for vasospasm, the constriction of intracranial blood vessels from smooth muscle contraction. It may occur suddenly and without warning, and usually begins in the vessel adjacent to the aneurysm. Depending on its intensity, it can spread through the major cerebral vessels, causing ischemia and possible infarction of involved areas with corresponding loss of neuromuscular function. Call the doctor immediately if you note hemiparesis, worsening of an existing motor deficit, visual disturbances, seizures, or altered level of consciousness.

After surgery, explain to the patient that he can gradually resume his normal activities. Focus your aftercare on measures to promote healing of the craniotomy. (See "Craniotomy," pages 253 to 256, for specific measures.)

Keep in mind that a patient with a cerebral aneurysm may be left with neurologic deficits that frustrate and possibly embarrass him and his family. Your positive, caring attitude and support can help them understand and cope with these problems.

Home care instructions

Emphasize the importance of returning for scheduled follow-up examinations and tests. (See "Craniotomy," pages 253 to 256, for additional home care instructions.)

Aspiration of an Intracranial Hematoma

An intracranial hematoma—epidural, subdural, or intracerebral—usually requires life-saving surgery to control bleeding and lower intracranial pressure (ICP). Even if the patient's life isn't in immediate danger, surgery is usually indicated to prevent irreversible damage from cerebral or brainstem ischemia.

The first priority in an epidural hematoma, which develops between the skull and the dura, is prompt aspiration and ligation of the bleeding site. Generally, this is done through a craniotomy; burr holes also may be drilled to relieve increased ICP.

A subdural hematoma, in which blood collects between the dura and the arachnoid membrane, is aspirated through either burr holes (if the clot is fluid) or a craniotomy (if it's solid). An acute or subacute subdural hematoma typically requires prompt aspiration. However, aspiration of a chronic (and sometimes a subacute) subdural hematoma depends on the patient's neurologic status. If it's stable or improving, surgery may be delayed. But if it's deteriorating and the hematoma is amenable to surgery, immediate aspiration is indicated.

An intracerebral hematoma, which involves bleeding in the subarachnoid space or brain parenchyma, also may require immediate aspiration through a craniotomy. But if the patient isn't in immediate danger, or if removal isn't feasible, surgery may be delayed or ruled out.

Hematoma aspiration carries the risk of severe infection and seizures as well as the physiologic problems associated with immobility during the prolonged recovery period. Even if hematoma removal is successful, associated head injuries and complications, such as cerebral edema, can produce permanent neurologic deficits, coma, or even death.

When caring for a patient undergoing hematoma removal, you'll need to provide preoperative teaching about the surgery and postoperative measures, such as the placement of drains in the surgical site. (Of course, in an emergency situation, you won't be able to provide such teaching.) You'll focus postoperative care on monitoring for complications and on taking steps to reduce their risk.

Purpose
To remove an intracranial hematoma, thereby relieving pressure on the cerebral vessels and preventing cerebral ischemia and brain tissue damage.

Preparation
If emergency aspiration is necessary, briefly explain the procedure to the patient, if possible. If immediate surgery isn't necessary, clarify the doctor's explanation and encourage the patient to ask questions. Then prepare the patient as you would for a craniotomy. (See "Craniotomy," pages 253 to 256.)

Procedure
Depending on the nature of the hematoma, the surgeon gains access to the bleeding site through either a craniotomy or burr holes.

If the hematoma is fluid, the surgeon uses a twist drill to burr holes through the skull, most commonly in the frontoparietal or temporoparietal areas. He drills at least two holes to delineate the extent of the clot and allow its complete aspiration. Once he reaches the clot, he inserts a small suction tip into the burr holes to aspirate the clot. He then inserts drains, which usually remain in place for 24 hours.

For a solid clot, or for a liquid one that can't be completely aspirated through burr holes, the surgeon performs a craniotomy. (For details, see "Craniotomy," pages 253 to 256.) After exposing the hematoma, he aspirates it with a small suction tip. He also may use saline irrigation to wash out parts of the clot. He then ligates any bleeding vessels in the hematoma cavity and closes the bone and scalp flaps. (If cerebral edema is severe, he may leave the craniotomy site exposed and replace the flaps only after edema subsides.) Usually, he places a drain in the surgical site.

Monitoring and aftercare
Perform a complete neurologic assessment and compare your findings to preoperative results. Carefully monitor the patient's vital signs and watch for signs of elevated ICP: headache, altered respirations, deteriorating level of consciousness, and visual disturbances. (See *Combating Increased ICP*, page 260.)

Take measures to prevent increased ICP, especially if the patient's hematoma was aspirated through burr holes. As ordered, and if the patient's condition permits, keep his head elevated about 30 degrees to promote venous drainage from the brain. Also as ordered, maintain fluid restrictions and administer osmotic diuretics or corticosteroids to decrease cerebral edema. Accurately record intake and output.

As ordered, give the patient an analgesic to relieve pain, antibiotics to prevent infection, and anticonvulsants to prevent seizures.

Regularly check the surgical dressing and the surrounding area for excessive bleeding or drainage. Evaluate drain patency by noting the amount of drainage. Although the surgeon may set specific guidelines, drainage usually shouldn't exceed 125 ml during the first 8 hours after surgery, 100 ml during

COMBATING INCREASED I.C.P.

Increased intracranial pressure (ICP), a dangerous complication of hematoma aspiration, can eventually lead to fatal brain herniation if unchecked. When caring for a patient with increased ICP, your first priority is to conduct a complete neurologic assessment. This will not only give you a clear picture of the patient's condition but will also provide you with a baseline against which you can compare subsequent changes in his neurologic status. Remember that changes in the patient's overall condition, rather than the onset of one specific symptom, signal increasing ICP.

Take precautionary measures
Keep resuscitation equipment on hand in case of a sudden deterioration in the patient's condition. Elevate the head of his bed 15 to 30 degrees to promote venous drainage from the brain. Don't place the patient in a jackknife position; this elevates intraabdominal and intrathoracic pressure, which in turn raises ICP. Place his head in a neutral position and support it with a cervical collar or neck rolls—especially when the patient's lying on his side. Also be sure to take seizure precautions, such as padding side rails.

Watch for ominous signs
Because altered level of consciousness is often the earliest sign of elevated ICP, assess frequently for restlessness, confusion, or unresponsiveness. If the patient lapses into unconsciousness, turn him onto his side to maintain airway patency and insert a nasogastric tube to prevent aspiration of vomitus and secretions.

Observe the patient closely for pupillary changes, such as unequal pupil size, constriction, dilation, or a brisk, sluggish, or absent response to light. If constriction occurs, notify the doctor immediately of this sign of impending brain herniation.

Frequently assess the patient's motor and sensory function. Increased pressure on motor and sensory tracts may cause partial or total loss of function.

Monitor vital signs at least every hour. You may see Cushing's triad: bradycardia, hypertension, and changes in respiratory pattern. Remember, increased ICP will at first stimulate and then depress the patient's respiratory and circulatory function. Be alert for widening pulse pressure.

Monitor pressure readings
Because small increases in ICP can escape detection during assessment, the doctor may decide to implant an ICP monitoring device. When caring for a patient with an ICP monitor, record pressure readings at least hourly and notify the doctor of any sudden increase.

Reduce fluid volume
Restrict fluids to 1,200 to 1,500 ml/day, thereby reducing total fluid volume and cerebral edema. Carefully record intake and output. If the patient is unresponsive or incontinent, you may need to insert an indwelling (Foley) catheter to obtain accurate measurements. The patient also may have a central venous line or a Swan-Ganz catheter inserted to aid in fluid management and an intraarterial line inserted to provide continuous blood pressure monitoring.

As ordered, administer a diuretic to further reduce fluid volume. To decrease cerebral edema, you also may administer a corticosteroid or perhaps I.V. lidocaine, a new treatment that shows promise in some patients.

Assist with other treatments
The doctor may order one or more treatments to reduce ICP:
● Administration of 100% oxygen, or controlled hyperventilation with mechanical ventilation, to reduce blood levels of carbon dioxide. Reducing carbon dioxide constricts cerebral vessels and reduces perfusion; these changes, in turn, lower ICP.
● I.V. barbiturates (usually pentobarbital or phenobarbital) to induce unresponsiveness or coma, thereby decreasing the metabolic rate, cerebral blood flow, and ultimately ICP. (See *Monitoring Patients in Barbiturate Coma*, page 274, for more details.)
● Implantation of a ventricular shunt to drain excess cerebrospinal fluid from the ventricular system, thereby lowering ICP. However, this treatment carries the risk of a sudden pressure drop that can cause brain herniation.

Throughout these treatments and during recovery, you'll continue to assess the patient closely for improvement or deterioration and report any changes in his condition.

the following 8 hours, and 75 ml over the next 8 hours. Report any abnormal drainage. Also ensure that the drainage is tested for glucose to detect any leakage of cerebrospinal fluid.

The patient will probably be restricted to bed rest for a prolonged period. To prevent decubiti formation and enhance circulation, turn him frequently and perform passive range-of-motion exercises for all his extremities.

Home care instructions

• Teach the patient and his family proper suture care techniques. Tell them to observe the suture line for signs of infection, such as redness and swelling, and to report any such signs immediately.

• Also instruct them to watch for and report any neurologic symptoms, such as altered level of consciousness and sudden weakness.

• Suggest that the patient wear a wig, hat, or scarf until his hair grows back. Advise using a lanolin-based lotion to help keep the scalp supple and decrease itching, but caution against applying lotion to the suture line.

• Remind the patient to continue taking prescribed anticonvulsant medications, as ordered, to minimize the risk of seizures. Also remind him to report any drug side effects, such as excessive drowsiness or confusion.

• Tell the patient he may take acetaminophen or another mild nonnarcotic analgesic for headaches.

Implantation of a Cerebellar Stimulator

[Cerebellar pacemaker]

A relatively new treatment, the cerebellar stimulator uses electrical impulses to regulate uncoordinated neuromuscular activity. Originally developed to prevent seizures in patients who didn't respond to drug therapy, the device also has been used successfully to reduce spasticity and provide better neuromuscular control in patients with cerebral palsy.

Basically, the cerebellar stimulator consists of two surgically implanted cerebellar electrodes attached to either an internal or an external power source and pulse generator. The pulse generator sends electrical impulses to the electrodes, stimulating the fibers of the cerebellar cortex. (See *How Cerebellar Stimulation Works*, page 262, for a more detailed explanation.)

Possible benefits of this device include reduced spasticity and abnormal movements, improved muscle and sphincter control, clearer speech, and decreased seizure activity. However, not all patients realize these benefits. And, in those who do, improvement may occur only over several months or even years.

Besides reinforcing the tentativeness of benefits, you'll need to provide support before this somewhat complex and often-frightening surgery. Postoperatively, you'll focus on monitoring for possible complications, such as infection or increased intracranial pressure, and on teaching the patient and his family how to care for the equipment.

Purpose

To electrically stimulate the cerebellum's inhibitory mechanisms, producing neuromuscular relaxation and decreased spasticity.

Preparation

When preparing the patient for electrode implantation, tailor your explanations and discussions to his age and level of understanding. Explain that the device regulates his brain's muscle control center much like a pacemaker regulates the heart, providing regularly timed electrical impulses that stimulate the muscles to function normally.

Explain the various components and how they work, stressing that the de-

HOW CEREBELLAR STIMULATION WORKS

The cerebellar stimulator system consists of two platinum and silicone electrode pads implanted on the cerebellar lobes and activated by one of two different power sources.

The monophasic *internal* system is powered by a self-contained lithium-iodine battery pack. Direct electrical current flows from this power source to the cerebellar electrodes.

The alternating-phase *external* system has a separate battery-operated transmitter and antenna along with a radio receiver that's implanted into the patient's neck or abdomen. The transmitter sends radio waves to the implanted receiver, which changes the current from alternating to direct and then relays it to the cerebellar electrodes.

In both systems, electronic pulses delivered at preset intervals stimulate the fibers of the cerebellar cortex. This activates inhibitory mechanisms in deep cerebellar, vestibular, and reticular areas of the brain, producing widespread neuromuscular relaxation.

INTERNAL SYSTEM

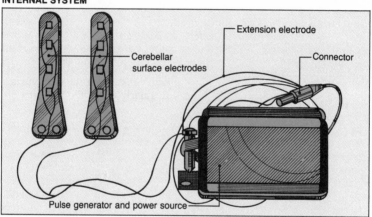

Cerebellar surface electrodes

Extension electrode

Connector

Pulse generator and power source

EXTERNAL SYSTEM

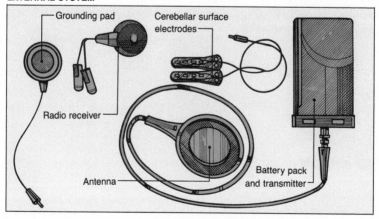

Grounding pad

Cerebellar surface electrodes

Radio receiver

Antenna

Battery pack and transmitter

vice's low-voltage electrical current cannot harm him. Briefly describe the implantation procedure. Explain that after he receives a general anesthetic, his head will be shaved and placed in a special headrest for the operation. Then the surgeon will make a total of four incisions for implanting the electrodes and other system components: two on the head, one on the neck, and one on the abdomen. Tell him that, upon awakening from the anesthetic, he'll feel the most pain from the neck incision but will receive medication to reduce his discomfort.

Discuss postoperative care measures, such as activity and fluid restrictions, progressive ambulation, and antibiotic therapy. Mention that you'll monitor him carefully to evaluate the device's effectiveness.

Before surgery, perform a complete neuromuscular evaluation to serve as a baseline.

Procedure

Before beginning implantation surgery, the surgeon makes a small scalp incision and drill hole through the skull in the right occipital area. (This hole will help relieve any postoperative intracranial hematoma or excessive edema.) Then he drills two burr holes in the suboccipital area and carefully places an electrode pad on the surface of each lobe of the cerebellum. He checks electrode placement with X-rays and adjusts the position, if necessary.

Once he's satisfied with electrode placement, the surgeon creates a subcutaneous pocket in the infraclavicular area or the right lower abdominal quadrant and implants the pulse generator and power source of the monophasic internal system. He then makes a subcutaneous tunnel running from the scalp incision down the side of the neck to the infraclavicular or abdominal pocket. Through this tunnel he threads the electrode leads and lead connectors. He then supervises the necessary hookups and testing of the unit's function and the patient's response.

Monitoring and aftercare

After surgery, carefully assess the patient's neurologic status and vital signs every hour for the first 24 hours, then once every 2 hours for the next few days. Watch for developing complications, such as increased intracranial pressure, infection, fluid imbalance, and aspiration pneumonia. Provide I.V. fluids, as ordered, if the patient experiences excessive nausea and vomiting because of cerebellar manipulation. Also observe for and record any seizure activity or spasticity to help the doctor evaluate the device's effectiveness.

Maintain the patient on bed rest until the second day after surgery. Keep his head elevated 15 to 30 degrees and turn him every 2 hours. Gradually increase his activities but make sure he avoids overexertion. Excessive activity can cause pooling of serous or cerebrospinal fluid in the subcutaneous pocket, possibly damaging the equipment.

Regularly check the patient's dressings for excessive bleeding or drainage, and change them as necessary. Assess suture lines for signs of infection and provide wound care. Administer antibiotics and analgesics, as ordered, but don't give the patient sedatives for sleep; they may skew neurologic findings.

Home care instructions

• Teach the patient and his family how to change a dressing. Tell them to change it about once every 2 days until the doctor removes the sutures (usually about 2 weeks after surgery).
• Also instruct them on proper wound care techniques for the suture lines.
• Warn them to watch for and report early signs of infection: fever and swelling or redness at the suture lines or subcutaneous pouch.
• Tell the patient that he can gradually resume his normal routine, but advise against excessive physical activity.
• Have the patient's family record the time, type, and duration of any seizures. Explain that this record will help the doctor evaluate the effectiveness of the cerebellar stimulator.

• Explain that the patient should keep regular follow-up appointments with his doctor to check on his condition and the unit's function.

Ventricular Catheter or Subarachnoid Screw Insertion

Besides monitoring intracranial pressure (ICP), the ventricular catheter and the subarachnoid screw allow drainage of cerebrospinal fluid (CSF) from the brain, thereby reducing ICP. Insertion of both devices is similar, through a twist-drill hole created in the skull. The ventricular catheter, inserted into a lateral ventricle, consists of a small polyethylene cannula and reservoir. The subarachnoid screw, inserted into the subarachnoid space, is a small hollow steel screw with a sensor tip. Both devices possess a built-in transducer that converts ICP to electrical impulses for constant monitoring. Both also have a drain to allow periodic removal of CSF. What's more, the ventricular catheter can be equipped with a continuous CSF drainage system.

Choice of device depends on several factors. The ventricular catheter provides more accurate ICP measurement and allows for continuous CSF drainage. The subarachnoid screw, although also providing accurate ICP measurements, can become occluded more readily. However, it's easier to insert, especially in patients with midline shifting or collapsed ventricles. Because the device requires a firm skull for anchoring, it isn't typically used in young children or in patients whose skull integrity may be compromised.

Whichever device the doctor chooses, your primary responsibilities are monitoring ICP and CSF drainage and preventing infection at the insertion site.

Purpose
• To monitor ICP
• To drain excessive CSF.

Preparation
If the patient is alert and communicative, tell him that the doctor will insert this device to check ICP and, if necessary, to drain excessive CSF. Briefly explain the insertion procedure and how the device works. Tell him his head will be shaved over the insertion site and that a sterile dressing will be placed over the site after the device is secured, to guard against infection. If a ventricular catheter is to be inserted, explain that the catheter will be sutured in place onto the scalp.

Point out that after insertion he'll probably be kept on strict bed rest, with constant monitoring of neurologic status, vital signs, ICP, and CSF drainage.

Procedure
After the insertion site is prepared, the surgeon uses a twist drill to create a hole in the appropriate area of the skull. To insert the ventricular device, he carefully introduces the soft polyethylene catheter into a lateral ventricle and sutures it in place onto the scalp. To insert a subarachnoid screw, he makes a small incision in the dura and locks the screw into place in the subarachnoid space.

Once the device is securely in place, the surgeon attaches a transducer and, if appropriate, a continuous CSF draining system with collection bag. The transducer picks up mechanical impulses generated by ICP and converts them into electrical energy. This energy, in turn, is transmitted to a recording instrument and converted to visible waveforms, which appear on a chart recorder or an oscilloscope.

Monitoring and aftercare
After insertion of the monitoring device, check the patient's ICP frequently. Notify the doctor of any changes. Also observe CSF drainage and note the amount, color, clarity, and presence of

any blood or sediment. If ordered, send daily drainage specimens to the laboratory for culture and sensitivity studies; white blood cell count; and protein, glucose, or chloride levels.

Take measures to prevent further increases in ICP. For example, keep the patient's room softly lit and quiet. Enforce bed rest and raise the patient's head 30 to 45 degrees to promote drainage. Instruct him to exhale while moving or turning in bed. Give stool softeners, as ordered, to prevent straining. Provide help if he needs to sit up, and instruct him not to flex his neck or hips or to push against the footboard with his legs. If you need to suction him, give him oxygen before starting and proceed carefully.

While the device is in place, perform regular neurologic checks. Be alert for early signs of increased ICP, such as headache, pupillary changes, vision disturbances, focal neurologic deficits, and changes in respiratory patterns.

Watch for signs of infection, and use strict aseptic technique when caring for the insertion site and the equipment. Administer prophylactic antibiotics, if ordered, and periodically check the patient's temperature.

Assist the doctor when he irrigates the insertion site. Don't use alcohol-containing saline solutions since these cause cortical necrosis. And never use heparin, which increases the risk of bleeding.

If a continuous CSF drainage system is used, check that the external drain stays at the correct height to maintain sufficient pressure for drainage (see *Hazards of CSF Drainage*). Check it at the beginning of each shift and whenever the patient changes his position. Also be sure to check the tubing for kinks or obstructions. Avoid putting pressure on the tubing to ensure adequate drainage and to prevent accidental dislodging.

When the patient's neurologic status has stabilized, the doctor will discontinue ICP monitoring and CSF drainage and remove the device. After he has

COMPLICATIONS

HAZARDS OF C.S.F. DRAINAGE

Supportive care for a patient with a ventricular catheter or subarachnoid screw involves careful monitoring for early signs of two life-threatening complications: infection and brain herniation. Here's what to look for, as well as ways to manage or help prevent these complications.

Both devices carry a high risk of infection, such as meningitis and ventriculitis. So be alert for signs of infection—redness and warmth around the insertion site, fever, elevated white blood cell count, and drainage from the wound—and call the doctor if any of these signs occur.

Help prevent infection by maintaining strict asepsis around the equipment and insertion site. When changing dressings, use aseptic technique. Teach the patient that this area must remain clean at all times, and warn him never to touch or manipulate the equipment or insertion site.

Brain herniation most commonly results from improper positioning of the device or from a sudden drop in ICP caused by excessive CSF drainage. Herniation involves displacement of the brain's structures, which raises ICP and eventually compresses the brain stem, causing death.

Because increasing ICP may herald herniation, carefully monitor the patient for the often subtle early signs of increased ICP: altered level of consciousness, increased restlessness, personality changes, and disorganized motor behavior (such as repetitive pulling at the gown); headache; visual disturbances; and vital sign changes, such as widened pulse pressure and irregular or decreased respiratory rate.

When draining CSF, help prevent herniation by checking the equipment carefully. Be sure all stopcocks are positioned correctly to prevent excessive CSF drainage.

done so, continue periodic neurologic assessments and maintain accurate intake and output records.

Home care instructions

Demonstrate aseptic technique to the patient and his family. Emphasize the need for proper care of the suture and insertion site until healing is complete.

Ventricular Shunting

Used for adult as well as pediatric patients, this surgical treatment for hydrocephalus involves insertion of a catheter into the ventricular system to drain cerebrospinal fluid (CSF) into another body space (usually the peritoneal sac) for absorption. The shunt extends from the cerebral ventricle to the scalp, where it's tunneled under the skin to the appropriate cavity.

Ventricular shunts treat both communicating hydrocephalus (excessive accumulation of CSF in the subarachnoid space) and noncommunicating hydrocephalus (blockage of normal CSF flow from the lateral ventricles to the subarachnoid space). By draining excessive CSF or relieving blockage, shunting can lower intracranial pressure (ICP) and prevent the brain damage caused by persistently elevated ICP.

When caring for a patient with a ventricular shunt, you'll need to carefully monitor for signs of infection and use strict aseptic technique when providing shunt and suture care. You may also be called upon to pump the shunt and check for any malfunction.

Besides infection, ventricular shunting carries a risk of ventricular collapse from improper catheter placement or faulty pumping techniques. And the shunt can become blocked or kinked—especially in growing children—resulting in elevated ICP.

Purpose
To relieve increased ICP by draining CSF from the brain's ventricles.

Preparation
Tell the patient or family that this procedure lowers ICP and helps prevent brain damage. Prepare the patient as you would for a craniotomy (see "Craniotomy," pages 253 to 256). Explain that he'll have dressings on his head and, depending on the site of drainage, on his abdomen or chest.

While the patient awaits surgery, carefully monitor his vital signs and neurologic status and watch for signs of increased ICP: headache, vomiting, irritability, visual disturbances, and decreased level of consciousness. If your patient's an infant, measure his head circumference daily to detect any increase. Also observe his fontanelles for bulging and tenderness.

Procedure
To implant a ventriculoperitoneal shunt, the surgeon peforms a craniotomy to gain access to the implantation site. He then inserts a catheter into the ventricular system, usually through a lateral ventricle. He tunnels the distal end of the catheter through subcutaneous tissue to a point below the diaphragm and inserts it into the peritoneal sac for CSF drainage.

The surgeon also performs a craniotomy to implant other types of ventricular shunts. For a ventriculoatrial shunt, he runs the catheter from the ventricle through the jugular vein to the right atrium of the heart. In an operation known as a third ventriculostomy, he elevates the frontal lobe to expose the third ventricle for catheter insertion. Then he passes the other end of the catheter into the cisterna chiasmatis of the subarachnoid space.

Unlike the other types of shunts, the ventriculocisternal shunt is usually temporary. It doesn't require a craniotomy; instead, the surgeon makes a small burr hole in the occipital region. He then inserts a catheter into a lateral ventricle and passes it under the dura and into the cisterna magna.

Monitoring and aftercare
Provide postoperative care as you would for a patient recovering from craniotomy. (See "Craniotomy," pages 253 to 256, for detailed care measures.) However, rather than elevate the patient's head after surgery, keep him flat

CARING FOR A VENTRICULAR SHUNT

Dear Parent,

Your child has had a shunt inserted to remove excess fluid from his brain. To help ensure the success of this treatment, you need to learn how to care for the shunt, how to pump it, and how to recognize signs of infection and shunt malfunction.

Caring for the shunt
• Bathe the shunt incision line as you normally bathe your child's skin.
• When picking up your child, be sure to support his buttocks. This prevents the drainage tube from moving from its proper position.
• Continue with your child's normal diet. To help prevent constipation, which can cause shunt malfunction, encourage him to eat soft foods and drink plenty of liquids.
• Be alert for signs of infection: rectal temperature above 101° F. (38.3° C.) for more than 6 hours, increased sleepiness, or warm, reddened skin at the incision site. Notify your doctor if you note any of these signs.

Keep in mind that reddened skin may be caused by lying on the shunt insertion side. Try to keep your child from lying on that side for prolonged periods.

Pumping the shunt
Your doctor may ask you to pump the shunt once or twice a day. If he does, locate the pump by feeling for the soft center of the device under the skin behind the ear.

Now, depress the center of the pump with your forefinger and then slowly release it. Pump only as many times as your doctor has ordered (usually between 25 and 50 times, once or twice a day).

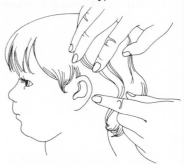

Checking for problems
Watch your child carefully for signs of shunt malfunction. Call your doctor immediately if you see bulging, tightness, and shining of the soft spots on your child's head. Also call him if your child seems unusually fussy or sleepy, if he refuses to eat, if he vomits forcefully, or if he has difficulty grasping objects.

for 3 to 5 days after shunt insertion. This will help him adjust to lowered ICP. Gradually raise his head in stages, about 20 degrees at a time. During this period, carefully check vital signs and neurologic status every 2 hours. Immediately report any signs of elevated ICP, which may indicate a blocked or malfunctioning shunt.

Check for and report any signs of infection, such as fever, headache, nuchal rigidity, and local pain and inflammation. If infection occurs, the doctor will probably order I.V. antibiotics. If the infection doesn't subside within 1 to 2 weeks, he'll remove and replace the shunt.

To avoid placing pressure on the shunt suture lines, position the patient on the nonoperative side. This will protect against suture abrasion and prevent local dependent edema.

If ordered, pump the shunt. Use proper technique to avoid excessive CSF drainage from the ventricular system, which can abruptly reduce ICP and lead to ventricular collapse or blood vessel rupture. While pumping, watch for signs of rapidly rising ICP, which may indicate ventricular collapse.

Home care instructions
• Teach the patient's family proper suture line care. Demonstrate how to mix a 1:1 hydrogen peroxide and saline solution, and how to use sterile technique when cleansing the suture line.
• Tell the family to report signs of infection or increased ICP immediately.
• Instruct them to have the patient avoid lying over the catheter's course for a prolonged period.
• If ordered, teach the family how to pump the shunt. (See *Caring for a Ventricular Shunt*, page 267.) Caution that excessive pumping can lead to serious complications.
• After shunt insertion, the doctor may order a 6- to 12-month course of anticonvulsant drug therapy. If so, reinforce the importance of complying with the medication schedule to prevent seizures. Also discuss possible drug side effects—especially those affecting the CNS and cardiovascular system—and the need to inform the doctor of any such effects.
• If the patient's a child, remind the parents that he'll need periodic surgery as he grows, to increase the shunt's length and modify its placement.

Myelomeningocele Repair

Surgical repair is the treatment of choice for myelomeningocele, a congenital spinal defect resulting from defective neural tube closure during the first trimester of pregnancy. This defect consists of a fragile saclike structure that protrudes over the spinal column and contains meninges, cerebrospinal fluid (CSF), and a portion of the spinal cord. CSF leakage from this sac can cause infection and can leave the infant with permanent neurologic deficits below the level of the lesion. For these reasons, most surgeons recommend prompt repair of the defect. Generally, surgery is delayed only when the infant is seriously debilitated or has associated defects that could complicate surgery.

Unfortunately, surgery can't reverse any existing neurologic deficits. It may, however, preserve existing function in the infant and prevent further deterioration.

When caring for an infant with this defect, you'll need to address both short- and long-term treatment goals. Your immediate goals include providing preoperative and postoperative nursing care, as well as teaching and support to help the infant's parents accept the diagnosis and its implications. Long-term goals include the prevention of complications caused by prolonged immobility, and parent teaching to help promote the infant's optimum neurologic function and development.

Purpose

To repair the congenital defect and prevent further neurologic compromise of the legs, bowel, and bladder.

Preparation

While the infant awaits surgery, take measures to protect the fragile defect from infection and damage. Keep it covered with sterile dressings moistened with sterile saline solution; cleanse it gently with sterile saline or a bactericidal solution, as ordered; and inspect it for signs of infection.

To prevent irritation of the sac, don't dress the infant in clothing or a diaper until after surgical correction; instead, keep him warm in an incubator. Position him on his side or abdomen to protect the fragile sac from rupture and minimize the risk of contamination from urine or feces. Put a diaper under him and change it often, and keep the anal and genital areas clean. Protect against skin breakdown by placing him on a sheepskin or foam pad and applying lotion to his knees, elbows, chin, and other pressure points.

Handle the infant carefully, and avoid placing any pressure on the defect. When holding him in your lap, lay him on his abdomen; teach his parents to do the same. Teach the parents to be cautious but unafraid of rupturing the sac, and encourage them to hold their baby often.

Before surgery, measure the child's head circumference. Also perform a baseline assessment of neuromuscular and sensory function below the defect. For instance, check the anal reflex by gently stroking the anal mucosa and checking for sphincter retraction.

Explain these preoperative care measures to the infant's parents, and reinforce the doctor's explanation of the surgical procedure, as necessary. They probably will feel anxious and concerned about the upcoming operation; help them cope with their feelings by answering their questions and listening to their concerns. Prepare them for the possibility that their child will have some physical and mental impairment, and make sure they understand that while the surgery may prevent further neurologic deterioration, it can't reverse existing neurologic damage. If necessary, recommend counseling for the parents.

Procedure

With the infant in a prone position and under general anesthesia, the surgeon isolates the neural tissue from the rest of the sac. After establishing this tissue's point of continuity with the spinal cord and nerve roots, he fashions a flap from the tissue. This flap protects the nerve junctions and eventually will become contiguous with the dura surrounding the spinal cord. He then sutures the skin closed over the defect and covers the wound with a sterile gauze dressing, then a waterproof covering to protect the dressing from contamination by feces or urine. Because the defect is usually relatively small, he rarely orders skin grafts for cosmetic repair.

Monitoring and aftercare

After surgery, carefully monitor the infant's vital signs and observe for signs of hydrocephalus and meningitis, which often follow such surgery. Measure head circumference regularly, and notify the doctor of any increase. Look for signs of increased intracranial pressure (ICP), especially bulging fontanelles and projectile vomiting. (Remember that excessive vomiting can lead to dehydration, which can prevent bulging fontanelles and thus mask this classic sign of increased ICP.) Also watch for fever; nuchal rigidity; opisthotonos; and even more subtle signs, such as irritability and refusal to eat.

Change the surgical dressing regularly, and check for drainage and wound infection. As before surgery, keep the infant positioned on his abdomen and protect his skin from breakdown. Place his hips in abduction and his feet in a neutral position. Frequently reposition his arms, legs, and

TRENDS IN PRENATAL CARE OF CONGENITAL SPINAL CORD DEFECTS

Two key advances in prenatal detection of spina bifida and related spinal cord defects—amniocentesis with alpha-fetoprotein testing and ultrasonography—are improving the prognosis for infants with these defects. How? By detecting defects early in gestation, these tests enable the doctor and parents to decide on the delivery method that will best protect the infant from damage.

Usually, they choose cesarean section. For a fetus with an external spinal cord defect, such as myelomeningocele or meningocele, compression of the cord during vaginal delivery can further compromise the cord and nerve roots and aggravate neuromuscular deficits. Cesarean delivery, which places little or no pressure on the fetus' spinal cord, is largely free of this risk.

If these defects are present, amniocentesis done at 14 to 16 weeks of gestation shows increased alpha-fetoprotein levels. In many cases, ultrasonography then visually confirms the defect.

Although amniocentesis can detect only open spinal cord defects, such as myelomeningocele and meningocele, this procedure is recommended for all high-risk pregnant women. This high-risk group includes women who previously have given birth to a child with a spinal cord defect or have a family history of such defects. It also includes pregnant women who are exposed to known or suspected teratogenic agents during the first 4 weeks of gestation.

head. If ordered, provide passive range-of-motion exercises, handling him very gently. Otherwise, keep handling to a minimum.

Monitor intake and output, and watch for decreased skin turgor, skin dryness, and other signs of dehydration. Check for urine retention and constipation resulting from decreased nerve function. If necessary, express urine manually to prevent urinary tract infection, and administer a mild laxative, as ordered, to prevent constipation.

As the infant recovers from surgery, periodically assess his neurologic function. Compare the findings to your preoperative baseline assessment.

Before discharge, prepare the infant's parents for their child's continuing care needs. Develop a patient-teaching plan for the parents; if possible, coordinate this plan with the nurse who will be providing visiting care after discharge. Begin parent teaching early to give them time to gain confidence in their ability to cope with their child's problems and meet long-range treatment goals. Throughout this teaching, provide support and encourage a positive attitude.

Home care instructions

• Teach the parents proper wound care techniques. Make sure they know how to recognize early signs of infection, such as redness or swelling. Tell them to keep the suture line clean and dry and to provide frequent diaper changes and cleansings. Explain that, if all goes well, the doctor will remove the sutures on the 10th day after surgery.

• Explain skin care measures to prevent breakdown, such as frequent repositioning, massage, and application of lotion to pressure areas.

• If necessary, teach the parents how to express urine manually from the child's bladder; instruct them to do this regularly. Encourage them to begin bladder training when their child reaches age 3.

• If the doctor has prescribed an antibiotic, teach the parents how to administer the drug and explain the need to follow the dosing schedule.

• Discuss the possibility of arranging for a visiting nurse to provide periodic in-home care.

• Remind them of the importance of regular neurologic assessments and physical examinations to evaluate their child's development.

• If appropriate, refer the parents for genetic counseling before they contemplate a future pregnancy. (See *Trends in Prenatal Care of Congenital Spinal Cord Defects.*) You also may want to refer them to a local support group.

MISCELLANEOUS TREATMENTS

Embolization of an Arteriovenous Malformation

Although surgical excision is the treatment of choice for an arteriovenous malformation (AVM), many of these congenital defects prove inaccessible to surgery. Embolization, a relatively new noninvasive technique, allows treatment of an AVM when surgical excision proves unsafe or impossible. In this technique, the doctor, guided by cerebral angiography, threads a flexible catheter to the AVM site. He then injects a quantity of small Silastic (heat-resistant silicone rubber) beads, which lodge in the feeder artery and occlude blood flow to the AVM. As an alternative, the doctor may insert a small balloon-tipped catheter in the feeder artery and inject a rapid-setting plastic polymer material into the AVM site.

Although this procedure rarely destroys the AVM, it may shrink the defect and usually decreases the risk of rupture and hemorrhage. It may also reduce pressure on adjacent brain tissue, possibly relieving existing neurologic abnormalities caused by the AVM.

When caring for a patient awaiting AVM embolization, you'll need to monitor him closely for any developing complications, including headache, focal or generalized tonic-clonic seizures, increased intracranial pressure, and focal neurologic signs, such as twitching or tremors. After treatment, you'll focus your care on monitoring his vital signs and neurologic status, as well as on taking measures to minimize the risk of complications, including AVM rebleeding and thrombosis, hematoma formation, or spasm in the affected artery.

Purpose

To occlude blood flow to the site of an AVM, reducing its size and helping prevent rupture.

Preparation

Explain to the patient that this procedure will shrink his AVM and decrease the risk of cerebral hemorrhage. Briefly describe the steps of the procedure. Tell him who will perform it and where, and that the entire procedure takes about 2 hours.

Tell the patient that he'll be placed on an X-ray table with his head immobilized and he'll be asked to lie still. Tell him that he'll receive a local anesthetic at the catheter insertion site. (Some patients, particularly children, may receive a general anesthetic.) Caution him that he'll probably feel a transient burning sensation during injection of the contrast medium, and that he may feel flushed and warm and experience nausea or vomiting, headache, and a salty taste in his mouth after injection. Reassure him that the injection of Silastic beads or polymer material is painless.

Check the patient's history for hypersensitivity to iodine, iodine-containing foods (such as shellfish), or other radiographic contrast media. Notify the doctor of any such hypersensitivities; he may need to order prophylactic medications or may choose not to perform the procedure.

Instruct the patient to fast for 8 to 10 hours before the procedure and to void just before it starts. Tell him to put on a hospital gown and to remove all jewelry, dentures, hairpins, and other radiopaque objects in the X-ray field. If ordered, administer a sedative and an anticholinergic 30 to 45 minutes before the procedure.

Make sure the patient or a responsible family member has signed a consent form.

HOW A.V.M. EMBOLIZATION WORKS

In this version of AVM embolization, small Silastic beads are injected through a catheter placed in the malformation's feeder artery. These beads lodge in the artery, forming an embolus that occludes blood flow to the malformation.

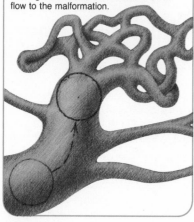

Procedure

If you're assisting with the procedure, begin by gathering the local anesthetic and catheterization equipment. Then place the patient on the X-ray table and instruct him to lie still. Confirm the catheter insertion site with the doctor, and position the patient so that the site is easily accessible. Shave the insertion site, if necessary, and clean it with alcohol and povidone-iodine.

Once the patient is prepared, the doctor will administer the local anesthetic and insert the catheter. Then he verifies catheter placement and injects the contrast medium to highlight the AVM site. Using angiographic guidance, he threads the catheter into the feeder artery as close as possible to the AVM and injects the Silastic beads or polymer material. After he's sure the material has flowed to and occluded the AVM, he removes the catheter.

Monitoring and aftercare

During contrast medium injection, keep emergency resuscitation equipment readily available. Monitor the patient for early signs of hypersensitivity: erythema, pruritus, thready pulse, sweating, and anxiety. If you detect any of these signs, inform the doctor immediately; he will stop the injection and, if necessary, begin emergency treatment.

After catheter removal, enforce bed rest and monitor the patient's vital signs and neurologic status every hour for the first 4 hours and then every 4 hours for the next 20 hours. Apply an ice bag to relieve pain and reduce swelling, and keep the site immobilized.

Check the insertion site for redness and swelling, indicating extravasation. Control any bleeding with firm pressure. If catheterization was done in the femoral artery, keep the affected leg still for 12 hours after the procedure. Watch for possible thrombus or hematoma formation by regularly checking all pulses distal to the insertion site and assessing the affected leg's temperature, color, and sensation.

If a carotid artery was used for catheterization, observe the patient for dysphagia and respiratory distress, which can result from extravasation. Also watch for signs of thrombosis, hematoma, or arterial spasm, such as disorientation and weakness or numbness in the extremities. Immediately notify the doctor if any of these develop.

To help reduce the risk of AVM bleeding after embolization, provide a quiet, softly lit environment and limit visitors. Administer analgesics and sedatives, as ordered, and provide a soft, high-fiber diet with stool softeners, as needed.

Home care instructions

Instruct the patient and his family to immediately report any abnormal symptoms, such as severe headache, weakness in the extremities, or deteriorating level of consciousness. Explain that these symptoms, which may indicate that the AVM is bleeding or increasing in size, require immediate medical evaluation.

Barbiturate Coma

When sustained or acute episodes of increased intracranial pressure (ICP) can't be corrected by such conventional treatments as fluid restriction, diuretic or corticosteroid therapy, or ventricular shunting, the doctor may order barbiturate coma. In this treatment, the patient receives high I.V. doses of a short-acting barbiturate (such as pentobarbital or phenobarbital) to produce coma. The drug reduces the patient's metabolic rate and cerebral blood flow, possibly relieving increased ICP.

Barbiturate coma is indicated only as a last resort for patients with acute ICP elevation above 40 mm Hg, persistent elevation above 20 mm Hg, or rapidly deteriorating neurologic status that's unresponsive to other treatments. If this treatment proves unsuccessful in lowering ICP, the patient's prognosis for recovery is poor.

Besides having only a marginal degree of effectiveness, barbiturate coma carries some serious risks. The most serious results from the small margin between therapeutic and toxic doses. On the one hand, a high dose is needed to induce coma; on the other, toxicity can produce severe, possibly fatal, CNS and respiratory depression. Even a therapeutic dose can cause complications, such as hypotension and arrhythmias. And overly abrupt withdrawal of barbiturates may produce convulsions or delirium.

Nursing care for a patient undergoing barbiturate coma will focus on supportive measures. You'll need to carefully monitor ICP, vital signs, and neurologic function. You'll also need to provide respiratory and nutritional support and to prevent complications resulting from prolonged immobility. And, finally, you should consider the patient's family; they'll probably have many fears and doubts about this treatment and will benefit greatly from your clear explanations and ongoing emotional support.

Purpose
To reduce the patient's metabolic rate and cerebral blood flow, relieving persistently increased ICP and preventing brain tissue damage.

Preparation
Because a patient who's undergoing barbiturate coma is severely compromised and thus uncommunicative, focus your attention on his family. They'll probably be frightened by the patient's condition and apprehensive about the treatment. Provide clear explanations of the procedure and its effects, and encourage them to ask questions. Convey a sense of optimism but provide no guarantees of the treatment's success. Because barbiturate coma represents a "last-ditch" effort to reduce ICP and save the patient's life, prepare them for the possibility that the patient may die or, if he survives, that he may be left with permanent neurologic impairment.

Also prepare the family for observable—and, to them, quite disturbing—changes in the patient's status during therapy, such as decreased respirations, hypotension, and loss of muscle tone and reflexes. Reassure them that despite the patient's disturbing appearance, he is being carefully monitored and provided with the necessary supportive care to ensure safe treatment. Briefly explain the various monitoring and supportive measures used during therapy.

Procedure
Before inducing barbiturate coma, the doctor orders an EEG and possibly brain stem auditory-evoked response testing to establish a reliable neurologic baseline. He also orders the patient placed on mechanical ventilation, ICP monitoring, and cardiac and intraarterial pressure monitoring.

He then administers a loading dose of barbiturate, 3 to 5 mg/kg via I.V.

COMPLICATIONS

MONITORING PATIENTS IN BARBITURATE COMA

A patient undergoing barbiturate coma therapy is at risk for numerous complications—some related to the drug's effects, others to prolonged inactivity and immobility. Use this chart to familiarize yourself with these complications, their causes, and the nursing interventions needed to prevent or manage them.

COMPLICATION	NURSING INTERVENTIONS
Hypotension from cardio-vascular instability and hypovolemia	• Continuously monitor arterial pressure, pulmonary artery pressure, EKG, and central venous pressure. • If the patient's systolic pressure falls below 90 mm Hg, administer a vasopressor, such as dopamine, as ordered. • Check urine output hourly.
Respiratory depression	• Maintain mechanical ventilation at ordered setting. • Assess the patient's breath sounds every 1 to 2 hours. • As appropriate, provide endotracheal tube or tracheostomy care. Suction every hour or as needed. • Suction nasopharyngeal secretions every 2 hours or more frequently if needed. • Check arterial blood gases daily or as ordered.
Fluid and electrolyte imbalance resulting from fluid restriction, diuretic therapy, or GI suctioning	• Periodically check serum osmolality; if it's greater than 320 mOsm, withhold diuretics and notify the doctor. • Check electrolyte, blood urea nitrogen, creatinine, and hematocrit levels at least daily. • Continuously monitor EKG and pulmonary artery pressure. • Measure urine output and specific gravity hourly. • Record intake and output; total them every 24 hours. • Observe the skin and mucous membranes for signs of dehydration.
GI depression (absence of bowel sounds, decreased motility)	• As ordered, insert a Salem sump or nasogastric tube to provide gravity drainage or intermittent suction. • Measure gastric drainage every shift or as appropriate. • Also during each shift, auscultate for bowel sounds, palpate the abdomen for distention, and check for fecal impaction. After bowel sounds return and tube feedings are initiated, check gastric contents regularly for absorption.
Loss of gag, swallow, and corneal reflexes	• Suction the oropharynx every hour or more frequently, if needed. • Position the patient on his side, not on his back. • Provide meticulous eye care, and instill liquid tears every 4 hours or as needed. If ordered, tape the patient's eyelids closed.
Susceptibility to infection	• Maintain strict asepsis at the infusion site. • Obtain culture specimens, as necessary.
Catabolic state from inadequate nutrition	• Provide a multivitamin with iron daily, as ordered. • Also as ordered, provide intravenous hyperalimentation.
Decubiti, contractures, and pulmonary congestion from prolonged immobility	• Institute appropriate preventive measures, such as frequent turning and repositioning, passive range-of-motion exercises, skin lotion and massage, and antiembolism stockings.

push, and watches the ICP monitor for a pressure decrease of at least 10 mm Hg within 10 minutes. If this drop doesn't occur, he may administer a second dose 2 hours later.

Once the loading dose lowers ICP significantly, the doctor orders hourly maintenance doses of 1 to 3 mg/kg or amounts sufficient to achieve a steady-state serum level of 2 to 4 mg/dl.

After the doctor determines that the patient's ICP has stabilized within acceptable limits (between 4 and 15 mm Hg), he discontinues therapy. He'll also order discontinuation if therapy proves unsuccessful at lowering ICP or if the patient shows signs of progressive neurologic impairment. To prevent side effects of abrupt withdrawal (including seizures and hallucinations), barbiturates are withdrawn gradually, at a rate based on the patient's condition and the doses administered during therapy.

Monitoring and aftercare
During barbiturate coma, closely monitor the patient's ICP, EKG, and vital signs. Notify the doctor of increased ICP, arrhythmias, or hypotension. Check serum barbiturate levels frequently, as ordered.

Because evaluation of the patient's neurologic function may be impossible while he's in a drug-induced coma, concentrate on providing supportive care. His respiratory function will be severely compromised, so ensure adequate ventilation and provide frequent suctioning to remove secretions. Provide adequate hydration and record intake and output. Monitor electrolyte levels and watch for signs of dehydration and hypokalemia, particularly if the doctor orders diuretics to help reduce cerebral edema. Because barbiturates depress GI function, provide nutritional support (including hyperalimentation, if ordered), and expect to insert a nasogastric tube to remove excessive gastric secretions.

Also take measures to prevent complications associated with prolonged immobility. Provide meticulous skin care, frequent repositioning, and passive range-of-motion exercises.

After discontinuation of therapy, and as the patient emerges from coma, watch him for signs of returning neurologic function. Begin by checking his gag reflex and assessing his response to painful stimuli, then work up to a full neurologic evaluation. Remember, however, that only after withdrawal is complete and the patient is fully conscious can you begin to determine the full extent of any neurologic impairment.

As barbiturates are discontinued, watch for sporadic elevations in ICP and for adverse effects of barbiturate withdrawal. If you note tremors, agitation, delirium or hallucinations, incoordination, or seizures, notify the doctor; place the patient in a quiet, darkened room; and keep him still. Take seizure precautions, such as padding the bed rails and keeping emergency equipment readily available.

Home care instructions
Tailor your home care instructions to the patient's specific neurologic impairments. For patients with preexisting neurologic dysfunction, remind the family that the elevated ICP may have caused additional impairment and that the patient's care may have to be adjusted accordingly.

Plasmapheresis
[Therapeutic plasma exchange (TPE)]

Plasmapheresis is the therapeutic removal of plasma from withdrawn blood and the reinfusion of formed blood elements. In this treatment, blood removed from the patient flows into a cell separator, where it's divided into plasma and formed elements. The plasma is collected in a container for disposal, while the formed elements are mixed with a plasma replacement solution and returned to the patient through a vein. In a newer method of plasmapheresis, the plasma is separated out, filtered to remove a specific disease mediator, and then returned to the patient.

Whichever method is used, plasmapheresis can be done on an inpatient or outpatient basis. The procedure, done under a doctor's supervision, requires a specially trained technician or nurse to operate the cell separator and a primary nurse to monitor the patient and provide supportive care.

By removing and replacing the plasma, plasmapheresis cleanses the blood of harmful substances, such as toxins, and of disease mediators, such as immune complexes and autoantibodies. Consequently, plasmapheresis has several neurologic applications, such as in Guillain-Barré syndrome, multiple sclerosis, and especially myasthenia gravis (MG). In MG, plasmapheresis removes circulating antiacetylcholine receptor antibodies. If successful, treatment may relieve symptoms for months; however, results vary. Plasmapheresis is used most commonly in patients with long-standing neuromuscular disease but may also be used to treat acute exacerbations. It may be performed as often as four times a week in acutely ill patients but is limited to about once every 2 weeks otherwise.

Plasmapheresis carries several possible complications: a hypersensitivity reaction to the ingredients of the replacement solution and hypocalcemia from excessive binding of circulating calcium to the citrate solution used as an anticoagulant in the replacement solution. Hypomagnesemia can follow repeated plasmapheresis, producing severe muscle cramps and tetany. And, because between 150 and 400 ml of the patient's blood is removed during treatment, the patient is at risk for hypotension and other complications of low blood volume.

Purpose

To remove disease mediators or toxic substances from circulating blood.

Preparation

Briefly explain the treatment and its purpose to the patient. Tell him that a needle will be inserted into one or both arms and that his blood will be pumped through a filtering machine, cleansed of harmful substances, then returned to his body. Explain that the procedure may take up to 5 hours. Inform him that, during treatment, frequent blood samples will be taken to monitor calcium and potassium levels, and his blood pressure and heart rate will be checked regularly. Instruct him to report any paresthesias.

Advise the patient to eat lightly before treatment and to drink milk before and during treatment to help reduce the risk of hypocalcemia. Because a full bladder may lead to mild hypotension as a result of fluid shift or vasovagal reaction, tell him to urinate before the procedure.

Before treatment begins, take vital signs for a baseline. As ordered, apply EKG leads to monitor heart rate. Also as ordered, draw blood samples for tests to determine baseline levels of hemoglobin, hematocrit, and other blood substances. If possible, give medications after treatment instead of before, to prevent their removal from the blood.

Procedure

If the patient doesn't have an I.V. line in place, perform one or more venipunctures in the antecubital veins, as ordered, to establish vascular access for blood withdrawal and reinfusion. Use large-bore needles to minimize resistance and prevent damage to blood cells. Once venous access is established, a technician or specially trained nurse connects the patient to the machine and starts it. The plasmapheresis process begins as whole blood is drawn into the cell separator's processing chamber, where it is mixed with a citrate anticoagulant. The blood is then separated into plasma and formed elements. The separated plasma is either collected for disposal or, in a newer technique, filtered to remove the disease mediator and then returned to the patient. The formed elements are mixed with a plasma replacement solution and then reinfused into the patient.

Monitoring and aftercare

As plasmapheresis begins, observe the patient for signs of hypersensitivity, such as respiratory distress, hives, diaphoresis, hypotension, or thready pulse. If any such signs occur, immediately notify the doctor, who will stop the procedure and provide emergency treatment.

During treatment, monitor vital signs every 30 minutes. (Don't take blood pressure readings in the arm being used for blood withdrawal and reinfusion, however.) Pay particular attention to temperature; reinfusion of blood that has cooled while in the cell separator can produce hypothermia.

Report any serious arrhythmias. Because arrhythmias can result from electrolyte imbalance or volume depletion, monitor blood levels of calcium and potassium and replace electrolytes, as ordered. Monitor intake and output to ensure adequate hydration. Also watch for signs of circulatory compromise. Compare levels of hematocrit, hemoglobin, electrolytes, antibody titers, and immune complexes with pretreatment levels.

If the patient is undergoing plasmapheresis for unstable MG, keep emergency equipment on hand and monitor blood pressure and pulse. Observe for symptoms of myasthenic crisis (dysphagia, ptosis, and diplopia), which this treatment can precipitate by removing antibodies or antimyasthenic drugs from the blood.

After completion of treatment and removal of needles, apply direct pressure on the puncture sites, then apply pressure dressings. Periodically assess the dressings for drainage and the puncture sites for signs of extravasation.

Home care instructions

• Tell the patient that he may feel tired for a day or two after plasmapheresis. (If he's undergoing repeated treatments, he may develop chronic fatigue.) Advise him to rest frequently during this period and to avoid strenuous activities. Unless contraindicated, instruct him to maintain a high-protein diet and to take a multivitamin with iron daily.

• If the patient is undergoing repeated treatments, tell him that he may require transfusions of fresh-frozen plasma to replace the normal clotting factors lost in his removed plasma.

• Because plasmapheresis can cause immunosuppression, warn the patient to avoid contact with persons with colds or other contagious viruses.

• Also instruct him to watch for and report any signs of hepatitis.

Selected References

Adams, Raymond, and Victor, Maurice. *Principles of Neurology.* New York: McGraw-Hill Book Co., 1985.

Fox, John L. *Intracranial Aneurysms,* vol. 3. New York: Springer-Verlag, 1983

Grant, Laura. "Hydrocephalus: An Overview and Update," *Journal of Neurosurgical Nursing* 16(6):313-18, December 1984.

Leatherlande, Jane, et al. "Cerebellar Implant: Care of the Cerebral Palsy Patient," *Association of Operating Room Nurses Journal* 39(7):1143-49, June 1984.

Marcotty, S., and Levin, A. "A New Approach in Epidural Intracranial Pressure Monitoring," *Journal of Neurosurgical Nursing* 16(1):54-59, February 1984.

7

Treating Musculoskeletal Dysfunction

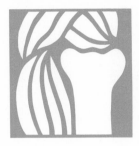

Treating Musculoskeletal Dysfunction

Introduction

Typically, patients with musculoskeletal disorders willingly seek treatment. That's because their two most common complaints, pain and impaired mobility, provide the necessary motivation. But how you respond to these complaints can shape the effectiveness of the overall treatment plan.

Relieving pain

Pain, of course, is a subjective complaint. You can't measure it quantitatively. Of course, you can help relieve it by giving prescribed analgesics. But you should also consider using nonpharmacologic measures, such as application of heat or cold, massage, transcutaneous electrical nerve stimulation (TENS), rest, and prescribed exercises. Employing these measures reduces reliance on drugs and gives the patient a feeling of control over his condition.

Restoring mobility

Loss of mobility can be especially frustrating for any patient. To help promote mobility, you'll need to stress a balanced program of exercise and rest. Exercise maintains joint mobility and muscle strength, whereas rest prevents undue fatigue. You may also need to teach your patient how to use a splint, brace, or other device to support a weakened or injured limb or joint.

Unfortunately, conservative treatments prove ineffective for some patients. That's when surgery may be necessary. For instance, it may be used to reshape deformed joints, to replace degenerated ones, or to repair traumatic injury. After surgery, the patient may require immobilization with a cast, brace, or other device, along with active or passive range-of-motion exercises to maintain mobility and prevent contractures.

New treatments, such as electrical bone growth stimulation, may also prove beneficial.

Combating complications

Despite continued improvements in medical and surgical treatments, many of their complications remain the same. Joint stiffness, for instance, can result from immobilization. Neurovascular compromise can arise from pressure exerted by an immobilization device on blood vessels and nerves. Infection may develop at wound or pin sites.

You can help prevent or minimize complications like these through careful monitoring and prompt intervention. For example, you'll need to assess the patient's neurovascular status regularly to detect signs of compromise. And you'll need to check and scrupulously care for pin insertion sites to prevent infection.

DRUG THERAPY

Nonsteroidal Anti-Inflammatory Drugs

This class of drugs includes *indomethacin, meclofenamate, mefenamic acid, oxyphenbutazone, phenylbutazone, piroxicam, sulindac,* and the propionic acid derivatives *fenoprofen, ibuprofen,* and *naproxen.* Because nonsteroidal anti-inflammatory drugs (NSAIDs) exert analgesic, antipyretic, and anti-inflammatory effects, they're useful in treating such conditions as acute bursitis, gouty arthritis, osteoarthritis, rheumatoid arthritis, and related disorders. Used correctly, they reduce pain and inflammation and enhance joint mobility.

For many patients with inflammatory joint disorders, NSAIDs represent an important adjunct or an alternative to salicylate therapy. In particular, the newer agents—fenoprofen, ibuprofen, naproxen, and piroxicam—prove useful for patients who are unable to tolerate the GI effects of salicylates. (The older NSAIDs, including indomethacin, oxyphenbutazone, and phenylbutazone, carry a high risk of GI upset and bleeding.)

NSAIDs, however, can't be used for every patient with an inflammatory condition. Although contraindications vary among these drugs, all NSAIDs should be used cautiously in patients with an allergy to salicylates or to other NSAIDs, asthma, GI disorders (especially peptic ulcer disease), blood dyscrasias, or cardiac, hepatic, or renal disease; and in children, pregnant patients, and the elderly.

Purpose and action

NSAIDs apparently act as prostaglandin inhibitors, relieving inflammation and pain by decreasing the effects of histamine and bradykinin precursors. They *do not* arrest the underlying disease or its sequelae, however. In rheumatoid arthritis, for instance, NSAIDs may reduce pain, redness, and swelling but do little to stop joint destruction.

Monitoring

Review the patient's drug regimen to avoid possible interactions. When combined with NSAIDs, aspirin and other nonnarcotic analgesics (especially diflunisal), diuretics, anticoagulants, antidiabetic drugs, and glucocorticoids can worsen such problems as GI upset, hypertension, bleeding tendencies, and platelet destruction.

Before long-term therapy, obtain baseline blood tests. At the start of therapy, be alert for indications of hypersensitivity, such as respiratory distress, pruritus, and cardiovascular compromise. Throughout therapy, watch for evidence of drug toxicity: fever, chills, rash, leukopenia, arthralgias, and abnormal renal or hepatic function test results.

If the patient complains of GI upset, administer the drug with food or milk.

Home care instructions

• If the patient's taking an NSAID, instruct him to immediately report rash, dyspnea, confusion, blurred vision, nausea, bloody vomitus, or black, tarry stools. These symptoms could indicate an overdose, acute hypersensitivity, or gastric bleeding.
• Advise the patient to take the drug with food, milk, or an antacid to minimize GI upset. Afterward, he should remain upright for 15 to 30 minutes to reduce esophageal irritation. If he experiences gastric burning or pain, tell him to notify the doctor. If he's taking fenoprofen or piroxicam, however, instruct him to take the drug on an empty stomach 1 hour before meals or 3 hours after them for best absorption.

SALICYLATES: FRONT-LINE DEFENSE AGAINST ARTHROPATHIES

Commonly used to reduce pain and fever, salicylates usually represent the drugs of choice for symptomatic treatment of rheumatoid arthritis, osteoarthritis, and other related rheumatic disorders. Given primarily for their anti-inflammatory effect, they must be administered to the point of maximum tolerance in many patients. However, not all patients can withstand such a high-dose regimen; some must seek other treatments.

How salicylates act
Salicylates produce analgesic and anti-inflammatory effects. Their mechanism of action isn't clearly understood, but they're believed to produce these effects by blocking transmission of pain impulses peripherally and by inhibiting prostaglandin synthesis. When given orally for arthropathies, salicylates are rapidly absorbed and achieve their peak effects in 1 to 2 hours for single doses. However, if exceptionally high doses are being given, salicylates may not achieve their peak effects for up to 1 week. Tinnitus and hearing loss, the first signs of toxicity, determine the maximum daily dose.

Cautions and contraindications
Salicylates should be used cautiously in patients with the triad of nasal polyps,

asthma, and aspirin-induced allergies, and in patients with renal dysfunction. They should be avoided in children with influenza or varicella because of the possible risk of Reye's syndrome. They should also be avoided in patients undergoing anticoagulant therapy because of the increased risk of bleeding.

Side effects: Sometimes severe
Oral salicylates are available as tablets, enteric-coated capsules, and elixirs. Regardless of their form, oral salicylates commonly cause GI disturbances, especially in the elderly and in patients with ulcer disease. What's worse, these drugs can cause gastric ulceration; signs of this complication may include severe abdominal cramps, bloody or tarry stools, and coffee-ground emesis.

To help forestall GI complications, instruct the patient to take the drug with a full glass of water and to maintain an upright position for 15 minutes. Taking the drug with food will decrease the rate of absorption but not the extent. If the patient's receiving high doses (more than 4 g/day), assess for nausea, vomiting, and gastric distress. Keep in mind that occult bleeding occurs in about 70% of patients routinely taking aspirin and that iron deficiency anemia may result after several months.

- Advise the patient to take a missed dose as soon as he remembers, unless it's almost time for the next dose—in which case he should skip the missed dose. Warn him to never double-dose.
- Remind him not to take the drug with aspirin, acetaminophen, or alcohol.

Corticosteroids

Intraarticular or, rarely, soft-tissue injection of the corticosteroids *betamethasone, cortisone, dexamethasone, hydrocortisone, prednisone,* or *triamcinolone* provides relief from local inflammation while causing minimal side effects. Used as adjunctive, short-term treatment, these drugs reduce

pain and improve joint mobility in rheumatoid arthritis, osteoarthritis, acute bursitis, acute gouty arthritis, epicondylitis, acute nonspecific tenosynovitis, and posttraumatic osteoarthritis. They provide symptomatic relief but do not halt the progression of the disease.

Because side effects are largely dose- or duration-dependent, corticosteroids should be given in the lowest possible dose over the shortest period necessary to control the patient's condition. Intraarticular injection fits these criteria well, allowing the doctor to administer the minimum therapeutic dose and thereby curtail systemic effects.

Because corticosteroids have been linked to placental and fetal abnormalities, they shouldn't be given during pregnancy.

UNDERSTANDING INTRAARTICULAR INJECTION

Intraarticular injection delivers medication directly into the synovial cavity of a joint in an attempt to reduce pain and inflammation, maintain mobility and function, and prevent contractures and muscle atrophy from disuse. Because of its invasive nature, this injection is contraindicated in patients with joint infection, joint instability or fracture, or systemic fungal infection.

The injection procedure itself, although painful, is relatively quick and uncomplicated. Begin by placing the patient in a comfortable position and stabilizing the affected joint. Then cleanse the injection

site, taking care to maintain aseptic technique, and drape the area. Next, the doctor administers a local anesthetic and usually withdraws a synovial fluid sample for laboratory analysis. Once he does so, he leaves the needle used for aspiration in place, removes the syringe containing aspirated fluid, and attaches a new syringe filled with medication. After injecting the medication into the joint, he withdraws the needle. Then he applies pressure on the injection site and massages the joint for a minute or two to enhance absorption.

**COMMON INTRAARTICULAR
INJECTION SITES**

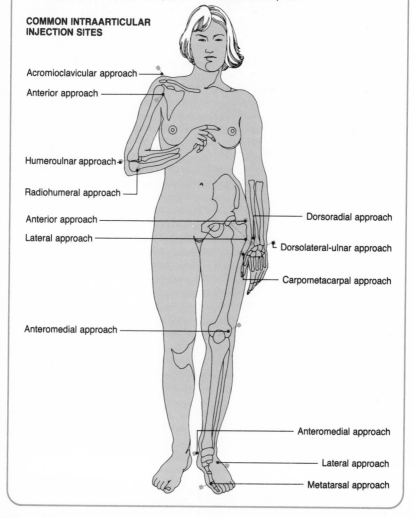

Acromioclavicular approach

Anterior approach

Humeroulnar approach

Radiohumeral approach

Anterior approach

Lateral approach

Anteromedial approach

Dorsoradial approach

Dorsolateral-ulnar approach

Carpometacarpal approach

Anteromedial approach

Lateral approach

Metatarsal approach

Purpose and action

Corticosteroids exert an anti-inflammatory effect by stabilizing cell membranes and inhibiting the release of proteolytic enzymes during the inflammatory reaction.

Monitoring

Before injection, check the patient's drug regimen for possible interactions. For instance, a patient taking indomethacin or aspirin requires careful monitoring during corticosteroid administration for signs of GI bleeding. A patient taking a barbiturate, phenytoin, or rifampin experiences decreased corticosteroid effects. What's more, estrogen-containing preparations, such as oral contraceptives, interfere with the protein-binding capability of glucocorticoids and can delay clearance. Consequently, a patient taking such preparations should be watched closely for toxic effects.

After intraarticular injection, apply pressure to the site and gently massage the area for 1 to 2 minutes to promote absorption. Observe the patient for signs of a hypersensitivity reaction or local allergic reaction.

If a local anesthetic was used to reduce injection pain, warn the patient that he may experience discomfort when the anesthetic wears off.

Home care instructions

• Instruct the patient to avoid heavy lifting or strenuous activity with the affected joint for 24 hours after injection. If a weight-bearing joint was treated, advise him to maintain bed rest for 24 to 48 hours, or as ordered. Explain to the patient that even though the drug has relieved pain and increased mobility, the underlying disease is still active and can cause further joint damage—especially if aggravated by stress or overuse.
• Tell him to promptly report blurred vision, hallucinations, frequent urination or increased thirst, rash or hives, or persistent pain at the injection site.
• Advise him to take antacids or eat a light snack to relieve GI distress.
• If the patient's receiving frequent, high-dose injections, warn him to avoid persons with known or suspected infections because of the drug's immunosuppressive effects.

Skeletal Muscle Relaxants

Skeletal muscle relaxants can be divided into two groups: those used as adjunctive treatment for painful muscle spasms resulting from acute, self-limiting disorders, such as sprains, strains, or fractures; and those used to treat severe spasticity associated with chronic disease, such as multiple sclerosis, or spasticity related to spinal cord transection. Drugs in the first group include *carisoprodol, chlorphenesin, chlorzoxazone, cyclobenzaprine, diazepam, methocarbamol, metaxalone*, and *orphenadrine*. The second group includes the more powerful drugs *baclofen* and *dantrolene*, as well as diazepam in high doses.

Prolonged therapy has a drawback: the risk of severe CNS depression. For this reason, skeletal muscle relaxants are contraindicated in patients with existing CNS depression and in those taking sedatives. Because these drugs are metabolized in the liver and excreted by the kidneys, they should be used cautiously in patients with impaired renal or hepatic function.

Besides these broad guidelines, specific contraindications and precautions apply to individual drugs. For example, carisoprodol is contraindicated in patients with hypersensitivity to related compounds (including meprobamate and tybamate) or intermittent porphyria; diazepam, in patients with acute-angle or chronic open-angle glaucoma, psychoses, or myasthenia gravis; metaxalone, in patients with a history of drug-induced hemolytic anemia or other anemias; and orphenadrine, in patients with prostatic hypertrophy or pyloric, duodenal, or bladder neck obstruction.

Baclofen and dantrolene usually are contraindicated in patients who require some degree of muscle spasticity to maintain motor function. In addition, baclofen should be used cautiously in patients with seizures because of the risk of increased seizure activity.

Purpose and action

Skeletal muscle relaxants produce their effects through somewhat different mechanisms. Carisoprodol, chlorphenesin, chlorzoxazone, cyclobenzaprine, metaxalone, methocarbamol, and orphenadrine reduce transmission of nerve impulses from the spinal cord to skeletal muscle. Dantrolene, though, acts directly on skeletal muscle to interfere with intracellular calcium movement. Diazepam appears to depress the CNS at the limbic and subcortical levels; besides relaxing skeletal muscle, it also produces anticonvulsive and sedative effects. Baclofen's mechanism of action isn't clear.

Monitoring

Review the patient's drug regimen for possible interactions. CNS depressants, such as monoamine oxidase inhibitors, narcotic analgesics, tricyclic antidepressants, and parenteral magnesium sulfate, can worsen CNS effects. The normally mild antimuscarinic effects of orphenadrine may be potentiated by atropine and related drugs; this combination may need to be avoided if effects, such as dry mouth and urinary difficulty, are severe.

Several drugs can interact with diazepam. Rifampin, for instance, speeds elimination of diazepam, possibly requiring a dosage increase. Cimetidine and isoniazid may delay diazepam clearance, potentiating sedative effects; dosage of one or both may need to be reduced.

During therapy, monitor the patient for adverse CNS effects, such as drowsiness, dizziness, light-headedness, and clumsiness, as well as for blurred or double vision. If severe side effects occur, take measures to protect the patient from injury, such as raising the side rails of his bed and assisting him with ambulation as necessary.

When discontinuing skeletal muscle relaxants, remember to withdraw the drug gradually. Abrupt withdrawal may produce rebound spasticity or milder symptoms, such as insomnia, headache, nausea, and abdominal cramps.

Home care instructions

• Instruct the patient never to take a skeletal muscle relaxant with alcohol or any over-the-counter CNS depressant, such as antihistamines or sleeping pills.

• Warn him to avoid driving or other tasks that require alertness and good psychomotor coordination and visual acuity until the CNS effects of the drug have been established.

• Advise the patient on baclofen, dantrolene, chlorphenesin, chlorzoxazone, or methocarbamol to take the drug with meals or a glass of milk to minimize GI distress. Explain that he can crush chlorzoxazone, metaxalone, or methocarbamol tablets and mix them with food or milk to ease swallowing. Tell the patient receiving diazepam to take the drug with food or a full glass of water and to swallow capsules whole, not to crush or chew them.

• Instruct the patient to make up a missed dose only if he remembers within an hour or so of the scheduled administration time. If more than an hour elapses, he should skip the missed dose and resume taking the drug with the next scheduled dose. Warn him to never double-dose.

• If the patient's on long-term therapy, stress the importance of regular follow-up examinations.

• As appropriate, explain that chlorzoxazone may produce orange or purple urine; methocarbamol may turn urine green, black, or brown. Reassure the patient that this effect is normal.

• Tell the patient taking orphenadrine to relieve dry mouth with ice chips or sugarless gum or candy. Instruct him to notify the doctor if this symptom persists for longer than 2 weeks.

• Advise the diabetic patient taking metaxalone that the drug may spuriously elevate urine glucose levels.

SURGERY

Amputation

Performed to preserve function in a remaining part or, at times, to prevent death, amputation represents a radical treatment for severe trauma, gangrene, cancer, vascular disease, congenital deformity, or thermal injury. It can take one of two basic forms. In a closed, or flap, amputation—the most commonly performed type—the surgeon uses skin flaps to cover the bone stump. In an open, or guillotine, amputation (a rarely performed emergency operation), he cuts the tissue and bone flush, leaving the wound open. A second operation completes repair and stump formation.

Purpose
To surgically remove all or part of a severely diseased or traumatized limb or digit.

Preparation
If time permits, review the doctor's explanation of the scheduled amputation, answering any questions the patient may have. Remember that the patient faces not only the loss of a body part, with an attendant change in body image, but also the threat of loss of mobility and independence. Keep in mind,

too, that loss of a limb or digit can be emotionally devastating to the patient; be sure to provide emotional support. If possible, arrange for the patient to meet with a well-adjusted amputee, who can provide additional reassurance and encouragement.

Discuss postoperative care and rehabilitation measures. Demonstrate appropriate exercises designed to strengthen the remaining portion of the limb and maintain mobility; such exercises may include active hip extension and abduction, and adduction for an above-the-knee amputation. Follow the doctor's or physical therapist's directions in explaining such exercises.

The patient may be fitted with a prosthesis while hospitalized, but most often he will require more time to heal and so will be discharged before being fitted. Explain to him that the duration between amputation and fitting of the prosthesis varies, depending on wound healing, muscle tone, and overall stump condition. Stress that good stump care can speed this process and help ensure a better fit for the prosthesis. If possible, show him the types of prostheses available for his type of amputation, and explain how they work.

Point out the possibility of phantom limb sensation, which commonly develops after a major amputation. Explain that he may "feel" sensations of pain, itching, or numbness in the area of amputation, even though the limb or digit has been removed. Reassure him that these sensations, although inexplicable, are common and should eventually disappear.

As ordered, administer broad-spectrum antibiotics to minimize the risk of infection.

Procedure
The patient receives a general anesthetic (or perhaps a local anesthetic for a finger or toe amputation). In the closed technique, the surgeon incises the tissue to the bone, leaving sufficient skin to cover the stump end. He usually controls bleeding with a tourniquet

COMMON LEVELS OF AMPUTATION

Amputation may be performed at a wide range of sites. Review this list for common types and levels of amputation:

Partial foot: removal of one or more toes and part of the foot

Total foot: removal of the foot below the ankle joint

Ankle (Syme's amputation): removal of the foot at the ankle joint

Below-the-knee: removal of the leg 5" to 7" (12.7 to 17.8 cm) below the knee

Knee disarticulation: removal of the patella with the quadriceps brought over the end of the femur, or fixation of the patella to a cut surface between the condyles (known as the Gritti-Stokes operation)

Above-the-knee: removal of the leg from 3" (7.6 cm) above the knee

Hip disarticulation: removal of both the leg and hip, or the leg and pelvis

Hemipelvectomy: removal of a leg and half of the pelvis

Fingers: removal of one or more fingers at the hinge or condyloid joints

Wrist disarticulation: removal of the hand at the wrist

Below-the-elbow: removal of the lower arm about 7" (17.8 cm) below the elbow

Elbow disarticulation: removal of the lower arm at the elbow

Above-the-elbow: removal of the arm from 3" (7.6 cm) above the elbow

surgeon may order a rigid dressing applied over the stump in the operating room. This enables immediate postoperative fitting of a prosthesis.

In an emergency, or guillotine, amputation, the surgeon makes a perpendicular incision through the bone and all tissue. He leaves the wound open, applying dressings only loosely.

Monitoring and aftercare

After the patient returns from surgery, monitor his vital signs every hour for the first 4 hours, every 2 hours for the next 4 hours, and then every 4 hours when stable. Watch particularly for bleeding through the dressing; keep a tourniquet at bedside in case massive hemorrhage occurs. If ordered, elevate the stump on a pillow or other support for 24 to 48 hours; however, this could lead to contractures. Check dressings frequently and change them as necessary. Assess drain patency and note the amount and character of drainage.

Assess for pain and provide analgesics and other pain control measures, such as heat application or whirlpool bath, as needed. Because movement may be painful and interfere with therapy, give analgesics about 30 minutes before scheduled exercises or ambulation. Distinguish stump pain from phantom limb sensation; severe, unremitting stump pain may indicate infection or other complications.

Keep the stump properly wrapped with elastic compression bandages. A properly applied bandage is essential to stump care: it supports soft tissue, controls edema and pain, and shrinks and molds the stump into a cone-shaped form to allow a good fit for the prosthesis. Rewrap the stump at least twice a day to maintain tightness. As an alternative to bandages, the doctor may order that the patient wear a stump shrinker—a custom-fitted elastic stocking that fits snugly over the stump.

If a rigid plaster dressing has been applied, care for it as you would a plaster cast for a fracture or severe sprain. Keep it from getting wet and observe

placed above the level of amputation. He then saws the bone (or resects a joint), files the bone ends smooth and rounded, and removes the periosteum up about ¼" from the bone end. After ligating all vessels and dividing the nerves, he sutures opposing muscles over the bone end and to the periosteum to provide better muscle control and circulation. Next, he sutures the skin flaps closed. Placement of an incisional drain and a soft dressing completes the procedure.

In a below-the-knee amputation, the

its margin for skin irritation and excessive or malodorous drainage, which may indicate infection. As the stump shrinks, the plaster dressing may loosen or fall off. If this occurs, notify the doctor and wrap the stump in an elastic compression bandage until he can replace the dressing.

Emphasize the need for proper body alignment and regular physical therapy to condition the stump and prevent contractures and deformity. If the patient has had a leg amputation, instruct him not to prop his stump on a pillow, to avoid hip flexion contracture. If he has had a below-the-knee amputation, tell him to keep the knee extended to prevent hamstring contracture. Instruct the patient with a partial arm amputation to keep his elbow extended and shoulder abducted. Encourage frequent ambulation, if possible, and a program of active or passive range-of-motion exercises, as ordered. If the patient is bedridden, encourage him to turn from side to side and to assume an alternate position—usually on his stomach—from time to time throughout the day. Frequent position changes will stretch the hip flexor muscles and prevent contractures.

If possible, give the patient information about available prostheses. Keep in mind the patient's age and physical condition, as well as the complexity and cost of the device. Generally, a child needs a relatively simple, inexpensive device that can be maintained easily and replaced at a reasonable cost when he outgrows it. An elderly patient may require a prosthesis that provides extra stability even if it means sacrificing some flexibility.

Throughout recovery and rehabilitation, encourage the patient to adopt a positive outlook toward resuming an independent life-style. Emphasize that the prosthesis should allow him to lead a full and active life, with few restrictions on activity. If he seems overly despondent or depressed, consider referring him to psychological counseling or social services.

Home care instructions

• Instruct the patient to examine his stump daily, using a hand-held mirror to visualize the entire area. Tell him to watch for and report swelling, redness, or excessive drainage, as well as increased pain. Also instruct him to note and report any skin changes on the stump, including rashes, blisters, or abrasions.

• Explain that good stump hygiene will prevent irritation, skin breakdown, and infection. Tell the patient to wash the stump daily with mild soap and water, then rinse and gently dry it. Suggest that he wash the stump at night, then bandage it when dry; advise against bandaging a wet stump since this may lead to skin maceration or infection. Also advise against applying body oil or lotion to the stump since this can interfere with proper fit of the prosthesis.

• Teach the patient how to apply a stump dressing. Instruct him to change dressings frequently, as necessary, and to maintain sterile technique. Explain that as the wound heals, he'll need to change the dressing less often.

• As appropriate, show the patient how to properly wrap his stump with elastic bandages or how to slip on a stump shrinker. If he's using bandages, show him how to apply them with even, moderate pressure, avoiding overtightness that could impair circulation. Suggest that he apply the bandages when he awakens in the morning and rewrap the stump at least twice a day to maintain proper compression. If he's using a shrinker, suggest that he have two available: one to wear while the other's being washed. Explain that he'll need to use elastic bandages or a stump shrinker at all times (except when bathing or exercising) until postoperative edema completely subsides and the prosthesis is properly fitted. Even after adjustment to the prosthesis, he may need to continue nighttime bandaging for many years.

• Instruct the patient to apply a clean stump sock before attaching his prosthesis. Advise him never to wear a stump sock that has any tears, holes, mends, or seams; these could cause skin irritation. Explain that as the stump shrinks over time, he may need to apply two stump socks to ensure a snug fit of the prosthesis. Tell him to notify the doctor if he needs more than two socks for proper fit or if his prosthesis feels loose for any other reason.

• Review proper care of the prosthesis. Instruct the patient never to immerse it in water, which could weaken its leather joints or hinges. Tell him to clean the device with soap and water each night before bedtime and to let it dry overnight.

• If necessary, refer the patient to a local support group.

Open Reduction and Internal Fixation

When closed reduction of a fracture or dislocation is impossible or inadvisable, open reduction and internal fixation may be necessary. This procedure involves surgical restoration of the normal position and alignment of bone fragments or a dislocated joint followed by insertion of internal fixation devices—pins, screws, nails, wires, rods, or plates—to maintain positioning until healing occurs.

Open reduction with internal fixation is typically indicated for patients with compound fractures, comminuted fractures (with the bone shattered into three or more fragments), impacted fractures (with one bone fragment forced into or onto another fragment), or a fracture or dislocation that has caused serious nerve or circulatory impairment. Most often performed in adults and adolescents, it's usually avoided in children because the handling of bones and placement of fixation devices can disrupt normal epiphyseal closure and interfere with

bone growth and development.

Timing is critical to the success of this operation. Best results are obtained when the bones are set and fixation applied as soon as possible after injury, before the bones have had a chance to set improperly. If necessary, skeletal traction may precede open reduction and fixation to reduce severe muscle spasm and help realign grossly angulated fracture fragments or dislocations. Usually, a cast or splint is applied after surgery to immobilize the injury site and aid healing. If severe tissue damage accompanies fracture or dislocation, cast application may be contraindicated and skin or skeletal traction may be used in its place.

Nursing care for a patient undergoing open reduction with internal fixation involves monitoring for potential complications, including infection, hypovolemia, and fat embolism, and taking steps to prevent or minimize them. It also involves encouraging the patient to maintain proper position and perform prescribed exercises.

Purpose

To restore displaced bone segments to their original position and maintain alignment with screws, rods, pins, plates, or other fixation devices.

Preparation

Keep the fracture site immobilized and raised, if appropriate, to reduce pain and swelling. Prepare the patient for X-rays to visualize the fracture and help the surgeon plan his approach. In a severe fracture with open wounds, apply direct pressure to control blood loss and, as ordered, administer fluid replacements (possibly including blood products) to prevent or treat hypovolemia. Observe for other possible complications of fracture—particularly for compartment syndrome, which can develop within 6 hours of injury. (See *Recognizing Complications of Fractures*, page 291.)

The patient will probably be in considerable pain. As ordered, administer

CLOSED REDUCTION:
PREFERRED TREATMENT FOR MOST FRACTURES

Closed reduction, or external fixation, refers to the nonsurgical restoration of bone fragments to their correct alignment. It's the treatment of choice for most fractures. However, it's contraindicated for open fractures, when soft tissue is interposed between bone fragments, and when nerve or circulatory damage exists.

With the patient under anesthesia (local for minor fractures and general for severe ones), the doctor performs closed reduction by manually applying traction to lock the ends of the bone fragments together and restore normal alignment. The maneuvers he uses during manipulation are traction and countertraction, angulation, and rotation. After closed reduction, X-ray films are taken to verify correct bone alignment, and a cast or other immobilization device is applied.

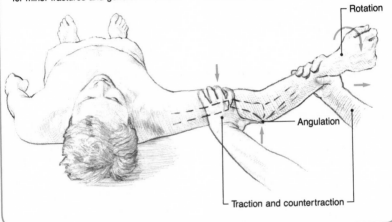

Rotation

Angulation

Traction and countertraction

a narcotic analgesic and sedative before surgery, and reassure him that analgesics will be made available after surgery as he needs them. Also, as ordered, begin prophylactic antibiotic therapy to guard against infection.

If time and the patient's condition permit, briefly explain the procedure and the type of fixation device the surgeon will use. Describe any cast, splint, or traction device the patient can expect after surgery.

Because this surgery typically requires general anesthesia, restrict food after midnight on the night before surgery. In an emergency, you may be asked to perform gastric lavage to empty the patient's stomach.

Procedure

With the patient under general anesthesia, the surgeon makes an incision through the skin and soft tissue and spreads the muscle to expose the fracture or dislocation. He realigns the fractured fragments or dislocated joint segments. Then he inserts one or more screws or another type of fixation device to immobilize the fragments in proper alignment. Next, he closes the incision and applies a cast, a splint, or traction, if necessary, to protect the surgical site and maintain alignment.

Monitoring and aftercare

If the patient has had a cast applied, observe its margin for drainage, foul odors, and signs of skin irritation. Promptly report any of these signs, which may signal infection. Also check for other signs of infection, such as fever and tachycardia. As ordered, begin antibiotic therapy to prevent or treat infection.

REVIEWING INTERNAL FIXATION METHODS

Fractures can be stabilized with a variety of internal devices: pins, nails, rods, or screwplates. Choice of a specific device depends on the location, type, and configuration of the fracture.

In a trochanteric fracture, for instance, a hip pin or nail (with or without plate) or screwplate may be used. In a subtrochanteric fracture, similar devices may be used. Because of the great stresses imposed on this area by weight bearing, strong control of both proximal and distal bone fragments is required. A pin or plate with extra nails stabilizes the fracture by impacting the bone ends at the fracture site.

In an uncomplicated fracture of the femoral shaft, an intramedullary rod may be used. This device permits early ambulation with partial weight bearing.

In an upper extremity fracture, a plate, rod, or nail may be used. Most radius and ulna fractures may be fixed with plates, whereas humerus fractures may be fixed with rods.

PINS IN HUMERUS

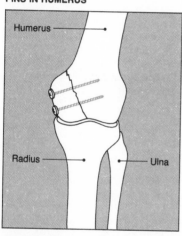

HIP PIN WITH SCREWPLATE

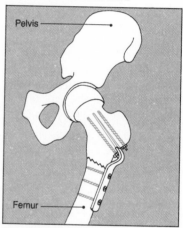

SCREWPLATE IN TIBIA

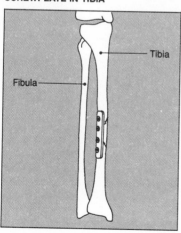

INTRAMEDULLARY ROD

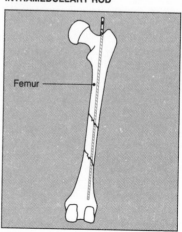

As appropriate, provide routine cast care. Maintain the affected body part in proper alignment and, if possible, support and elevate it to reduce swelling and the risk of circulatory impairment. Check for and report signs of impaired circulation in distal areas: skin mottling or discoloration and numbness, tingling, or coldness in the extremities. Such complications may require cast adjustment.

If the patient has suffered a major fracture that requires long-term immobilization with traction, be sure to reposition him often to prevent pressure sores and enhance his comfort. Encourage coughing and deep breathing to prevent pulmonary complications and adequate fluid intake to prevent urinary stasis and constipation.

As instructed by the doctor or physical therapist, assist the patient with active or passive range-of-motion exercises to prevent muscle atrophy and contractures. Encourage the patient to get out of bed and move about as soon as possible after surgery; assist with ambulation as necessary.

Home care instructions

• Review prescribed activity restrictions with the patient. In particular, focus on weight-bearing restrictions for the affected limb. As appropriate, demonstrate proper use of crutches.
• Encourage compliance with prescribed physical therapy to maintain muscle tone and promote mobility.
• Instruct the patient to watch for and report signs of wound infection, including fever, fatigue, and increased pain at the incision site.
• Tell him that pain in the affected bone may persist for up to several months; advise him to take analgesics as prescribed.
• If the patient is discharged with a cast in place, make sure he understands all aspects of cast care. Tell him to watch for signs of skin irritation around the cast edges and to report severe irritation, foul odor, or dis-

RECOGNIZING COMPLICATIONS OF FRACTURES

A major open fracture can cause severe complications, such as compartment syndrome, hypovolemic shock, and fat embolism. To detect compartment syndrome, be alert for intense cramping pain, extreme muscle tension, and swelling in the fracture area, and numbness, erythema, and loss of pulse in the limb. If these signs occur, loosen restrictive dressings and keep the limb flat to relieve pressure and enhance circulation. Notify the doctor.

A patient with a severe open fracture of a large bone, such as the femur, is at particular risk for hypovolemic shock. Assess this patient's vital signs frequently and report hypotension, narrowed pulse pressure, decreased level of consciousness, tachycardia, rapid and shallow respirations, and cold, pale, clammy skin.

Fat embolism, a potentially fatal complication, may follow the release of fat droplets from the bone marrow or the release of catecholamines after trauma, which mobilizes fatty acids. Fat emboli can lodge in the lungs or the brain. They typically develop within 24 hours after a fracture, but may be delayed for up to 72 hours. Suspect this complication if you detect diaphoresis, cyanosis, and a characteristic petechial rash on the patient's chest and shoulders. Does the patient seem apprehensive or dyspneic? Does he have a fever? Decreased level of consciousness or overt seizure activity? Report any of these signs immediately to prevent irreversible damage.

charge. Also instruct him to immediately report signs of impaired circulation, such as numbness, tingling, and skin discoloration or coldness. Warn him against getting the cast wet or inserting foreign objects under it to scratch his skin.
• If the patient's discharged with a removable splint, teach him how to apply and remove the device.
• To promote healing, instruct the patient to maintain a balanced diet with generous amounts of protein, calcium, and vitamin C, and to drink plenty of fluids.

Laminectomy and Spinal Fusion

In laminectomy, the surgeon removes one or more of the bony laminae that cover the vertebrae. Most commonly performed to relieve pressure on the spinal cord or spinal nerve roots resulting from a herniated disk, laminectomy also may be done to treat compression fracture or dislocation of vertebrae or a spinal cord tumor.

After removal of several laminae, spinal fusion—grafting of bone chips between vertebral spaces—is often performed to stabilize the spine. It also may be done apart from laminectomy in some patients with vertebrae seriously weakened by trauma or disease. Usually, spinal fusion is done only when more conservative treatments—including prolonged bed rest, traction, or the use of a back brace—prove ineffective.

This complex and delicate surgery carries the risk of several potentially serious complications. The most common include herniation relapse, arachnoiditis, chronic neuritis caused by adhesions and scarring, and problems associated with prolonged immobility, such as urinary retention, paralytic ileus, and pulmonary complications. And even though surgery may relieve pressure on the nerves, reducing pain and improving mobility, it can't reverse existing nerve or muscle damage from chronic disorders.

When caring for a patient undergoing laminectomy or spinal fusion, your primary responsibilities involve maintaining the patient's spine in proper alignment after surgery to promote healing, enhancing his comfort, and monitoring for and taking steps to prevent or minimize complications. As recovery progresses, you'll assist with rehabilitation to speed healing and restore function.

Purpose
- *For laminectomy*: To repair spinal cord defects, such as a herniated disk.
- *For spinal fusion*: To strengthen and stabilize the spine.

Preparation
The patient will probably be extremely apprehensive of the scheduled surgery. Whether he expresses his fears or not, he'll have many questions. Try to ease his fears by answering his questions clearly and matter-of-factly. Try to anticipate information that he may want to know but is reluctant to ask about.

Discuss postoperative recovery and rehabilitation. Point out that surgery won't relieve back pain immediately and that pain may even worsen after the operation. Explain that relief will come only after chronic nerve irritation and swelling subside, which may take up to several weeks. Reassure him that analgesics and muscle relaxants will be available during recovery.

Tell the patient that he'll return from surgery with a dressing over the incision and that he'll be kept on bed rest for the duration prescribed by the doctor. Explain that he'll be turned often to prevent pressure sores and pulmonary complications. Show him the logrolling method of turning, and explain that he'll use this method later to get in and out of bed by himself.

Just before surgery, perform a baseline assessment of motor function and sensation in the patient's lower trunk, legs, and feet. Carefully document the results for comparison with postoperative findings.

Procedure
The patient is given a general anesthetic and placed in a prone position. To perform a laminectomy, the surgeon makes a midline vertical incision and strips the fascia and muscles off the bony laminae. He then removes one or more sections of laminae to expose the spinal defect. For a herniated disk, the surgeon removes part or all of the disk. For a spinal cord tumor, he incises the

dura and explores the cord for metastasis. Then he dissects the tumor and removes it, using suction, forceps, or dissecting scissors.

To perform spinal fusion, the surgeon exposes the affected vertebrae, then inserts bone chips obtained from the patient's iliac crest or, rarely, from a bone bank. For optimum strength, he wires these bone grafts into several vertebrae surrounding the area of instability. Then he closes the incision and applies a dressing. After completion of the operation, external traction (such as a halo device, if surgery involved the cervical spine) may be applied.

Monitoring and aftercare

After surgery, keep the head of the patient's bed flat for at least 24 hours. Urge the patient to remain in the supine position for the prescribed period to prevent any strain on the involved vertebrae. When he's able to assume a side-lying position, make sure he keeps his spine straight with his knees flexed and drawn up toward his chest. Insert a pillow between his knees to relieve pressure on the spine from hip adduction.

Inspect the dressing frequently for bleeding or cerebrospinal fluid leakage; report either immediately. The surgeon will probably perform the initial dressing change himself; you may be asked to perform subsequent changes.

Assess motor and neurologic function in the patient's trunk and lower extremities and compare the results with baseline findings. Also evaluate circulation in his legs and feet and report any abnormalities. Give analgesics and muscle relaxants, as ordered.

Every 2 to 4 hours, assess urine output and auscultate for the return of bowel sounds. If the patient doesn't void within 8 to 12 hours after surgery, notify the doctor and prepare to insert a catheter to relieve retention. If the patient can void normally, assist him in getting on and off a bedpan while maintaining proper alignment.

ALTERNATIVES TO LAMINECTOMY

Percutaneous automated diskectomy and chemonucleolysis represent alternatives to the traditional surgical treatment of a herniated disk.

Percutaneous automated diskectomy
In this technique, the doctor uses a suction technique and X-ray visualization to remove only the disk portion that's causing pain. Typically used for smaller, less severe disk abnormalities, percutaneous automated diskectomy has an unimpressive 50% success rate, perhaps because it doesn't involve direct visualization of the operative site. One report indicates a high incidence of postoperative diskitis with this method.

Nursing care of the patient after diskectomy is similar to that after laminectomy; he's generally allowed out of bed in 48 hours, and he can ambulate without assistance within 4 days.

Chemonucleolysis
This treatment involves injection of the drug chymopapain or collagenase to destroy the disk. Usually performed with radiographic visualization, it eliminates the need for surgery.

Chemonucleolysis isn't without risks, however. Studies indicate disk space narrowing after chemonucleolysis, leading to irreversible osteoarthritis-like changes.

Nursing care after chemonucleolysis involves monitoring the patient for changes in neurologic status, such as worsened back pain or decreased sensation below the injection site. This may suggest bleeding into the disk space (most common) or an antigenic reaction to the drug.

Home care instructions

● Teach the patient and his caregiver proper incision care measures. Tell them to check the incision site often for signs of infection—increased pain and tenderness, redness, swelling, and changes in the amount and character of drainage—and to report any such signs immediately. Instruct the patient to avoid soaking his stitches in a tub bath until healing is complete. Also advise him to shower with his back facing away from the stream of water.

• Make sure the patient understands the importance of resuming activity gradually after surgery. As ordered, instruct him to start with short walks and to slowly progress to longer distances. Review any prescribed exercises, such as pelvic tilts, leg raises, and toe pointing. Advise him to rest frequently and avoid overexertion.

• Review any prescribed activity restrictions. Usually, the doctor will prohibit sitting for prolonged periods, lifting heavy objects or even bending over, and climbing long flights of stairs. He may also impose other restrictions, depending on the patient's condition.

• Teach the patient proper body mechanics to lessen strain and pressure on his spine. Instruct him to lie on his back, with his knees propped up with pillows, or on his side with his knees drawn up and a pillow placed between his legs. Warn him against lying on his stomach or on his back with legs flat. When sitting, he should place his feet on a low stool to elevate his knees above hip level. He should use a firm, straight-backed chair and sit up straight with his lower back pressed flat against the chair back. When standing for prolonged periods, he should alternate placing each foot on a low stool to straighten his lower back and relieve strain. When bending, he should keep his spine straight and bend at his knees and hips rather than at his waist.

• Instruct the patient to sleep only on a firm mattress. If necessary, advise him to purchase a new one or to insert a bed board between his existing mattress and box spring.

Joint Replacement

[Arthroplasty]

Total or partial replacement of a joint with a synthetic prosthesis restores mobility and stability and relieves pain. In fact, recent improvements in surgical techniques and prosthetic devices have made joint replacement an increasingly common treatment for patients with severe chronic arthritis, degenerative joint disorders, and extensive joint trauma. All joints except the spine can be replaced with a prosthesis; hip and knee replacements are the most common. The benefits of joint replacement include not only improved, pain-free mobility but also an increased sense of independence and self-worth.

Purpose
To replace a diseased or damaged joint with a prosthesis, restoring normal function.

Preparation
Because of joint replacement's complexity, patient preparation begins long before the day of surgery with extensive tests and studies. In fact, by the time the patient enters the hospital for surgery, the doctor will have explained the procedure to him in detail. However, the patient still may have questions about the surgery and its expected outcome. And because the patient is likely to be elderly, his family may have questions that you'll need to address. Answer them as completely as you can.

Discuss postoperative recovery with the patient and his family. Mention that the patient will probably remain in bed for up to 5 or 6 days after surgery. Explain that even while he's confined to bed, he'll begin an exercise program to maintain joint mobility. As appropriate, show him range-of-motion exercises or demonstrate the continuous passive motion (CPM) device that he'll use during recovery.

Prepare the patient for an extended period of rehabilitation. Point out that he may not experience pain relief immediately after surgery and that, in fact, pain actually may worsen for several weeks. Reassure him that pain will diminish dramatically once edema subsides. Reassure him that analgesics will be available as needed.

Ensure that the patient or a responsible family member has signed a consent form.

Procedure

The details of the joint replacement procedure vary slightly, depending on the joint and its condition. In a total hip replacement, for instance, the patient is placed in a supine or lateral position and given a general anesthetic. The surgeon then makes an incision to expose the hip joint. As necessary, he incises or excises the hip capsule, then dislocates the joint to expose the acetabulum and the head of the femur. Next, he reams and shapes the acetabulum to accept the socket part of the ball-and-socket hip prosthesis and secures the device in place with methyl methacrylate adhesive. He then repeats this process on the head of the femur for the ball portion of the prosthesis. Once the parts of the prosthesis are in place, he fits them together to restore the joint. Then he closes the incision in layers and applies a dressing.

Monitoring and aftercare

When the patient returns from surgery, keep him on bed rest for the prescribed period. Maintain the affected joint in proper alignment. If traction is used, periodically check the weights and other equipment.

Assess the patient's level of pain and provide analgesics, as ordered. If you're administering narcotic analgesics, be alert for signs of toxicity or oversedation.

During the recovery period, monitor for complications of joint replacement. In particular, watch for hypovolemic shock from massive blood loss during surgery. Assess the patient's vital signs frequently and report hypotension, narrowed pulse pressure, tachycardia, decreased level of consciousness, rapid and shallow respirations, or cold, pale, clammy skin.

Also watch for signs of a fat embolism, a potentially fatal complication caused by release of fat molecules in

---

RECONSTRUCTION ALTERNATIVES

Arthroplasty is a surgical technique intended to restore motion to a stiffened joint. Joint replacement is one option. Other options include *joint resection* or *interpositional reconstruction.*

Joint resection involves careful excision of bone portions, creating a 2-cm gap in one or both bone surfaces of the joint. Fibrous scar tissue eventually fills in the gap. Although this surgery restores mobility and relieves pain, it decreases joint stability.

Interpositional reconstruction involves reshaping the joint and placing a prosthetic disk between the reshaped bony ends. The prosthesis used for this procedure may be composed of metal, plastic, fascia, or skin. However, with repeated injury and surgical reshaping, total joint replacement may be necessary.

---

response to increased intermedullary canal pressure from the prosthesis. Fat embolism usually develops within 72 hours after surgery and is characterized by apprehension, diaphoresis, fever, dyspnea, pulmonary effusion, tachycardia, cyanosis, seizures, decreased level of consciousness, and a petechial rash on the chest and shoulders.

Inspect the incision site and dressing frequently for signs of infection. Change the dressing as necessary, maintaining strict aseptic technique. Periodically assess neurovascular and motor status distal to the site of joint replacement. Immediately report any abnormalities.

Be sure to reposition the patient often to enhance comfort and prevent pressure sores. Encourage frequent coughing and deep breathing to prevent pulmonary complications and adequate fluid intake to prevent urinary stasis and constipation.

As ordered, have the patient begin exercising the affected joint soon after surgery. (Some doctors routinely order physical therapy to begin on the day of surgery.) The doctor may prescribe CPM, which involves use of a machine or a system of suspended ropes and pulleys, or a series of active or passive range-of-motion (ROM) exercises. (See "Range-of-Motion Exercises" in this chapter for further details.)

Home care instructions

• Reinforce the doctor's and physical therapist's instructions for the patient's exercise regimen. Remind him to stick closely to the prescribed schedule and not to rush rehabilitation, no matter how good he feels.

• Review prescribed limitations on activity. Depending on the location and extent of surgery, the doctor may order the patient to avoid bending or lifting, extensive stair climbing, or sitting for prolonged periods (including long car trips or plane flights). He also will caution against overusing the joint—especially weight-bearing joints.

• The patient who has undergone knee replacement may be instructed to wear a knee brace or an immobilizer. If so, make sure he knows how to apply it properly.

• If the patient has undergone hip replacement, instruct him to keep his hips abducted and not to cross his legs when sitting, to reduce the risk of dislocating the prosthesis. Tell him to avoid flexing his hips more than 90 degrees when arising from a bed or chair. Encourage him to sit in chairs with high arms and a firm seat and to sleep only on a firm mattress.

• Before the patient with a knee or hip replacement is discharged, make sure that he has a properly sized pair of crutches and knows how to use them properly.

• If the patient has undergone shoulder joint replacement, instruct him to keep his arm in a sling until postoperative swelling subsides, then to slowly begin the prescribed exercise program when healing is complete—usually about 6 weeks after surgery.

• Caution the patient to promptly report signs of possible infection, such as persistent fever and increased pain, tenderness, and stiffness in the joint

and surrounding area. Remind him that infection may develop even several months after joint replacement.

• Tell the patient to report a sudden increase of pain, which may indicate dislodgment of the prosthesis.

Carpal Tunnel Release

If rest, splinting, and corticosteroid injections fail to relieve carpal tunnel syndrome, surgery may be necessary to decompress the median nerve. This surgery involves sectioning the entire transverse carpal tunnel ligament and possibly performing neurolysis as well. It almost always relieves pain and restores function in the wrist and hand.

Although this surgery is relatively simple and generally risk-free, certain complications may arise. These include hematoma formation, infection, painful scar formation, and tenosynovitis.

Purpose

To decompress the median nerve within the carpal tunnel, thereby relieving pain and restoring function.

Preparation

Reinforce the purpose of the planned surgery. Tell the patient that the procedure should relieve the pain in his wrist and help him regain full use of his hand. Outline the steps of surgery, tailoring your explanation to the particular procedure the doctor has chosen as well as to the patient's level of understanding.

Explain to the patient that before surgery, the affected arm will be shaved and cleansed and he'll be given a local anesthetic. Reassure him that although he may feel some pressure, the anesthetic will ensure a pain-free operation.

Discuss postoperative care measures. Point out that he'll have a dressing wrapped around his hand and lower arm, which usually will remain in place for 1 to 2 days after surgery. Explain that he may experience pain once the anesthetic wears off but that analgesics will be available.

Teach him the rehabilitative exercises that he'll be asked to do during the recovery period: gentle range-of-motion exercises with the wrist and fingers to prevent muscle atrophy. Demonstrate these exercises and have him perform them. Keep in mind, however, that severe pain may prevent him from doing so.

Procedure
The surgeon can choose from several approaches to carpal tunnel release. Whichever technique he chooses, though, must involve complete transection of the transverse carpal tunnel ligament to ensure adequate medial nerve decompression.

In one of the more popular techniques, the surgeon makes an incision around the thenar eminence to expose the flexor retinaculum, which he then transects to relieve pressure on the median nerve. Depending on the extent of nerve compression, he also may perform neurolysis to free flattened nerve fibers.

Monitoring and aftercare
After the patient returns from surgery, monitor his vital signs and carefully assess circulation and sensory and motor function in the affected arm and hand. Keep the hand elevated to reduce swelling and discomfort.

Check the dressing often for unusual drainage or bleeding, which may indicate infection. Assess for pain and provide analgesics as needed. Report severe, persistent pain or tenderness, which may point to tenosynovitis or hematoma formation.

Encourage him to perform his wrist and finger exercises daily, to improve circulation and enhance muscle tone. If these exercises are painful, have him perform them with his wrist and hand

immersed in warm water. (Have him wear a surgical glove if his dressing's still in place.)

Home care instructions
• Instruct the patient to keep the incision site clean and dry. Tell him to cover it with a surgical or rubber glove when immersing it in water for exercises or when taking a bath or shower.
• Teach him how to change the dressing. Instruct him to do so once a day until healing is complete.
• Tell him to notify the doctor if redness, swelling, pain, or excessive drainage persists at the operative site.
• Encourage the patient to continue daily wrist and finger exercises. However, warn him against overusing the affected wrist or against lifting any object heavier than a thin magazine.
• If the patient's carpal tunnel syndrome is job-related, suggest that he seek occupational counseling to help him find more suitable employment.

FLUID ASPIRATION

Arthrocentesis

Commonly used as an adjunctive treatment for orthopedic disorders, such as joint trauma or septic arthritis, arthrocentesis involves insertion of a needle into the joint space to aspirate excessive synovial fluid or blood, or to instill corticosteroids or other anti-inflammatory drugs. It also may be performed to obtain a specimen for diagnostic testing.

Most commonly performed on the knee, arthrocentesis also may be done on the elbow, shoulder, or other joints. It's often combined with two related procedures: arthroscopy, which allows endoscopic visualization of the joint, and arthrography, an X-ray showing joint tissue and structure.

Arthrocentesis is performed under strict aseptic technique to avoid infecting the joint or contaminating the specimen. Other possible complications include intraarticular or soft-tissue hemorrhage, tendon rupture, and temporary nerve palsy.

Purpose
• To remove excessive fluid from the joint space
• To instill anti-inflammatory drugs
• To obtain a specimen for laboratory analysis.

Preparation
Review the procedure with the patient, reinforcing and clarifying the doctor's explanation as necessary. Explain that he needs to keep his joint extended and motionless throughout the procedure, to aid the doctor and minimize the risk of complications. Point out that, although he'll receive a local anesthetic, he may feel some pain as the needle is introduced into the joint space. Reassure him that this pain should resolve quickly, however, and that he should be able to resume his normal activities soon after the procedure.

If the patient is undergoing arthrocentesis to withdraw a synovial fluid sample for glucose analysis, restrict foods or fluids for the prescribed length of time before the procedure.

Make sure the patient or a responsible family member has signed a consent form. Check the patient's history for hypersensitivity to iodine compounds (such as povidone-iodine), procaine, lidocaine, or other local anesthetics. Administer a sedative, as ordered.

Assemble the necessary equipment, including a corticosteroid suspension, if necessary.

Procedure
Position the patient as ordered. After cleansing and sterilizing the puncture site, the doctor injects or sprays a local anesthetic at the site. He then inserts the appropriate needle and aspirates at least 10 to 15 ml of synovial fluid from the joint. To aid aspiration, he may wrap an elastic bandage around the joint above and below the puncture site; this compresses the fluid into the site and ensures maximum aspiration.

If the doctor will be injecting medication into the joint space, he leaves the needle in the joint, detaches the fluid-filled syringe, attaches a drug-filled syringe, and injects the medication. After withdrawing the needle, he applies direct pressure over the puncture site for 2 minutes, then applies a sterile pressure dressing to control bleeding. If a large amount of fluid has been aspirated from the knee, an elastic bandage may be applied to improve joint stability and inhibit further fluid accumulation.

Monitoring and aftercare
After treatment, monitor the puncture site for excessive bleeding, and take steps to control it if necessary. Elevate the affected limb and apply ice or cold packs to the joint for 24 to 36 hours to decrease pain and swelling.

Assess for signs of infection, such as fever or increased joint pain. Report such signs promptly, and prepare to initiate antibiotic therapy as ordered. To minimize the risk of infection, handle all dressings and linens carefully, and keep the puncture site clean.

Home care instructions
• Advise the patient that he can resume normal activities soon after the procedure. However, warn him to avoid overusing the affected joint for several days, to prevent increased pain, swelling, and stiffness.
• Instruct the patient to immediately report increased pain, redness, swelling, or fever; explain that these signs may indicate infection, which requires prompt medical attention.
• Remind him to keep follow-up medical appointments so that the doctor can evaluate the effectiveness of treatment.

EXERCISE AND MOVEMENT

Range-of-Motion Exercises

Range-of-motion (ROM) exercises are designed to move the patient's joints through as full a range of motion as possible. When performed properly, they help improve or maintain joint mobility, enhance muscle tone, and prevent contractures and subsequent deformity.

ROM exercises may be active or passive. *Active ROM exercises* are performed by the patient himself, either alone or with the assistance of a nurse or physical therapist. They're indicated for patients who have a good degree of neuromuscular function.

Passive ROM exercises are performed manually by a nurse, a physical therapist, a member of the patient's family or another caregiver, or with the aid of a CPM machine. They're indicated for patients experiencing temporary or permanent loss of function, paralysis, or unconsciousness. They require recognition of the patient's mobility limitations and the support of all joints during movement.

Contraindications to ROM therapy include severe arthritic joint inflammation, septic joint, recent trauma with possible occult fracture or internal injuries, thrombophlebitis, severe pain, and a stiff or immovable joint. Forced passive stretching—movement of a joint that's immobile because of disuse, disease, or injury—must be specially ordered and performed by a doctor or physical therapist.

Potential complications of active ROM include exacerbation of inflammation from overmanipulation, and joint or muscle injury from forced or excessive movement. For passive ROM, possible complications include joint instability and effusion from hyperextension and even joint dislocation or bone fracture from rough handling during exercise. To help prevent these complications, keep in mind three cardinal rules of ROM therapy: stop the exercise at once if the patient complains of pain, exercise only one extremity at a time, and never force any movement.

Purpose
To maintain or restore normal joint movement and muscle tone, preventing stiffness and contractures, improving circulation, and possibly speeding return of function.

Preparation
Assess the patient for disability and weakness in the involved extremity, and compare your findings against those from a baseline neuromuscular assessment. If you note any deterioration in neuromuscular function, consult the doctor or physical therapist, who may order changes in the patient's exercise regimen.

If the patient's alert and responsive, explain the exercises to him; if not, explain them to a family member or whomever will be the patient's primary caregiver after discharge. For passive ROM, explain that you'll move his extremities, one at a time, through their normal range of motion in a prescribed pattern to maintain function and prevent stiffening.

If the patient is to perform active ROM, describe and demonstrate the prescribed exercises. Explain that he will perform the exercises at least twice a day, but warn him against overextension or overexertion, which can lead to complications.

Before passive ROM therapy, raise the patient's bed to a comfortable working height, and position the patient properly—if possible, flat on his back, without a pillow, with hands at his sides and his feet together.

CONTINUOUS PASSIVE MOTION

Continuous passive motion (CPM) uses an electrically powered or manually operated machine to automatically move a joint through its normal range of motion for an extended duration. An alternative to nurse-assisted passive range-of-motion exercise, CPM is most commonly used in patients recovering from total hip or knee replacement, internal fixation of knee or ankle fractures, or removal of the synovial membrane in the knee or other major joints.

Nursing responsibilities for patients undergoing CPM include setting up the machine and positioning the patient in it, monitoring therapy, and ensuring patient comfort.

Performing CPM
• Attach the machine to the patient's bed and set the degree of flexion and extension prescribed.
• Fasten the patient's extremity securely in the frame.
• Run the machine through one cycle and double-check the degree of flexion and extension. Adjust as necessary.
• Restart the machine and continue operation for the prescribed duration.

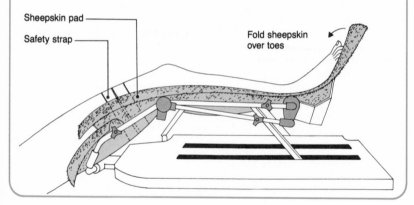

Sheepskin pad

Safety strap

Fold sheepskin over toes

Procedure

Depending on the mobility and condition of the joints being exercised, ROM therapy will include some or all of the following movements: flexion and extension, internal and external rotation, abduction and adduction, supination and pronation, and eversion and inversion.

When performing passive ROM, support the extremity at the joint and move the joint slowly, smoothly, and gently through its normal range of motion. If the joint is painful to the touch, as in arthritis, support the extremity as close to the joint as possible without causing pain. If the patient reports pain during any movement, stop immediately and document this in your notes.

If the patient is to perform active ROM, make sure he understands the prescribed exercises and the recommended frequency. Tell him to move the involved joints slowly and smoothly through their range-of-motion, and to stop and notify you if he feels any unusual pain or stiffness.

Monitoring and aftercare

While performing passive ROM exercises, assess for degree of mobility in the joint and for the level of pain the movements elicit. Stiffness, immobility, or pain may indicate joint irritation resulting from overuse. If these occur, consult the doctor or therapist, who may need to reevaluate therapy.

After completing passive ROM, position the patient comfortably in bed and urge him to relax. If pain develops after exercise, administer analgesics, as ordered.

Observe the patient performing active ROM to ensure proper movement. Make sure that he performs all the prescribed exercises; by the same token, watch that he doesn't overdo it. Again, if the patient complains of pain and stiffness during or after the exercises, consult with the doctor or therapist about possible changes in his program.

Home care instructions
• Before discharge, make sure the patient and a family member or caregiver, if appropriate, fully understand each aspect of the prescribed exercise program and the need for strict compliance. Provide written, illustrated, or tape-recorded instructions, if possible, to enhance their understanding and improve compliance.
• To demonstrate understanding and the ability to do the exercises, have the patient or caregiver perform each aspect of prescribed ROM therapy to your satisfaction before discharge.
• Instruct the patient or caregiver to report any complications associated with ROM exercise, such as increased joint or muscle pain, stiffness, or immobility.
• Stress the need for regular follow-up examinations to evaluate the patient's progress and the effectiveness of the exercise program.

Bone Growth Stimulation
[Galvanic therapy]

This therapy involves the application of a mild electrical current to bone fracture fragments to help stimulate new bone growth and speed healing. It isn't routinely used to treat fractures. In-

stead, it's reserved for patients with fractures that fail to heal within 6 to 9 months of injury (about 3% of all skeletal fractures).

Three types of electrical bone growth stimulators are currently used. The *fully implantable direct-current stimulator* consists of a power generator and titanium cathodes implanted at the fracture site. The *semi-invasive percutaneous stimulator* uses one to four Teflon-coated implanted cathode pins and an external anode skin pad and battery pack. A noninvasive device, the *pulsating electromagnetic fields* (PEMFs) system, uses external wire coils and a generator to produce the therapeutic electrical current.

Selection of a bone growth stimulator depends on such factors as the fracture's type and location, the doctor's preference, and perhaps most important, the patient's ability to comply with treatment. Although the invasive device requires little or no patient intervention, the semi-invasive and PEMFs systems require that the patient manage his own treatment schedule as well as maintain the system.

Purpose
To electrically stimulate new bone growth in areas of fracture and speed healing.

Preparation
If the patient's scheduled for surgical insertion of a fully implantable stimulator, explain the device (show it to him, if possible) and reassure him that it carries no risk of electrocution. Describe the implantation procedure and mention that he'll have a cast applied after surgery. Review the basics of cast care, including keeping the cast well-supported and away from water until it's completely dry.

If the patient will have a semi-invasive stimulator implanted, show him the device and explain how it works. Identify the implantation site and discuss his responsibilities during therapy, such as changing the anode

COMPARING ELECTRICAL BONE STIMULATORS

TYPE	CONTRAINDICATIONS AND COMPLICATIONS	PATIENT TEACHING
Noninvasive pulsating electromagnetic fields (PEMFs)	• Contraindicated in pseudarthrosis or presence of a pacemaker or magnetic metal fixation device. • No known complications.	• Tell the patient to use PEMFs 10 to 12 hours each day. He'll need a 110-volt outlet to provide electrical current. • Mention that treatment usually lasts 5 months. • Caution him to avoid weightbearing until the doctor gives consent.
Semi-invasive percutaneous stimulator	• Contraindicated in systemic infection, infection at nonunion site or adjacent bone or soft tissue, thrombophlebitis, osteomyelitis, sensitivity to nickel or chromium, synovial pseudarthrosis, and pathologic fractures caused by benign or malignant tumors. • Complications include local skin irritation from anode pad or cathodes and breakage of cathode pins.	• Instruct patient to change anode pad every 48 hours. • Caution him to avoid weightbearing for duration of treatment, which is usually 3 months.
Fully implantable direct current stimulator	• Don't use diathermy over the implant site or electrical surgical equipment. • Complications are the same as for bone surgery.	• Instruct the patient to follow the doctor's advice on weightbearing and activity. • Tell him that treatment usually lasts 5 to 6 months.

pad every 48 hours and providing cast care. Reassure him that the electrical current poses no danger.

If the patient will be using the PEMFs system, briefly explain how it works and identify the application site. Tell him that the device will be applied after he has been fitted with a cast to maintain alignment of the fracture fragments. Reinforce the need for cast care. Point out that once the device is in place, he should avoid placing any weight on the involved limb until healing is completed.

Procedure

For insertion of a fully implantable stimulator, the patient receives a general anesthetic and the doctor makes one incision over the fracture site and another into a nearby healthy muscle. After exposing the fracture fragments, he further separates them, if necessary, to accommodate the cathode. He then reams out the medullary canal of one fragment and inserts the cathode. Next, he implants the generator between two opposing muscle groups near the fracture site and creates a connecting pathway between the cathode and the generator through which he threads a lead wire encased in a Teflon tube. He then places a coiled titanium wire on either side of the fracture site and fits bone grafts between the coils.

For insertion of a semi-invasive percutaneous stimulator, also implanted with the patient under general anesthesia, the doctor places a cathode just inside the margin of each bone at the fracture site. He then wraps the cathodes with gauze saturated with an antimicrobial solution, then wraps the surgical area with cast padding. After trimming the protruding cathode wires and securing them to the negative wires of the battery pack, the doctor applies an anode pad to the skin and connects it to the battery pack via a lead wire. Finally, he applies a non-weight-bearing cast over the battery pack.

For application of PEMFs, the patient first is fitted with a snug plaster cast. The doctor then measures the cast's circumference at the fracture site. The measurement guides the distance between coils, as well as the amount of voltage required for the generator. Using a locator block, the doctor places coils around the circumference of the cast. After X-rays confirm proper coil placement in relation to the fracture site, the locator block is incorporated into the cast, and a Velcro strap applied to hold the coils in place.

Monitoring and aftercare
For a patient with an implantable or semi-implantable device, check vital signs and assess neurovascular status in the affected limb. Watch for signs of infection, such as fever and swelling, redness, tenderness, and discharge at or near the implantation site.

For all types of devices, reinforce the doctor's instructions regarding weight-bearing restrictions.

Home care instructions
• Tell the patient to report any signs of infection at the treatment site.
• Make sure he understands how to care for the cast.
• As ordered, tell the patient when he can place weight on the affected leg. Generally, this will be after X-rays confirm complete healing.
• Stress having regular follow-up exams to evaluate therapy and healing.

• Instruct the patient using PEMFs to wear the coils 10 to 12 hours a day, in intervals no shorter than 1 hour. Suggest that he wear the coils while sleeping to provide a long period of uninterrupted therapy. Also instruct him to test the unit regularly and to call the doctor if it doesn't work properly or if the generator alarm signals.

Immobilization

Commonly used to maintain proper alignment and limit movement, immobilization devices also relieve pressure and pain. These devices include plaster and synthetic *casts* applied after closed or open reduction of fractures or after other severe injuries; *splints* to immobilize fractures, dislocations, or subluxations; *slings* to support and immobilize an injured arm, wrist, or hand, or to support the weight of a splint or hold dressings in place; *skin or skeletal traction*, using a system of weights and pulleys to reduce fractures, treat dislocations, correct deformities, or decrease muscle spasms; *braces* to support weakened or deformed joints; and *cervical collars* to immobilize the cervical spine, decrease muscle spasms, and possibly relieve pain.

All types of immobilization devices help heal not only injured bones but also surrounding soft tissue.

Purpose
To maintain proper alignment and limit movement, thereby promoting healing or providing support.

Preparation
Explain to the patient the purpose of the immobilization device the doctor has chosen. If possible, show him the device before application and demonstrate how it works. Tell him approximately how long the device will remain in place. Explain that he can anticipate

UNDERSTANDING TYPES OF IMMOBILIZATION

TYPE AND DESCRIPTION	INDICATIONS
Braces Support devices of metal, leather, and hard plastic usually worn externally. Common types include the Milwaukee brace, the Parvis brace, and the Somi brace.	• To limit movement and enhance stability of an injured or weakened joint. • To help correct neuromuscular defects in cerebral palsy, other spastic disorders, and scoliosis.
Casts Made of plaster or synthetic material, casts may be applied virtually anywhere on the body from a single finger to full body coverage. Types include the Minerva jacket, spica cast, and extremity fixation with plaster of Paris.	• To maintain proper alignment and immobilization during healing. Casts are used for traumatic injuries and correction of congenital deformities. Examples of their use include severe ligament rupture, extremity or spinal fractures, club foot, and congenital hip dysplasia. If necessary, casts may used with traction to enhance immobilization.
Collars Made of soft foam or metal and plastic components that fit around the neck and under the chin. Common collars include the Philadelphia collar, doll's collar, Camp Victoria collar, and soft or hard cervical collar.	• To support an injured or weakened cervical spine and maintain alignment during healing. Common indications include cervical osteoarthritis, muscle strain, herniated disk, cervical spondylosis, and torticollis.
Skeletal traction Involves placement of a pin through the bone, to which the traction apparatus is attached. Common types include Gardner-Wells and Crutchfield tongs; halo vest; pin placement through the femur, lower tibia, calcaneus, ulna, radius, or wrists; Kirschner wire; and Steinmann pin.	• To immobilize bones and allow healing of fractures, correction of congenital abnormalities, or stabilization of spinal degeneration.
Skin traction Applied to the skin and soft tissue, thereby indirectly pulling on the skeletal system. This immobilization system typically consists of weights, ropes, pulleys, and slings. Common types include Buck's traction, Alvik traction, Hamilton-Russell traction, Bryant's traction, and Cotrel's traction.	• To relieve muscle spasms. • To restrict movement and provide proper alignment in cervical disk disease, pelvic fractures of the extremities, and spinal deformities.
Slings Composed of a soft fabric material or elastoplast fabric. Common types include the Gisson sling, Synder sling, and Velpeau bandage.	• To support an injured arm, hand or wrist. • To treat other upper extremity problems, such as fractures of the scapula or clavicle and shoulder dislocation, along with other types of immobilization.
Splints Made of leather, metal, and hard plastic components. Common splints include the Denis Brown splint, McKibbee splint, Thomas splint, Bell-Grice splint, Shrewsbury splint, Foster-Brown splint, Girdlestone mermaid splint, Nissen splint, Hodgen splint, and Brain-Thomas working splint.	• To provide support for injured or weakened limbs or digits. • To help correct deformities, such as mallet finger. • To help treat spinal tuberculosis, inflammatory lesions of the hip, spine, or shoulder, hip dislocation or dysplasia, long-bone fractures, scoliosis, and footdrop.

NURSING CONSIDERATIONS

• Check the condition of the brace daily for worn or malfunctioning components.
• Frequently assess the skin under the brace for breakdown and abrasions.

• Check carefully for proper fit, keeping in mind that any fluctuation in the patient's weight may alter the device's fit.

• Support a plaster cast with pillows while it's drying (for up to 72 hours, depending on cast size) to maintain proper shape. Keep the cast dry at all times.
• Demonstrate to the patient proper body mechanics for movement with larger casts.
• Perform regular neurovascular checks.

• Tell the patient to report extreme pain or pressure beneath the cast. Note any drainage or fever, which may point to infection under the cast.
• Check the skin along the edges of the cast and protect it as necessary.

• Check carefully for proper fit. You should be able to slip only one finger beneath the edge of the collar.
• Regularly inspect the skin under the collar for abrasions and breakdown.
• Keep the collar clean.

• Because the patient's head movement will be restricted, assist him with eating and other activities as necessary.
• Remove a Philadelphia collar one half at a time, with the patient lying flat.

• Perform pin care daily with water and normal saline or hydrogen peroxide.
• Observe the pin insertion site for signs of infection.
• Check the pin for proper fit, making sure that it doesn't move in the bone.
• Teach the patient how to use the trapeze to lift himself off the bed, if permitted.
• If cervical traction is being used, check the occipital area of the head for skin breakdown.

• When caring for a patient in a halo vest, bathe under the vest daily. *Never* move the patient by grasping the tongs. Instead, stabilize him on his back before opening the vest. Then open it one side at a time.
• Teach the patient how to ambulate with an altered center of gravity and show him how to adapt his clothes to fit over the vest. Remind him not to bend over, but to use an assistive device for reaching. Also, tell him to change the vest liner, as needed.

• Periodically check to ensure that weights, ropes, and pulleys are in proper alignment and functional. Check the skin application for proper placement.
• Do not manipulate the weights yourself;

consult the doctor if you suspect the need for any adjustments.
• Show the patient how to move in bed without disturbing the traction.

• Check for proper placement to ensure support of the weakened or injured area.
• Perform frequent neurovascular checks to detect circulatory or nerve impairment.
• Stress the need to wear the sling for the

prescribed period, to prevent further injury or delayed healing.
• Regularly perform passive range-of-motion exercises, as ordered.

• Check to ensure proper fit and alignment of the device. Frequently inspect the splint for cleanliness and overall condition.
• Regularly assess for skin breakdown un-

der the splint.
• Clean leather components daily with saddle soap to keep them soft and supple.

discomfort initially, but reassure him that this will resolve as he becomes accustomed to the device.

If the patient is in pain, give analgesics and muscle relaxants, as ordered.

Procedure

Application procedures vary depending on the type of immobilization device. (See *Understanding Types of Immobilization*, pages 304 and 305, for details on common devices.)

Monitoring and aftercare

Take steps to prevent complications of immobility, especially if the patient is in traction or requires long-term bed rest. For instance, reposition him frequently to enhance comfort and prevent pressure sores. As ordered, assist with active or passive ROM exercises to maintain muscle tone and prevent contractures. Encourage regular coughing and deep breathing to prevent pulmonary complications, and adequate fluid intake to prevent urinary stasis and constipation.

Encourage the bedridden patient to engage in hobbies or other activities to relieve boredom. This will help him maintain the positive mental outlook that's important to recovery. Encourage ambulation, and provide assistance as necessary.

Provide analgesics, as ordered. If you're administering narcotics, watch for signs of toxicity or oversedation.

Home care instructions

• Instruct the patient to promptly report signs of complications, including increased pain, drainage, or swelling in the involved area.
• Stress the need for strict compliance with activity restrictions while the immobilization device is in place.
• If the patient has been given crutches to use while a leg or ankle cast, splint, or knee immobilizer's in place, make sure he understands how to use them.
• If the patient has a removable device, such as a knee immobilizer, make sure

he knows how to apply it correctly.
• Advise him to keep scheduled medical appointments to evaluate healing.

BASIC CARE

Foot Care

Essential to prevent or correct complications of impaired pedal circulation, meticulous foot care especially benefits patients with diabetic neuropathy, traumatic injury, prolonged immobilization, or peripheral vascular disease. An effective foot care regimen restores or maintains skin integrity and enhances circulation to rejuvenate or maintain peripheral sensory function and, if necessary, aid healing.

Many patients are discharged with orders to follow a daily foot care routine at home. Such patients need thorough teaching to promote compliance.

Purpose

To maintain cleanliness, control odor, prevent infection, and improve circulation in the feet.

Preparation

Discuss the purpose of foot care with the patient, and explain all the steps. If he'll be performing foot care after discharge, instruct him to pay close attention and to ask questions.

Gather the equipment: bath blanket, large basin, bath thermometer, soap, washcloth and towel, linen-saver pad, toenail clippers, orangewood stick, emery board, cotton-tipped swabs or cotton balls, lotion, and water-absorbent powder. Fill the basin halfway with warm water and test the temperature with a thermometer. Keep in mind that a patient with impaired peripheral circulation could immerse his feet in water hot enough to cause burns while feeling no pain.

Procedure

Begin by carefully inspecting the patient's feet. Look for blisters, bruises, cracks, open lesions, corns, calluses, and areas of dry or reddened skin. Pay particular attention to bony prominences, which are subject to rubbing from ill-fitting shoes, and to the areas between the toes. Observe the color, shape, and texture of the toenails; note any abnormalities.

Next, wash the patient's feet. Cover him with a bath blanket and fanfold the top linen to the foot of the bed. Place a linen-saver pad and a towel under the patient's feet and position the water-filled basin on the pad. Place a pillow under the patient's knees to provide support, and place the edge of the towel over the rim of the basin to provide a cushion for the patient's lower legs. Now immerse one foot in the basin, wash it with soap, and allow it to soak for 5 to 10 minutes. Next, rinse the foot, remove it from the basin, and pat it dry; avoid rubbing, which could damage the skin. Pay special attention to the areas between the toes; any moisture there can cause skin breakdown. If necessary, apply powder between the toes to absorb moisture.

Empty the basin, refill it with clean warm water, and cleanse the other foot.

Now carefully clean the toenails on the dry foot with a cotton-tipped swab or cotton ball. Then gently remove any dirt or debris from under the nails with an orangewood stick, taking care to avoid injuring the delicate subungual skin. Trim the nails as necessary, cutting straight across to prevent ingrown nails. Next, file the nails with an emery board to remove any rough edges and prevent scratching.

After the second foot has soaked for 5 to 10 minutes, remove it from the basin, dry it, and perform a pedicure. Finally, apply lubricating lotion to both feet to prevent dryness and cracking.

Monitoring and aftercare

Watch for and report any redness, bruising, drying or cracking, blisters, open wounds or other lesions, and ingrown or abnormal toenails—especially if the patient has impaired peripheral circulation. Because such a patient is especially susceptible to infection and gangrene, he requires prompt attention.

Home care instructions

● If the patient will be performing regular foot care at home, be sure to review all the steps before discharge. Have him demonstrate each step.
● Caution against oversoaking the feet; explain that this may increase the risk of infection and skin damage.
● Encourage the patient to see his podiatrist regularly.

Selected References

Browner, C., et al. "Halo Immobilization Brace Care," *Journal of NeuroScience Nursing* 19(1):24-29, February 1987.
D'Ambrosia, R. *Musculoskeletal Disorders: Regional Examination and Differential Diagnosis,* 2nd ed. Philadelphia: J.B. Lippincott Co., 1986.
Diagnostics, 2nd ed. Nurse's Reference Library. Springhouse, Pa.: Springhouse Corp., 1986.
Jones, A., et al. "Metrizimide Myelography and Lumbar Laminectomy," *Journal of* *NeuroScience Nursing* 19(2):90-94, April 1987.
Nursing88 Drug Handbook. Springhouse, Pa.: Springhouse Corp., 1988.
Pritchett, J.W., and Clark, J.M. "Prosthetic Replacement for Dislocations of the Shoulder," *Clinical Orthopaedics* (216):89-93, March 1987.
Schlegel, M. "Helping Your Patient Recover from a Lumbar Laminectomy," *NursingLife* 6(5):31-32, September/October 1986.

8

Treating Renal and Urologic Dysfunction

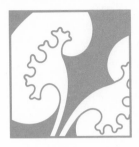

Treating Renal and Urologic Dysfunction

Introduction

The sheer diversity of treatments for renal and urologic disorders will certainly challenge your nursing skills. However, despite their differences, many of these treatments pose similar nursing problems.

Ensuring urine flow
Because the renal and urologic systems produce, transport, and excrete urine, any dysfunction typically impairs elimination of waste products and disrupts fluid, electrolyte, and acid-base balance, often with serious consequences. As a result, treatment may often involve insertion or creation of a temporary or permanent urinary diversion—either a mechanical device, such as an indwelling (Foley) catheter, or a surgically created diversion, such as a ureterostomy or an ileal conduit—to facilitate elimination.

Before insertion of such a device, you'll need to prepare the patient for the procedure. For example, before insertion of a Foley catheter, you'll need to tell the patient that he'll feel slight pressure or discomfort during insertion and that the catheter will produce a sense of bladder fullness or the urge to void. You'll also need to tell him that he must take care not to dislodge the catheter after insertion and that the collection bag must remain below bladder level to promote drainage.

If the patient's being discharged with the catheter in place, you'll need to teach him how to care for the catheter and collection appliance, including periodic irrigation to ensure catheter patency and the proper procedure for emptying and reattaching a collection bag. You also may teach him how to perform self-catheterization to help control incontinence.

Caring for the surgical patient
Surgery is commonplace for many renal and urologic disorders. It may be necessary to sustain life, such as a kidney transplant in renal failure. Or it may be needed to correct a medical problem that can prove devastating to a patient's self-image, such as an undescended testis in a young boy or stress incontinence in an older woman.

Surgery may be necessary when conservative treatments fail to control the patient's disorder. For instance, transurethral resection of the prostate or prostatectomy may need to be performed to relieve urinary obstruction in benign prostatic hypertrophy, a common disorder in men over age 50.

If your patient will be undergoing surgery, you'll need to prepare him thoroughly beforehand. After surgery, you'll need to provide an ongoing assessment to detect any complications, thereby allowing prompt intervention.

DRUG THERAPY

Antispasmodics

Flavoxate, oxybutynin, and *propantheline* inhibit smooth muscle spasm in the urinary tract. These antispasmodics are widely used to relieve contractions in neurogenic bladder and to provide symptomatic relief of dysuria, urinary frequency and urgency, nocturia, incontinence, suprapubic

TREATING URINARY RETENTION WITH BETHANECHOL

A potent cholinergic drug, bethanechol is widely used to treat urinary retention caused by neurogenic bladder. It's also used to relieve acute postoperative and postpartum nonobstructive retention. Typically the initial treatment for these disorders, bethanechol may preclude the need for invasive measures, such as bladder drainage or permanent urinary diversion.

Administration tips
Because bethanechol is highly potent, it requires careful administration and close monitoring of the patient's response. It's usually given orally in high doses (up to 100 mg) to relieve retention; S.C. test doses may be administered to determine the minimal effective dose. However, the drug should never be given I.M. or I.V.; doing so could precipitate hypotension, severe abdominal cramping, bloody diarrhea, and even shock, circulatory collapse, or cardiac arrest.
When giving bethanechol, monitor the patient's vital signs, noting especially his respiratory rate and pattern. Keep atropine readily available and be prepared to initiate respiratory support, if needed. Watch closely for signs of drug toxicity, such as abdominal cramps and diarrhea, especially during S.C. administration.

pain, and bladder and ureteral spasm in various urologic disorders.

Because of their spasmolytic effects, these drugs should be given cautiously in suspected glaucoma, pyloric or duodenal obstruction, intestinal lesions or ileus, or urinary tract obstruction.

Purpose and action
Flavoxate exerts a direct spasmolytic effect on the smooth muscles of the urinary tract. What's more, it provides local anesthetic and analgesic effects. *Oxybutynin* exerts both a direct spasmolytic effect and an anticholinergic-like effect on the smooth muscles of the urinary tract but has little effect on vascular smooth muscle. This drug increases bladder capacity and provides local anesthetic and mild analgesic effects. *Propantheline,* a quaternary anticholinergic, acts at the parasympathetic ganglia and at smooth muscle receptors by competitively inhibiting the effects of acetylcholine, thus decreasing bladder contractility.

Monitoring
Review the patient's drug regimen for possible interactions. Concurrent use of anticholinergics, for instance, enhances the effects of both drugs.

Periodically monitor vital signs during therapy, watching especially for tachycardia and fever. Notify the doctor if these untoward signs occur. Observe for signs of drug hypersensitivity, such as rash, pruritus, and urticaria. If these develop, stop the drug and alert the doctor; he may need to reduce the dosage or change the drug.

Monitor intake and output to assess drug effectiveness and detect urinary retention. Encourage fluids to help prevent retention and constipation.

Assess for visual disturbances, such as eye pain, blurred vision, and photophobia; these may require ophthalmologic evaluation. Report any changes in mental status, such as confusion, memory loss, and paradoxical excitement. Elderly patients are especially prone to these effects.

Home care instructions

• If the patient's taking oxybutynin or flavoxate, tell him to take the drug with milk or food to help reduce GI upset. (He can take it with water on an empty stomach if he doesn't experience any discomfort.) Tell him that if he misses a dose, he should take it as soon as possible. However, if it's almost time for the next dose, he should skip the missed dose. Warn him never to double-dose.

• If the patient's taking propantheline, instruct him to take the drug at least 30 minutes before meals to maximize absorption. If he misses a dose, he should skip it and resume his schedule with the next dose.

• Because antispasmodics can cause dizziness or drowsiness, warn against performing activities that require alertness, coordination, and clear vision until the patient's response to the drug has been determined.

• Also warn against using alcohol and other CNS depressants, which can increase the drug's sedative effects.

• Because antispasmodics interfere with perspiration and thermoregulation, advise the patient to avoid prolonged exercise or strenuous activity, especially in hot weather, to prevent drug-induced heatstroke.

• Suggest that he use sugarless gum, hard candy, or ice chips to relieve dry mouth and throat. Tell him to report excessive dryness that lasts longer than 2 weeks.

• Instruct the patient to report any eye problems, such as blurred vision, pain, or abnormal sensitivity to light. Advise him to wear sunglasses when outdoors.

• Tell the patient to report rash, flushing, hives, and CNS effects, such as dizziness, drowsiness, anxiety, impaired coordination, agitation, or hallucinations. He should also report difficulty breathing, shortness of breath, or a rapid or irregular pulse.

• Explain that he can minimize constipation, another common side effect, by drinking plenty of fluids and eating high-fiber foods.

External Sphincter Relaxants

The powerful skeletal muscle relaxants *baclofen* and *dantrolene*, customarily used to relieve spasticity in multiple sclerosis, spinal cord injury, or other neuromuscular disorders, are today being used for yet another therapeutic purpose: to relax the external urinary sphincter and ease voiding. In fact, successful treatment with these drugs may preclude the need for sphincterotomy to restore urine flow and promote adequate bladder emptying.

These drugs can't be used for every patient with voiding difficulty, however. Baclofen should be used cautiously in the elderly and in patients with renal impairment, cerebrovascular accident, seizures, psychiatric disturbances, or peptic ulcers. Dantrolene should be used cautiously in patients with cardiopulmonary impairment and in all patients over age 35 because of an increased risk of hepatotoxicity. It's contraindicated during lactation and in patients with hepatic disease or spasticity resulting from rheumatoid arthritis. Because both drugs relax skeletal muscles, they're contraindicated in patients who need some degree of spasticity for motor function.

Purpose and action

Both dantrolene and baclofen relax all skeletal muscles, including the external urinary sphincter. But they do so in entirely different ways. Dantrolene acts directly on skeletal muscle to interfere with intracellular calcium movement. Baclofen acts indirectly, through an as-yet-unclear mechanism, to decrease nerve impulse transmission from the spinal cord to the skeletal muscles.

Monitoring

Before giving dantrolene, ensure that the patient undergoes baseline liver function studies (serum glutamic-pyruvic transaminase, serum glutamic-oxaloacetic transaminase, and serum alkaline phosphatase). Before giving baclofen, weigh the patient and review his drug regimen for possible interactions. Concurrent use of baclofen and monoamine oxidase inhibitors, for instance, can potentiate the action of both drugs; you may need to decrease the dosage of one or both drugs.

During therapy with either drug, carefully monitor vital signs; watch especially for hypotension and tachycardia. Check for CNS effects, such as drowsiness and dizziness. Keep in mind that elderly patients are at higher risk for CNS effects. Assess the patient for GI effects, such as diarrhea, constipation, nausea or vomiting, and abdominal cramps, and for signs of hypersensitivity. Report any of these effects to the doctor; he may decide to reduce the dosage or stop the drug.

Monitor the amount and character of urine output. Report decreased output, dark or bloody urine, and complaints of difficult or painful urination, urinary frequency, or incontinence.

During dantrolene therapy, observe the patient for signs of hepatitis (such as fever and jaundice), severe diarrhea, or weakness. If any of these occur, hold the dose and notify the doctor. Because of the risk of hepatotoxicity, make sure the patient undergoes periodic liver function tests during therapy.

During baclofen therapy, weigh the patient regularly and assess for other signs of fluid retention.

Home care instructions

● Instruct the patient to promptly report confusion, dizziness, weakness, drowsiness, nausea, difficulty urinating, swollen ankles and weight gain (with baclofen), rapid heart rate, and constipation or diarrhea. Also tell him to watch for and report rash, pruritus, or respiratory distress, which may indicate drug hypersensitivity.

● Warn the patient to avoid alcohol and other CNS depressants, including antihistamines, to prevent increased sedation.

● Instruct him to avoid driving and other activities that demand alertness and good coordination until his CNS response to the drug has been determined.

● Provide instructions for missed doses: if the patient can't make up a missed dose within an hour or so of the scheduled administration time, he should skip the dose and take the next one as scheduled. He should never double-dose.

● If the patient has difficulty swallowing dantrolene capsules, advise him to open the capsule and mix the powder with fruit juice. Tell him to stir the mixture thoroughly and drink it right away.

● If dantrolene causes photosensitivity, advise the patient to wear protective clothing and apply a sunscreen when exposed to sunlight.

● Remind the patient taking dantrolene to see the doctor regularly for evaluation of the drug's effectiveness and its effect on liver function.

● If the patient's taking baclofen, warn him never to stop taking the drug abruptly but rather to withdraw it slowly, as ordered. Tell him to report any withdrawal symptoms, such as hallucinations, rebound spasticity, seizures, mood swings, nervousness, or restlessness.

SURGERY

Nephrectomy

Nephrectomy, the surgical removal of a kidney, represents the treatment of choice for advanced renal cell carcinoma that's refractory to chemotherapy and radiation. It's also used to harvest a healthy kidney for transplantation. And when conservative treatments fail, nephrectomy may be used to treat renal trauma, infection, hypertension, hydronephrosis, and inoperable renal calculi.

Nephrectomy may be unilateral or bilateral. Unilateral nephrectomy, the more commonly performed procedure, usually doesn't interfere with renal function as long as one healthy kidney remains. However, bilateral nephrectomy (or the removal of a lone kidney) requires lifelong dialysis or transplantation to support renal function.

Four major types of nephrectomy are performed: partial nephrectomy, involving resection of only a portion of the kidney; simple nephrectomy, removal of the entire kidney; radical nephrectomy, resection of the entire kidney and the surrounding fat tissue; and nephroureterectomy, removal of the entire kidney, the perinephric fat, and the entire ureter. Except for variations in the extent of tissue resection, the surgical approach remains basically the same.

Nephrectomy, of course, can cause serious complications. The most common include infection, hemorrhage, atelectasis, pneumonia, deep vein thrombosis, and pulmonary embolism.

Purpose
● To remove one or both kidneys to help treat renal carcinoma or other renal disease
● To obtain a healthy organ for transplantation.

Preparation
As with any organ excision, the patient will have many concerns and questions. First and foremost, he'll probably want to know how the surgery will affect his kidney function. If the patient's having unilateral nephrectomy, reassure him that one healthy kidney is all he'll need for adequate function. If the patient's scheduled for bilateral nephrectomy or the removal of his only kidney, prepare him for radical changes in his life-style, most notably the need for regular dialysis. If appropriate, discuss the possibility of a future kidney transplant to restore normal function.

Describe postoperative measures to the patient. Tell him that he'll return from surgery with an indwelling (Foley) catheter in place to allow precise measurement of urine output and a nasogastric tube in place to prevent abdominal pain, distention, and vomiting. Explain that he won't receive food or fluids by mouth after surgery until bowel sounds have returned, but that he'll receive I.V. fluids to maintain hydration. He'll also have a dressing and possibly a drain at the incision site. Prepare him for frequent dressing changes.

Stress the need for postoperative deep breathing and coughing to prevent pulmonary complications. Demonstrate these exercises and have him practice them before surgery.

Ensure that the patient or a responsible family member has signed a consent form.

Procedure
To perform a unilateral nephrectomy, the surgeon first makes a flank incision to expose the kidney. (Alternatively, he may make a thoracicoabdominal or transthoracic incision if extensive renovascular repair or radical excision of the kidney and surrounding structures is necessary or if the patient suffers from respiratory or cardiac dysfunction.) He then mobilizes the kidney and frees it of fat and adhesions, releases the lower pole, and locates the ureter and frees its upper third. He orders the ureter double-clamped and then cuts between the clamps and ligates both ends. Next, he frees and double-clamps the vascular pedicle and then removes the kidney distal to the clamps. After resecting surrounding perinephric fat and the ureter, if necessary, he inserts a flank catheter and Penrose drain and sutures the wound closed.

Monitoring and aftercare

After surgery, provide routine I.V. line, nasogastric tube, and Foley catheter care. Carefully monitor the rate, volume, and type of I.V. fluids. Keep in mind that mistakes in fluid therapy can be particularly devastating for a patient who has only one kidney. Measure and record urine output and notify the doctor if it falls below 50 ml/hour. Assess for signs of electrolyte imbalance and fluid overload.

Check the patient's dressing and drain every 4 hours for the first 24 to 48 hours, then once every shift to assess the amount and nature of drainage. Maintain drain patency.

Unless otherwise ordered, the doctor will perform the first dressing change after surgery. Thereafter, change the dressing whenever it becomes wet or once a day, using sterile technique and taking care not to dislodge the drain. During dressing changes, assess the suture line for swelling, redness, and purulent drainage.

Maintain food and fluid restrictions, as ordered. Periodically auscultate for bowel sounds; when they return and the patient is able to pass flatus, usually by the 4th day after surgery, notify the doctor and prepare to resume oral feedings. When oral intake is permitted, encourage fluids—up to 3,000 ml a day.

Encourage coughing, deep breathing, incentive spirometry, and position changes. Regularly assess the patient's respiratory status. Be alert for signs of pulmonary embolism, especially 5 to 10 days after surgery. Watch for dyspnea, tachypnea, pleuritic chest pain, and hemoptysis; if these develop, immediately notify the doctor, raise the head of the patient's bed at least 30 degrees, and administer oxygen.

To reduce the risk of deep vein thrombosis, encourage early and regular ambulation and apply antiembolism stockings, as ordered. Assess for signs and symptoms of deep vein thrombosis, such as leg pain, edema, and erythema.

Monitor for signs of hemorrhage and shock. Keep in mind that the risk of hemorrhage is greatest 8 to 12 days after surgery, owing to tissue sloughing.

Home care instructions

• Teach the patient how to monitor intake and output at home, and explain how this helps assess renal function. Instruct him to call the doctor immediately if he detects any significant decrease in urine output, a reliable sign of renal failure.

• Tell the patient to notify the doctor if he experiences fever, chills, hematuria, or flank pain. Explain that these signs and symptoms may indicate urinary tract infection, a potentially serious complication.

• If the patient has undergone nephrectomy to treat renal cell carcinoma, convey the importance of reporting any weight loss, bone pain, altered mental status, and paresthesias in the extremities—possible signs of tumor metastasis.

• Emphasize the importance of following the doctor's guidelines on fluid intake and dietary restrictions.

• Explain to the patient that he may experience incisional pain and fatigue for several weeks after discharge; reassure him that these are normal postoperative effects. Encourage him to refrain from doing any strenuous exercise or heavy lifting and from sexual activity until his doctor grants permission to engage in them.

• Stress the need for regular follow-up examinations to evaluate kidney function and to assess for possible complications.

Kidney Transplant

Ranking among the most commonly performed and most successful of all organ transplants, kidney transplant represents an attractive alternative to dialysis for many patients with otherwise unmanageable end-stage renal disease. It also may be necessary to sustain life in a patient who has suffered traumatic loss of kidney function or in whom dialysis is contraindicated. Kidney transplant, however, isn't performed on all patients who seemingly could benefit from it. For instance, severely debilitated, diabetic, elderly, or young patients generally aren't considered good candidates.

In this transplant, a healthy kidney harvested from a living relative or cadaver donor is implanted in the recipient's iliac fossa and anastomosed in place. The recipient's own kidneys usually aren't removed unless they're structurally abnormal, infected, greatly enlarged, or causing intractable hypertension. They're left in place to increase circulating hematocrit levels and to ease dialysis management and reduce blood transfusion requirements in case of transplant rejection.

The major obstacle to successful transplantation is rejection of the donated organ by the recipient's body. However, careful tissue matching between donor and recipient decreases this risk. Blood relatives make the most compatible donors. In fact, a kidney donated by a recipient's identical twin can be transplanted successfully 95% of the time; a kidney transplanted from any other sibling has about an 80% success rate. Parent-child transplants have a success rate of about 75%. Most transplanted kidneys, however, come from cadavers. Such transplants possess a much lower success rate (just over 50% after 1 year) despite continued improvements in surgical techniques, histocompatibility procedures, and immunosuppressive therapy.

A patient undergoing kidney transplantation requires comprehensive nursing care. Preparatory care focuses on promoting both physical and emotional readiness for surgery, including pointing out the possibility of transplant rejection and the need to return to dialysis. Important postoperative care measures include maintaining fluid and electrolyte balance, ensuring indwelling (Foley) catheter patency, monitoring for complications, and preparing the patient for discharge and perhaps a life free from dialysis.

Purpose

To restore renal function by implanting a healthy donor kidney.

Preparation

The patient will understandably find the prospect of kidney transplantation confusing and frightening. He may have ambivalent emotions about the operation: on the one hand, he may feel elated that a donor kidney is finally available; on the other hand, he may feel apprehensive about the surgery and its outcome. You can help the patient cope with such emotions by preparing him thoroughly for transplantation and a prolonged recovery period and by offering ongoing emotional support.

Encourage the patient to express his feelings. If he's concerned about rejection of the donor kidney, explain that if this happens and cannot be reversed, he will simply resume dialysis and wait for another suitable donor organ. Reassure him that transplant rejection normally isn't life-threatening.

Describe the routine preoperative measures, such as a thorough physical examination and a battery of laboratory tests to detect any infection (followed by antibiotic therapy to clear it up), electrolyte studies, abdominal X-rays, an EKG, a cleansing enema, and shaving of the operative area. Tell him he'll undergo dialysis the day before surgery to cleanse his blood of unwanted fluid and electrolytes. Also point out that he may need dialysis for a few days after surgery if his transplanted kidney doesn't start functioning immediately.

Review the transplant procedure itself, supplementing and clarifying the doctor's explanation as necessary. Tell the patient that he'll receive a general anesthetic before surgery and that the procedure should take about 4 hours. Next, explain what the patient can expect after he awakens from anesthesia, including the presence of I.V. lines, a Foley catheter, an arterial line, and possibly a respirator. Describe routine postoperative care, including frequent checks of vital signs, monitoring of intake and output, and respiratory therapy. Prepare him for postoperative pain and reassure him that analgesics will be made available. If possible, arrange for him to tour the recovery room and intensive care unit.

Teach the patient the proper methods of turning, coughing, deep breathing, and, if ordered, incentive spirometry. Discuss the immunosuppressive drugs he'll be taking and explain their possible side effects. Point out that these drugs increase his susceptibility to infection; as a result, he'll be kept temporarily isolated after surgery, either in his hospital room or in a reverse-isolation unit.

As ordered, begin giving immunosuppressive drugs, such as azathioprine, cyclosporine, and corticosteroids. You may begin oral azathioprine as early as 5 days before surgery. In contrast, you'll usually begin slow I.V. infusion of cyclosporine 4 to 12 hours before surgery; when doing so, closely monitor the patient for anaphylaxis, especially during the first 30 minutes of administration. If anaphylaxis occurs, give epinephrine, as ordered.

Ensure that the patient or a responsible family member has signed a consent form.

Procedure

With the patient under general anesthesia, the surgeon makes a curvilinear incision in the right or left lower quadrant, extending from the symphysis pubis to the anterior superior iliac spine and up to just below the thoracic cage. He exposes the iliac fossa with a self-retaining retractor, then performs segmental separation, ligature, and division of perivascular tissue. Next, he clamps the iliac vein and artery in preparation for anastomosis to the donor kidney's renal vein and artery.

Meanwhile the donor kidney is prepared for transplantation. If a cadaver kidney is being used, it's removed from cold storage or a perfusion preparation machine. If the kidney's from a living donor, it's harvested in an adjacent operating room via nephrectomy and placed in cold Ringer's lactate solution. Before transplantation, the donor kidney's renal artery is flushed with cold heparinized Ringer's lactate solution to prevent clogging. Then the surgeon positions the kidney in a sling over the implantation site. (He never holds the kidney in his hands, since this would warm it and possibly cause necrosis.)

The surgeon then implants the kidney in the retroperitoneal area of the iliac fossa, where it's protected by the hip bone. If a donor's left kidney is being used, the surgeon implants it in the recipient's right side; conversely, he implants a donor's right kidney in the recipient's left side. Doing so permits the renal pelvis to rest anteriorly and allows the new kidney's ureter to rest in front of the iliac artery, where the ureter's more accessible.

Once the kidney is in place, the surgeon anastomoses its renal vein to the recipient's iliac vein and the renal artery to the recipient's internal iliac artery (see *Understanding Kidney Transplant*). He then removes the venous and arterial clamps and checks for patency of the anastomoses. Next, he attaches the donor kidney's ureter to the recipient's bladder, taking care to ensure a watertight closure. When the transplant's complete, the surgeon sutures the incision and sends the patient to the recovery room.

Monitoring and aftercare

Keep in mind that you're caring for a patient whose immune system has been suppressed by medication and who consequently runs a high risk of contracting an infection. First and foremost, you need to take special precautions to reduce this risk. For instance, use strict aseptic technique when changing dressings and perform-

UNDERSTANDING KIDNEY TRANSPLANT

In kidney transplant, the donated organ is implanted in the iliac fossa. The organ's vessels are then connected to the internal iliac vein and internal iliac artery, as shown in the illustration. Typically, the patient's own kidneys are left in place.

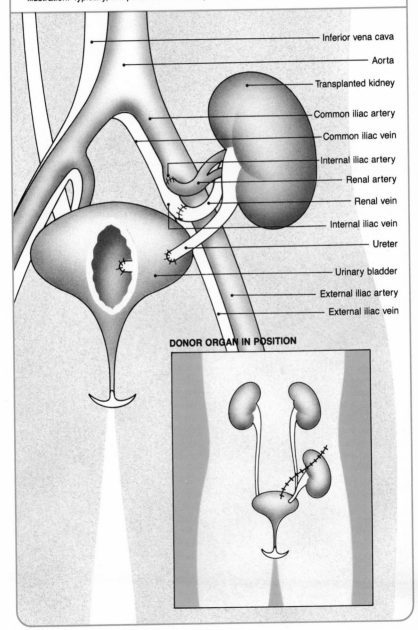

Inferior vena cava

Aorta

Transplanted kidney

Common iliac artery

Common iliac vein

Internal iliac artery

Renal artery

Renal vein

Internal iliac vein

Ureter

Urinary bladder

External iliac artery

External iliac vein

DONOR ORGAN IN POSITION

MANAGING TRANSPLANT REJECTION

Transplant rejection can occur immediately after surgery or not until years later. But whenever rejection occurs, it demands prompt intervention.

Hyperacute rejection

Hyperacute rejection occurs several minutes to hours after transplantation as the patient's circulating antibodies attack the donor kidney. Renal perfusion plummets and the organ rapidly becomes ischemic and dies.

If the patient experiences hyperacute rejection, prepare him for removal of the rejected kidney. Provide emotional support to help lessen his disappointment. Also provide support for the donor, if possible, who may feel dejected.

Acute rejection

This type of rejection may occur 1 week to 6 months after transplantation of a living donor kidney or 1 week to 2 years after transplantation of a cadaver kidney. It's caused by an antigen-antibody reaction, which produces acute tubular necrosis.

Acute rejection may be reversible with prompt treatment. Be alert for its characteristic indicators: signs of infection (fever, rapid pulse, lethargy, elevated white blood cell count), oliguria or anuria, hypertension, or a weight gain of more than 3 lb in a day.

If the patient displays signs of acute rejection, reassure him that this complication is common and often reversible. As ordered, prepare him for dialysis.

Chronic rejection

This irreversible complication can start several months or even years after transplantation. It's caused by long-term antibody destruction of the donor kidney. Typically, it's detected by serial laboratory studies that show a declining glomerular filtration rate accompanied by rising blood urea nitrogen and serum creatinine levels.

If the patient's experiencing chronic rejection, inform him that complete destruction of the donor kidney may not occur for several years. Prepare him for a renal scan, renal biopsy, and other tests, as ordered. Administer increased dosages of immunosuppressive drugs and adjust his dietary and fluid regimen, as ordered. When necessary, prepare him for dialysis or another transplant, as ordered.

ing catheter care. Also, limit the patient's contact with staff, other patients, and visitors, and have all people in the patient's room wear surgical masks for the first 2 weeks after surgery. Monitor the patient's white blood cell (WBC) count; if it drops precipitously, notify the doctor, who may order isolation.

Throughout the recovery period watch for signs and symptoms of tissue rejection. Observe the transplant site for redness, tenderness, and swelling. Does the patient have a fever or an elevated WBC count? Decreased urine output with increased proteinuria? Sudden weight gain or hypertension? Elevated serum creatinine and blood urea nitrogen (BUN) levels? Report any of these untoward effects immediately.

Assess the patient for pain and provide analgesics, as ordered. Look for a significant decrease in pain after 24 hours.

Carefully monitor urine output; promptly report output of less than 100 ml/hour. In a living donor transplant, urine flow often begins immediately after revascularization and connection of the ureter to the recipient's bladder. In a cadaver kidney transplant, anuria may persist for anywhere from 2 days to 2 weeks; dialysis will be necessary during this period.

Connect the patient's Foley catheter to a closed drainage system to prevent overextension of the bladder. Observe his urine color; it should be slightly blood-tinged for several days and then should gradually clear. Irrigate the catheter, as ordered, using strict aseptic technique.

Review daily the results of renal function tests, such as creatinine clearance and BUN, hematocrit, and hemoglobin levels. Also review results of tests that assess renal perfusion, such as urine creatinine, urea, sodium, potassium, pH, and specific gravity. Monitor for hematuria and proteinuria.

Assess the patient's fluid and electrolyte balance. Watch particularly for signs of hyperkalemia, such as weakness and pulse irregularities. If they develop, notify the doctor and give calcium carbonate I.V., as ordered. Weigh the patient daily and report any rapid gain, a possible sign of fluid retention.

Periodically auscultate for bowel sounds, and notify the doctor when they return. He'll then order gradual resumption of a normal diet, perhaps with some restrictions. For instance, he may order a low-sodium diet if the patient's receiving corticosteroids, to prevent fluid retention.

Home care instructions

• Instruct the patient to carefully measure and record intake and output to monitor kidney function. Teach him how to collect 24-hour urine samples, and tell him to notify the doctor if output falls below 20 oz (600 ml) during any 24-hour period. Tell him to drink at least 1 qt (or liter) of fluid a day unless the doctor orders otherwise.
• Have the patient weigh himself at least twice a week and report any rapid gain. Explain that such gain may indicate fluid retention.
• Direct him to watch for and promptly report any signs and symptoms of infection or transplant rejection, including redness, warmth, tenderness, or swelling over the kidney; fever exceeding 100° F. (37.8° C.); decreased urine output; and elevated blood pressure.
• Because the patient has an increased risk of infection, advise him to avoid crowds and contact with persons with known or suspected infections for at least 3 months after surgery.
• Stress strict compliance with all prescribed medication regimens. Remind the patient that he needs to continue immunosuppressive therapy for as long as he has the transplanted kidney, to prevent rejection. If ordered, instruct him to take an antacid immediately before a corticosteroid to combat its ulcerogenic effects. Also instruct him to report any side effects.
• Encourage a program of regular, moderate exercise. Tell the patient to begin slowly and increase the amount of exercise gradually. Recommend that

he avoid excessive bending, heavy lifting, or contact sports for at least 3 months or until the doctor grants permission for such activities.
• Also warn him against activities or positions that place pressure on the new kidney—for example, long car trips and lap-style seat belts.
• Advise the patient to wait at least 6 weeks before engaging in sexual activity. Because pregnancy poses an additional risk to a new kidney, provide the female patient with appropriate information on birth control.
• Stress the importance of regular follow-up doctor's visits to evaluate renal function and transplant acceptance.

Urinary Diversion Surgery
[Ureterostomy, ileal conduit]

A urinary diversion provides an alternate route for urine excretion when pathology impedes normal flow through the bladder. Most commonly done in patients who've undergone total or partial cystectomy, diversion surgery also may be performed in patients with a congenital urinary tract defect; a severe, unmanageable urinary tract infection that threatens renal function; an injury to the ureters, bladder, or urethra; an obstructive malignancy; or a neurogenic bladder.

Several types of urinary diversion surgery can be performed; the two most common are cutaneous ureterostomy and ileal conduit. In *cutaneous ureterostomy*, the simplest type of urinary diversion, one or both ureters are dissected from the bladder and brought out through the skin surface on the flank or the anterior abdominal wall to form one or two stomas. The surgeon can choose among five basic approaches to this procedure: unilateral, bilateral, flank loop, and double-barrel ureterostomy and transureteroureterostomy. (See *Reviewing Types of Urinary Diversion* for descriptions and illustrations of these approaches.)

Cutaneous ureterostomy offers several advantages over other urinary diversion surgeries. Besides being a shorter and easier-to-perform surgery, it can be done successfully on chronically dilated, thick-walled ureters. Unlike an ileal conduit, it doesn't involve intestinal anastomoses and thus carries little risk of peritoneal and intestinal complications caused by intestinal absorption of urinary constituents.

Ileal conduit, the most common urinary diversion, involves anastomosis of the ureters to a small portion of the ileum excised especially for the procedure, followed by the creation of a stoma from one end of the ileal segment. Because use of the ileum allows for a much larger stoma than can be created from a ureter, an ileal conduit is generally easier to care for than a ureterostomy.

Regardless of the type of surgery performed, urinary diversion demands ongoing patient cooperation to ensure its success. Because urine flow is constant, the patient must wear an external collection device at all times, emptying and reapplying it regularly, using the proper technique. What's more, the patient must practice meticulous stoma and peristomal care to help prevent stomal stenosis and skin excoriation.

Nursing care of the patient undergoing urinary diversion surgery focuses on teaching proper collection and stoma management techniques. It also aims to improve the prospects of his compliance by providing emotional support as he adjusts to changes in his self-image brought about by the stoma and the collection device.

Purpose
To provide an alternate route for urine excretion when bladder dysfunction or removal doesn't allow normal drainage.

Preparation
Review the planned surgery with the patient, reinforcing the doctor's explanations as necessary. Try using a simple anatomic diagram to enhance your discussion, and provide printed information from the United Ostomy Association or other sources, if possible. Explain to the patient that he'll receive a general anesthetic and have a nasogastric tube in place after surgery.

Prepare the patient for the appearance and general location of the stoma. If he's scheduled for an ileal conduit, explain that the stoma will be located somewhere in the lower abdomen, probably below the waistline. If he's scheduled for a cutaneous ureterostomy, explain that the exact stoma site often is chosen during surgery, based on the length of patent ureter available.

Review the enterostomal therapist's explanation of the urine collection device the patient will use after surgery. Encourage the patient to handle the device to help ease his acceptance of it. Reassure him that he'll receive complete training on how to use it after he returns from surgery.

If possible, arrange for a visit by a well-adjusted ostomy patient, who can provide a firsthand account of the operation and offer some insight into the realities of ongoing stoma and collection device care. And, as appropriate, be sure to include the patient's family in all aspects of preoperative teaching—especially if they'll be providing much of the routine care after discharge. Ensure that the patient or a responsible family member has signed a consent form.

Before surgery, prepare the bowel to reduce the risk of postoperative infection from intestinal flora. As ordered, maintain a low-residue or clear liquid diet and administer a cleansing enema and an antimicrobial drug, such as erythromycin or neomycin. Other possible measures may include I.V. hyperalimentation or fluid replacement therapy for debilitated patients and prophylactic I.V. antibiotics.

REVIEWING TYPES OF URINARY DIVERSION

Urinary diversion can be done in several ways: ileal conduit, unilateral or bilateral ureterostomy, double-barrel ureterostomy, transureteroureterostomy, or flank loop ureterostomy.

ILEAL CONDUIT

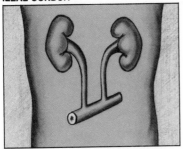

Both ureters are anastomosed to a small segment of ileum, one end of which is brought to the surface of the lower abdomen to form a stoma.

UNILATERAL URETEROSTOMY

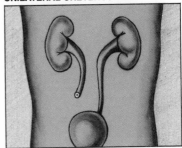

One ureter is dissected from the bladder and brought to the skin surface to form a stoma.

BILATERAL URETEROSTOMY

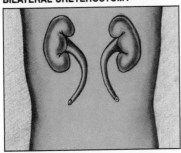

Both ureters are brought to the skin surface to form two widely separated stomas.

DOUBLE-BARREL URETEROSTOMY

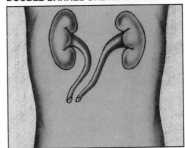

Both ureters are brought to the skin surface to form side-by-side stomas.

TRANSURETEROURETEROSTOMY

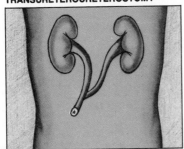

One ureter is anastomosed to the other and brought to the skin surface to form a single stoma.

FLANK LOOP URETEROSTOMY

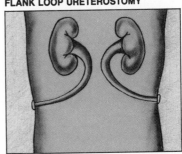

The ureters are brought in loops to the skin surface of the flanks to form two stomas.

Procedure

The surgeon makes a midline or para-medial abdominal incision.

To construct an ileal conduit, he excises a 6" to 8" segment of the ileum (also taking its mesentery to help preserve tissue viability) and then anastomoses the remaining ileal ends to maintain intestinal integrity. Next, he dissects the ureters from the bladder and implants them in the ileal segment. He then sutures one end of the ileal segment closed and brings the other end through the abdominal wall to form a stoma.

In a unilateral ureterostomy, the surgeon dissects one ureter from the bladder and brings it to the skin surface of the flank or upper abdomen to form a stoma. In a bilateral ureterostomy, he dissects both ureters and brings them out in opposite directions to form two widely separated stomas. In a double-barrel ureterostomy, a better alternative, he forms two side-by-side stomas out of the ureters.

In a transureteroureterostomy, the surgeon anastomoses one ureter to the other, then brings it out to form a single stoma. In a flank loop ureterostomy, he doesn't dissect the ureters from the bladder, but rather brings each one in a loop to the skin surface of each flank to form a stoma.

Monitoring and aftercare

After the patient returns from surgery, monitor his vital signs every hour until they're stable. Carefully check and record urine output; report any decrease, which could indicate obstruction from postoperative edema or ureteral stenosis. Observe urine drainage for pus and blood; keep in mind that urine is often blood-tinged initially but should rapidly clear.

Record the amount, color, and consistency of drainage from the incisional drain and nasogastric tube. Notify the doctor of any urine leakage from the drain or suture line; such leakage may point to developing complications, such as hydronephrosis. Watch for signs of peritonitis (fever, abdominal distention and pain), which can develop from intraperitoneal urine leakage.

Check dressings frequently and change them at least once each shift. (The doctor will probably perform the first dressing change.) When changing dressings, check the suture line for redness, swelling, and drainage.

Maintain fluid and electrolyte balance and continue I.V. replacement therapy, as ordered. Provide I.V. hyperalimentation, if necessary, to ensure adequate nutrition.

Perform routine ostomy maintenance. Make sure the collection device fits tightly around the stoma; allow no more than a 1/8-inch margin of skin between the stoma and the device's faceplate. Regularly check the appearance of the stoma and peristomal skin. The stoma should appear bright red; if it becomes deep red or bluish, suspect a problem with blood flow and notify the doctor. It should also be smooth; report any dimpling or retraction, which may point to stenosis. Check the peristomal skin for irritation or breakdown. Remember that the main cause of irritation is urine leakage around the edges of the collection device's faceplate. If you detect leakage, change the device, taking care to properly apply the skin sealer to ensure a tight fit.

If skin breakdown occurs, cleanse the area with warm water and pat it dry, then apply a light dusting of karaya powder and a thin layer of protective dressing. If you detect severe excoriation, notify the doctor.

Provide emotional support throughout the recovery period to help the patient adjust to the stoma and collection pouch. Assure him that the pouch shouldn't interfere with his life-style and that he can eventually resume all of his former activities.

Home care instructions

• Make sure the patient and his family understand and can properly perform stoma care and change the ostomy pouch.

• Instruct them to watch for and report signs of complications, such as fever, chills, flank or abdominal pain, and pus or blood in the urine.

• Stress the importance of keeping scheduled follow-up appointments with the doctor and enterostomal therapist to evaluate stoma care and make any necessary changes in equipment. For instance, stoma shrinkage, which normally occurs within 8 weeks after surgery, may require a change in pouch size to ensure a tight fit.

• Tell the patient that he should be able to return to work soon after discharge; however, if his job requires heavy lifting, tell him to talk to his doctor before resuming work. Explain that he can safely participate in most sports, even such strenuous ones as skiing, skydiving, and scuba diving. Do, however, suggest that he avoid contact sports, such as football and wrestling.

• If the patient expresses doubts or insecurities about his sexuality related to the stoma and collection device, refer him for sexual counseling.

• Assure the female ostomate that pregnancy should cause her no special problems. But urge her to consult with her doctor before she becomes pregnant.

• Refer the patient to a support group, such as the United Ostomy Association.

Transurethral Bladder Resection

A relatively quick and simple procedure, transurethral resection of the bladder (TURB) involves insertion of a resectoscope through the urethra and into the bladder to remove lesions. (It can also be performed using a Yag laser.) Most commonly done to treat superficial and early bladder carcinoma, TURB also may be used to remove benign papillomas or relieve fibrosis of the bladder neck. This treatment isn't indicated for large or infiltrating tumors or for metastatic bladder cancer.

When used to remove superficial tumors, TURB may need to be performed a dozen or more times. A typical schedule might involve treatment every 3 months for the first 2 years, then every 6 months for the next 3 years.

Potential complications include hematuria, urinary retention, bladder perforation, and urinary tract infection. The risk of complications can be reduced by careful monitoring and indwelling (Foley) catheter care.

Purpose
• To remove superficial tumors or papillomas from the bladder wall
• To relieve bladder neck fibrosis.

Preparation
Briefly explain the procedure. Tell the patient that he'll receive a local anesthetic and be awake during treatment. Reassure him that he should experience little or no discomfort, and that such posttreatment effects as hematuria and a burning sensation during urination should quickly subside. Point out, however, that he may experience painful bladder spasms; at the same time reassure him that analgesics will be available. Also reassure him that TURB will not interfere with normal genitourinary function.

Explain care after TURB. Tell the patient that he'll have a Foley catheter in place for 1 to 5 days after the procedure to ensure urine drainage. Also tell him that the doctor may order continuous bladder irrigation for 24 or more hours after treatment. As ordered, prepare the patient for intravenous pyelography to evaluate renal function and rule out tumors elsewhere in the urinary tract; cytoscopy and biopsy to evaluate the location and size of the lesion; and a bone scan to detect any metastasis.

Procedure
With the patient placed in a lithotomy position, the doctor administers a local

UNDERSTANDING T.U.R.B.

In transurethral bladder resection, the doctor inserts a resectoscope through the urethra into the bladder to remove small superficial lesions.

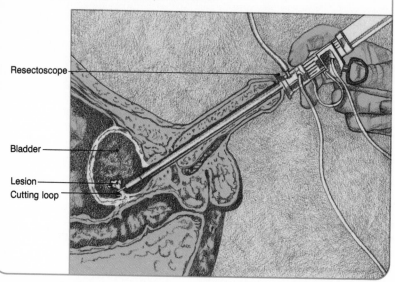

Resectoscope

Bladder

Lesion
Cutting loop

anesthetic. He then introduces a resectoscope into the urethra and passes it into the bladder. Next, he fills the bladder with a clear, nonconducting irrigating solution, locates the lesion, and positions the resectoscope's cutting loop in place. He turns on an electric current, which runs through the loop, to cut or cauterize the lesion. Finally, he removes the resectoscope.

Monitoring and aftercare

Focus your care on maintaining Foley catheter patency and monitoring for possible complications. Maintain adequate fluid intake and provide meticulous catheter care, including frequent irrigation. (The doctor may prescribe continuous or intermittent irrigation, especially if the removal of a large vascular lesion has compromised hemostasis.) Check urine output and assess for abdominal pain or distention, looking for signs of catheter obstruction from blood clots. If you cannot clear an obstruction promptly, notify the

doctor. Also notify the doctor if the patient's unable to urinate within 6 hours of TURB despite adequate fluid intake.

Observe urine drainage for the presence of blood. Remember that slight hematuria normally occurs directly after TURB. However, notify the doctor immediately of any frank bleeding. If hematuria seems excessive, observe the patient for signs of hypovolemic shock, including increased pulse and respiratory rates, hypotension, pallor, and diaphoresis.

Assess for signs and symptoms of bladder perforation: abdominal pain and rigidity, fever, and decreased urine output despite adequate hydration. If you suspect perforation, notify the doctor and hold all fluids.

Carefully assess the level and location of any pain the patient is experiencing to help detect its source. Try to distinguish between the pain of bladder spasms, catheter irritation (intermittent, spasmodic pain in the urethra), and obstruction (severe, persistent pain in the suprapubic area). As ordered, administer antispasmodics for bladder spasm and analgesics for pain from any source.

Home care instructions
• Tell the patient to expect slight hematuria for several weeks after TURB. However, he should promptly report bleeding or hematuria that lasts longer than several weeks.
• Advise the patient to drink plenty of water (10 glasses daily) and to void every 2 to 3 hours to reduce the risk of clot formation, urethral obstruction, and urinary tract infection. Emphasize that he shouldn't ignore the urge to urinate.
• Instruct him to report fever, chills, or flank pain, which may indicate urinary tract infection.
• To promote healing and reduce the risk of bleeding from increased intraabdominal pressure, advise the patient to refrain from sexual or other strenuous activity, not to lift anything heavier than 10 lb, and to continue taking a stool softener or other laxative until the doctor orders otherwise.
• Emphasize the importance of regular follow-up examinations to evaluate the need for repeat treatments. Explain that early detection and removal of bladder tumors through TURB may prevent the need for cystectomy.

Cystectomy

Partial or total removal of the urinary bladder and surrounding structures may be necessary to treat advanced bladder cancer or, rarely, other bladder disorders, such as interstitial cystitis. In most patients with bladder cancer, combined use of radiation therapy and surgery yields the best results. In metastatic bladder cancer, cystectomy and radiation therapy may provide palliative benefits and prolong life.

Cystectomy may be partial, simple, or radical. *Partial*, or segmental, cystectomy involves resection of cancerous bladder tissue. Commonly preserving bladder function, this surgery is most often indicated for a single, easily accessible tumor. *Simple*, or total, cystectomy involves resection of the entire bladder, with preservation of surrounding structures. It's indicated for multiple or extensive carcinoma, advanced interstitial cystitis, and related disorders.

Radical cystectomy is generally indicated for muscle-invasive, primary bladder carcinoma. In men, the bladder, prostate, and seminal vesicles are removed. In women, the bladder, urethra, and usually the uterus, fallopian tubes, ovaries, and a segment of the vaginal wall are excised. It also may involve bilateral pelvic lymphadenectomy. Because this surgery is so extensive, it typically produces impotence in men and sterility in women. A permanent urinary diversion is needed in both radical and simple cystectomy.

Like any complicated surgery, cystectomy carries the risk of many complications. Radical and simple cystectomy can also cause psychological problems relating to changes in the patient's body image and loss of sexual or reproductive function.

Purpose
To surgically remove malignant or diseased tissue in the bladder and, as necessary, in surrounding structures.

Preparation
Review the surgery with the patient and his family, if appropriate. Pay special attention to the patient's emotional state since he'll probably be anxious. Help allay his fears by listening to his concerns and answering his questions. If the patient's undergoing simple or radical cystectomy, he'll also be concerned about the effects of a urinary diversion on his life-style. Reassure him that such diversion needn't interfere with his normal activities, and arrange for a visit by an enterostomal therapist, who

can provide additional information.

If the patient's scheduled for radical cystectomy, you'll need to address concerns about the inevitable loss of sexual or reproductive function. As appropriate, refer the patient for psychological and sexual counseling.

Explain to the patient that he'll awaken in an intensive care unit (ICU) after surgery. Mention that he'll have a nasogastric (NG) tube, a central venous catheter, and an indwelling (Foley) catheter in place and a drain at the surgical site. Tell him that he won't be able to eat or drink until the return of bowel function, and that he'll be given I.V. fluids during this period. After that, he can resume oral fluids and eventually progress to solids. If possible, arrange for the patient and his family to visit the ICU before surgery to familiarize themselves with the unit and meet the staff.

About 4 days before surgery, begin full bowel preparation to help prevent infection. Maintain a low-residue diet for 3 days and then infuse high-calorie fluids on the 4th day. As ordered, administer antibiotics—usually erythromycin and neomycin—for 24 hours before surgery. On the night before surgery, administer an enema to clear fecal matter from the bowel.

Procedure

In a partial cystectomy, the surgeon makes a suprapubic incision and opens the bladder at a point away from the tumor. Next, he resects the tumor and attached fat and perineum, taking a 1-1/4 inch (3.2 cm) margin of healthy tissue. He then closes the wound, leaving a Penrose drain and suprapubic catheter in place.

In a simple cystectomy, the surgeon makes a vertical or transverse incision and separates the bladder's posterior and lateral connective tissue. He then opens the bladder near its neck and resects the bladder walls and surrounding tissue. After suturing the bladder neck closed and inserting a drainage catheter, he brings the ureters

to the skin to form a urinary diversion.

In a radical cystectomy, the surgeon makes a lateral incision extending from the pubis to the epigastrium. He makes the incision slightly off the midline, on the side opposite the planned urinary diversion stoma. After exposing the bladder and surrounding organs, he palpates and inspects the organs for signs of metastasis, gallstones, or suspicious nodes. He usually does bilateral lymphadenectomy at this time to detect and remove nodal metastases. If he detects extensive metastasis, he may reconsider going ahead with surgery, weighing the chance of cure against any perceived palliative benefits.

If the surgeon decides to proceed, he ligates and divides the ureters deep in the pelvis and resects the entire bladder, surrounding adipose tissue, and overlying pelvic peritoneum, along with the prostate and seminal vesicles in males and the urethra, uterus, fallopian tubes, ovaries, and part or all of the vagina in females. He then inserts and inflates an indwelling urethral catheter to control bleeding from the urogenital diaphragm, inserts an abdominal drain, and brings the ureters to the skin surface to form a urinary diversion—most commonly an ileal conduit.

Monitoring and aftercare

After the patient returns from surgery, monitor the amount and character of urine drainage every hour. Report output of less than 30 ml/hour, which may indicate retention. (Other signs of retention may include bladder distention and spasms.) If output is low, check the patency of the Foley catheter or stoma, as appropriate, and irrigate as ordered.

Monitor vital signs closely. Watch especially for signs of hypovolemic shock: increased pulse and respiratory rate, hypotension, diaphoresis, and pallor. (Be especially alert for hemorrhage if the doctor has ordered anticoagulant therapy to reduce the risk of pulmonary embolism.) Periodically inspect the stoma and incision site for bleeding, and observe urine drainage for frank hematuria and clots. Slight hematuria normally occurs for several days after surgery but should clear thereafter. Test all drainage from the NG tube, abdominal drains, Foley catheter, and urine collection appliance for blood, and notify the doctor of positive findings.

Observe the wound site and all drainage for signs of infection. Change abdominal dressings frequently, using sterile technique.

Periodically ask the patient about incisional pain and, if he has had a partial cystectomy, ask about bladder spasms, too. Provide analgesics, as ordered. You also may be asked to administer an antispasmodic, such as oxybutynin.

To prevent pulmonary complications associated with prolonged immobility, encourage frequent position changes, coughing and deep breathing and, if possible, early ambulation. Assess respiratory status regularly. Also provide scrupulous stoma care and teach the patient (or a family member, if appropriate) proper management techniques for use after discharge.

Continue to offer the patient emotional support throughout the recovery period to help him accept changes in body image and, if appropriate, sexual function. If possible, refer the patient and his family for psychological and sexual counseling to further aid this adjustment.

Home care instructions

• Explain to the patient that incisional pain and fatigue will probably last for several weeks after discharge. Tell him to notify the doctor if these effects persist or worsen.

• Instruct the patient to watch for and report any signs of urinary tract infection (fever, chills, flank pain, and decreased urine volume) or wound infection (redness, swelling, and purulent drainage at the incision site). Also tell him to report persistent hematuria.

• Make sure the patient or a family member understands how to care for his stoma and where to obtain needed supplies. If needed, arrange for visits by a home care nurse, who can reinforce stoma care measures and provide emotional support. You also may want to refer the patient to a support group, such as a local chapter of the United Ostomy Association.

• Stress the importance of follow-up examinations to evaluate healing and recurrence of cancer.

Cystostomy

This type of urinary diversion involves transcutaneous insertion of a catheter through the suprapubic area into the bladder, with connection of the device to a closed drainage system. Typically, cystostomy provides temporary urinary diversion after certain gynecologic procedures, bladder surgery, or prostatectomy and relieves obstruction from calculi, severe urethral strictures, or pelvic trauma. Less often, it may be used to create a permanent urinary diversion, thereby relieving obstruction from an inoperable tumor.

In certain patients, cystostomy represents an attractive alternative to urethral catheterization. For instance, it provides a more comfortable means of drainage and decreases the potential for some of the problems inherent in urethral catheterization, including meatal irritation and urinary tract infection. It's often useful in infants and young children, whose narrow urethras may hinder insertion of an indwelling catheter.

Cystostomy isn't without potential complications. It can lead to urinary retention from catheter obstruction, bladder infection, and skin breakdown. Fortunately, these complications can usually be prevented by regularly checking catheter patency and providing meticulous skin care.

COMPARING CYSTOSTOMIES

Percutaneous cystostomy involves the introduction of a cystostomy tube through a trocar into the bladder via a simple abdominal incision. Open suprapubic cystostomy requires a transverse incision above the pubic symphysis and insertion of a Malecot catheter into the bladder. The catheter is brought out to the skin surface through the skin incision or a stab wound above the site.

PERCUTANEOUS CYSTOSTOMY

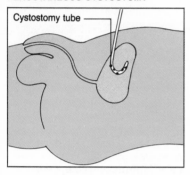

Cystostomy tube

OPEN SUPRAPUBIC CYSTOSTOMY

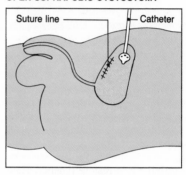

Suture line — Catheter

Purpose

To provide an alternate route for urinary drainage when urethral catheterization is contraindicated.

Preparation

Tell the patient (or his parents) that the doctor will insert a soft plastic tube through the skin of the abdomen and into the bladder, then connect the tube to an external collection bag. Explain that the procedure is done under local anesthesia, that it causes little or no discomfort, and that it takes 15 to 45 minutes.

Teach the patient about postoperative care of the catheter, collection bag, and surrounding skin. If possible, arrange for a visit by an enterostomal therapist, who can provide the patient with more information.

Ensure that the patient or a responsible family member has signed a consent form.

Procedure

To perform a *percutaneous cystostomy*, the surgeon makes a stab wound in the area above the pubic symphysis, inserts a trocar and cannula, and advances them into the bladder until he detects urine return. Next, he passes the cystostomy tube through the cannula into the bladder and anchors it in place on the skin surface with several nonabsorbable sutures.

To perform an *open suprapubic cystostomy*, the surgeon makes a short (6 to 8 cm) transverse incision above the pubic symphysis. He divides the anterior fascia and separates the rectus muscles to expose the anterior bladder wall. Next, he introduces a Malecot catheter into the bladder and brings the catheter out to the skin surface through the skin incision or, more commonly, through a stab wound above the incision. He also may insert a Penrose drain in the incision. After closing the incision, he sutures the catheter in place and secures it with tape.

Monitoring and aftercare

Provide routine postoperative care: monitor vital signs, intake and output, and fluid status and encourage coughing, deep breathing, and early ambulation. In addition, focus on providing tube care and assessing for possible complications.

To ensure adequate drainage and tube patency, check the cystostomy tube at least hourly for the first 24 hours after insertion. Carefully document the color and amount of drainage from the tube; note particularly any color changes. Assess tube patency by checking the amount of urine in the drainage bag and by palpating for bladder distention. Make sure the collection bag is below bladder level to enhance drainage and prevent backflow, which can lead to infection.

Irrigate the cystostomy tube as ordered, using the same technique as you would for irrigating an indwelling urinary catheter. Check the tube frequently for kinks or obstruction. If a blood clot or mucus blocks the tube, try milking it to restore patency. However, if you can't clear the obstruction promptly, notify the doctor.

To prevent kinks in the tube, curve it gently but don't bend it. Tape the tube securely in place on the abdominal skin to reduce tension and prevent dislodgment. However, if the tube does become dislodged, immediately notify the doctor; he may be able to reinsert the tube through the original tract.

As ordered, perform a voiding trial by closing the stopcock (or clamping the tube) for 4 hours, asking the patient to attempt urination, then reopening the tube and measuring residual urine.

Check dressings often and change them at least once a day or as ordered. Observe the skin around the insertion site for signs of infection and encrustation.

Home care instructions
• Teach the patient or his parents how to change the dressing and how to empty and reattach the collection bag.
• Tell the patient or his family to promptly notify the doctor of signs of infection or encrustation, such as discolored or foul-smelling discharge, impaired drainage, and swelling, redness, or tenderness at the tube insertion site.

• Encourage the patient to drink plenty of fluids to reduce the risk of complications.
• Stress the importance of regular follow-up examinations to allow early detection of possible complications. Encourage visits with the enterostomal therapist to help manage urinary diversion.

Marshall-Marchetti-Krantz Procedure

When stress incontinence in women doesn't respond to pubococcygeus muscle exercises or sympathomimetic drugs, surgery may help restore urinary sphincter competence. The Marshall-Marchetti-Krantz procedure, the most common surgery for stress incontinence, involves the creation of a vesicourethral suspension by elevating the anterior vaginal wall. This relatively simple surgery eliminates stress incontinence in most patients and carries a minimal chance of recurrence. It does, however, carry the risk of several complications, including urethral obstruction with resultant urinary retention and infection caused by leakage of urine into the vagina. These complications can often be prevented or corrected by careful postoperative monitoring, prompt intervention, and comprehensive patient teaching.

Purpose
To eliminate stress incontinence by restoring the normal posterior vesicourethral angle.

Preparation
Review the procedure with the patient and answer any questions she may have. Explain that she'll probably have an indwelling urethral catheter or cystostomy tube in place for 2 to 4 days after surgery to drain urine and promote healing. Prepare her for the pres-

ence of a lower abdominal drain and the need for frequent dressing changes. Reassure her that her need for privacy will be respected during catheterization and dressing changes. Ensure that she has signed a consent form.

Procedure

With the patient under general anesthesia and placed in a modified lithotomy position, the surgeon makes a transverse suprapubic incision and frees the bladder neck, urethra, and anterior vaginal wall. He then suspends the urethra and bladder neck by suturing both sides of the anterior vaginal wall to the periosteum of the pubic bones and to the lower rectal fascia. (If the periosteum is in poor condition, as in many elderly patients, he may use Cooper's ligament in the bladder neck region.) He typically completes the procedure by inserting a drain in the retropubic space and an indwelling urethral catheter or a cystostomy (suprapubic) tube, closing the incision, and applying a sterile dressing.

Monitoring and aftercare

Check the incisional drain and dressing every 4 hours for the first 24 hours and then once every shift thereafter. Keep in mind that a small amount of serosanguineous drainage is normal. Change the dressing when it becomes wet or as ordered, remembering to use sterile technique and taking care not to dislodge the incisional drain or cystostomy tube (if one's in place).

Monitor the amount and color of urine drainage from the urethral catheter or cystostomy tube. Remember that blood-tinged urine normally occurs for 24 to 48 hours after surgery. However, notify the doctor if the urine appears bright red or if hematuria persists for longer than 48 hours. Also report signs of urinary retention, and be prepared to institute intermittent catheterization, as ordered, to drain the bladder and prevent complications.

If the patient continues to experience difficulty voiding, you may need to teach her intermittent self-catheterization. (Refer to the entry "Bladder Training" in this chapter for detailed instructions.) Generally, intermittent catheterization isn't necessary once healing is complete and edema subsides.

Home care instructions

• Explain to the patient that weakness, fatigue, and incisional pain may persist for up to several weeks. Advise her to get plenty of rest and to avoid strenuous activity during this period.
• If the patient requires intermittent catheterization after discharge, provide her with written instructions on self-catheterization technique.
• Instruct her to report signs of urinary tract infection, such as fever, chills, flank pain, and hematuria. Also tell her to report signs of wound infection, such as severe pain, redness, and swelling at the incision site.

Prostatectomy

When chronic prostatitis, benign prostatic hypertrophy (BPH), or prostate cancer fails to respond to drug therapy or other treatments, total or partial prostatectomy may be necessary to remove diseased or obstructive tissue and restore urine flow through the urethra. Depending on the disease, one of four approaches is used. Transurethral resection of the prostate (TURP), the most common approach, involves insertion of a resectoscope into the urethra. Open surgical approaches include suprapubic, retropubic, and radical perineal prostatectomy. (See *Comparing Types of Prostatectomy,* pages 332 and 333, for indications, advantages, and drawbacks of each approach.)

Whichever approach is used, prostatectomy requires thorough teaching about the surgery and the expected course of recovery. A primary part of this preparation involves emotional and psychological support for the patient to help him overcome the fears and anxieties associated with this surgery. After prostatectomy, nursing care focuses on preventing or promptly detecting complications, which may include hemorrhage, infection, and urinary retention.

Purpose
To treat chronic prostatitis, BPH, or prostate cancer.

Preparation
Begin by reviewing the planned surgery, paying special attention to what the patient knows about the procedure and its aftermath. Encourage him to ask questions. After all, he probably has heard many things about prostatectomy, some of which may be misleading or erroneous. Provide honest answers and straightforward information to help clear up any misconceptions he may have.

Be sure to consider the patient's emotional state as well. Most likely he'll be worried about the surgery and its effects on his life-style. Encourage him to express his fears; help to allay them by emphasizing the positive aspects of the surgery, such as improved urination and prevention of further complications.

Keep in mind that some types of prostatectomy may result in the patient's becoming impotent. Typically, the doctor will discuss this possibility with the patient before surgery. If necessary, arrange for sexual counseling to help the patient cope with this often devastating loss. Or, if the patient's scheduled for TURP, mention that this procedure often causes retrograde ejaculation but no other impairment of sexual function.

Before surgery, as ordered, shave and cleanse the surgical site (unless the patient's scheduled for TURP) and administer a cleansing enema. Explain to the patient that a catheter will remain in place for several days after surgery to ensure proper urine drainage.

Procedure
In *TURP*, the patient is placed in a lithotomy position and anesthetized. The surgeon then introduces a resectoscope into the urethra and advances it to the prostate. After instilling a clear irrigating solution and visualizing the obstruction, he uses the resectoscope's cutting loop to resect prostatic tissue and restore the urethral opening.

In a *suprapubic prostatectomy*, the patient is given a general anesthetic and placed in a supine position. The surgeon begins by making a horizontal incision just above the pubic symphysis. After instilling fluid into the bladder to distend it, he makes a small incision in the bladder wall to expose the prostate. He then shells the obstructing prostatic tissue out of its bed with his finger. After clearing the obstruction and ligating all bleeding points, he usually inserts a suprapubic drainage tube and a Penrose drain.

In a *retropubic prostatectomy*, the patient is anesthetized and placed in a supine position. The surgeon makes a horizontal suprapubic incision and approaches the prostate from between the bladder and the pubic arch. He then makes another incision in the prostatic capsule and removes the obstructing tissue. After controlling any bleeding, he usually inserts a suprapubic tube and a Penrose drain.

In a *radical perineal prostatectomy*, the patient is anesthetized and placed in the perineal position, an exaggerated lithotomy position in which the knees are drawn up against the chest and the buttocks slightly elevated. The surgeon makes an inverted U-shaped incision in the perineum, then removes the entire prostate and the seminal vesicles. He anastomoses the urethra to the bladder and closes the incision, leaving a Penrose drain in place.

Monitoring and aftercare
Carefully observe the patient for complications. Monitor his vital signs closely, looking for indications of possible hemorrhage and shock. Fre-

quently check the incision site (unless the patient underwent TURP) for signs of infection and change dressings as necessary. Also watch for and report signs of epididymitis: fever, chills, groin pain, and a tender, swollen epididymis.

Check and record the amount and nature of urine drainage. Maintain Foley catheter patency through intermittent or continuous irrigation, as ordered. Watch for catheter blockage from kinking or clot formation, and correct as necessary.

Maintain the patency of the suprapubic tube, if inserted, and monitor the amount and character of drainage. Drainage should be amber or slightly blood-tinged; report any abnormalities. Keep the collection container below the level of the patient's bladder to promote drainage, and keep the skin around the tube insertion site clean and dry.

Expect and report frank bleeding the 1st day after surgery. If bleeding is venous, the doctor may order increasing the traction on the catheter or increasing pressure in the catheter's balloon end. However, if bleeding is arterial (bright red with numerous clots and increased viscosity), the doctor may need to control it surgically.

As ordered, administer antispasmodics to control painful bladder spasms and analgesics to relieve incisional pain. If necessary, offer sitz baths to reduce perineal discomfort.

Watch for signs of dilutional hyponatremia, characterized by altered mental status, muscle twitching, and seizures. If these occur, raise the side rails of the patient's bed to prevent injury. Then notify the doctor, draw blood for serum sodium determination, and prepare hypertonic saline solution for possible I.V. infusion.

If the patient has had a radical perineal prostatectomy, provide emotional support because this procedure usually causes impotence. If possible, arrange for psychological and sexual counseling during the recovery period.

COMPARING TYPES OF PROSTATECTOMY

PROCEDURE AND INDICATIONS	ADVANTAGES
Perineal prostatectomy • Prostate cancer • Benign prostatic hypertrophy (BPH) if the prostate is too large for transurethral resection and the patient is no longer sexually active	• Allows direct visualization of gland • Permits drainage by gravity • Low mortality and decreased incidence of shock
Retropubic prostatectomy • BPH if the prostate is too large for transurethral resection • Prostate cancer when total removal of gland is necessary	• Allows direct visualization of gland • Avoids bladder incision • Short convalescence period • Patient may remain potent
Suprapubic prostatectomy • BPH if the prostate is too large for transurethral resection • Prostate cancer when total removal of gland is necessary • Bladder lesions	• Allows exploration of wide area, such as into lymph nodes • Simple procedure
Transurethral resection of prostate • BPH • Moderately enlarged prostate • Prostate cancer, as a palliative measure to remove obstruction	• Safer and less painful and invasive than other prostate procedures • Doesn't require surgical incision • Short hospital stay • Little risk of impotence

DISADVANTAGES	POSTOPERATIVE DRAINAGE

- High incidence of impotence and incontinence
- Risk of damage to rectum and external sphincter
- Restricted operative field

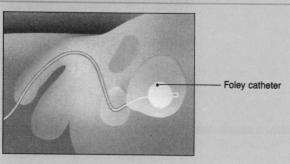

— Foley catheter

— Incisional drain

- Can't be used to treat associated bladder pathology
- Increased risk of hemorrhage from prostate venous plexus

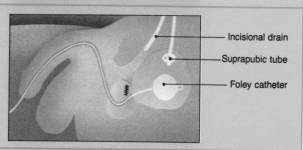

— Incisional drain
— Suprapubic tube
— Foley catheter

- Requires bladder incision
- Hemorrhage control difficult
- Urinary leakage common around suprapubic tube
- Prolonged and uncomfortable recovery

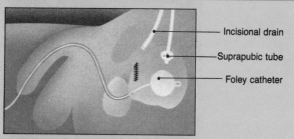

— Incisional drain
— Suprapubic tube
— Foley catheter

- Urethral stricture and delayed bleeding may occur
- Not a curative surgery for prostate cancer

— Foley catheter

Home care instructions

• Tell the patient to drink 10 glasses of water a day, to void at least every 2 hours, and to notify the doctor promptly if he has trouble voiding.

• Explain to the patient that he may experience transient urinary frequency and dribbling after catheter removal. Reassure him that he'll gradually regain control over urination. Teach him how to perform perineum-tightening exercises (Kegel exercises) to speed the return of sphincter control. Suggest that he avoid caffeine-containing beverages, which produce mild diuresis.

• Reassure the patient that slightly blood-tinged urine normally occurs for the first few weeks after surgery. Instruct him to report bright-red urine or persistent hematuria, however.

• Tell him to watch for and immediately report any signs of infection, such as fever, chills, and flank pain.

• Warn the patient against engaging in sexual relations, lifting any object heavier than 10 lb, performing strenuous exercise (short walks are usually permitted), and taking long car trips until the doctor gives permission. Explain that these activities should usually be delayed for several weeks because of the risk of bleeding.

• Advise him to keep taking prescribed medications, such as antibiotics, antispasmodics, and stool softeners. Encourage periodic sitz baths, if necessary, to relieve perineal discomfort.

• Remind the patient of the importance of having yearly prostate examinations—unless, of course, he has undergone a radical prostatectomy.

Hydrocelectomy

Hydrocelectomy may be necessary if needle aspiration fails to resolve a persistent hydrocele—a collection of fluid in the tunica vaginalis of the testicle or along the spermatic cord. In this simple surgery, the hydrocele is excised or pli-

cated through a small scrotal incision. Hydrocelectomy is characteristically reserved for males older than age 1; in infants, the hydrocele often regresses spontaneously. It seldom causes complications if meticulous wound care is provided.

Purpose

To remove a persistent hydrocele through surgical excision or plication.

Preparation

Briefly explain the procedure to the patient (or to his parents, if the patient's a young boy). Tell him that the procedure involves a small scrotal incision and application of a dressing, and, depending on the surgical procedure used, may include insertion of an incisional drain. Explain that the drain prevents fluid buildup, helping to prevent infection and promote healing.

Inform the patient that he'll receive a local anesthetic before surgery and should experience no discomfort during it. Point out that scrotal swelling and pain may develop after surgery but that analgesics and a scrotal supporter will be provided to relieve symptoms. Prepare him for frequent dressing changes and reassure him that his need for privacy will be respected.

Keep in mind that a patient scheduled for testicular surgery is bound to be anxious and apprehensive. To allay his concerns, reassure him that the surgery will not impair sexual or reproductive function and may actually enhance it by removing a source of discomfort and a possible cause of low sperm production.

Procedure

After the patient receives a local anesthetic and assumes the supine position, the surgeon makes a small horizontal incision between the visible blood vessels in the scrotal skin. He gently separates the hydrocele from the scrotal sac, excises it close to the testicle, and achieves hemostasis with ligation and fulguration. He then inserts

ASPIRATING A HYDROCELE

Typically attempted before surgery, needle aspiration represents a common treatment for chronic hydrocele. In this procedure, the doctor injects a sclerosing solution, such as urea or quinine hydrochloride, into the hydrocele and subsequently aspirates the fluid. However, if aspiration fails to correct the condition, hydrocelectomy may be necessary to prevent compression of testicular tissue and loss of function.

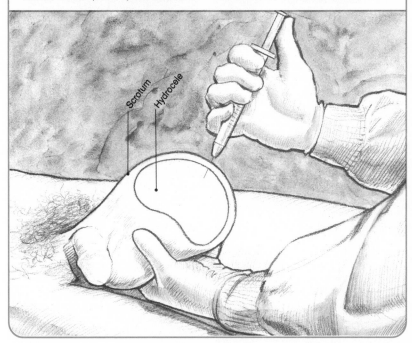

a small incisional drain, closes the wound, and applies a dressing and a scrotal support or suspensory.

Alternatively, the surgeon may plicate the hydrocele (Lord's procedure), permanently collapsing its walls and preventing refilling. After plication, no incisional drain is required.

Monitoring and aftercare

Check the dressing every 2 to 4 hours for the first 24 hours after surgery. Expect moderate to heavy serosanguineous drainage during this period. Change the dressing as necessary, using sterile technique and taking care not to dislodge the incisional drain.

Observe for frank bleeding from the drain or the suture line. Assess for signs of internal scrotal hemorrhage, including increased pain, swelling, and tenderness and systemic signs of infection.

Keep the scrotum elevated to minimize swelling and snugly supported to enhance comfort. Provide extra scrotal supporters and change the support when it becomes saturated with drainage. As ordered, administer anti-inflammatory drugs to reduce scrotal swelling.

Home care instructions

• Inform the patient that scrotal swelling may persist for up to a month after surgery. Reassure him that swelling will gradually subside.
• Instruct him to watch for and report signs of possible infection, including

fever, chills, and worsening scrotal pain, tenderness, or swelling.

• Tell the patient to avoid taking baths until all wound drainage has ceased and healing is complete.

• Warn the patient to avoid heavy lifting or straining for at least 6 weeks to reduce the risk of incisional hernia.

• Also warn the postpubescent patient to refrain from sexual activity until his doctor advises him otherwise.

Orchiopexy

This surgical procedure secures the testis in the scrotum. It's indicated for the patient with cryptorchidism (undescended testis) or testicular torsion. In cryptorchidism, orchiopexy is usually performed between ages 1 and 6 (but the patient may be older) and when other treatments, such as hormonal therapy with human chorionic gonadotropin, fail. When successful, this surgery reduces the risk of sterility, testicular cancer, and testicular trauma from abnormal positioning. It also precludes harmful psychological effects caused by poor sexual image.

In testicular torsion, which can affect males of all ages, orchiopexy is indicated when the testis remains viable. However, if the testis can't be saved, an orchiectomy (removal of the testis) may be performed.

Complications, though uncommon, include hemorrhage and dysuria.

Purpose
To correct cryptorchidism or testicular torsion.

Preparation
If the patient has testicular torsion, briefly explain the surgery to him and, if appropriate and time permits, to his parents. Tell them that the surgeon will untwist and permanently stabilize the spermatic cord. If this isn't possible, he'll remove the twisted appendage.

If the patient has an undescended testis, review the doctor's explanation of the surgery, using terms the patient can understand. If appropriate, try using simple diagrams or anatomically detailed models to enhance your explanation. If the patient's a child, include his parents in your explanation.

Reassure the postpubescent patient that surgery shouldn't impair sexual performance and reproductive function. In fact, it may actually enhance them by correcting a potential source of problems and improving the appearance of his sexual organs. Also reassure the patient that recovery should be rapid and that he'll be able to resume most normal activities within a week.

Procedure
After the patient receives a general anesthetic, the surgeon makes the incision. If the patient has testicular torsion, the surgeon makes an incision in the scrotal skin and attempts to untwist and stabilize the spermatic cord. He may also remove a hydrocele, if present. However, if he's unable to save the testis, he performs an orchiectomy.

If the patient has an undescended testis, the surgeon makes an incision in the inguinal area or lower abdomen to expose the testis, and a small incision in the scrotal skin to open the scrotum. He then frees the testis and lowers it into the scrotal sac, where he secures it in place with sutures. If bilateral cryptorchidism is present, he repeats this procedure for the other testis.

In two-stage orchiopexy, an alternate procedure, the surgeon brings the testis down into the scrotal sac and sutures it to the thigh. Then, 2 or 3 months later, he imbeds it in the scrotal sac. However, if the spermatic cord's too short to accommodate repositioning of the testis, the surgeon may perform the Fowler-Stephens procedure, in which he discontinues the spermatic cord before placing the testis in the scrotal sac. After completing the procedure, the surgeon sutures the incision and applies a dressing.

Monitoring and aftercare

Monitor the patient's vital signs, looking for evidence of hemorrhage or infection. Check the incision site and dressing frequently for redness, inflammation, and bleeding. Frequently change the dressing.

Carefully monitor and record the patient's intake and output. Watch for urinary retention or dysuria, which may result from postsurgical edema or the effects of the anesthetic.

Take measures to promote patient comfort, such as applying an ice pack or a scrotal support. Administer analgesics, as ordered.

Home care instructions

• Instruct the patient to promptly report increased scrotal pain or swelling or other changes in the testis. Explain that these symptoms may indicate infection or ischemia and require immediate medical attention.

• Advise him to gradually resume normal activities beginning about 1 week after surgery but to avoid heavy lifting and other strenuous activities until the doctor advises otherwise.

• Encourage the patient to wear a scrotal support to enhance comfort and control edema.

• Advise the adult patient to refrain from sexual activity for 6 weeks after surgery or for the duration recommended by the doctor.

• Teach the patient how to perform testicular self-examination. Advise him to regularly examine both testes and to report any lumps or unusual findings. For as-yet-unclear reasons, the patient with cryptorchidism has an increased risk for testicular cancer.

Circumcision

Surgical removal of the foreskin from the glans penis may be performed on an adult patient to treat phimosis (abnormal tightening of the foreskin around the glans) or paraphimosis (inability to return the foreskin to its normal position after retraction). Most commonly, circumcision is performed on neonates 2 or 3 days after birth.

There is much controversy currently concerning routine neonatal circumcision. Its proponents contend that circumcision helps reduce the risk of future penile cancer and of cervical cancer in female sexual partners. However, most authorities, including the American Academy of Pediatrics, find no medical justification for routine circumcision. Nevertheless, it remains the most commonly performed of all pediatric surgeries. That's largely the result of circumcision's religious significance. In the Jewish faith, for instance, circumcision is a religious ritual called a *brith*, performed by a *mohel* on the 8th day after birth.

Although circumcision is a relatively minor and safe operation, it can cause bleeding or, less commonly, infection and urethral damage, such as meatal stenosis or urethral fistulae.

Purpose

• To correct foreskin disorders
• To remove the foreskin for religious reasons.

Preparation

Review the procedure with the patient or with his parents. Make sure they know what to expect before, during, and after surgery and that they've signed a consent form.

If the patient's undergoing circumcision to relieve a foreskin disorder, reassure him that surgery will not interfere with urinary, sexual, or reproductive function.

If you'll be assisting with the procedure, prepare the necessary equipment, including circumcision clamps or a plastic circumcision bell, as appropriate, and, for the neonate, a restraining board with arm and leg restraints. (Because of the risk of respiratory complications, no anesthetic is used for neonatal circumcision, and the infant must be restrained during this procedure.) Make sure the neonate hasn't been fed for at least 1 hour before surgery to reduce the risk of vomiting.

Procedure

The surgeon can choose from several different procedures. If he's using a plastic circumcision bell (Plastibell), he slides the device between the foreskin and glans penis and then tightly ties a length of suture around the foreskin at the glans' coronal edge. The foreskin distal to the suture first becomes ischemic and then atropic. After 5 to 8 days it drops off to leave a clean, well-healed line of excision.

If the surgeon's using a Gomco clamp, he stretches the foreskin forward over the glans and applies the clamp on the penis distal to the glans. He then excises the foreskin, removes the clamp, and sutures around the base of the glans to control bleeding.

If the surgeon's performing a sleeve resection, the preferred method for an adult patient, he incises and dissects the inner and outer surfaces of the foreskin, then puts sutures in place to approximate the skin edges. He may use electrocoagulation to control bleeding, if necessary, and usually applies a compression dressing.

Monitoring and aftercare

Monitor vital signs after surgery, and check for bleeding every 15 minutes for the first hour and every hour for the next 24 hours. Control slight bleeding by applying pressure with sterile gauze sponges. However, notify the doctor if bleeding is heavy or persistent.

Periodically examine the dressing, suture line, and glans penis for swelling, redness, or purulent exudate. Report any signs of possible infection and obtain a specimen of the exudate for culture and analysis.

Check for or encourage voiding after surgery. If the patient hasn't voided within 6 hours, notify the doctor.

Take steps to promote healing and enhance the patient's comfort. Change

dressings often, as ordered, and apply antibiotic ointment, petrolatum, or petrolatum gauze. Position the patient on his side and, if necessary, use a bed cradle to keep bed linen from exerting pressure on the penis. Diaper the neonate loosely to prevent irritation.

As ordered, provide analgesics to relieve incisional pain. For the older patient—who is more subject to pain from pressure exerted on the suture line by an erection—use a topical anesthetic ointment or spray, as needed. Provide a sedative, if ordered, to help prevent nocturnal penile tumescence.

Home care instructions

• Teach the patient or his parents proper wound care, including, if appropriate, how to change a dressing. Tell them to watch for and report any renewed bleeding or signs of infection.
• Advise the adult patient that he can resume normal sexual activity as soon as healing is complete, usually after a week or so.
• Encourage the use of prescribed analgesics to relieve discomfort.

DIALYSIS

Hemodialysis

Hemodialysis removes toxic wastes and other impurities from the blood of a patient with renal failure. In this technique, the blood is removed from the body through a surgically created access site, pumped through a dialyzing unit to remove toxins, and then returned to the body. The extracorporeal dialyzer works through a combination of osmosis, diffusion, and filtration (see *How Hemodialysis Works*). By extracting byproducts of protein metabolism—notably urea and uric acid—as

HOW HEMODIALYSIS WORKS

Within the dialyzer, the patient's blood flows between coils, plates, or hollow fibers of semipermeable material, depending on the machine being used. Simultaneously, the dialysis solution—an aqueous solution typically containing low concentrations of sodium, potassium, calcium, magnesium cations, and chloride anions and high concentrations of acetate (which the body readily converts to bicarbonate) and glucose—is pumped around the other side under hydrostatic pressure.

Pressure and concentration gradients between blood and the dialysis solution remove toxic wastes and excess water. Because blood has higher concentrations of hydrogen ions and other electrolytes than dialysis solution, these solutes diffuse across the semipermeable material into the solution. Conversely, glucose and acetate are more highly concentrated in the dialysis solution and so diffuse back across the semipermeable material into the blood. Through this mechanism, hemodialysis removes excess water and toxins, reverses acidosis, and amends electrolyte imbalances.

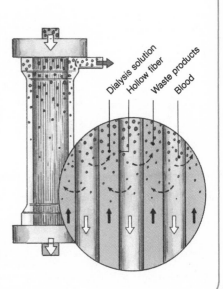

Dialysis solution Hollow fiber Waste products Blood

well as creatinine and excess water, hemodialysis helps restore or maintain acid-base and electrolyte balance and prevent the complications associated with uremia.

Hemodialysis can be performed in an emergency in acute renal failure or as regular long-term therapy in end-stage renal disease. In chronic renal failure, the frequency and duration of treatments depend on the patient's condition; up to several treatments a week, each lasting up to 6 hours, may be required. Rarely, hemodialysis is done to treat acute poisoning or drug overdose.

Specially trained nurses usually perform the procedure in a hemodialysis unit. If the patient is too ill to be moved, it can be performed at bedside, using portable equipment.

Purpose
To remove toxic wastes from the blood until renal failure resolves, kidney transplant can be performed, or the patient dies.

Preparation
If the patient is undergoing hemodialysis for the first time, begin by explaining its purpose and what to expect during and after treatment. Explain that he first will undergo surgery to create vascular access. (See *Reviewing Hemodialysis Access Sites,* page 340, for information on how the doctor creates the different types of accesses.)

After vascular access has been created and the patient is ready for dialysis, weigh him and take his vital signs. Be sure to take the patient's blood pressure in both supine and standing positions.

As ordered, prepare the hemodialysis equipment, following the manufacturer's and your hospital's protocols and maintaining strict aseptic technique to prevent the introduction of

REVIEWING HEMODIALYSIS ACCESS SITES

Hemodialysis requires vascular access. The site and type of access selected vary, depending on the expected duration of dialysis, the surgeon's preference, and the patient's condition.

ARTERIOVENOUS FISTULA

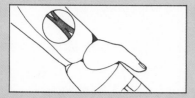

The surgeon makes an incision into the patient's wrist, then a small incision in the side of an artery and another in the side of a vein. He sutures the edges of these incisions together to make a common opening 3 to 7 mm long.

ARTERIOVENOUS SHUNT

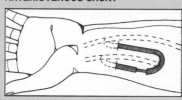

The surgeon makes an incision in the patient's wrist (or rarely, an ankle). He then inserts a 6" to 10" (15.2 to 25.4 cm) transparent Silastic cannula into an artery and another into a vein. Finally, he tunnels the cannulas out through stab wounds and connects them with a short piece of Teflon tubing.

ARTERIOVENOUS VEIN GRAFT

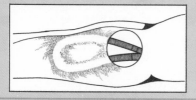

The surgeon makes an incision in the patient's forearm, upper arm, or thigh. He then tunnels a natural or synthetic graft under the skin and sutures the distal end to an artery and the proximal end to a vein.

SUBCLAVIAN VEIN CATHETERIZATION

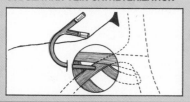

Using the Seldinger technique, the surgeon inserts an introducer needle into the subclavian vein. He then inserts a guide wire through the introducer needle and removes the needle. Using the guide wire, he then threads a 5" to 12" (12.7 to 30.5 cm) plastic or Teflon catheter (with a Y hub) into the vein.

FEMORAL VEIN CATHETERIZATION

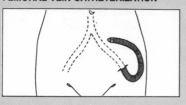

Using the Seldinger technique, the surgeon inserts an introducer needle into the left or right femoral vein. He then inserts a guide wire through the introducer needle and removes the needle. Using the guide wire, he then threads a 5" to 12" plastic or Teflon catheter into the vein. He may use a single catheter with a Y hub or two catheters, one for inflow and another placed about 1/2 inch distal to the first for outflow.

pathogens into the patient's bloodstream during treatment.

Place the patient in a supine position and make him as comfortable as possible. Keep the venous access site well supported and resting on a sterile drape or sterile barrier shield.

Procedure

Hemodialysis begins with connection of the blood lines from the dialyzer to the needles that have been placed in the venous access site. After all connections have been made, blood samples are drawn for laboratory analysis.

The dialyzer's pump is then switched on, and hemodialysis is begun at a blood flow rate of 90 to 120 ml/minute. If heparinization is being used, a loading dose of 1,000 to 3,000 units is injected in the port on the arterial line. Blood pressure and vital signs are checked periodically; if stable, the blood flow rate is gradually increased to about 300 ml/minute and maintained at this level for the duration of treatment, unless complications arise. Depending on the patient's condition, dialysis is continued for 3 to 6 hours.

To end the treatment, more blood samples are taken and checked, the blood remaining in the dialyzer is returned to the patient, and the needles are removed from the venous access site.

Monitoring and aftercare

Monitor the patient throughout dialysis. Once every 30 minutes check and record vital signs to detect possible complications. Fever may point to infection from pathogens in the dialysate or equipment; notify the doctor, who may prescribe an antipyretic and/or an antibiotic. Hypotension may indicate hypovolemia or a drop in hematocrit level; give blood or fluid supplements I.V., as ordered. Rapid respirations may signal hypoxemia; give supplemental oxygen, as ordered.

About every hour, draw a blood sample for analysis of clotting time. Using the dialyzing unit's bed scale or a portable scale, check the patient's weight regularly to ensure adequate ultrafiltration during treatment. Also periodically check the dialyzer's blood lines to make sure all connections are secure, and monitor the lines for clotting.

Assess for headache, muscle twitching, backache, nausea or vomiting, and seizures, which may indicate disequilibrium syndrome caused by rapid fluid removal and electrolyte changes. If this syndrome occurs, notify the doctor immediately; he may reduce the blood flow rate or stop dialysis. Muscle cramps also may result from rapid fluid and electrolyte shifts. As ordered, relieve cramps by injecting normal saline solution into the venous return line.

Observe the patient carefully for signs of internal bleeding: apprehension; restlessness; pale, cold, clammy skin; excessive thirst; hypotension; rapid, weak, thready pulse; increased respirations; and decreased body temperature. Report any of these signs immediately and prepare to decrease heparinization; the doctor also may order blood transfusions.

Be especially alert for signs of air embolism—a potentially fatal complication characterized by sudden hypotension, dyspnea, chest pain, cyanosis, and a weak, rapid pulse. If these signs develop, turn the patient onto his left side and lower the head of the bed (to help keep air bubbles on the right side of his body, where they can be absorbed by the pulmonary artery), and call the doctor immediately.

After completion of hemodialysis, monitor the venous access site for bleeding. If bleeding is excessive, maintain pressure on the site and notify the doctor.

To prevent clotting or other problems with blood flow, make sure that the arm used for venous access isn't used for any other procedure, including I.V. line insertion, blood pressure monitoring, and venipuncture. At least four times a day, assess circulation at the access site by auscultating for bruits and palpating for thrills.

Keep an accurate record of the patient's food and fluid intake, and encourage him to comply with prescribed restrictions, such as limited protein, potassium, and sodium intake, increased caloric intake, and decreased fluid intake.

Home care instructions

• Teach the patient how to care for his venous access site. Tell him to keep the incision clean and dry to prevent infection and to cleanse it with hydrogen peroxide solution daily until healing is complete and the sutures are removed (usually 10 to 14 days after surgery).

• Tell him to notify the doctor of pain, swelling, redness, or drainage in the accessed arm. Teach him how to use a stethoscope to auscultate for bruits.

• Explain that once the access site has healed, he may use the arm freely. In fact, exercise is beneficial because it helps stimulate vein enlargement. Remind him not to allow any treatments or procedures on the accessed arm, including blood pressure monitoring or needle punctures. Also tell him to avoid putting excessive pressure on the arm; he shouldn't sleep on it, wear constricting clothing on it, or lift heavy objects or strain with it. He also should avoid showering, bathing, or swimming for several hours after dialysis.

• Teach him exercises for the affected arm to promote venous dilation and enhance blood flow. Explain the exercise routine as follows: 1 week after surgery, squeeze a small rubber ball or other soft object for 15 minutes, four times a day; 2 weeks after surgery, apply a tourniquet on the upper arm above the fistula site, making sure it's snug but not tight. With the tourniquet in place, squeeze the rubber ball for 5 minutes; repeat four times daily. After the incision has healed completely, perform the exercise with the arm submerged in warm water.

• If the patient will be performing hemodialysis at home, make sure he thoroughly understands all aspects of the procedure. Give him the phone number of the dialysis center and encourage him to call if he has any questions about the treatment. Also encourage him to arrange for another person to be present during dialysis in case any problems develop.

• Encourage the patient to contact the National Association of Patients on Hemodialysis and Transplantation or the National Kidney Foundation for information and support.

Peritoneal Dialysis

Like hemodialysis, peritoneal dialysis removes toxins from the blood of a patient with acute or chronic renal failure who doesn't respond to other treatments. But unlike hemodialysis, it uses the patient's peritoneal membrane as a semipermeable dialyzing membrane. In this technique, a hypertonic dialyzing solution is instilled through a catheter inserted into the peritoneal cavity. Then, by diffusion, excessive concentrations of electrolytes and uremic toxins in the blood move across the peritoneal membrane into the dialysis solution. Next, by osmosis, excessive water in the blood does the same. After an appropriate dwelling time, the dialysis solution is drained, taking toxins and wastes with it.

Peritoneal dialysis may be performed manually, by an automatic or semiautomatic cycler machine, or as continuous ambulatory peritoneal dialysis (CAPD). In manual dialysis, the nurse, the patient, or a family member instills dialyzing solution through the catheter into the peritoneal cavity, allows it to dwell for a specified time, and then drains it from the peritoneal cavity. Typically, this process is repeated for 6 to 8 hours at a time, five or six times a week.

The cycler machine requires sterile set-up and connection technique, and then it automatically completes dialysis.

CAPD is performed by the patient himself. He fills a special plastic bag with dialyzing solution and then instills the solution through a catheter into his peritoneal cavity. While the solution remains in the peritoneal cavity, the patient can roll up the empty bag, place it under his clothing, and go about his normal activities. After 6 to 8 hours of dwell time, he drains the spent solution into the bag, removes and discards the full bag, and attaches a new bag and instills a new batch of dialyzing solution. He repeats the process to ensure continuous dialysis 24 hours a day, 7 days a week. As its name implies, CAPD allows the patient to be out of bed and active during dialysis, and thus only minimally disrupts his life-style.

Some patients use CAPD in combination with an automatic cycler, in a treatment called continuous-cycling peritoneal dialysis (CCPD). In CCPD, the cycler performs dialysis at night while the patient sleeps, and the patient performs CAPD in the daytime.

Peritoneal dialysis has several advantages over hemodialysis—it's simpler, less costly, and less stressful. What's more, it's nearly as effective as hemodialysis while posing fewer risks.

Peritoneal dialysis can cause severe complications, however. The most serious one, peritonitis, results from bacteria entering the peritoneal cavity through the catheter or the insertion site. Other complications include catheter obstruction from clots, lodgment against the abdominal wall, or kinking, hypotension, and hypovolemia from excessive plasma fluid removal.

Purpose

To remove toxic wastes from the blood of a patient with renal failure until the disease resolves, a kidney transplant is performed, or the patient requires hemodialysis.

Preparation

For the first-time peritoneal dialysis patient, explain the purpose of the treatment and what he can expect during and after the procedure. Tell him that first the doctor will insert a catheter into his abdomen to allow instillation of dialyzing solution; explain the appropriate insertion procedure (see *Catheters for Peritoneal Dialysis*, pages 344 and 345).

Before catheter insertion, take and record the patient's baseline vital signs and weight. (Be sure to check blood pressure in both the supine and standing positions.) Ask him to urinate to reduce the risk of bladder perforation and increase comfort during catheter insertion. If he can't urinate, perform straight catheterization, as ordered, to drain the bladder.

While the patient's undergoing peritoneal catheter insertion, warm the dialysate to body temperature in a warmer, heating pad, or water bath. The dialysate may be a 1.5%, 2.5%, or 4.25% dextrose solution, usually with heparin added to prevent clotting in the catheter. The dialysate should be clear and colorless. Add any prescribed medication at this time.

Next, put on a surgical mask and prepare the dialysis administration set. Place the drainage bag below the patient to facilitate gravity drainage, and connect the outflow tubing to it. Then connect the dialysis infusion lines to the bags or bottles of dialyzing solution, and hang the containers on an I.V. pole at the patient's bedside. Maintain sterile technique during solution and equipment preparation to avoid introducing pathogens into the patient's peritoneal cavity during treatment.

When the equipment and solution are ready, place the patient in a supine position, have him put on a surgical mask, and tell him to relax. Prime the tubing with solution, keeping the clamps closed, and connect one infusion line to the abdominal catheter.

To test the catheter's patency, open the clamp on the infusion line and rapidly instill 500 ml of dialyzing solution into the patient's peritoneal cavity. Immediately unclamp the outflow line and let fluid drain into the collection bag; outflow should be brisk. Once you've established catheter patency, you're ready to start dialysis.

Procedure

To begin dialysis, open the clamps on the infusion lines and infuse the prescribed amount of dialyzing solution over a period of 5 to 10 minutes. When the bottle is empty, immediately close the clamps to prevent air from entering the tubing.

Allow the solution to dwell in the peritoneal cavity for the prescribed length of time (usually between 10 minutes and 4 hours) so that excess water, electrolytes, and accumulated wastes can move from the blood through the peritoneal membrane and into the solution. At the completion of the prescribed dwelling time, open the outflow clamps and allow the solution to drain from the peritoneal cavity into the collection bag.

Repeat the infusion-dwell-drainage cycle, using new solution each time, until you've instilled the prescribed amount of solution and completed the prescribed number of cycles. When dialysis is completed, put on sterile gloves and clamp the catheter with a small, sterile plastic clamp. Disconnect the inflow line from the catheter, taking care not to dislodge or pull on the catheter, and place a sterile protective cap over the catheter's distal end. Apply povidone-iodine or antibiotic ointment to the catheter insertion site with a sterile gauze sponge, then place two split-drain sponges around the site and secure them with tape.

Monitoring and aftercare

During dialysis, monitor the patient's vital signs every 10 minutes until they stabilize, then every 2 to 4 hours or as ordered. Report any abrupt or significant changes. Also periodically check the patient's weight and report any gain. Using aseptic technique, change the catheter dressing every 24 hours or whenever it becomes wet or soiled.

CATHETERS FOR PERITONEAL DIALYSIS

The first step in any type of peritoneal dialysis is insertion of a catheter to allow instillation of dialyzing fluid. The surgeon may insert one of three different catheters, as described below.

TENCKHOFF CATHETER

To implant a Tenckhoff catheter, the surgeon inserts the first 6¾ inches (17 cm) of the catheter into the patient's abdomen. The next 2¾-inch (7-cm) segment, which has a Dacron cuff at each end, is imbedded subcutaneously. Within a few days after insertion, the patient's tissues grow around these Dacron cuffs, forming a tight barrier against bacterial infiltration. The remaining 3⅞ inches (10 cm) of the catheter extends outside of the abdomen and is equipped with a metal adapter at the tip to allow connection to dialyzer tubing.

GORE-TEX CATHETER

To insert a Gore-Tex catheter, the surgeon positions its flanged collar just below the dermis so that the device extends through the abdominal wall. He keeps the distal end of the cuff from extending into the peritoneum, where it could cause adhesions.

COLUMN-DISK PERITONEAL CATHETER (CDPC)

To insert a CDPC, the surgeon rolls up the flexible disk section of the implant, inserts it into the peritoneal cavity, and retracts it against the abdominal wall. The implant's first cuff rests just outside the peritoneal membrane, while its second cuff rests just beneath the skin. Because the CDPC doesn't float freely in the peritoneal cavity, it keeps inflowing dialyzing fluid from being directed at sensitive organs—which increases patient comfort during dialysis.

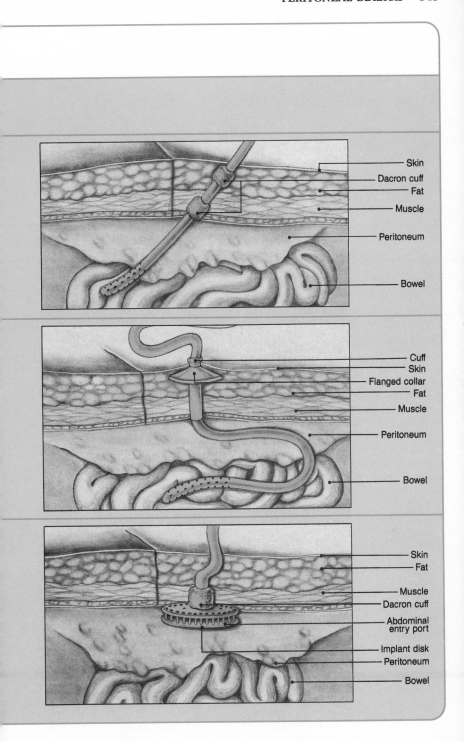

Skin
Dacron cuff
Fat
Muscle

Peritoneum

Bowel

Cuff
Skin
Flanged collar
Fat
Muscle

Peritoneum

Bowel

Skin
Fat

Muscle
Dacron cuff
Abdominal
entry port
Implant disk
Peritoneum
Bowel

Watch closely for developing complications. Peritonitis may be manifested by fever, persistent abdominal pain and cramping, slow or cloudy dialysis drainage, swelling and tenderness around the catheter, and an increased white blood cell count. If you detect these signs and symptoms, notify the doctor and send a dialysate specimen to the laboratory for smear and culture.

Observe the outflow drainage for blood. Keep in mind that drainage is commonly blood-tinged after catheter placement but should clear after a few fluid exchanges. Notify the doctor of bright red or persistent bleeding.

Watch for respiratory distress, which may indicate fluid overload or leakage of dialyzing solution into the pleural space. If it's severe, drain the patient's peritoneal cavity and call the doctor.

To help prevent fluid imbalance, calculate the patient's fluid balance at the end of each dialysis session or after every 8-hour period in a longer session. Include both oral and I.V. fluid intake, as well as urinary output, wound drainage, and perspiration. Record and report any significant imbalance, either positive or negative.

Periodically check the outflow tubing for clots or kinks that may be obstructing drainage. If you cannot clear an obstruction, notify the doctor.

Have the patient change position frequently. Provide passive range-of-motion exercises and encourage deep breathing and coughing. This will improve patient comfort, reduce the chance of skin breakdown and respiratory problems, and enhance dialysate drainage.

Maintain adequate nutrition, following any prescribed diet. Keep in mind that the patient loses protein through the dialysis procedure and so requires protein replacement.

Home care instructions
● If the patient will perform CAPD or CCPD at home, make sure he thoroughly understands and can do each step of the procedure. Normally, he'll go through a 2-week training program before beginning treatment on his own.
● Instruct the patient to wear a Medic Alert bracelet or carry a card identifying him as a dialysis patient. Also tell him to keep the phone number of the dialysis center on hand at all times in case of an emergency.
● Tell the patient to watch for and report signs of infection and fluid imbalance. Make sure he knows how to take his vital signs to provide a record of response to treatment.
● Stress the importance of follow-up appointments with the doctor and dialysis team to evaluate the success of treatment and detect any problems.
● If possible, introduce the patient to other patients on peritoneal dialysis, to help him develop a support system. Arrange for periodic visits by a home care nurse to assess his adjustment to CAPD.

CALCULI REMOVAL OR DESTRUCTION

Calculi Basketing

When ureteral calculi are too large for normal elimination, removal with a basketing instrument represents the treatment of choice, helping to relieve pain and prevent infection and renal dysfunction. In this technique, a basketing instrument is inserted through a cystoscope or ureteroscope into the ureter to capture the calculus and then is withdrawn to remove it.

When performed properly, basketing causes few complications. However, because of the risk of ureteral perforation, basketing is generally contraindicated for a calculus whose diameter exceeds that of the ureteral lumen and for a calculus with extremely sharp or rough edges.

Purpose
To remove obstructing ureteral calculi.

Preparation
Review the procedure with the patient and explain why it's necessary. Prepare him for tests to determine calculi location and renal status. Such tests typically include abdominal X-rays and intravenous pyelography.

Tell the patient that after calculi removal, he'll have an indwelling (Foley) catheter inserted to ensure normal urine drainage. Explain that the catheter probably will remain in place for 24 to 48 hours and that he'll receive I.V. fluids during and immediately after the procedure to maintain urine output and prevent complications, such as hydronephrosis and pyelonephritis.

As ordered, give a broad-spectrum antibiotic to prevent infection.

Procedure
The patient is placed in a lithotomy position on an X-ray table, and a lower

---

UNDERSTANDING CALCULI BASKETING

In this technique for removing ureteral calculi, a basketing instrument housed within a flexible rod (such as a Dormia or a Johnson extractor) is inserted through a cystoscope or ureteroscope into the ureter and advanced to the calculus. Once the apparatus is adjacent to the calculus, the doctor pushes the wire basket through the rod and beyond the calculus, allowing the flexible wires to spread out within the ureter. Then he slowly pulls back the wire basket to capture the calculus. Next, he carefully withdraws the entire apparatus.

EXTRACTOR IN PLACE

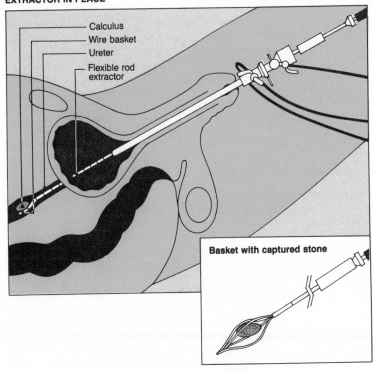

- Calculus
- Wire basket
- Ureter
- Flexible rod extractor

Basket with captured stone

abdominal X-ray is taken to locate the obstructing calculus. A general or spinal anesthetic is then administered, depending on the doctor's preference.

After inserting a cystoscope or ureteroscope into the urethra, the surgeon passes the basketing instrument through the scope, into the ureter, and past the calculus. He then opens the basket to engage the calculus and carefully withdraws the instrument to remove it. (See *Understanding Calculi Basketing*, page 347.)

After calculus removal, the surgeon usually inserts a ureteral catheter or stent into the kidney to drain urine into the bladder. He also inserts a Foley catheter to aid bladder drainage.

The calculus is examined and compared with the X-ray film to determine whether it has been totally removed.

Monitoring and aftercare

After the procedure, monitor the patient's vital signs and intake and output. Promote fluids to maintain a urine output of 3 to 4 liters a day. Observe the color of urine drainage from the Foley catheter; it should be slightly blood-tinged at first, gradually clearing within 24 to 48 hours. However, notify the doctor if frank or persistent hematuria occurs. Irrigate the catheter, as ordered, using sterile technique.

Observe for and report any signs of septicemia, which may result from ureteral perforation during basketing. If you suspect infection, obtain blood and urine samples, as ordered, and send them to the laboratory for analysis. Check drainage from the ureteral catheter, if one is implanted. Keep the catheter taped securely to the patient's thigh to prevent dislodgment or undue traction.

As ordered, administer analgesics to control pain.

Home care instructions

• Teach the patient and his family the importance of following prescribed dietary and medication regimens to prevent recurrence of calculi.

• For the same reason, encourage him to drink 3 to 4 qt of fluid a day, unless contraindicated.

• Advise the patient to take prescribed analgesics, as needed.

• Tell him to immediately report signs and symptoms of recurrent calculi (flank pain, hematuria, nausea, fever, and chills) or acute ureteral obstruction (severe pain and inability to void).

• Encourage regular follow-up examinations to assess for formation of new calculi.

Extracorporeal Shock-Wave Lithotripsy

A revolutionary noninvasive technique for removing obstructive renal calculi, extracorporeal shock-wave lithotripsy (ESWL) uses high-energy shock waves to break up calculi and allow their normal passage. In this treatment, the patient is anesthetized and placed in a water tank. His affected kidney is positioned over an electric spark generator, which creates high-energy shock waves that shatter calculi without damaging surrounding tissue. Afterward, the patient is easily able to excrete the fine gravel-like remains of the calculi.

ESWL may be performed as a preventive measure in a patient with potentially obstructive calculi or as an emergency treatment for an acute obstruction. Because ESWL is noninvasive, the patient usually requires a maximum of only 2 to 3 days in the hospital after treatment and can resume normal activities immediately after discharge. ESWL also minimizes many of the potentially serious complications associated with invasive methods of calculi removal, such as infection and hemorrhage.

ESWL isn't suitable for all patients, however. For instance, it may be contraindicated during pregnancy or in a patient with a pacemaker (because of potential electrical interference), urinary tract obstruction distal to the calculi (which would prevent passage of fragments), renal carcinoma, and calculi that are fixed to the kidney or ureter or located below the level of the iliac crest. Repeat treatments may be necessary for large or multiple calculi.

Purpose
To break obstructive renal calculi into fine, easily eliminated particles.

Preparation
As necessary, review the doctor's explanation of ESWL with the patient. If he has received a preadmission information packet, go over the material with him and answer any questions. Explain who will perform the treatment and where and that it should take 30 minutes to 1 hour. Tell him that he'll receive a general or epidural anesthetic, depending on the doctor's preference, and that the treatment should be painless. Tell the patient that he'll have an I.V. line and indwelling (Foley) catheter in place after ESWL.

If possible, arrange for the patient to see the ESWL device before his first scheduled treatment. Explain its components and how they work.

Procedure
Before undergoing ESWL, the patient receives a general or epidural anesthetic and has an I.V. line and Foley catheter inserted and EKG electrodes attached. He's then placed in a semireclining position on the machine's hydraulic stretcher and lowered into the water tank. In the tank, the patient's position is adjusted so that the shockwave generator focuses directly on the calculi. Biplane fluoroscopy confirms proper positioning.

The generator is then activated to direct high-energy shock waves through the water at the calculi. To prevent disruption of the patient's cardiac rhythm, the shock waves are synchronized to the patient's R waves and fired during diastole. The number of waves fired depends on the size and composition of the stone; the patient may receive 500 to 2,000 shocks during a treatment.

After the shocks are delivered, the patient's removed from the tub and the EKG electrodes are removed.

Monitoring and aftercare
Check the patient's vital signs every 4 hours for the first 24 hours after treatment, then every 8 hours until discharge. Notify the doctor of any abnormal findings

Maintain Foley catheter and I.V. line patency, and closely monitor intake and output. Strain all urine for calculi fragments and send these to the laboratory for analysis. Note urine color and test pH. Remember that slight hematuria normally occurs for several days after ESWL. However, notify the doctor if you detect frank or persistent bleeding.

Encourage ambulation as early as possible after treatment to aid passage of calculi fragments. For the same reason, increase fluid intake, as ordered.

To help remove any particles lodged in gravity-dependent kidney pockets, instruct the patient to lie face down with his head and shoulders over the edge of the bed for about 10 minutes. Have him perform this maneuver twice a day. To enhance its effectiveness, encourage fluids 30 to 45 minutes before starting.

Assess for pain on the treated side, and administer analgesics, as ordered. Keep in mind that severe pain may indicate ureteral obstruction from new calculi; promptly report such findings to the doctor.

Home care instructions
• Instruct the patient to drink 3 to 4 qt of fluid each day for about a month after treatment. Explain that this will aid passage of fragments and help prevent formation of new calculi.
• Teach the patient how to strain his urine for fragments. Tell him to strain all urine for the 1st week after treat-

ment, to save all fragments in the container you've provided, and to bring the container with him on his first follow-up doctor's appointment.

• Discuss expected side effects of ESWL, including pain in the treated side as fragments pass, slight redness or bruising on the treated side, blood-tinged urine for several days after treatment, and mild GI upset. Reassure the patient that these effects are normal and are no cause for concern. However, tell him to report severe unremitting pain, persistent hematuria, inability to void, fever and chills, or recurrent nausea and vomiting.

• Encourage him to resume normal activities, including exercise and work, as soon as he feels able (unless, of course, the doctor instructs otherwise). Explain that physical activity will enhance the passage of calculi fragments.

• Stress the importance of complying with any special dietary or drug regimen designed to reduce the risk of new calculi formation.

Percutaneous Ultrasonic Lithotripsy

In this relatively new lithotripsy technique, an ultrasonic probe inserted through a nephrostomy tube into the renal pelvis generates ultrahigh-frequency sound waves to shatter calculi, while continuous suctioning removes the fragments. Like extracorporeal shock-wave lithotripsy (ESWL), percutaneous ultrasonic lithotripsy (PUL) greatly reduces the patient's recovery time compared to major renal surgery. PUL may be used in place of ESWL or may be performed after it to remove residual fragments. It's particularly useful for radiolucent calculi lodged in the kidney, which aren't treatable by ESWL.

Because PUL is an invasive procedure, it carries many of the risks associated with older lithotripsy methods. Besides possibly causing hemorrhage and infection, it may lead to renal damage from nephrostomy tube insertion and ureteral obstruction from incomplete passage of calculi fragments.

Purpose
To shatter renal calculi and remove their fragments by suction.

Preparation
Explain all facets of the procedure to the patient, including insertion of the nephrostomy tube and the lithotripsy technique. Some doctors prefer to perform PUL in two stages, with nephrostomy tube insertion on the 1st day followed by lithotripsy a day or two later, after intrarenal bleeding has subsided and the calculi can be better visualized. If the doctor has scheduled two-stage PUL, explain this to the patient.

Tell the patient that he may experience discomfort from the nephrostomy tube but otherwise the treatment should be painless. Reassure him that analgesics will be given if needed.

Describe posttreatment care measures, including increased fluid intake, frequent nephrostomy tube irrigations, and straining of urine to capture passed calculi fragments and allow laboratory analysis of their composition. Explain that if no complications develop, he may be discharged 2 to 4 days after treatment.

The day before scheduled treatment, as ordered, prepare the patient for intravenous pyelography or lower abdominal X-rays to locate the calculi. After midnight, withhold all foods and fluids.

Procedure
The patient receives a local or general anesthetic, depending on the surgeon's preference. Then the surgeon establishes a nephrostomy tract with a needle puncture performed under fluoroscopic guidance. He then threads an angiographic wire through the nee-

PERCUTANEOUS ULTRASONIC LITHOTRIPTOR

In percutaneous ultrasonic lithotripsy, the lithotriptor's ultrasonic probe breaks up calculi by vibration and continuously suctions the fragments from the kidney.

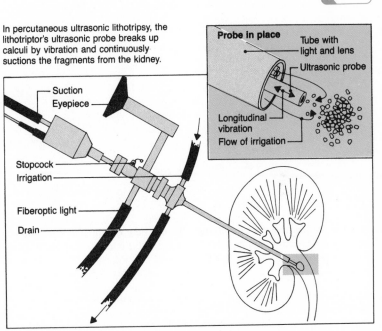

Suction
Eyepiece
Stopcock
Irrigation
Fiberoptic light
Drain

Probe in place
Tube with light and lens
Ultrasonic probe
Longitudinal vibration
Flow of irrigation

dle and passes various-sized nephrostomy tubes over the wire to progressively dilate the tract. When the tract is sufficiently dilated, he removes the tube and inserts a nephroscope to visualize the calculus.

Next (or a day or two later, if PUL is being performed in two stages), the surgeon inserts a working tube resembling a small cystoscope through the nephrostomy tract and into the kidney's collecting system. He then passes an ultrasonic probe through the tube and positions it against the calculus. When the probe's in position, he turns on the device, producing ultrahigh-frequency sound waves that shatter the calculus into fragments. He then uses suction or, if necessary, irrigation or a basketing instrument to remove the fragments.

Once treatment is complete, the sur-

geon withdraws the probe and the working tube. Then he reinserts the nephrostomy tube.

Monitoring and aftercare

After treatment, check the volume of nephrostomy tube drainage hourly for the first 24 hours and then every 4 hours or so thereafter. Report absent or decreased drainage, which could indicate obstruction from retained calculi fragments. Also note urine color and test pH. Keep in mind that slight hematuria occurs normally for several days after PUL. However, if you detect frank or persistent bleeding, notify the doctor. Strain all urine for calculi and send any fragments to the laboratory for analysis.

Assess the patient for pain and administer analgesics, as needed. Keep in mind that severe pain accompanied by decreased drainage may indicate obstruction from unremoved fragments; promptly report such findings to the doctor. Also watch for and report signs of hemorrhage or infection.

As ordered, gently irrigate the nephrostomy tube to ensure its patency. Maintain sterile technique and use no more than 10 ml of normal saline solution. Never clamp the tube; the resultant pressure increase could cause renal damage.

To aid passage of retained calculi fragments and hinder formation of new calculi, maintain the patient on high fluid intake—up to 4,000 ml a day, as ordered. For the same reason, encourage early ambulation.

A day or two after treatment, prepare the patient for nephrotomography to check for retained fragments. If no fragments are revealed, the doctor usually will remove the nephrostomy tube. Occasionally a patient will be discharged with the tube in place.

Home care instructions
• Instruct the patient to drink 3 to 4 qt (or liters) of fluid each day for about a month after treatment. Explain that this will aid passage of any unremoved calculi fragments and help prevent formation of new calculi.
• Tell him to promptly report persistent bloody or cloudy, foul-smelling urine, an inability to void, fever and chills, or severe, unremitting flank pain. He should also report redness, swelling, or purulent drainage from the nephrostomy tube insertion site.
• Teach the patient how to strain his urine for calculi fragments. Tell him to strain all urine for the 1st week after treatment, to save all fragments in the container you've provided, and to bring the container with him on his first follow-up doctor's appointment.
• Encourage him to avoid strenuous exercise, sexual activity, heavy lifting, or straining until his doctor instructs otherwise. Do, however, encourage him to take short walks as he's able. Explain

that mild physical activity will help aid passage of any retained calculi fragments.
• Review with the patient any prescribed dietary or drug regimen to help prevent formation of new calculi.
• If the patient is discharged with a nephrostomy tube in place, outline proper tube care.

BLADDER MANAGEMENT

Bladder Training

A conservative treatment for managing incontinence resulting from neurologic or mechanical dysfunction, bladder training attempts to teach the patient how to empty the bladder and minimize urinary retention. Several techniques can be used in such a program, including continuous catheterization, perineal muscle–strengthening exercises, and even biofeedback training. Most bladder-training programs currently center around teaching the patient to perform intermittent self-catheterization at home.

Almost any patient with some degree of manual dexterity can learn to perform self-catheterization. However, this technique isn't suitable for the patient who demonstrates an inability or unwillingness to care for himself.

Purpose
To correct incontinence.

Preparation
Tell the patient that periodic self-catheterization is necessary to drain urine from his bladder, preventing complications from urinary retention, such as infection and incontinence. Explain all aspects of self-catheterization. Tell him that after washing his hands and

cleansing the urinary meatus and surrounding area, he'll insert the catheter into the urethra and advance it into the bladder until urine begins to drain. After all urine has drained into the measuring container, he'll slowly remove the catheter and wash, rinse, and dry it before storing it for subsequent use. Then he'll carefully record the amount of urine drainage, noting the date and time and any unusual characteristics, such as strong odor or discoloration.

The patient may feel uneasy and possibly overwhelmed by the prospect of self-catheterization. Reassure him that you'll demonstrate the procedure and assist him as necessary until he can confidently perform it himself.

Now, gather all the necessary equipment: a straight catheter (preferably clear plastic), a graduated measuring container, a catheter insertion tray, sterile gloves (for sterile technique only), and a hand-held mirror (to help the female patient visualize the urinary meatus).

Procedure

Have the patient attempt to void. If necessary, use Credé's maneuver to promote urination.

Next, have the patient assume a comfortable position suitable for catheterization. A male patient may sit on the edge of the bed or on the toilet. A female patient may find a semireclining position with her knees flexed more effective. Remember to consider the patient's need for privacy.

With the patient positioned comfortably, perform straight catheterization, using sterile technique. As you do so, thoroughly explain each step to the patient, encouraging questions. Go through the entire catheter insertion and removal process, including recording the amount and characteristics of drainage and cleaning and storing the equipment.

Next, have the patient try self-catheterization. Provide assistance and reassurance, as necessary, to prevent him from becoming discouraged by clumsy or unsuccessful initial attempts. Encourage deep breathing and other relaxation methods to aid passage of the catheter.

Monitoring and aftercare

Have the patient perform self-catheterization until he can master the technique. Provide positive reinforcement after each successful attempt.

To help devise an optimum catheterization schedule, measure and record urine output after each catheterization. Typically, the output from each catheterization should be between 100 and 300 ml. If output is consistently less than 100 ml, increase the interval between catheterizations; if it's more than 300 ml, decrease the interval.

Observe for and report signs of urinary tract infection, including a low-grade fever and blood or pus in the urine. Begin antibiotic therapy, if ordered.

Assess the patient's emotional status. In particular, watch for frustration, anger, or depression. If appropriate, suggest psychological counseling to help him learn to cope with such feelings.

Home care instructions

• Make sure the patient thoroughly understands and can perform self-catheterization. Give him written instructions. Also, remember to provide him with a list of local stores where he can purchase the necessary supplies.
• Explain the direct relationship between fluid intake and urine output. Instruct the patient not to drink anything after his evening meal to reduce nocturnal urinary retention and delay the need for catheterization until the morning.
• Tell him to promptly report any signs of urinary tract infection.
• Remind the patient to take extra catheterization equipment with him on extended trips, including antiseptic premoistened towelettes in case washing facilities aren't available.

Catheterization

The insertion of a drainage device into the urinary bladder, catheterization may be intermittent or continuous.

Intermittent catheterization drains urine remaining in the bladder after voiding. It may be used postoperatively and for patients with urinary incontinence, urethral strictures, cystitis, prostatic obstruction, neurogenic bladder, or other disorders that interfere with bladder emptying. In this technique, a nurse inserts a sterile straight catheter through the urethra into the bladder, leaves it in place only long enough to drain residual urine, and withdraws it when urine flow stops.

An indwelling catheter (also known as a Foley or retention catheter) is inserted in the same manner as a straight catheter but is left in the bladder for continuous drainage of urine. After catheter insertion, a balloon at the proximal end is inflated to secure the catheter in place.

Indwelling catheterization helps relieve bladder distention caused by such conditions as urinary tract obstruction and neurogenic bladder. It also allows continuous urinary drainage in patients with a urinary meatus swollen from surgery, local trauma, or childbirth. What's more, indwelling catheterization can provide accurate monitoring of urine output when normal voiding is impaired.

Purpose
• To relieve urinary retention
• To provide postoperative urine drainage
• To obtain a urine sample for laboratory analysis
• To allow accurate measurement of urine output.

Preparation
Thoroughly review the procedure with the patient. Tell him that you'll insert a slender tube into the urinary meatus and advance it through the urethra and into the bladder. As appropriate, explain that the urine will drain into a measuring container or into a collection bag. If indwelling catheterization is scheduled, tell him that drainage tubing will be taped to his abdomen or thigh to hold the catheter in place.

Reassure the patient that although catheterization may produce slight discomfort, it shouldn't be painful. Explain that you'll stop the procedure if he experiences severe discomfort.

Assemble the necessary equipment. If possible, use a prepackaged sterile catheterization kit (preferably a closed-type system, with a preconnected catheter and dependent drainage bag, to minimize the risk of urinary tract infection). If you can't use a kit, gather the following equipment: a sterile indwelling catheter (latex or silicone #10 to #22 French, as ordered); a sterile syringe filled with 5 to 8 ml of sterile normal saline solution; a washcloth, towel, and soap and water; two linen-saver pads; a sterile plain drape and fenestrated drape; sterile gloves; povidone-iodine or other sterile cleansing solution; sterile cotton-tipped applicators (or cotton balls and plastic forceps); sterile water-soluble lubricant; a urine receptacle or sterile drainage collection bag; adhesive tape or a catheter tube holder; and a light source.

If possible, arrange for another nurse to assist you with the procedure.

Procedure
Ensure privacy for the patient and adequate lighting to provide maximum visualization of the urinary meatus. Place the female patient in the supine position, with her knees flexed and separated and her feet flat on the bed. If she finds this position uncomfortable, have her flex only one knee and keep the other leg flat on the bed. Position the male patient supine with his legs flat and extended. Instruct the patient to maintain this position throughout the procedure and to relax.

Thoroughly cleanse the patient's genitalia and perineum with soap and water, if necessary. Dry the area, then wash your hands.

Place the linen-saver pads between the patient's legs and tuck them under the hips. To create a sterile field, open the prepackaged kit and place it between the patient's legs. Put on the sterile gloves. Slide the plain drape under the patient's hips and place the fenestrated drape over the patient's lower abdomen and thighs so that only the genitals are exposed. Be careful not to contaminate your sterile gloves.

Carefully inspect the catheter; a roughened or cracked catheter can injure the delicate urethral mucosa during insertion, predisposing the patient to urinary tract infection. If you're inserting a Foley catheter, inflate the balloon tip with 8 to 10 ml of sterile water or normal saline solution and check for leaks. If you don't detect any leaks, withdraw the fluid to deflate the balloon, leaving the syringe attached to the catheter's inflation port.

Next, lubricate the catheter tip and 2″ to 3 ″ (5 to 7.6 cm) of the shaft with water-soluble lubricant. Place the lubricated catheter in the bottom of the sterile tray. Open the packet of cleansing solution and saturate the cotton balls or applicators with it, taking care not to spill any solution on the equipment.

If you're catheterizing a female patient, expose the urinary meatus by separating the labia majora and labia minora with the thumb and forefinger of one hand. (Be sure to keep the labia well separated throughout the procedure so that they do not fall back into position and obscure the meatus or contaminate the insertion site once it's cleansed.) With your free hand, pick up a saturated cotton-tipped applicator (or use plastic forceps to grasp a saturated cotton ball) and wipe one side of the urinary meatus in a single downward stroke. Wipe the other side of the meatus and then the meatus itself in the same manner, using a new applicator or cotton ball each time. During this cleansing procedure, take care not to contaminate your sterile glove; if you do, be sure to change the glove before proceeding.

If you're catheterizing a male patient, grasp his penis in your nondominant hand. If he's uncircumcised, gently retract the foreskin to expose the urinary meatus. With your free hand, use a saturated cotton-tipped applicator or a cotton ball held in forceps to cleanse the glans penis. Clean in a circular motion, starting from the meatus and working outward. Then repeat the cleansing procedure with a new applicator or cotton ball, taking care not to contaminate your glove.

Once cleansing is complete, you're ready to insert the catheter. Pick up the catheter with your free hand, holding it about 3″ (7.6 cm) from the tip, and carefully insert it into the urinary meatus. To aid insertion, ask the patient to cough as you do this. (Coughing temporarily relaxes the urinary sphincter.)

Slowly advance the catheter into the urethra—about 3″ for a female patient and 6″ to 7″ (15 to 18 cm) for a male, or until urine begins to flow. As you do so, instruct the patient to relax and breathe deeply and slowly to further relax the sphincter and prevent spasms. To aid insertion in the male patient, gently stretch and straighten the penis to create slight traction and then elevate it to an angle of 60 to 90 degrees to straighten the urethra. After urine starts to flow, replace an uncircumsized male's foreskin to prevent swelling and compromised circulation.

Remember to never force the catheter forward during insertion—if you encounter resistance, gently maneuver the catheter while the patient coughs. If you still meet resistance, stop the procedure and notify the doctor, who may have to insert the catheter using size-graduated dilating instruments.

If you're draining residual urine, collect the urine in a measuring container. When urine flow stops, slowly withdraw the catheter, taking care to main-

COMPLICATIONS

COMBATING CATHETER PROBLEMS

What should you do if your patient's indwelling (Foley) catheter won't drain? Here are some tips to help you find the cause of poor drainage and correct the problem.

First, help the patient into a different position—one that promotes drainage by the force of gravity. Then have him cough and bear down slightly. Often, this will be enough to clear the obstruction.

However, if the obstruction persists, you may need to irrigate the catheter. (Be sure to obtain the doctor's permission before you perform irrigation.) To do so, clamp the drainage tubing behind the catheter's sampling port, then inject 30 to 100 ml of sterile normal saline solution through the port. Now unclamp the tubing to allow the saline solution to flow back through the catheter, and check for clearing. *Caution*: Don't inject more than 100 ml of irrigating solution at one time to avoid painful bladder distention.

Next, check catheter placement to ensure that the balloon tip is still in the bladder. Gently push on the catheter to see if you can move it into the bladder, then pull back slightly to seat the balloon in the bladder. If obstruction is still present, notify the doctor, who may order insertion of a new catheter.

pull back on the catheter until you meet slight resistance. This seats the balloon correctly in the bladder.

Position the collection bag below bladder level to enhance drainage and prevent urine reflux into the bladder, which can cause infection.

Finally, secure the catheter in position to prevent traction on the bladder and maintain normal direction of urine flow. Tape or strap the catheter to a female patient's thigh to prevent tension in the urogenital area. In males, secure the catheter to the thigh or lower abdomen. Attaching it to the lower abdomen prevents pressure on the urethra at the penoscrotal junction, which can cause formation of urethrocutaneous fistulae.

Monitoring and aftercare

During catheterization, note the difficulty or ease of insertion, any patient discomfort, and the amount and nature of urine drainage. Document this information, and notify the doctor if you observe hematuria or extremely foul-smelling or cloudy urine. During urine drainage, monitor the patient for pallor, diaphoresis, and painful bladder spasms. If these occur, clamp the catheter tubing and call the doctor.

To ensure proper drainage, maintain proper position of the drainage system. Coil the tubing on the bed and secure it to the bedsheet with a safety pin (taking care, of course, not to puncture the tube). Ensure that the tubing remains free of kinks. Keep the collection bag at a level lower than the patient's bladder, taking care that it doesn't come in contact with the floor.

Maintain good catheter care throughout the course of treatment. Cleanse the urinary meatus and catheter junction at least daily, more often if you note buildup of exudate. Expect a small amount of mucous drainage at the catheter insertion site from irritation of the urethral wall, but notify the doctor of excessive, bloody, or purulent drainage.

Frequently assess the patient's intake

tain sterile technique.

If you've inserted a Foley catheter, also collect the urine in a measuring container. But when the urine stops flowing, use the saline-filled syringe to inflate the catheter's balloon tip and keep the catheter in place within the bladder. *Caution*: Never inflate the balloon until you've established urine flow to ensure that you've inserted the catheter into the bladder and not left it in the urethral channel. If you can't elicit urine flow, palpate the bladder to check whether it's empty. If the bladder is empty, make sure you've advanced the catheter at least 6″ to 7″ before inflating the balloon, to avoid any injury to the urethra.

After inflating the balloon, gently

and output. Encourage fluids (up to 3,000 ml/day, if necessary) to maintain continuous urine flow through the catheter and decrease the risk of infection and clot formation. Note the color and amount of urine drainage; dark, concentrated urine may indicate the need for increased fluid intake.

To help prevent infection, avoid separating the catheter and tubing unless absolutely necessary. Use the collection port to secure specimens and instill medications. However, if you must separate the catheter and the tubing, maintain strict asepsis and wipe the connection with an antiseptic solution before and after the procedure.

Throughout treatment, remain alert for signs of urinary tract infection, including low-grade fever, possibly with chills; meatal or scrotal swelling and tenderness; flank pain; and cloudy, foul-smelling urine. Report these signs to the doctor, and prepare to take samples for culture and sensitivity testing.

Monitor for signs of catheter obstruction. Watch for decreased or absent urine output (less than 30 ml/hour); severe, persistent bladder spasms; urine leakage around the catheter insertion site; and bladder distention. If you suspect obstruction, try to clear it yourself (see *Combating Catheter Problems*); if you're unsuccessful, promptly notify the doctor.

Home care instructions

● Instruct the patient to drink at least 2 qt (or liters) of water a day, unless the doctor orders otherwise.
● Teach the patient how to minimize the risk of infection by performing daily periurethral care.
● Stress the need for thorough handwashing before and after handling the catheter and collection system.
● If the patient has an indwelling catheter, ensure that he knows how to secure the tubing and the leg bag. Tell him to alternate legs every other day to prevent skin irritation. As appropriate, teach him how to switch from the leg bag to the closed-system drainage bag for nighttime use. Instruct him to keep the leg bag or closed-system drainage bag lower than the level of the bladder to facilitate drainage. Explain that he should empty the bag when it's about half-full, and teach him how to empty it. Also demonstrate how to apply a new bag.
● Tell the patient that he may take showers but should avoid tub baths while the catheter's in place.
● Instruct the patient to notify the doctor if he notices urine leakage around the catheter. Also instruct him to report any signs of urinary tract infection, such as fever, chills, flank or urinary tract pain, and cloudy or foul-smelling urine.

Selected References

Abrams, J. *Abdominal Stomas.* Boston: PSG Pub. Co., 1984.

Brenner, B., and Rector, F., eds. *The Kidney,* 2 vols., 2nd ed. Philadelphia: W.B. Saunders Co., 1981.

Cubler, A.J., and Whalen-Myers, M.A. "Ureteroscopy: Using Endoscopes for Ureterolithotripsy," *AORN Journal* 42(6):853-58, December 1985.

Glenn, J. *Urologic Surgery,* 3rd ed. Philadelphia: J.B. Lippincott Co., 1983.

Hanno, P., and Wein, A. *A Clinical Manual of Urology.* East Norwalk, Conn.: Appleton & Lange, 1987.

McConnell, E., and Zimmerman, M. *Care of Patients with Urologic Problems.* Philadelphia: J.B. Lippincott Co., 1982.

Richard, C. *Comprehensive Nephrology Nursing.* Boston: Little, Brown & Co., 1986.

Smith, D. *General Urology,* 11th ed. East Norwalk, Conn.: Appleton & Lange, 1984.

Young, M. "Lithotripsy: A Revolutionary Technique with Implications for Nursing Care," *Journal of Nephrology Nursing* 3(1):34-41, January/February 1986.

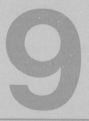

9 Treating Obstetric and Gynecologic Dysfunction

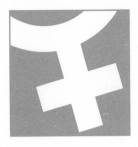

Treating Obstetric and Gynecologic Dysfunction

Introduction

To provide effective obstetric and gynecologic care, you'll need an in-depth knowledge of current drug therapy, surgery, and related treatments. What's more, you'll need a clear understanding of the social and psychological aspects of women's health. After all, any treatment that affects reproductive or sexual function may lead to feelings of embarrassment, vulnerability, and even guilt and disillusionment in your patient. That's an important reason for you to maintain a supportive, nonjudgmental attitude toward your patient—whether she's undergoing dilatation and evacuation or artificial insemination.

Drug therapy

Drugs provide the core treatment for many gynecologic problems. For instance, naproxen and other nonsteroidal anti-inflammatory drugs help treat dysmenorrhea. Progestins help manage dysfunctional uterine bleeding, and estrogens treat a wide range of disorders associated with estrogen deficiency. Fertility agents, such as clomiphene, can provide new hope for a childless couple. And uterine relaxants may correct cervical incompetence, thereby sparing a fetus from premature delivery.

Despite the benefits these drugs may have, their effects require close monitoring. Estrogens, for example, can lead to thromboembolic disorders, especially if the patient smokes.

Surgery

Gynecologic surgery may leave the patient with disfigurement or an altered body image. As a result, you'll need to provide strong emotional support and give her the opportunity to express her concerns. For example, you'll need to help the mastectomy patient express her feelings about changes in her appearance and sexual image, social isolation, tumor recurrence, and death.

In obstetric surgeries, such as cesarean section, you'll need to provide vigilant monitoring to prevent complications, such as maternal bleeding and fetal respiratory depression.

Treating infertility

Artificial insemination proves emotionally taxing for the patient and her spouse. By the time treatment is attempted, the couple has typically undergone unpleasant and sometimes uncomfortable tests and procedures to identify the problem and attempt to correct it.

To help the childless couple, provide ongoing emotional support. Be realistic, though, about the prospects of pregnancy. Unfounded expectations can prove especially damaging.

Nonsteroidal Anti-Inflammatory Drugs

In treating obstetric and gynecologic conditions, nonsteroidal anti-inflammatory drugs (NSAIDs) are used primarily for their analgesic and anti-inflammatory effects. NSAIDS, such as *naproxen* and *ibuprofen,* relieve mild to moderate pain in primary dysmenorrhea, in premenstrual syndrome, and after episiotomy. Because NSAIDS have different chemical structures, they vary in their onset of action, duration of effect, and method of metabolism and excretion. As a result, the selection of a specific NSAID depends on the patient's response.

The chief side effects of NSAIDS include GI irritation, hepatotoxicity, nephrotoxicity, and headache. These drugs are contraindicated in hypersensitivity to other anti-inflammatory drugs, in pregnancy, and in peptic ulcer. They should be used cautiously in patients with renal or hepatic impairment. Naproxen sodium should be used cautiously in patients with restricted sodium intake.

Purpose and action
NSAIDs are thought to relieve pain by inhibiting prostaglandin synthesis. Prostaglandins appear to stimulate uterine hyperactivity, thus causing pain.

Monitoring
Before administering NSAIDS, check the patient's history for previous hypersensitivity reactions to other NSAIDS and for any disorders that may contraindicate use of these drugs.

During therapy, ask the patient about GI side effects, such as nausea, diarrhea, or tarry stools. Also ask about CNS effects, such as headache, drowsiness, and dizziness, and renal effects, such as hematuria and dysuria. If any of these untoward effects occur, report them to the doctor. He'll probably reduce the dosage.

Check for edema and elevated blood pressure, especially in hypertensive patients; NSAIDS may cause sodium or fluid retention. In long-term therapy, monitor renal and liver function studies, complete blood count, and prothrombin time. Notify the doctor of any abnormalities.

Also assess the patient for visual disturbances or rash.

Home care instructions
- Instruct the patient to take the drug with meals or milk to help prevent GI upset.
- Warn her to avoid driving or operating machinery until she knows her response to the drug. Tell her the drug may cause drowsiness or dizziness.
- If the patient misses a dose, advise her to take it as soon as she remembers. However, if the next dose is less than 4 hours away, she should skip the missed dose and return to her regular schedule. She shouldn't double-dose.
- Tell the patient to notify the doctor immediately if she experiences GI upset, visual disturbances, rash, unexplained weight gain, or swollen ankles or feet.
- Tell her to avoid alcohol while she's taking the drug because it may increase the risk of GI ulcers and bleeding.

Progestins

The progestins, the natural hormone progesterone and its synthetic derivatives, transform a proliferative endometrium into a secretory one. They also inhibit the release of pituitary gonadotropins, which in turn prevents follicular maturation and ovulation. What's more, the progestins inhibit spontaneous uterine contraction and may demonstrate some estrogenic, anabolic, or androgenic activity.

Progestins effectively treat gynecologic conditions that respond to changes in the body's steroid hormone balance. In menstrual disorders caused by hormonal imbalance, *hydroxyprogesterone*, *progesterone* (both given I.M.), or *norethindrone* (given orally) can induce a normal menstrual cycle. These drugs can also be given to stop dysfunctional uterine bleeding arising from a hyperplastic, nonsecreting endometrium. In addition, norethindrone helps treat endometriosis and progesterone suppositories help treat premenstrual syndrome. *Norgestrel*, used as a contraceptive drug, isn't as commonly prescribed as estrogen-progesterone combinations because of its higher incidence of breakthrough bleeding and pregnancy. However, it may be used in patients in whom estrogens are contraindicated.

Because progesterone is relatively inactive in its oral form, the synthetic progestins are more commonly prescribed. In varying degrees, their effects are similar to those of progesterone.

The chief side effects of progestins include breakthrough bleeding, spotting, changes in menstrual flow, amenorrhea, edema, and weight loss or gain. Progestins can also produce cholestatic jaundice, pruritic or nonpruritic rash, acne, chloasma, depression, breast tenderness or discharge, alopecia, hirsutism, and changes in the cervix, such as erosion and abnormal secretions.

Progestins are contraindicated in patients with thrombophlebitis, thromboembolic disorders, cerebral hemorrhage, or impaired liver function. They're also contraindicated in known or suspected breast cancer, cancer of the genitalia, undiagnosed vaginal bleeding, or missed abortion. In addition, the synthetic progestins shouldn't be used during the first 4 months of pregnancy.

Progestins should be used cautiously in diabetes mellitus, seizure disorders, migraine headache, cardiac or renal disease, asthma, or mental illness.

Purpose and action

Progestins help correct menstrual disorders and dysfunctional uterine bleeding by balancing the effects of estrogen in the menstrual cycle. They inhibit the release of luteinizing hormone from the anterior pituitary, inducing secretory changes in the endometrium, relaxing uterine smooth muscle, and thickening cervical mucus. They also reduce the probability of follicular maturation and ovulation by suppressing secretion of pituitary gonadotropins.

Monitoring

Before administering progestins, check the patient's history for hypersensitivity to these drugs or for disorders that may contraindicate their use. Give I.M. injections of progestins deep in the gluteal muscle, and watch for sterile abscess formation.

Because progestins can cause emboli, you'll need to be alert for calf tenderness, dyspnea, pleuritic pain, visual disturbances, or paresthesias. Also observe and palpate the patient's breasts for any changes.

Home care instructions

• Instruct the patient to immediately report severe or sudden headache, loss of coordination, slurred speech, visual changes, and severe depression or irritability. She should also report pain in her chest, groin, or legs or any shortness of breath, especially if it's not related to exertion.

• Tell her to report menorrhagia, metrorrhagia, or absence of bleeding for 45 or more days.

• Advise the patient to take the drug after meals to reduce GI upset.

• If she smokes, warn her that smoking

increases the risk of thromboembolic disorders; encourage her to stop.
• Teach her how to perform breast self-examination. Suggest that she do this monthly and report any abnormalities.
• Ensure that the patient knows the signs of pregnancy, and tell her to return to her doctor for a pregnancy test if she suspects she's pregnant, since progestins can harm the fetus.
• If the patient is taking mini-pill progestins as a contraceptive, instruct her to take the pill every day at about the same time to maintain an effective blood level of the drug.

If she misses a dose, she should take it as soon as she remembers and should take the next pill according to her regular schedule. Advise her to use an alternate method of contraception (such as a contraceptive foam, with her partner wearing a condom) whenever she misses a dose. If she misses two doses, she should take only one of the missed pills, then resume her regular schedule and use an alternate method of contraception until her next period.
• Instruct her to inform other health care providers that she's taking progestins. Tell her to make an appointment every 6 to 12 months for a pelvic and breast examination and a Papanicolaou test.

Estrogens

Estrogens refer to naturally occurring hormones or to synthetic steroidal and nonsteroidal compounds that possess estrogenic activity. The steroidal estrogens include the natural estrogens, such as *estradiol, conjugated and esterified estrogens*, and the semisynthetic estrogen *ethinyl estradiol*. The nonsteroidal estrogens include *chlorotrianisene, dienestrol, diethylstilbestrol*, and *quinestrol*.

Natural and synthetic estrogens help treat a wide variety of conditions associated with endogenous estrogen deficiency, such as female hypogonadism, primary ovarian failure, vasomotor symptoms in menopause, atrophic vaginitis, and kraurosis vulvae. Conjugated estrogens also help treat abnormal uterine bleeding caused by hormonal imbalance. Short-acting forms of these synthetic agents are used together with increased calcium intake and physical therapy to retard bone loss and the progression of osteoporosis in postmenopausal patients. Longer-acting preparations help treat breast cancer (see Chapter 13, "Treating Cancer," for details on these estrogens). The synthetic estrogen diethylstilbestrol provides postcoital contraception.

Estrogens are administered orally, parenterally, intravaginally, or topically. Short-acting oral and parenteral forms are typically used for cyclic replacement therapy (3 weeks on and 1 week off the drug, for example).

Estrogens can cause side effects in most body systems. What's more, these drugs are contraindicated in patients with thrombophlebitis, thromboembolic disorders, or abnormal or undiagnosed vaginal bleeding. They should be used cautiously in patients with hypertension, gallbladder disease, blood dyscrasias, migraine headaches, seizure disorders, diabetes mellitus, amenorrhea, heart failure, hepatic or renal dysfunction, or a family history of breast or genital tract cancer.

Purpose and action
Estrogens restore normal hormonal balance by replacing absent or deficient endogenous hormones. As oral contraceptives, in combination with progestins, estrogens suppress anterior pituitary secretion of gonadotropins through a negative feedback mechanism. They slow the progress of osteoporosis by increasing calcium deposition in the bone.

Monitoring
Before giving estrogens, review the patient's history for any disorders that may contraindicate their use. During

administration, you'll need to be alert for numerous side effects. These may include headache, dizziness, hypertension, edema, thromboembolism, nausea, or worsening of myopia or astigmatism. The patient may also experience increased appetite, hyperglycemia, acne, and breast tenderness and enlargement. You'll also need to watch for changes in vaginal bleeding patterns, such as amenorrhea, spotting, or breakthrough or persistent bleeding.

If you're administering the drug I.M., give the injection slowly and deeply into a large muscle, such as the upper outer quadrant of the buttock.

Home care instructions

• Review the package insert with the patient and answer any questions she may have.

• Instruct her to seek emergency treatment immediately if she experiences sudden or severe headache, sudden loss of coordination or change in vision, pains in her chest, groin, or leg (especially her calf), shortness of breath, sudden slurring of speech, or weakness or numbness in an arm or leg.

• Advise her to report swollen ankles or feet, changes in vaginal bleeding, breast lumps or discharge, abdominal or flank pain, rash, yellowing of her skin or eyes, or dark urine.

• Suggest that she take the drug with food if she develops nausea during the first few weeks of therapy. Explain that nausea usually disappears with continued therapy.

• Instruct her to take a missed dose as soon as she remembers. However, tell her to stop taking the drug and to check with her doctor if she suspects she's pregnant.

• If the patient is using the transdermal form of estradiol, instruct her to apply the patch to a clean section of her abdomen (but not to her breasts or to any areas where the patch might be rubbed loose). Tell her to apply the patch to a different area each day and to wait for at least a week before she applies the patch in the same area.

• If she's receiving cyclic therapy for postmenopausal symptoms, explain that withdrawal bleeding may occur during the week off the drug but that she can't become pregnant.

• If the patient smokes, encourage her to stop. Warn her that smoking during estrogen therapy increases the risk of serious cardiovascular effects, especially if she's over age 35.

• Teach her how to perform a breast

self-examination. Advise her to perform this examination monthly and to report any abnormalities to the doctor.
• Instruct the patient to schedule a yearly pelvic and breast examination and a Papanicolaou test.

Fertility Drugs

Used to stimulate ovulation in an anovulatory patient who wishes to become pregnant, fertility drugs include clomiphene, menotropins, and human chorionic gonadotropin. The synthetic steroid *clomiphene,* the fertility drug of choice, enhances secretion of follicle-stimulating hormone (FSH) and luteinizing hormone (LH), which stimulate follicular maturation in the ovary. Drug dosages may begin at 50 mg/day, increasing up to 250 mg/day if ovulation doesn't occur. Typically, ovulation occurs 4 to 10 days after the last day of treatment.

If clomiphene fails to induce ovulation after three trials, *menotropins* (human menopausal gonadotropin) and *human chorionic gonadotropin* (HCG) may be given. Menotropins must be used with HCG to stimulate ovulation, which should occur within 18 hours after administration. HCG may also be used 7 to 10 days after clomiphene therapy.

The use of fertility drugs may lead to multiple births. The incidence varies from 5% with clomiphene to 20% with HCG.

Fertility drugs are contraindicated in undiagnosed vaginal bleeding, fibroid tumors, ovarian cysts, hepatic dysfunction, or thrombophlebitis. They should be used cautiously in patients with asthma, seizure disorders, or heart disease.

Purpose and action
• *For clomiphene:* To stimulate follicular maturation in the ovary. It achieves this effect by acting on the hypothalamic-pituitary axis to enhance secretion of FSH and LH.
• *For menotropins:* To promote growth and maturation of ovarian follicles by mimicking the action of FSH and LH.
• *For HCG:* To stimulate ovulation of a menotropins-prepared follicle by serving as a substitute for LH. (See *How Fertility Drugs Work.*)

Monitoring
Starting 1 week after treatment begins, measure estrogen levels daily to help detect excessive ovarian stimulation. In addition, the doctor may perform a pelvic examination to evaluate ovarian size when estrogen levels begin to rise. Enlargement indicates excessive ovarian stimulation, requiring a decreased dosage or discontinuation of the drug for several days to weeks with a dosage reduction during the next course of therapy.

Be alert for and report signs of severe ovarian hyperstimulation, such as ascites, pleural effusion, electrolyte imbalance, and hypovolemia with oliguria and hypotension. Also be alert for signs of mild ovarian hyperstimulation, such as abdominal distention and weight gain.

Home care instructions
• Instruct the patient to immediately report bloating or abdominal pain, indicating excessive ovarian stimulation.
• Inform her that the fertility drugs may cause visual difficulties, dizziness, or light-headedness. Tell her to avoid driving until she knows how she responds to the drug.
• Advise her that the possibility of multiple births increases if she becomes pregnant while taking a fertility drug.
• Instruct the patient to take a missed dose as soon as she remembers or to double the dose if she doesn't remember until the time of her next dose. Tell her to inform the doctor if she misses more than one dose.
• Reinforce the importance of having intercourse as the doctor prescribes (usually every day or every other day

HOW FERTILITY DRUGS WORK

In the anovulatory patient, the fertility drug *clomiphene* binds to estrogenic receptors, thereby decreasing the number of available estrogenic receptors. A false signal is sent to the hypothalamus and pituitary gland that estrogen levels are low, and they respond by increasing the secretion of luteinizing hormone (LH), follicle-stimulating hormone (FSH), and gonadotropins. In this hormonal environment, the ovarian follicle matures and ovulation occurs.

If clomiphene fails to induce ovulation, *menotropins* may be administered. This drug mimics the effects of FSH by stimulating ovarian follicular growth and development; however, its LH effects aren't sufficient to stimulate ovulation. For ovulation to occur, *human chorionic gonadotropin* (HCG) must be given after menotropins has stimulated the follicle. HCG substitutes for LH, contributing to follicular growth and maturation, thereby triggering ovulation.

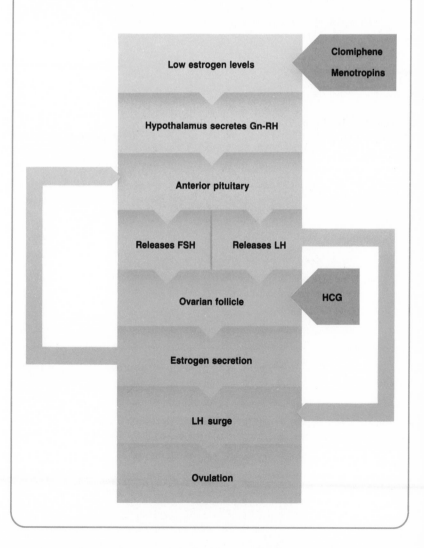

during the patient's fertile period).
• Teach her to take her basal body temperature and to chart it on a graph. Suggest that she also use an ovulatory predictor test kit.
• Explain the importance of keeping follow-up appointments so that her response to therapy can be monitored.
• Instruct the patient to bring a first-morning urine specimen for testing at each follow-up visit.
• Tell her that the first course of treatment is usually effective. However, if she doesn't become pregnant, the doctor may try another course of therapy.

Uterine Relaxants

The beta agonists *ritodrine*, *terbutaline*, and *isoxsuprine* relax uterine muscles to suppress premature labor. These relaxants are used when conservative treatments, such as hydration or bed rest, fail to halt contractions. Specifically, they're used when diagnosis of premature labor is certain, gestation is less than 34 weeks, the cervix is dilated less than 4 cm, and no contraindications exist for their use.

Currently, only ritodrine has Food and Drug Administration approval for inhibiting preterm labor. However, terbutaline was used before the introduction of ritodrine, and it's still preferred by some doctors. Both drugs prove equally effective and cause similar side effects. In contrast, isoxsuprine causes more frequent and severe cardiovascular effects.

Beta agonists usually are administered by I.V. infusion until contractions stop. Then after discharge, the patient may continue with oral doses until the delivery of a mature infant is assured. Alternatively, some doctors prescribe a 5-day treatment course, which they believe is equally effective and avoids prolonged maternal and fetal exposure. I.V. infusion may be repeated if premature labor recurs.

The adverse cardiovascular and metabolic effects of these drugs are most severe with I.V. administration. They occur in both the mother and the fetus, but they can usually be controlled by reducing the drug dosage.

Uterine relaxants shouldn't be used in any condition in which continuation of the pregnancy presents a greater hazard than premature delivery. Such conditions include pregnancy-induced hypertension, hemorrhage, intrauterine fetal death, maternal cardiac disease, or hypothyroidism. They should be used cautiously in cardiovascular disease, diabetes mellitus, and hyperthyroidism and with concurrent administration of corticosteroids.

Purpose and action
Uterine relaxants decrease the frequency, intensity, and duration of uterine contractions by direct stimulation of beta$_2$-receptors. This decreases the sensitivity of myometrial cells to oxytocin and prostaglandins.

Monitoring
Careful monitoring is essential throughout therapy. If a uterine relaxant will be given I.V., perform a baseline EKG and connect the patient to a fetal monitor. Also collect serum samples for a complete blood count and electrolyte and glucose studies, as ordered. During therapy, monitor these laboratory studies, usually at 6-hour intervals, to detect hypokalemia, hypoglycemia, or decreased hematocrit. Report abnormal findings to the doctor.

Monitor the patient's cardiac status continuously and report any arrhythmias. Also check her blood pressure and pulse every 10 to 15 minutes initially, then every 30 minutes or as ordered. Notify the doctor if her pulse rate exceeds 140 beats/minute or if her blood pressure falls 15 mm Hg or more. Tachycardia and hypotension may be the first signs of drug intolerance, signaling the need for a dosage adjustment. Be sure the patient remains in the left lateral position to provide increased blood flow to the uterus.

If the patient complains of palpitations or chest pain or tightness, decrease the drug dosage and notify the doctor immediately. Keep emergency resuscitation equipment nearby.

Assess pulmonary status every hour during I.V. therapy, and monitor intake and output. Fluid overload may lead to pulmonary edema, especially if the patient is receiving corticosteroids along with ritodrine. Auscultate her lungs and report any rales or increased respirations. Also notify the doctor if urinary output drops below 50 ml/hour. If signs of pulmonary edema develop, place the patient in a high Fowler position, administer oxygen as ordered, and notify the doctor.

Check the patient's temperature every 4 hours during I.V. infusion. Report any fever to the doctor.

Note the frequency and duration of the contractions. Check the fetal heart rate on the monitor every 10 to 15 minutes initially and then every 30 minutes, or as ordered. Immediately notify the doctor if the fetal heart rate exceeds 180 or falls below 120 beats/minute.

For 1 to 2 hours after I.V. therapy, monitor the patient's vital signs, intake and output, and fetal heart sounds. Perform serial EKGs, as ordered, and assess for uterine contractions. Immediately report tachycardia, hypotension, decreased urinary output, or diminished or absent fetal heart sounds.

Home care instructions
● Reassure the patient that drug effects on her baby should be minimal—for example, mild hypoglycemia for the first 24 hours after birth.
● Tell the patient to notify the doctor immediately if she experiences sweating, chest pain, or increased pulse rate. Teach her to check her pulse before oral administration. If her pulse exceeds 130 beats/minute, she shouldn't take the drug and should notify the doctor.
● Also emphasize the importance of immediately reporting any contrac-

tions, low back pain, cramping, or increased vaginal discharge.
● Instruct her to report other side effects, such as headache, nervousness, tremors, restlessness, nausea, or vomiting, to the doctor; he'll probably reduce the drug dosage. Also have her notify the doctor if her urinary output decreases or if she gains more than 5 lb in a week.
● Tell her to take her temperature every day and to report any fever to the doctor. This may be a sign of infection.
● Advise her to take oral doses of the drug with food (to avoid GI upset) and to take the last dose several hours before bedtime (to avoid insomnia).
● Instruct her to remain in bed as much as possible and not to prepare her breasts for nursing until about 2 weeks before her due date, because this can stimulate the release of oxytocin and initiate contractions.
● Emphasize the importance of keeping follow-up appointments so that the doctor can monitor her progress with laboratory tests and fetal monitoring.

Oxytocic Drugs

The endogenous hormone oxytocin stimulates the uterus and induces contraction of the myoepithelium of the lacteal glands. It also exerts a vasopressive, an antidiuretic, and a transient relaxing effect on vascular smooth muscle. Uterine sensitivity to this hormone increases gradually during gestation, then increases sharply before parturition.

Oxytocic agents (synthetic oxytocin preparations) are primarily given by I.V. infusion to induce or stimulate labor. They're also used to control postpartum bleeding and may be given I.V., I.M., or P.O. at this time. The nasal form of oxytocin can be given to stimulate lactation, and thus relieve breast engorgement.

In the antepartum period, oxytocin

PREVENTING THE PERILS OF OXYTOCIN ADMINISTRATION

Oxytocin infusion can cause uterine stimulation and fluid overload. To help you forestall these complications, follow these guidelines.

Excessive uterine stimulation
Drug overdose or hypersensitivity may cause excessive uterine stimulation, leading to hypertonicity, tetany, rupture, cervical and perineal lacerations, premature placental separation, fetal hypoxia, or rapid forceful delivery.

To prevent these complications, always administer oxytocin by piggyback infusion so that the drug may be discontinued, if necessary, without interrupting the main I.V. line. Every 15 minutes, monitor uterine contractions, intrauterine pressure, fetal heart rate, and the character of blood loss.

If contractions occur less than 2 minutes apart, last 90 seconds or longer, or exceed 50 mm Hg, stop the infusion, turn the patient onto her side, preferably the left, and notify the doctor. Contractions should occur every 2½ to 3 minutes, followed by a period of relaxation.

Keep magnesium sulfate (20% solution) available to relax the myometrium.

Fluid overload
Oxytocin's antidiuretic effect increases renal reabsorption of water. This can cause fluid overload, leading to seizures and coma.

To identify this complication, monitor the patient's intake and output, especially in prolonged infusion of doses above 20 mU/minute. The risk of fluid overload also increases when oxytocin is given after abortion in hypertonic saline solution.

emia, nausea and vomiting, and pelvic hematoma. What's more, an overdose or a hypersensitivity to the drug may lead to uterine hypertonicity, tetanic contractions, or uterine rupture. In the fetus, the drug may cause bradycardia, neonatal jaundice, and an anaphylactic reaction.

Oxytocin is contraindicated in significant cephalopelvic disproportion, unfavorable fetal position or presentation, obstetric emergencies requiring intervention, fetal distress when delivery isn't imminent, prolonged uterine inertia, severe toxemia, or hypertonic uterine patterns. It shouldn't be given to a patient who has received a sympathomimetic, such as epinephrine or phenylephrine, since severe hypertension or intracranial hemorrhage could occur.

Oxytocin must be used cautiously if the patient has a history of cervical or uterine surgery, grand multiparity, uterine sepsis, or traumatic delivery; if the uterus is overdistended; or if the patient is over age 35 and in her first pregnancy. The drug must be used with extreme caution during the first and second stages of labor since cervical laceration, uterine rupture, and maternal and fetal death can occur.

Purpose and action
- To induce or stimulate labor by initiating or enhancing contractions of uterine smooth muscle
- To stimulate lactation by inducing contraction of the myoepithelium of the lacteal glands.

Monitoring
Monitor the patient continuously during oxytocin infusion. Check her blood pressure and pulse every 15 minutes; high doses may cause an initial drop in blood pressure followed by a sustained elevation. If the patient's receiving cyclopropane anesthesia, though, concurrent administration of oxytocin may produce severe hypotension.

Monitor uterine contractions and watch closely for signs of fluid over-

may be infused in patients with complications from Rh incompatibility or maternal diabetes, pregnancy-induced hypertension, premature membrane rupture, or inevitable or incomplete abortion. It may also be used in some patients with uterine inactivity.

Adverse maternal reactions to oxytocin include fluid overload, hypertension or hypotension, postpartum hemorrhage, arrhythmias, premature ventricular contractions, afibrinogen-

load. (See *Preventing the Perils of Oxytocin Administration.*)

If the patient is using oxytocin nasal spray to promote lactation, instruct her to clear her nasal passages first. Then, with her head upright, she should eject the solution into her nostril.

Home care instructions

Because oxytocin is given only in a hospital, it doesn't require any directions for home use.

SURGERY

Mastectomy

Primarily performed to remove malignant breast tissue and any regional lymphatic metastases, mastectomy is commonly combined with radiation therapy and chemotherapy. Until recently, radical mastectomy was the treatment of choice for breast cancer. Now, six different types of mastectomy can be performed, depending on the size of the tumor and the presence of any metastases.

A *partial mastectomy*, also called a lumpectomy, tylectomy, or segmental resection, is indicated for Stage I lesions, which are small and peripherally located. This approach leaves a cosmetically satisfactory breast but may fail to remove all malignant tissue or to detect metastases in axillary lymph nodes.

In the patient with a central, noninvasive tumor, a *subcutaneous mastectomy* may be used. It's also used for chronic cystic mastitis, multiple fibroadenomas, or hyperplastic duct changes.

If a tumor is confined to breast tissue, a *simple mastectomy* may be performed. It's also used palliatively for advanced, ulcerative malignancy and as treatment for extensive benign disease.

A *modified radical mastectomy*, the standard surgery for Stage I and II lesions, removes small, localized tumors. Besides causing less disfigurement than a radical mastectomy, it also reduces postoperative arm edema and shoulder problems.

A *radical mastectomy* controls the spread of larger, metastatic lesions. Later, breast reconstruction may be performed, using a portion of the latissimus dorsi. Rarely, an *extended radical mastectomy* may be used to treat malignancy in the medial quadrant of the breast or in subareolar tissue. It's used to prevent possible metastasis to the internal mammary lymph nodes.

In any type of mastectomy, infection and delayed healing are possible. However, the major complication of radical mastectomy and axillary dissection is lymphedema, occurring soon after surgery and persisting for years. Dissection of the lymph nodes draining the axilla may interfere with lymphatic drainage of the arm on the affected side.

Purpose

• To remove a malignant breast tumor
• To treat chronic cystic mastitis, multiple fibroadenomas, or hyperplastic duct changes.

Preparation

Mastectomy may prove more threatening to a woman's self-image than any other surgery. As a result, be sure to explore the patient's feelings about it. Typically, she'll be afraid and anxious. She may have many questions, but she may feel too confused or upset to pose them. Be a supportive, caring listener and help her to express her concerns. Discuss her sexuality and her relationship with her sex partner to identify possible conflicts about the surgery and the degree of support she can expect from him afterward.

Review the surgeon's explanation of

the procedure. In addition, prepare the patient for her postoperative care. Explain that a catheter and suction may be used to drain the incision and that the arm on her affected side will be elevated. She'll have to sit up and turn in bed by pushing up with her unaffected arm, but not pulling. Tell her that she'll start arm and shoulder exercises shortly after surgery. Demonstrate them and have her repeat them.

Provide other information, too, such as the types of breast prostheses available. Most women, however, will need to concentrate on dealing with the upcoming procedure and the immediate recovery period. So defer discussion of rehabilitation until after surgery.

Take arm measurements on both sides to provide baseline data. If the patient will be having a radical mastectomy, explain that the skin on the anterior surface of one thigh may be shaved and prepared in case she needs a graft.

Ensure that the patient has signed a consent form.

Procedure

In a *partial mastectomy*, the surgeon removes the entire tumor mass along with at least 1″ (2.5 cm) of the surrounding healthy tissue. In a *subcutaneous mastectomy*, he removes all breast tissue but preserves the overlying skin and nipple. He may also insert a prosthesis, depending on his decision and the patient's wishes. In a *simple mastectomy*, he removes the entire breast without dissecting the lymph nodes. He may apply a skin graft, if necessary.

If the surgeon's performing a *modified radical mastectomy*, he may employ one of several techniques to remove the entire breast. He also resects all axillary lymph nodes, while leaving the pectoralis major intact. He may or may not remove the pectoralis minor. If the patient has small lesions and no metastases, the surgeon may perform breast reconstruction immediately or a few days later.

In a *radical mastectomy*, the surgeon removes the entire breast, the axillary lymph nodes, the underlying pectoral muscles, and adjacent tissues. During the operation, he covers skin flaps and exposed tissue with moist packs for protection and, before closure, he irrigates the chest wall and axilla.

In an *extended radical mastectomy*, the surgeon removes the breast, underlying pectoral muscles, axillary contents, and the upper internal mammary (mediastinal) lymph node chain.

After closing the mastectomy site, he may make a stab wound and insert a catheter. The catheter removes blood that may collect under the skin flaps, prevent healing, and predispose the patient to infection. Less commonly, he may use large pressure dressings instead.

If a graft was needed to close the wound, he'll probably place a pressure dressing over the donor site.

Monitoring and aftercare

When the patient returns to the unit, elevate her arm on a pillow to enhance circulation and prevent edema. Periodically check the suction tubing to ensure proper function and observe the drainage site for erythema, induration, and drainage. Using aseptic technique, measure and record drainage every 8 hours. Keep in mind that the drainage should change from sanguineous to serosanguineous fluid. After 2 or 3 days, you may need to "milk" the drain periodically to prevent clots from occluding the tubing.

As ordered, teach the patient arm exercises to prevent muscle shortening and contracture of the shoulder joint and to facilitate lymph drainage. The surgeon will determine the optimal time for initiating these exercises, based on the degree of healing, the presence of a drainage tube, and the tension placed on skin flaps and sutures with movement. You can usually initiate arm flexion and extension on the first postoperative day and then add exercises each day, depending on the patient's needs and the procedure performed.

Plan an exercise program with the patient. Such exercises may include climbing the wall with her hands, arm swinging, and rope pulling.

To prevent lymphedema, make sure that no blood pressure readings, injections, or venipunctures are performed on the affected arm. Place a sign bearing this message at the head of the patient's bed.

Because mastectomy causes emotional distress, you'll need to teach the patient to conserve her energy and to recognize the early signs of fatigue. Gently encourage the patient to view the operative site by describing its appearance and allowing her to express her feelings. Be sure to be present when she looks at the wound for the first time.

Arrange for a volunteer who's had a mastectomy to talk with the patient. Contact the American Cancer Society's rehabilitation program, Reach to Recovery.

After 2 or 3 days, initiate a fitting for a temporary breast pad. Soft and lightweight, the pad may be inserted into a bra without stays or underwires.

If appropriate, explain breast reconstruction. (See *Reconstructing a Breast.*)

Home care instructions

● Inform the patient that prevention of lymphedema is critical. Explain that swelling may follow even minor trauma to the arm on her affected side. Tell her to promptly wash cuts and scrapes on the affected side and to contact the doctor immediately if erythema, edema, or induration occurs.

● Advise her to use the arm as much as possible and to avoid keeping it in a dependent position for a prolonged period.

● Reinforce the importance of performing range-of-motion exercises daily. She must do them with both arms to maintain symmetry and prevent additional deformities.

● Emphasize the importance of not al-

RECONSTRUCTING A BREAST

Breast reconstruction, or reconstruction mammoplasty, can help relieve the emotional distress caused by mastectomy. As a result, it can improve the patient's self-image and restore her sexual identity.

Breast reconstruction isn't for every mastectomy patient. For instance, it's contraindicated when metastasis is possible, if healing is impaired, or if the patient has unrealistic expectations. But even when breast reconstruction is feasible, some women choose not to undergo it. They're comfortable, active, and well-adjusted without it. Or they may not consider the burden of additional surgery, anesthesia, pain, or expense worthwhile.

How it's done
In breast reconstruction, the surgeon places an implant filled with silicone or saline solution under the skin. He may bank the patient's own nipple on her inner thigh or inguinal area and salvage it at the appropriate time. (Its color may darken in the immediate postoperative period, but this should fade.) Or he may reconstruct a nipple from labial tissue.

How you can help
If the surgeon offers the patient the option of breast reconstruction, review the procedure with her and answer any questions she may have. Give her ample time to express her concerns.

Encourage the patient to contact the local chapter of the American Cancer Society for additional information. You'll also want to ask a volunteer from the Reach to Recovery program to talk with the patient.

---

lowing any blood pressure readings, injections, or venipunctures on the affected arm.

● Remind the patient that her energy level will wax and wane. Instruct her to be alert for signs of fatigue and to rest frequently during the day for the first few weeks after discharge.

● Stress the importance of monthly self-examination of the remaining breast and the mastectomy site. Demonstrate the correct technique and have the patient repeat it.

● Explain the importance of keeping

scheduled postoperative appointments.
- If necessary, provide information regarding a permanent prosthesis. This can be fitted 3 to 4 weeks after surgery. Prostheses are available in a wide range of styles, skin tones, and weights from lingerie shops, medical supply stores, and department stores.
- Reassure the patient that she can wear the same type of clothing she wore before her surgery.

Dilatation and Curettage or Evacuation

The most commonly performed gynecologic procedures, dilatation and curettage (D & C) and dilatation and evacuation (D & E) involve cervical expansion or dilatation to allow access to the endocervix and uterus. In a D & C, a curette is used to scrape endometrial tissue; in a D & E, suction is applied to extract the uterine contents.

A D & C provides treatment for an incomplete abortion, controls abnormal uterine bleeding, and can secure an endometrial or endocervical tissue sample for cytologic study. A D & E can also be used for an incomplete or a therapeutic abortion, usually up to 12 weeks of gestation but occasionally as late as 16 weeks.

Potential complications of these surgeries include uterine perforation, hemorrhage, and infection. If cervical trauma occurs during these procedures, subsequent pregnancies may be affected. In fact, such trauma can lead to spontaneous abortion, cervical incompetence, or premature birth.

Both gynecologic surgeries should be avoided in acute infection or if pregnancy is desired.

Purpose
For a D & C:
- To remove tissue after an incomplete, early abortion

- To control abnormal uterine bleeding
- To explore the uterus and confirm pathology
- To obtain tissue for cytologic study.
For a D & E:
- To perform a therapeutic abortion or to treat an incomplete abortion occurring late in the first trimester or early in the second trimester.

Preparation
Review the procedure with the patient and answer her questions. Inform her that afterward she'll have some vaginal drainage and a perineal pad in place. Explain that temporary abdominal cramping and pelvic and low back pain are normal symptoms after the procedure.

Ensure that preliminary studies have been completed, including a medical history, physical examination, urinalysis, Papanicolaou test, and hematocrit and hemoglobin measurements. Call the doctor's attention to any abnormalities.

Be sure that the patient has followed preoperative directions for fasting and used an enema to empty the colon before admission. Remind her that she'll be groggy after the procedure and won't be able to drive. Make sure that she has arranged transportation.

Ask the patient to void before you administer any preoperative medications, such as meperidine or diazepam. Start I.V. fluids, as ordered (either 5% dextrose in water or normal saline solution), to facilitate administration of the anesthetic. For D & C or D & E, the patient may receive a general anesthetic, a regional paracervical block, or a local anesthetic.

Make sure that the patient has signed a consent form.

Procedure
After receiving an anesthetic, the patient is placed in the dorsal lithotomy position. The surgeon performs a preliminary bimanual pelvic examination. Then he exposes the cervix and checks the depth and direction of the

uterine cavity. (In a D & E, this confirms gestational size.) He then dilates the cervical canal.

In a *D & C*, he next explores the uterine cavity, removing any polyps. If he suspects any cervical or uterine malignancy, he obtains biopsy specimens from the endocervical canal. Then he performs standard curettage to remove the superficial layer of the endometrium, taking biopsy specimens from the four quadrants of the cervix. If a D & C is used to treat an incomplete abortion, he also removes the remaining products of conception.

In a *D & E* , the surgeon uses a suction curette to extract the contents of the uterus. He then explores the uterine cavity to ensure complete removal of the products of conception.

Monitoring and aftercare

After surgery, administer analgesics, as ordered. Expect moderate cramping and pelvic and low back pain, but be sure to report any continuous, sharp abdominal pain that doesn't respond to analgesics; this may indicate perforation of the uterus.

You'll also need to monitor the patient for hemorrhage and signs of infection, such as purulent, foul-smelling vaginal drainage. Also check the color and volume of urine; hematuria indicates infection. Report any of these untoward signs immediately.

Administer fluids, as tolerated, and allow food if the patient requests it. Keep the bed's side rails raised and help the patient walk to the bathroom, if appropriate.

Home care instructions

• Instruct the patient to report any signs of infection. Tell her to use analgesics to control pain but to report any unrelenting sharp pain.
• Inform her that spotting and discharge may last a week or longer. Tell her to report any bright red blood.
• Instruct her to schedule an appointment with the doctor for a routine checkup.

• Tell her to resume activity as tolerated, but remind her to follow her doctor's instructions for vigorous exercise and sexual intercourse. They're usually discouraged until after the follow-up visit.
• Advise her to seek birth control counseling, if needed, and refer her to an appropriate center.

Hysterectomy

Hysterectomy refers to the excision of the uterus. Although it can be performed using a vaginal or an abdominal approach, the latter approach allows better visualization of the pelvic organs and a larger operating field. The vaginal approach may be used to repair relaxed pelvic structures, such as cystocele or rectocele, at the same time as hysterectomy.

Hysterectomy may be classified as total, subtotal, or radical. A *total* hysterectomy (panhysterectomy) involves removal of the entire uterus, whereas a *subtotal* one removes only a portion of the uterus, leaving the cervical stump intact. Both surgeries are commonly performed for uterine myomas or endometrial disease. They may also be performed postpartum if the placenta fails to separate from the uterus after a cesarean delivery or if amnionitis is present. A *radical* hysterectomy, the treatment of choice for cervical carcinoma, involves removal of all the reproductive organs.

In general, complications of hysterectomy reflect the surgical approach. With a vaginal hysterectomy, complications are few, although perineal infection is possible. More serious complications may occur with the abdominal approach, including infection, urinary retention, abdominal distention, thrombophlebitis, atelectasis, and pneumonia. Major complications of a radical hysterectomy include the formation of ureteral fis-

UNDERSTANDING ABDOMINAL HYSTERECTOMY

In an abdominal hysterectomy, the surgeon makes an incision in the midline, from the umbilicus to the symphysis pubis, and identifies major organs and structures.

He then severs the round ligament to gain access to the fallopian tubes and ovaries if the chosen procedure calls for their removal.

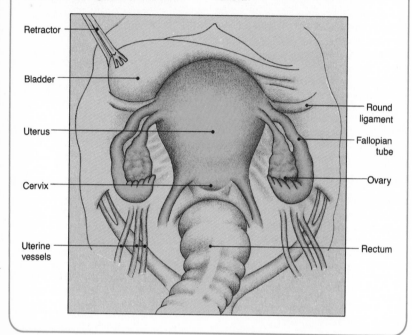

Retractor

Bladder

Uterus

Cervix

Uterine vessels

Round ligament

Fallopian tube

Ovary

Rectum

tulas and cystic lymphangiomas, pelvic infection, and hemorrhage.

Purpose
• To treat uterine myomas and endometrial disease
• To treat cervical carcinoma
• To remove the placenta if it fails to separate from the uterus.

Preparation
The patient may enter the hospital 1 to 2 days before surgery. This gives you time to explore her expectations about her menstrual and reproductive status after surgery.

Review the surgical approach and the extent of the excision. To prepare the patient for an abdominal hysterectomy, tell her to expect a cleansing enema and a douche the evening before surgery and a shower with an antibacterial soap. Explain that urinary retention commonly occurs after surgery, requiring an indwelling (Foley) catheter. If she develops abdominal distention, she may have a nasogastric tube or a rectal tube inserted.

Tell the patient scheduled for a vaginal hysterectomy to expect abdominal cramping and moderate amounts of drainage postoperatively and that she'll have a perineal pad in place.

Inform the patient that after surgery she'll lie supine or in a low to mid-Fowler position. Demonstrate the exercises that she'll need to do to prevent venous stasis.

Ensure that the patient has signed a consent form.

Procedure

For an abdominal approach, the surgeon makes an incision in the midline from the umbilicus to the symphysis pubis. For a vaginal approach, he makes an incision above and around the cervix.

In a radical hysterectomy, the surgeon removes the fallopian tubes, the ovaries, the uterus, adjacent lymph nodes, and part of the vagina. He may preserve some ovarian tissue in the premenopausal patient.

In a total hysterectomy, the surgeon removes both the body of the uterus and the cervix, leaving the ovaries and fallopian tubes intact. In a subtotal procedure, he removes only part of the uterus, leaving intact the cervical stump, fallopian tubes, and ovaries.

After hysterectomy, the surgeon closes the peritoneal cavity and applies a pad or dressing.

Monitoring and aftercare

If the patient has had a vaginal hysterectomy, change her perineal pad frequently. Provide analgesics to relieve cramps. As ordered, change dressings.

If the patient has had an abdominal hysterectomy, tell her to remain supine or in a low to mid-Fowler position. Encourage her to perform the prescribed exercises to prevent venous stasis. And monitor her urine output since retention commonly occurs.

If abdominal distention develops, relieve it by inserting a nasogastric or rectal tube, as ordered. Note bowel sounds during routine assessment.

Home care instructions

• If the patient has had a vaginal hysterectomy, instruct her to report severe cramping, heavy bleeding, or hot flashes to her doctor immediately.
• If she has had an abdominal procedure, tell her to avoid heavy lifting, rapid walking, or dancing, which can cause pelvic congestion. Encourage her to walk a little more each day and to avoid sitting for a prolonged period. Tell her that swimming is permissible.

• Advise the patient to eat a high-protein, high-residue diet to avoid constipation, which may increase abdominal pressure. Her doctor may also order increased fluids (3,000 ml/day).
• Advise her to express her feelings about her altered body image and to contact the doctor if she has questions about any changes.
• Mention that the doctor will inform her when she can resume sexual activity (usually 6 weeks after surgery).
• Explain to the patient and her family that she may feel depressed or irritable temporarily because of abrupt hormonal fluctuations. Encourage family members to respond calmly and with understanding.

Laparoscopy and Laparotomy

Various laparoscopic procedures and laparotomy allow removal of endometrial implants. Treatment selection depends on the size and extent of the lesions, the severity of symptoms, the patient's age, and her desire to have children.

Laparoscopy permits visualization of pelvic and upper abdominal organs and peritoneal surfaces to identify endometrial implants. The laparoscope also allows passage of surgical instruments, permitting removal of small lesions with a laser beam or a cryosurgical or an electrocautery device.

If endometrial implants are too large for removal by laparoscopy, a laparotomy may be performed. Laparoscopy also allows resection of ovarian cysts containing endometrial tissue, thereby averting the risk of rupture.

Possible complications of laparoscopic procedures include excessive bleeding, abdominal cramps, and shoulder pain. These effects may occur as a result of the abdomen's being inflated with carbon dioxide. Compli-

COMPARING PROCEDURES FOR REMOVING ENDOMETRIAL IMPLANTS

TREATMENT	PURPOSE AND EFFECTS	PROCEDURE
Laparoscopy		
Argon laser therapy	Uses thermal radiation to ablate widespread, deep-seated (1 to 2 mm) endometrial implants. The laser destroys specific lesions while sparing adjacent tissues. It causes minimal scarring.	The surgeon passes the argon laser through a flexible quartz fiberoptic wave guide. He then uses the laser to deliver a scattered beam of radiation to destroy endometrial implants.
Carbon dioxide (CO_2) laser therapy	Removes shallow endometrial implants by penetrating tissue to a depth of 0.1 to 1.2 mm with minimal effect on surrounding tissue. The CO_2 beam achieves this effect by raising the temperature of intracellular water to a flash boiling point, causing the explosion and vaporization of target tissue.	The surgeon uses a focused CO_2 laser beam, which is transmitted through the laparoscope, to cause a surface burn at the point of contact. The beam's intense heat coagulates vessels as it cuts through them to destroy endometrial implants. Suction applied through the laparoscope removes the vapor produced during the procedure.
Cryosurgery	Destroys endometrial tissue by local freezing without injuring adjacent healthy tissue. Causes intracapillary thrombosis and tissue necrosis in the frozen area with minimal bleeding.	The surgeon introduces a probe through the laparoscope into the pelvic cavity. He then passes a refrigerant, such as liquid nitrogen, Freon, or CO_2, from a vacuum container through an insulated tube to the tip of the probe. (All but the tip is insulated.) This causes a ball of frozen endometrial tissue to gradually form around the uninsulated tip.
Electrocautery	Destroys a small amount of endometrial tissue on contact and coagulates blood vessels by using extreme heat. Doesn't cause bleeding.	In this procedure, the surgeon uses laparoscopy to apply a small, heated wire loop to endometrial implants. The loop is heated by a steady, direct electric current.
Laparotomy		
Cyst resection	Removes a cyst that contains endometrial implants, thereby relieving dysmenorrhea, abnormal bleeding, and dyspareunia. Cyst resection preserves normal tissue to maintain reproductive function. Scarring and adhesions are minimal.	After entering the pelvic cavity through an abdominal incision, the surgeon aspirates the ovarian cyst, which contains endometrial tissue and blood. He then palpates the ovary to determine the depth of cystic tissue, and cuts the cyst from the ovarian cortex.

cations of laparotomy may include infection or other complications associated with abdominal surgery.

Laparoscopy should be avoided in a patient with intestinal obstruction, abdominal cancer, acute abdominal tuberculosis, or ruptured ectopic pregnancy with massive hemorrhage. Laparotomy is contraindicated if endometrial implants extend deep into the wall of the bowel, bladder, or ureter.

Purpose
• *For laparoscopy and laparotomy:* To remove endometrial implants
• *For laparatomy:* To resect ovarian cysts containing endometrial tissue.

Preparation
Explain laparotomy or the specific laparoscopic procedure to the patient and answer any questions she may have. If she'll be undergoing laparoscopic surgery, mention that she'll be discharged the same day, after she recovers from the procedure. If she'll be undergoing laparotomy, prepare her as you would for abdominal surgery. If she'll be having an ovarian cyst resected, determine if she has followed the prescribed preoperative regimen. She may have been given danazol to promote endometrial atrophy, thereby reducing the extent of resection required. Ensure that the patient has signed a consent form.

Procedure
For details on laparoscopic procedures and laparotomy, see *Comparing Procedures for Removing Endometrial Implants*.

Monitoring and aftercare
After laparoscopy, check for excessive vaginal bleeding, which may indicate hemorrhage; minor bleeding is normal. Ask the patient about abdominal cramps or shoulder pain and provide analgesics, as ordered. If the patient complains of bloating or abdominal fullness, explain that the feeling will subside as the gas in her abdomen is absorbed into the bloodstream, ex-

changed in the lungs, and exhaled.

After laparotomy, provide care as you would for a patient who has undergone abdominal surgery.

Home care instructions
• If the patient has undergone laparoscopy, emphasize the importance of reporting bright red vaginal bleeding. If she has undergone laparotomy, tell her about activity restrictions.
• Explain that she should return for follow-up visits since endometrial implants tend to recur.

Cervical Suturing
[Cerclage]

Using a purse-string suture, this surgery reinforces an incompetent cervix to maintain pregnancy. Typically performed between the 14th and 18th week of gestation, when the major risk of spontaneous abortion has passed, cervical suturing is indicated for patients with a history of premature delivery caused by an incompetent cervix.

Two cervical suturing procedures are commonly used. The *modified Shirodkar technique* involves elevating the vaginal mucous membrane and threading and tying a Mersilene band around the internal cervical os. The *McDonald procedure*, which is similar, places a nonabsorbable suture around the cervix, high on the mucosa. Both techniques are successful in maintaining pregnancy for about 90% of patients.

Cervical suturing can cause complications, such as preterm labor, hemorrhage, or sepsis. It's contraindicated if the patient has vaginal bleeding or uterine cramping.

Purpose
To maintain closure of the internal cervical os until term, preventing premature labor and delivery.

Preparation

Explain to the patient that an incompetent cervix means premature dilation of the cervix and doesn't imply any deficiency on her part. Inform her that she'll receive a general anesthetic and be hospitalized for 2 or 3 days. Explain that the procedure involves the surgical placement of a suture around the cervix so that the pregnancy can continue until the mature fetus is delivered. Show the patient pictures of the procedure. Tell her that the suture will be surgically removed when labor begins. If

THE McDONALD PROCEDURE

In a patient with an incompetent cervix, the cervical canal partially dilates, allowing membrane prolapse. To help correct this and allow a pregnancy to continue, the doctor may perform the McDonald procedure. In this procedure, he places a nonabsorbable suture in the cervix near the level of the internal os. He then encircles the body of the cervix with a purse-string suture, pulling it tight. Next, he places a dilator at the level of ligation to maintain canal patency while tying the suture.

BEFORE SUTURING

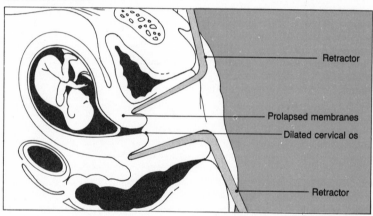

- Retractor
- Prolapsed membranes
- Dilated cervical os
- Retractor

SUTURE IN POSITION

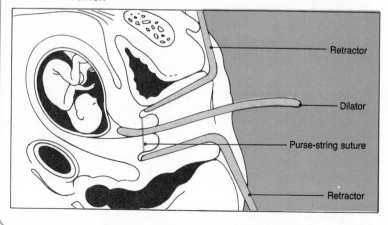

- Retractor
- Dilator
- Purse-string suture
- Retractor

she's to have a cesarean section, though, the suture may be left in place until the infant is delivered.

Assure the patient that she and the fetus will be monitored closely throughout the procedure and for several hours afterward. Tell her that she may be attached to a fetal monitor.

Make sure a thorough obstetric history has been completed. And continue to assess the patient to be sure her membranes are intact and the cervix isn't effaced more than 50%. Promptly report increasing dilation and effacement, contractions, fever, membrane rupture, or bleeding. If such complications develop, cervical suturing is contraindicated and supportive therapy, such as antibiotics or surgery, may be required. Or delivery may be necessary.

Before cervical suturing, ensure that the patient has signed a consent form.

Procedure

The patient receives a general anesthetic. Then, if the surgeon's using the modified Shirodkar technique, he retracts the vaginal walls and elevates the vaginal mucous membrane. After making an incision, he weaves a narrow nonabsorbable suture, such as Mersilene, around the internal cervical os. He then tightens the suture to close the os, restores the vaginal mucosa to its original position, and sutures it in place, usually with an absorbable suture. He removes the retractors and puts a perineal pad in place.

For information on the McDonald procedure, see *The McDonald Procedure.*

Monitoring and aftercare

Continuously monitor fetal heart rate during the procedure and at least every 30 minutes afterward, or as ordered. Notify the doctor immediately if uterine contractions occur or if the membranes rupture. The suture material may need to be removed and uterine relaxant drugs, such as ritodrine, given.

Note the amount of blood on the perineal pad. Spotting is normal, but immediately report any bright red blood.

Home care instructions

● Instruct the patient to immediately report uterine contractions, membrane rupture, vaginal bleeding, fever, or pain.
● Tell the patient to expect some spotting from the cervical incision for several days but to immediately report bright red blood or excessive bleeding to the doctor.
● Instruct her to change the perineal pad as needed or at least every 8 hours. Mention that she may find tiny pieces of suture on the pad. Reassure her that these come from the absorbable suture used to close the cervical incision, not from the suture holding the cervix closed.
● Tell her to abstain from intercourse or douching until she has had her postoperative checkup.

Cesarean Section

When vaginal delivery is unsafe for the mother or the fetus, cesarean section may be performed to remove the fetus from the uterus. Although cephalopelvic disproportion is the most common reason for cesarean delivery, other indications may include severe pregnancy-induced hypertension, placenta previa, fetal distress, premature separation of the placenta, breech presentation, prolapsed umbilical cord, previous uterine surgery, and abnormal labor caused by uterine dysfunction.

Several approaches may be used. The procedure of choice, lower segment cesarean delivery, involves a vertical or horizontal abdominal incision as well as an incision in the lower uterine segment. This characteristically leads to less maternal blood loss and a stronger uterine scar than the classic procedure, which involves vertical incisions in

QUESTIONS MOTHERS ASK AFTER CESAREAN DELIVERY

Will my next baby have to be delivered by cesarean, too?

Not necessarily. In the past, women who had one cesarean delivery were almost automatically given a cesarean at later births. Recently, however, normal labor and vaginal delivery have been allowed in some later pregnancies. Whether your next delivery will be vaginal or cesarean depends on the reason for your first cesarean and if you still have that condition, and on the type of incision. It also depends on your health and the health of the fetus at the time of delivery. If you've had two or more cesarean deliveries, your next delivery usually will be cesarean, too.

Can I breast-feed after a cesarean?

Certainly. In fact, it promotes uterine contractions, which help reduce the size of your uterus. But because of your surgery, you may need help positioning the baby.

Is it safe for me to exercise?

Check with your doctor before you start an exercise program. He'll probably permit isometric exercises and walking. But you shouldn't do more strenuous exercises until after your 6-week postpartum checkup.

In cesarean section, key nursing responsibilities include providing emotional support and patient teaching, assisting in the delivery, and providing antepartum and postpartum care for the mother and the fetus. Monitoring is crucial to prevent, detect, or manage complications. Maternal complications may include infection, hemorrhage, and wound dehiscence. Fetal complications may include hypoxia, acidosis, respiratory distress, and prematurity.

Purpose

To manage or prevent maternal or fetal complications resulting from conditions that make vaginal delivery hazardous or impossible.

Preparation

If time permits, allow the patient to express her concerns about the well-being of the fetus. Although some childbirth classes provide preparation for cesarean delivery, the patient may be beset with misconceptions and fears.

Prepare the patient for an I.V. infusion to provide hydration, fluid replacement, and access for medication. Also inform her that she'll have an indwelling (Foley) catheter in place to prevent bladder damage and allow access to the uterus.

Explain to the patient that she will be transported to the surgical area in a semi-Fowler's position or with her uterus tilted to the left. She shouldn't lie supine because the weight of the uterus compresses the inferior vena cava and aorta, resulting in decreased venous return and cardiac output.

Tell her that a spinal or an epidural anesthetic, rather than a general anesthetic, is usually given to lower the risk of aspiration, minimize neonatal respiratory depression, and facilitate earlier bonding. (Some patients may need a general anesthetic because it works faster and gives the anesthesiologist better control of cardiopulmonary function. Also, the duration from induction to delivery is reduced to help prevent altered placental cir-

both the abdomen and uterus.

Extraperitoneal cesarean section avoids entry into the peritoneal cavity, instead approaching the uterus through the space above the bladder. It involves an incision in the lower uterine segment. This approach, which is slow and difficult, is used only when necessary to avoid spreading infection from the uterus into the peritoneum.

culation, fetal hypoxia and acidosis, and neonatal respiratory depression.)

Before cesarean section, ensure that the patient has signed a consent form. If her partner will be allowed in the operating room, have him scrub and dress according to hospital policy.

Procedure

To begin, the surgeon makes an abdominal incision, retracts the bladder, and incises the uterus. He then removes the retractor and delivers the fetal head. Next, he suctions the infant's nose and mouth with a bulb syringe to clear the airway. Then he completes the delivery. After he clamps and cuts the umbilical cord, the surgeon transfers the infant to the neonatal team.

Next, the surgeon administers I.V. oxytocin to contract the uterus. This helps reduce blood loss and promotes delivery of the placenta. Then he closes the incision. Finally, the fundus is palpated and massaged to help contract the uterus, since uterine relaxation may cause hemorrhage.

Immediately after delivery, the infant is evaluated by obtaining an Apgar score at 1 and 5 minutes after birth. The doctor performs a physical examination, and the infant is taken to the nursery or intensive care unit, depending on his condition.

Monitoring and aftercare

After a cesarean section, palpate the fundus. Its height in the abdomen may help you detect uterine relaxation. Usually positioned below or at the level of the umbilicus, the uterus should be firm, indicating contraction. However, if the uterus is deviated to the left or is higher than the umbilicus, check the patency of the Foley catheter.

Monitor the patient's vital signs to detect shock and infection. Record intake and output to help determine the rate of fluid replacement. After removal of the Foley catheter, check for dysuria and decreased output.

Evaluate the lochia. Initially, it contains clots. Note its color (red for the first 3 or 4 days postpartum), amount (moderate is normal; a heavy discharge may indicate excessive bleeding), and odor (if unusual, suspect infection).

If the patient received a spinal or an epidural anesthetic, explain that she'll experience tingling when sensation returns. If she received a spinal anesthetic, explain that she may have a headache. Preventive measures include adequate hydration and lying flat in bed for 8 hours postoperatively.

Check the dressing for bleeding and the wound for signs of infection and hematoma formation.

To promote bonding, provide for early mother-infant contact, if appropriate. Allow the patient to express any anger, guilt, or grief she may feel over not experiencing vaginal delivery or over the condition of her infant.

Home care instructions

• Tell the patient to immediately report hemorrhage, chest or leg pain (possible thrombosis), dyspnea, or separation of the wound's edges. She should also report signs of infection, such as fever, difficult urination, or flank pain.
• Remind her to keep her follow-up appointment. At that time, she can talk to the doctor about contraceptive measures and resumption of intercourse.

ARTIFICIAL INSEMINATION

In Vivo Fertilization

In vivo fertilization involves the placement or instillation of seminal fluid into the vaginal canal or cervix. This controversial treatment for infertility may be attempted in obstruction of the male genital tract or if sperm are inadequate in number or function. It may also be used if an abnormality in the female

UNDERSTANDING IN VITRO FERTILIZATION

When the patient's fallopian tubes are absent, blocked, or damaged, in vitro fertilization offers an alternative method to achieve pregnancy. Although certain religious groups oppose this practice, many couples see it as a last resort for having children. Here's how this controversial treatment works.

Inducing ovulation

In vitro fertilization begins with the administration of a hormone to stimulate the development of an ovarian follicle. Measurement of serum estradiol confirms this.

Next, ultrasonography determines the best time to administer human chorionic gonadotropin (HCG), used to induce ovulation.

Retrieving the ovum

Ovum retrieval can occur 36 hours after HCG administration. The surgeon performs laparoscopy to visualize and aspirate the ovum. He then punctures the mature follicle with a needle and transfers the ovum and fluid into a sterile test tube.

Fertilizing the ovum

The surgeon places the aspirated ovum in a culture dish containing maternal serum and a culture medium, which is a mixture of amino acids, carbohydrates, and vitamins. After the ovum incubates in this medium for 24 hours at 98.6° F. (37° C.), sperm is added to the dish. (The husband or a donor provides a semen sample 2 hours after ovum retrieval, and the sperm is frozen until needed.) After another incubation period, this time for 36 hours, the oocyte divides if fertilization has occurred.

Transferring the embryo

With the patient in the knee-chest position, the surgeon uses a small catheter to transfer the embryo into the fundus of the cervix. Typically, this causes no cervical dilation or pain.

Immediately after the patient receives the embryo, she's given progesterone I.M. To prevent loss of the embryo, she must maintain the knee-chest position for at least 8 hours. Afterward, she may return home.

Providing home care

At home, the patient will need daily I.M. doses of progesterone to help implant the ovum in the uterine wall. Teach the patient's husband how to give this injection.

Tell the couple to return for a follow-up appointment after hormonal therapy has been completed. At that time, the patient will have a pregnancy test.

reproductive tract prohibits sperm from reaching the ovum.

The in vivo technique achieves fertilization differently than the in vitro technique, which uses a culture medium in a laboratory to bond ovum and sperm. (See *Understanding In Vitro Fertilization.*)

The in vivo technique can use the husband's sperm (if he's fertile) or a donor's. If the husband's sperm is of poor quality or motility, several samples are collected from him. The sper-matozoan-rich first portion, called a split ejaculate, is used. These samples are frozen, using liquid nitrogen, and later pooled to increase the sperm count.

The in vivo technique achieves conception in about 70% of patients when the husband's sperm is used. When donor sperm is used, the success rate stands at about 50% after 2 months and almost 90% after 6 months. However, multiple trials may be necessary before correctly timing insemination and ovulation.

In vivo fertilization causes few complications. Multiple births are possible but are usually welcomed by a childless couple. However, concern is growing over the use of donor semen because of the risk of spreading acquired immune deficiency syndrome (AIDS). To help reduce this risk, sperm banks now screen for the human immunodeficiency virus antibody.

Purpose
To achieve fertilization of a healthy ovum by viable sperm.

Preparation
Be supportive yet realistic as the couple approaches this treatment. Expect emotions to run high. After all, the couple has experienced many disappointments and frustrations over their inability to have a child and have thus far undergone a number of tests and procedures. Explain to them that this technique makes pregnancy possible but doesn't guarantee it. Mention, however, that most patients do become pregnant. Point out that multiple inseminations may be necessary to achieve conception and that these will be coordinated with ovulation. Teach the patient how to track her basal body temperature and cervical mucus or how to use an ovulatory predictor test kit.

Explain to the patient that she'll have to remain in the knee-chest position after the procedure. Inform her that the doctor may apply a cervical cap to prevent leakage of the instilled semen into the vagina.

Procedure
The doctor either places the semen at the cervical os with a cannula and a syringe within a day or two of the estimated time of ovulation, or injects the semen into a plastic cervical cap that he places around the cervix. The cap retains the specimen at the cervix and is removed several hours later.

The doctor repeats the procedure on alternate days until the patient's basal body temperature indicates that ovulation has occurred.

If fertilization fails to occur the 1st month, the doctor repeats the procedure the next month.

Monitoring and aftercare
Instruct the patient to remain in the knee-chest position for the prescribed period.

Provide support for the couple as they go through artificial insemination. Keep in mind that they may feel that this treatment represents their last chance to have a child of their own.

Home care instructions
● Encourage counseling for couples who are having difficulty communicating their feelings or who express uncontrollable anger or grief.
● Advise the couple to return for follow-up appointments, as necessary.

Selected References

Jensen, M., and Bobak, I. *Maternity and Gynecologic Care: The Nurse and The Family*, 3rd ed. St. Louis: C.V. Mosby Co., 1985.

Long, B., and Phipps, W. *Essentials of Medical-Surgical Nursing: A Nursing Process Approach*. St. Louis: C.V. Mosby Co., 1985.

Neeson J., and May, K. *Comprehensive Maternity Nursing*. Philadelphia: J.B. Lippincott Co., 1986.

Nursing88 Drug Handbook. Springhouse, Pa.: Springhouse Corp., 1988.

Pritchard, J., et al. *Williams Obstetrics*, 17th ed. East Norwalk, Conn.: Appleton & Lange, 1984.

Reeder, J., et al. *Maternity Nursing*, 16th ed. Philadelphia: J.B. Lippincott Co., 1987.

10 Treating Sexual Dysfunction

Treating Sexual Dysfunction

Introduction

Perhaps no health problem is as deeply personal, as emotionally devastating, or as difficult to overcome as sexual dysfunction. That's why helping a patient overcome this problem will certainly challenge your nursing skills.

How will you recognize the patient who needs sex therapy? Sometimes, he may be hospitalized specifically for treatment of sexual dysfunction; for example, he may be scheduled for implantation of a penile prosthesis. Or he may be hospitalized for a disorder that impairs sexual function, such as spinal cord injury, diabetes, or multiple sclerosis. He may even be hospitalized for an unrelated disorder and incidentally disclose that he's having sexual problems.

Fortunately, you're in an ideal position to help the patient—primarily through education and counseling. In many cases, he may feel more comfortable bringing up a sexual problem with you than with his doctor.

A diversified role

In the treatment of sexual dysfunction, you'll probably play several roles. For example, you may be called upon to teach the patient and his partner about the causes of the dysfunction while correcting any misconceptions they have about sexuality. Or you may be called upon to describe therapeutic techniques, such as how to inject vasoactive drugs to achieve an erection. To help a couple explore alternate ways of giving and receiving sexual pleasure, you may need to suggest use of sexual aids, such as vibrators. Above all, you'll need to be a supportive, nonjudgmental listener as the patient shares his concerns and frustrations with you.

A word about obstacles

No matter what kind of sexual dysfunction the patient is experiencing, you're likely to encounter a few obstacles to his successful treatment. For example, the patient may be reluctant to discuss his sex life with anyone, including his partner. Or he may feel inhibited and embarrassed about performing a specific therapy, such as the squeeze technique. Because therapy is often long and arduous, the patient or his partner may become discouraged and lose the commitment necessary to resolve the problem.

Inadvertently, you may also pose an obstacle to successful treatment. To effectively help the patient, you'll need to be comfortable discussing his sexual concerns and truly knowledgeable about the causes and treatment of sexual dysfunction. Only then will you be able to help rebuild the patient's self-esteem and confidence and restore the health of his intimate relationships.

DRUG THERAPY

Drug-Induced Erection

Injection of vasoactive drugs, such as papaverine and phentolamine, into the corpora cavernosa of the penis may produce an erection in patients with organic or psychogenic impotence. These drugs increase arterial flow through the penis, allowing blood to fill the sinuses as in a normal erection. The erection usually occurs 5 to 10 minutes after injection and lasts from 15 minutes to 6 hours. Rarely, the erection lasts longer, requiring an irrigation of epinephrine and normal saline solution to relax the penis. Drug-induced erection is successful in most patients; however, it may be of little or no benefit if the blood vessels supplying the penis are damaged.

When the patient's scheduled for this treatment, you'll need to provide reassurance as the injection will undoubtedly seem unpleasant or even frightening to him. By reinforcing the doctor's instructions, though, you can help the patient gain the confidence necessary to perform self-injection at home.

Purpose
To treat erectile dysfunction through the injection of vasoactive drugs into the corpora cavernosa.

Preparation
Explain to the patient that he'll receive a physical examination, have a sexual history taken, and undergo nocturnal penile tumescence monitoring before this treatment to determine if erection is physiologically possible. Prepare him for additional studies, including vascular and neuropsychiatric testing, and serum hormone levels, if ordered.

Encourage the patient's partner to accompany him to the doctor's office for the trial injection. Explain that if the injection produces an erection, the erection will last longer than a natural one and will not subside after ejaculation. However, the erection should gradually subside within 6 hours after injection as the medication stops working. Also, unlike priapism, this unusually prolonged erection probably won't be painful.

Mention to the patient that the injection will not affect his ability to ejaculate. If he was able to ejaculate before treatment, he will be able to do so after it. Likewise, if he was unable to ejaculate, he will not regain that ability.

Procedure
Initially, the doctor performs a trial injection in his office. After cleansing the base of the penis with an alcohol swab, he inserts the needle at a 90-degree angle into one corpus cavernosum and injects 30 mg of papaverine and 1 to 2 mg of phentolamine. If erection occurs, he sends the patient and his partner home to attempt intercourse.

On a follow-up visit, the doctor gives the patient the option of learning self-injection technique for practice at home. (See *How to Achieve a Drug-Induced Erection.*)

Monitoring and aftercare
During the trial injection, assess the patient for side effects, including dizziness, a metallic taste, and tingling along the shaft of the penis.

After the doctor teaches the injection technique to the patient, reinforce the instructions and answer any questions the patient or his partner may have.

Home care instructions
● After a successful trial injection, tell the patient to keep track of how long the erection lasts. If an erection lasts longer than 6 hours or if swelling sub-

HOW TO ACHIEVE A DRUG-INDUCED ERECTION

Dear Patient:

To help you overcome impotence, the doctor wants you to inject a vasoactive drug into your penis. This drug will produce an erection within 5 to 10 minutes that lasts from 15 minutes to 6 hours.

Follow these steps to correctly inject the drug.

1

Gather the medication, a syringe with needle, and an alcohol swab. Next, wash your hands thoroughly and dry them with a clean towel. Then sit on a firm chair or bed. Be sure you have plenty of light.

2

Mix the medication by gently tipping it from side to side. Don't shake the bottle.

3

Clean the top of the bottle with an alcohol swab and remove the needle's cap. Now pull back on the plunger until you reach the mark on the syringe that equals the amount of medication your doctor has prescribed. With the bottle upright, inject an equal amount of air into the bottle. This avoids creating a vacuum in the bottle and makes withdrawing the medication easier.

4

Turn the bottle and the syringe upside down and withdraw the correct amount of medication. If you see air bubbles in the syringe after you fill it, tap the syringe gently to remove them. Then remove the needle from the bottle and carefully replace the cap.

5

Hold the shaft of your penis between the thumb and index finger of one hand. With the other hand, clean the underside and sides of your penis with an alcohol swab.

6

Remove the needle's cap and insert the needle into the base of one of the corpora cavernosa, located midshaft along the penis. Take care to avoid the urethra and the small vessels that you see on the skin. Pull back on the plunger slightly to check for blood backflow. If there's none, slowly inject the

(continued)

388

HOW TO ACHIEVE A DRUG-INDUCED
ERECTION *(continued)*

medication over 1 to 3 minutes. Expect a slight tingling sensation within your penis; this will disappear in a few minutes.

CROSS SECTION OF PENIS

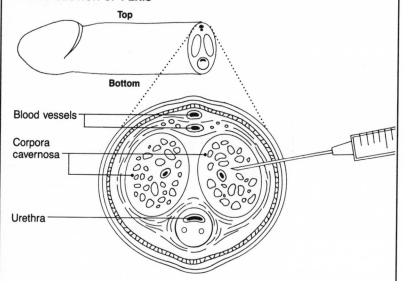

7

Remove the needle. Using an alcohol swab, apply pressure over the injection site for 2 or 3 minutes. Then dispose of the needle and syringe.

A few precautions

If the injection produces an erection, you may attempt intercourse. The erection should then subside slowly over the next 6 hours. If it lasts beyond 6 hours, call your doctor. If the injection doesn't produce an erection, you can try again after 24 hours.

Unless your doctor orders

otherwise, limit injections to 3 per week. Also, remember to rotate injection sites. Use the diagram below; after you use a site, cross it off and mark the date.

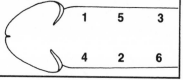

sequently occurs, instruct him to notify his doctor at once. Also, have him evaluate the quality of the erection.

• Mention that mild bruising occurs normally after injection. Also mild pain may occur at times during intercourse.

• When the patient begins self-injection, advise him to limit it to three times per week and to rotate injection sites to avoid tissue damage. Teach him and his partner the signs of tissue damage, including cyanosis, pain, and edema. Have him report any of these signs to his doctor immediately.

PROSTHETIC AND MECHANICAL AIDS

Vaginal Dilation

The treatment of choice for vaginismus, dilation involves introducing one or two fingers or a series of graduated plastic dilators into the vagina. Both types of dilation help the patient systematically correct involuntary vaginal muscle spasms. When combined with sensate focus therapy and psychotherapy, dilation can usually correct vaginismus unless an irreversible organic pathology exists.

As a nurse, you'll be responsible for teaching or reinforcing how to perform digital or instrumental dilation. Your support and reassurance can contribute much to the treatment's success.

Purpose
To treat vaginismus by gradually reducing the patient's anxiety about vaginal penetration.

Preparation
To decrease anxiety and allay feelings of guilt, explain to the patient and her partner that vaginal spasms are real and involuntary. Also, clear up any questions about female anatomy and physiology. Then teach the patient how to practice deep breathing and other relaxation techniques.

Procedure
Teach the patient how to perform digital or instrumental dilation, or reinforce the instructions given by the doctor or sex therapist. Instruct the patient to begin by inserting one lubricated finger or the smallest in a series of graduated plastic dilators into the vagina and to hold it there for a few minutes. Have her perform deep breathing or another relaxation technique to ease insertion. After she successfully completes this exercise, instruct her to introduce two fingers or the next size dilator into her vagina. Have her continue gradually increasing the size of the dilator introduced until it approximates the size of a penis.

Next, instruct the patient to repeat digital or instrumental dilation with her partner observing, but not participating. Inform her that it may take several days to weeks before she's comfortable enough to complete dilation in front of him. Once she does so, however, have her guide her partner's fingers, and later his penis, into her vagina. Stress that she should play this dominant role to maintain her sense of control. Advise her to use a water-soluble jelly to ease insertion and not to attempt intercourse until she feels ready. Also, recommend lying on top of her partner during intercourse until they achieve painless intromission.

Monitoring and aftercare
Answer any questions the patient or her partner may have about dilation. Ask the patient if she felt anxious during the insertion procedure. If so, reinforce relaxation techniques.

Home care instructions
• Reinforce that intromission is painless, and encourage the patient to master deep breathing and relaxation techniques.

• Suggest participation in sensate focus therapy or psychotherapy, as indicated.

Penile Prosthesis

Helpful in treating both organic and psychogenic erectile dysfunction, a penile prosthesis consists of a pair of semirigid rods or inflatable cylinders surgically implanted in the corpora cavernosa of the penis. For patients with organic dysfunction, a prosthesis may be the only treatment feasible. For those with psychogenic dysfunction, though, it's usually a last resort. Organic dysfunction may result from diabetes, arteriosclerosis, multiple sclerosis, spinal cord injury, or use of alcohol or drugs, such as antihypertensives. Psychogenic dysfunction may result from sexual performance anxiety, low self-esteem, or past failures in sustaining an erection.

Of the two types of penile prostheses, the semirigid device costs less and allows easier implantation. This device is especially beneficial for the patient with limited hand or finger function because its use doesn't demand manual dexterity. However, its major disadvantage is constant semierection, which may embarrass the patient. Also, some couples complain that the semirigid prosthesis produces an erection that isn't sufficiently stiff to be sexually satisfying.

Compared to the semirigid device, the inflatable prosthesis more closely mimics a normal erection. The patient controls erection by simply squeezing a pump in the scrotum that releases radiopaque fluid from a reservoir into the implanted cylinders. (See *How Penile Prostheses Work.*) However, implantation of this prosthesis is contraindicated in patients with iodine sensitivity.

Both types of prostheses place the patient at risk for infection, although the incidence ranges from only 1% to 4%. Rarely, the inflatable prosthesis may also leak fluid, or the tubing connecting the pump, reservoir, and cylinders may become kinked.

Before surgery, you'll be responsible for answering the couple's questions and allaying their fears about how the prosthesis may affect their sex life. After surgery, you'll need to reinforce how to use the prosthesis correctly and teach the patient how to recognize postoperative complications.

Purpose
To correct erectile dysfunction through the surgical implantation of semirigid rods or inflatable cylinders into the corpora cavernosa of the penis.

Preparation
Reinforce the doctor's explanation of the surgery and clear up any questions. Note that the prosthesis will not affect ejaculation or orgasmic pleasure; if the patient experienced either before surgery, he'll remain capable after it. Recognize that the patient and his partner are likely to be anxious before surgery, so provide emotional support, too.

Instruct the patient to shower the evening before and the morning of the surgery, using an antimicrobial soap. Tell him that he'll be shaved in the operating room to reduce the risk of infection. If ordered, begin antibiotic therapy.

Procedure
Typically, the prosthesis is implanted in the operating room under general anesthesia; however, the semirigid device may also be implanted on an outpatient basis under local anesthesia.

To implant a semirigid prosthesis, the doctor makes an incision in the middle of the scrotum, then dilates one corpus cavernosum to create a space for one rod. After introducing the rod, he dilates the other corpus cavernosum to house the second rod.

To implant an inflatable prosthesis, the doctor performs these same steps

HOW PENILE PROSTHESES WORK

Two types of penile prostheses are available: a semirigid device and an inflatable one. The semirigid prosthesis consists of a pair of rods inserted into the corpora cavernosa through a scrotal incision. With this prosthesis, the patient always maintains a partial erection.

The inflatable prosthesis consists of two cylinders, a reservoir containing radiopaque fluid, a pump, and a release valve. By squeezing the pump, the patient releases fluid from the reservoir into the inflatable cylinders, producing an erection. He then presses the release valve to return fluid to the reservoir and thus lose the erection.

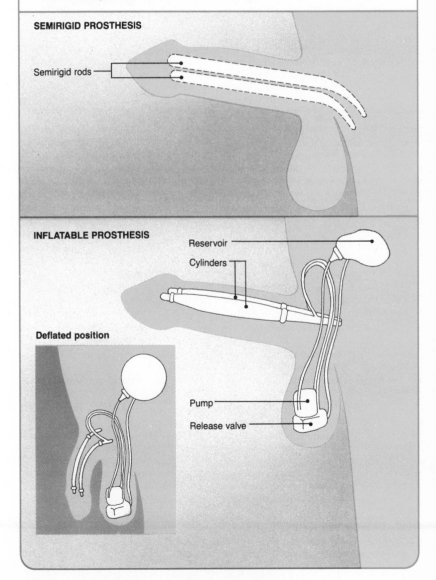

SEMIRIGID PROSTHESIS

Semirigid rods

INFLATABLE PROSTHESIS

Reservoir

Cylinders

Deflated position

Pump

Release valve

to position the cylinders. Then he makes an abdominal and a perineal incision and places a reservoir, filled with 60 ml of radiopaque fluid, through the external inguinal ring. Next, he places a pump in the lateral portion of the scrotum and connects the cylinders, reservoir, and pump with tubing. By squeezing the pump, he tests the function of the prosthesis. Finally, he completes the surgery by inserting a Jackson Pratt drain.

Monitoring and aftercare
Apply ice packs to the patient's penis for 24 hours after surgery. Empty the drain when it's full, or as ordered, to reduce the risk of infection. If the patient has an inflatable prosthesis, tell him to pull the scrotal pump downward to ensure proper alignment. With the doctor's approval, encourage the patient to practice inflating and deflating the prosthesis when the pain subsides. Pumping promotes healing of the tissue sheath around the reservoir and the pump.

Home care instructions
• Stress the importance of returning for all follow-up appointments to ensure that the incision is healing properly.
• Instruct the patient to wash the incision daily with an antimicrobial soap. Also instruct him to watch for signs of infection and to report them immediately to his doctor.
• Tell the patient and his partner that scrotal swelling and discoloration may last up to 3 weeks.
• Remind the patient to pull the scrotal pump downward to ensure proper alignment.
• Warn the couple that they may experience dyspareunia when they're permitted to resume sexual activity—usually about 6 weeks after surgery. This may result from an inability to have intercourse for a prolonged period before surgery. Suggest use of a water-soluble jelly to minimize or avoid discomfort. Also, emphasize the need for gentleness and prolonged foreplay to allow for sufficient vaginal lubrication, especially in older women whose lubrication normally decreases with age.

SEX THERAPY

Seman's Technique

Also called the "start-stop" technique, Seman's technique can successfully treat premature ejaculation in many patients. In this technique, the partner manually stimulates the patient's penis, halting just before ejaculation so that the patient becomes more aware of his sexual response. Typically, Seman's technique is combined with sensate focus therapy—nongenital touching between the patient and his partner—to increase communication and reduce sexual anxiety.

By reinforcing how to correctly perform Seman's technique, you can contribute to the successful treatment of premature ejaculation. What's more, your understanding can help the patient cope with a problem that might otherwise devastate his self-esteem.

Purpose
To help the patient gradually regain control over ejaculation through serial "stop-start" penile stimulation.

Preparation
Begin by reinforcing the instructions given to the patient and his partner by the doctor, psychologist, or sex therapist. Then, to avoid discouragement, emphasize that the patient and his partner may need to practice this technique for up to several months before the patient can avoid ejaculating prematurely. Note that even as he makes strides, he'll also experience setbacks.

Procedure

To perform Seman's technique, instruct the partner to stimulate the patient's penis with her hands until he feels the urge to ejaculate. Tell her to then stop stimulation and wait for this urge to pass before stimulating his penis again. Have her repeat penile stimulation four times, each time stopping short of ejaculation. Next, instruct her to stimulate his penis one more time, allowing him to ejaculate.

Explain to the couple that once they've mastered this controlled manual stimulation, they can proceed to intercourse. Suggest that the partner lie on top of the patient so that she can easily raise or lower her body. In this way she can control the depth of penetration and degree of penile excitation. Once the patient regains control of ejaculation, encourage the couple to use whatever sexual positions they find most satisfying.

Monitoring and aftercare

Review the instructions for performing Seman's technique, as necessary, to ensure that the couple will practice it correctly at home.

Home care instructions

- Stress the importance of setting aside time to satisfy the sexual needs of the patient's partner.
- Encourage the patient and his partner to attend follow-up counseling sessions to discuss their progress in using Seman's technique.

Squeeze Technique

Developed by the sex therapists Masters and Johnson, the squeeze technique is the treatment of choice for premature ejaculation. In this technique, the patient's partner briefly squeezes the penis just below and above the coronal ridge when the patient feels the urge to ejaculate. This delays ejaculation and

so helps the patient gradually gain more awareness and control over ejaculation. Because the technique's success depends on proper timing and hand placement, you'll need to frequently reinforce how to perform the technique. You'll also need to provide encouragement and support, since the couple may have to practice the technique for months before achieving success.

Purpose

To prevent premature ejaculation, thus improving the patient's self-esteem and sexual relationships.

Preparation

Begin by reviewing the anatomy of the penis and the physiology of erection and ejaculation. Then reinforce the instructions given to the couple by the doctor, psychologist, or sex therapist. Reassure them that this technique is painless and has a good success rate. However, tell them that it may take up to several months before they achieve success. Mention that they'll require follow-up counseling—perhaps for up to 2 years—since relapses commonly occur.

Procedure

To perform this technique, instruct the partner to manually stimulate the patient's penis and to have him let her know when he feels the urge to ejaculate. Tell the partner to then position her fingers around the penis and to squeeze firmly for 3 or 4 seconds. (See *The Squeeze Technique: Position and Pressure Important*, page 394.) This will cause slight flaccidity and forestall ejaculation.

Tell the couple to wait 15 to 30 seconds before resuming penile stimulation. Each time the patient nears ejaculation, have his partner apply the squeeze technique until he can control ejaculation on his own. Once he achieves this, tell him to progress to inserting his penis into her vagina—but to avoid thrusting. As he develops

THE SQUEEZE TECHNIQUE: POSITION AND PRESSURE IMPORTANT

To forestall ejaculation using the squeeze technique, the patient's partner will have to position her fingers correctly around the penis and apply the right amount of pressure. When the patient feels the urge to ejaculate, she should place her thumb on the frenulum of the penis and her index and middle fingers above and below the coronal ridge, as shown here. Tell her to squeeze the penis from front to back. How firmly she should squeeze will depend on the erection's stiffness: more firmly for a stiff penis and less firmly for a partially flaccid one. The patient will feel pressure but no pain.

ANATOMIC STRUCTURES

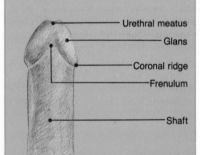

- Urethral meatus
- Glans
- Coronal ridge
- Frenulum
- Shaft

HAND POSITION

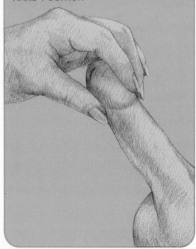

control, he can attempt thrusting, gradually increasing speed. Have his partner use the squeeze technique, as necessary, to delay ejaculation to the optimal time.

Monitoring and aftercare

Stress the importance of performing the squeeze technique, as instructed. Note that proper timing and hand placement are the keys to success.

Home care instructions

- Warn the patient that the squeeze technique may cause temporary impotence, although this is uncommon. Also, have him watch for and report symptoms of prostatitis, including chills and fever; lower back, abdominal, rectal, or perineal pain; and bloody, painful, frequent, or urgent urination.
- Stress the importance of setting aside time to satisfy the sexual needs of the patient's partner.
- Encourage the patient and his partner to attend follow-up counseling sessions to discuss their progress in using the squeeze technique.

Sensate Focus Therapy

Helpful in treating a variety of sexual disorders, sensate focus therapy encourages a couple to relax and express intimacy through nongenital and genital touching exercises. Initially, vaginal penetration is prohibited during these exercises to encourage each partner to focus on sensual feelings without being burdened by preset goals or performance anxiety. As a result, many couples discover or renew a deep sense of intimacy.

Besides explaining sensate focus exercises to the couple, you'll need to encourage them to be assertive and take responsibility for their sexual pleasure by frankly discussing what they find enjoyable—and what they find unpleasant. What's more, you'll need to stress the importance of progressing through the exercises at their own pace to ensure success.

Purpose
To decrease sexual anxiety by increasing a couple's awareness of touch and sexual intimacy.

Preparation
Tell the couple that they may feel uncomfortable or embarrassed when they first practice sensate focus exercises; however, with time, they'll overcome these inhibitions. Stress the importance of letting each other know what feels good and what doesn't.

Procedure
Explain how to perform sensate focus exercises so the couple can practice them at home. To begin, instruct the couple to remove all their clothes. Then tell one partner to touch and explore the other's body, except for the genitals and breasts. Suggest touching with the hands to start, then blowing, sucking, and stroking with objects, such as a feather, for variety and spice. Encourage the other partner to concentrate on the pleasurable sensations of being touched. Next, have the couple reverse roles so that each person gives and receives pleasurable sensations. Although such touching may be sexually stimulating, emphasize that they

mustn't attempt intercourse. After the exercise, tell them to share their feelings about what they enjoyed and, equally important, what they found uncomfortable or unpleasant. Encourage the couple to practice this exercise until they feel at ease performing it.

Once they're comfortable performing this exercise, tell them to include touching the genitals and breasts. Remind them to avoid intercourse until they feel fully at ease. When they are, mention that intromission without thrusting is the next step. However, they should check with their therapist before taking this step and the next one: intromission with thrusting.

Monitoring and aftercare
Clear up any questions the couple may have about sensate focus exercises. Then remind them to set aside an uninterrupted time during the day or evening when they feel relaxed to practice these exercises.

Home care instructions
● Instruct the couple not to rush sensate focus exercises. Encourage them to repeat each exercise until they feel completely at ease, before moving on to the next one. Stress that each couple must progress at their own pace, depending on their needs.
● Because many couples attempt intercourse too early during therapy, emphasize the importance of concentrating on touch and intimacy in a relaxed, nondemanding atmosphere.

Selected References

Annon, Jack. *Behavioral Treatment of Sexual Problems.* Honolulu: Enabling Systems, 1975.

Hoffman, D., et al. "Treatment for Impotence: Penile Implants," *Today's OR Nurse* 6(8):16-21, August 1984.

Hogan, Rosemary. *Sexuality: A Nursing Perspective,* 2nd ed. East Norwalk, Conn.: Appleton-Lange, 1984.

Kaplan, H. *The New Sex Therapy: Active Treatment of Sexual Dysfunctions.* New York: Brunner-Mazel, 1974.

LoPiccolo, Joseph, and LoPiccolo, Leslie, eds. *Handbook of Sex Therapy.* New York: Plenum Pubs., 1978.

Masters, William, and Johnson, Virginia. *Human Sexual Response.* Boston: Little, Brown & Co., 1966.

11 Treating Endocrine Dysfunction

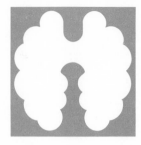

Treating Endocrine Dysfunction

Introduction

With endocrine disorders, treatment characteristically focuses on one of two major areas: either replacing the deficient hormone, in the case of endocrine hypofunction, or reducing hormonal excess, in the case of endocrine hyperfunction.

Treating hypofunction
For endocrine *hypofunction*, the patient may require replacement hormones, such as thyroid hormones. Or he may require drugs such as oral sulfonylureas: diabetic agents that alter the body's regulatory response.

Diet therapy plays an important role as well. In diabetes mellitus, for example, diet helps minimize the effects of deficient insulin secretion. In hypoparathyroidism, a high-calcium, low-phosphorus diet helps the patient maintain calcium-phosphorus balance.

New therapies have also improved the quality of life for many patients with endocrine disorders. For instance, many insulin-dependent diabetic patients can maintain excellent blood glucose control using blood glucose monitors, purified insulins, or continuous subcutaneous insulin infusion.

Treating hyperfunction
For endocrine *hyperfunction*, surgery is often the answer. The patient with thyroid disease, for example, may initially be treated with antithyroid drugs or radioactive iodine to curb excess thyroid hormone secretion. But if these treatments fail or are contraindicated, subtotal thyroidectomy becomes the treatment of choice. Similarly, adrenalectomy, hypophysectomy, pancreatectomy, or parathyroidectomy may be indicated to reduce excessive hormonal secretion or to treat malignancy. Fortunately, new microsurgical techniques and improved instruments have made total removal of any of these glands rare. Today, the surgeon is more likely to remove only the tumor or problem area, allowing some return of gland activity.

Careful teaching crucial
Your role in caring for patients with endocrine disorders goes far beyond patient preparation and postoperative care. Patient teaching, for example, is crucial. After all, many patients who have endocrine hypofunction or who have undergone gland resection or removal need lifelong hormone replacement therapy to avoid such potentially lethal conditions as myxedema coma, adrenal crisis, and diabetic ketoacidosis. If these patients fail to fully understand their condition, they may be tempted to stop taking their medication or to ignore their dietary restrictions.

DRUG THERAPY

Adrenocorticosteroids

Synthetic adrenocorticosteroids help correct adrenal insufficiency: the deficiency or absence of endogenous corticosteroids. These drugs can be broadly classified as glucocorticoids or mineralocorticoids. The major glucocorticoids include *hydrocortisone* and *cortisone* (short-acting corticosteroids), *prednisone* and *prednisolone* (intermediate-acting), and *dexamethasone* (long-acting); *desoxycorticosterone* and *fludrocortisone* represent the major mineralocorticoids. These drugs may be given alone or in combinations, depending on the patient's condition. In adrenal crisis, I.V. hydrocortisone is usually ordered. In primary adrenal insufficiency, a glucocorticoid and a mineralocorticoid are typically needed, whereas secondary adrenal insufficiency usually requires a glucocorticoid and a high-sodium diet.

The chief side effects of corticosteroids depend on the duration of therapy and the dosage. Long-term therapy causes cushingoid symptoms, such as moon face, hirsutism, and buffalo hump. In addition, it can cause cataracts, increased intraocular pressure, and peptic ulcers. High corticosteroid doses can cause psychotic behavior.

Corticosteroids should be given with extreme caution to patients with peptic ulcers, heart disease, infections, psychoses, diabetes mellitus, osteoporosis, or glaucoma.

Purpose and action

Adrenocorticosteroids restore hormonal and metabolic balance by replacing deficient or absent endogenous corticosteroids.

Monitoring

Before beginning therapy, weigh the patient to establish a baseline. During therapy, weigh him regularly to detect any increases caused by corticosteroid-induced appetite stimulation and fluid retention. Check also for edema, thinning of the extremities, and elevated blood pressure. Notify the doctor if the patient gains weight rapidly or develops edema or hypertension.

Observe the patient's skin for petechiae and bruising and monitor serum electrolyte and glucose levels to detect hypokalemia, hypernatremia, and hyperglycemia. If ordered, give potassium supplements and place the patient on a salt-restricted diet.

Assess the patient's mental status, especially if he's taking high doses. Report sudden mood swings to the doctor.

If the patient has recently had surgery, monitor the wound for dehiscence and evisceration because corticosteroids may delay healing. Watch for such signs of infection as diminished breath sounds and rhonchi because corticosteroids may mask expected signs.

Review the patient's medication regimen for possible interactions. Concurrent use of indomethacin or aspirin, for example, increases the risk of GI distress and bleeding. Barbiturates, phenytoin, and rifampin decrease corticosteroid effects.

If the patient complains of GI upset, give antacids, as ordered, to counteract the hyperacidity caused by corticosteroids. Also, give the drug with milk or food.

Home care instructions

• If the patient's receiving a daily dose, instruct him to take it in the morning, thereby mimicking the secretory pattern of endogenous corticosteroids, which peaks in the morning and reaches its nadir in the evening. If he's taking a divided dose, explain that the doctor has ordered the larger amount for the morning dose.

• Provide directions for missed doses. If the patient's on an alternate-day

ANABOLIC STEROIDS: SIDE EFFECTS SIGNIFICANT

Anabolic steroids, synthetic derivatives of testosterone, produce both androgenic and muscle-building effects by promoting protein synthesis and positive nitrogen balance. These drugs are mainly used to treat aplastic anemias, Fanconi's syndrome, severe debilitation, and growth problems resulting from pituitary dysfunction. Unfortunately, their side effects can be severe and include hepatotoxicity, fluid and sodium retention, and hypercalcemia. What's more, women may experience virilization with menstrual abnormalities, hirsutism, hoarseness, and reversible clitoral enlargement. Prepubertal males may experience premature epiphyseal closure, acne, priapism, growth of body and facial hair, and phallic enlargement. Postpubertal males, in turn, may experience testicular atrophy, oligospermia, impotence, gynecomastia, and male pattern baldness.

Obviously, these drugs must be prescribed cautiously and monitored carefully. And yet, despite their hazards, they continue to be popular with athletes, especially weight lifters and others who rely upon muscle mass and strength. Anabolic steroids *do* build muscle mass—but they apparently *don't* cause an increase in muscle strength proportional to muscle bulk, making their use highly questionable even without the added problem of their side effects.

To help reduce the incidence of anabolic steroid abuse in athletes, many collegiate and tournament regulations now require screening tests before or after major competitions to detect the presence of these drugs.

schedule, tell him to take the missed dose if he remembers later that morning; otherwise, he should take the dose the next morning and then skip the following day, resuming an alternate-day schedule. If the patient's on a daily schedule, tell him to make up the missed dose as soon as he remembers, unless it's almost time for the next dose; tell him *not* to double-dose. If he takes his medication several times daily, tell him to take a missed dose as soon as he remembers and to double up if it's time for his next dose.

• Tell him that if he vomits within 1 hour of taking his dose, he should take another dose. However, he should call his doctor if vomiting persists.

• Warn him to promptly report signs of adrenal insufficiency: headache, abdominal pain, anorexia, weakness, restlessness, and agitation. Stress that he should *never* stop taking his medication because this may precipitate adrenal insufficiency or life-threatening adrenal crisis.

• Advise him to report minor stress or illness, such as a cold, or a dental extraction so that the doctor can increase the dosage. Explain that he'll require hospitalization and parenteral steroids

if he suffers a major illness or requires an invasive procedure.

• If the patient has primary adrenal insufficiency, remind him to maintain a liberal salt intake because his decreased aldosterone levels may cause sodium and fluid depletion. Advise him to be especially careful during hot weather because perspiration increases sodium excretion.

• Warn the patient not to take any other drugs, including aspirin, without his doctor's approval.

• Tell him to wear a Medic Alert bracelet, which will advise emergency personnel of his condition and medication regimen. If ordered, instruct him to carry prefilled syringes or an emergency kit containing a syringe and vial of the appropriate corticosteroid.

Subcutaneous Insulin Injection

First used in the 1920s, insulin injection remains the treatment of choice for Type I (insulin-dependent) diabetes.

The insulins also treat Type II (non-insulin-dependent) diabetes when affected patients experience acute infection or excessive stress.

Although the indications for insulin use have remained the same, commercial preparations of this drug have undergone many changes since their introduction. For instance, U-80 insulin has been replaced by U-100 insulin, by far the most commonly used strength. And U-500 insulin is available for patients with severe insulin resistance.

What's more, conventional insulins, made primarily from beef and pork pancreases, have been supplemented by semisynthetic and recombinant DNA human insulins and by "purified" insulins—beef or pork insulins with

COMPARING DRUGS

COMPARING INSULIN PREPARATIONS

Insulins come in a wide variety of types and purities. Most are derived from beef or pork, but Humulin is a recombinant DNA human product and Novolin is a semisynthetic human product. Insulins also have varying times of onset and peak effect and varying durations

PREPARATION	PURIFIED	ONSET (hours)	PEAK EFFECT (hours)	DURATION OF ACTION (hours)
Rapid-acting insulins				
Insulin injection (regular, crystalline zinc)				
Regular Iletin I	No	½ to 1	2 to 4	6 to 8
Regular Insulin	No	½	2½ to 5	8
Pork Regular Iletin II	Yes	½ to 1	2 to 4	6 to 8
Beef Regular Iletin II	Yes	½ to 1	2 to 4	6 to 8
Regular (concentrated) Iletin II	Yes	½	—	24
Velosulin	Yes	½	1 to 3	8
Purified Pork Insulin	Yes	½	2½ to 5	8
Humulin R	N.A.	½ to 1	2 to 4	6 to 8
Novolin R	N.A.	½	2½ to 5	8
Prompt insulin zinc suspension (semilente)				
Semilente Iletin I	No	1 to 3	3 to 8	10 to 16
Semilente Insulin	No	1½	5 to 10	16
Semilente Purified Pork Prompt Insulin	Yes	1½	5 to 10	16
Intermediate-acting insulins				
Isophane insulin suspension (NPH)				
NPH Iletin I	No	2	6 to 12	18 to 26
NPH Insulin	No	1½	4 to 12	24
Beef NPH Iletin II	Yes	2	6 to 12	18 to 26
Pork NPH Iletin II	Yes	2	6 to 12	18 to 26
NPH Purified Pork Isophane Insulin	Yes	1½	4 to 12	24
Insulatard NPH	Yes	1½	4 to 12	24
Humulin N	N.A.	1 to 2	6 to 12	18 to 24
Novolin N	N.A.	1½	4 to 12	24

less than 10 parts per million (ppm) of the byproduct proinsulin, as compared with less than 25 ppm for conventional insulins. These newer insulins reduce the risk of allergic reactions. They're recommended for patients who have never received insulin; for Type II diabetic patients who need insulin during a period of stress or illness; for patients with gestational diabetes; and for nondiabetic patients who are receiving I.V. hyperalimentation.

Besides coming from various sources, insulins vary in their durations of action. (See *Comparing Insulin Preparations* for details.) They may also be prescribed in a "split and mix" regimen, in which the patient takes two or three insulins with different durations of action, thereby improving his

of action. The doctor may prescribe any of the insulins shown below for your patient, or he may prescribe a mixture of them. Make sure you're familiar with these preparations.

PREPARATION	PURIFIED	ONSET (hours)	PEAK EFFECT (hours)	DURATION OF ACTION (hours)
Intermediate-acting insulins *(continued)*				
Insulin zinc suspension (lente)				
Lente Iletin I	No	2 to 4	6 to 12	18 to 26
Lente Insulin	No	2½	7 to 15	24
Beef Lente Iletin II	Yes	2 to 4	6 to 12	18 to 26
Pork Lente Iletin II	Yes	2 to 4	6 to 12	18 to 26
Lente Purified Pork Insulin	Yes	2½	7 to 15	22
Humulin L	N.A.	1 to 3	6 to 12	18 to 21
Novolin L	N.A.	2½	7 to 15	22
Isophane (NPH) 70%, regular insulin 30%				
Mixtard	Yes	½	4 to 8	24
Long-acting insulins				
Protamine zinc insulin suspension				
Protamine Zinc & Iletin I	No	4 to 8	14 to 24	28 to 36
Beef Protamine Zinc & Iletin II	Yes	4 to 8	14 to 24	28 to 36
Pork Protamine Zinc & Iletin II	Yes	4 to 8	14 to 24	28 to 36
Extended insulin zinc suspension (ultra-lente)				
Ultralente Iletin I	No	4 to 8	14 to 24	28 to 36
Ultralente Insulin	No	4	10 to 30	36
Ultralente Purified Beef Insulin	Yes	4	10 to 30	36

N.A. indicates not applicable.

GIVING YOURSELF A SUBCUTANEOUS INSULIN INJECTION

Dear Patient:

To inject insulin subcutaneously, wash your hands thoroughly and remove your prescribed insulin from the refrigerator if it's stored there. Then follow these steps.

1

Warm and mix the insulin by rolling the vial between your palms.

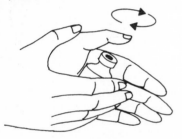

Caution: Never shake the vial. Check the expiration date; then read the label to make sure the medication is the correct strength and type. Use an alcohol swab to cleanse the rubber stopper on top of the vial.

2

Select an appropriate site. (Refer to the guide your nurse gave you, showing you how to rotate your injection sites correctly. To help you remember which site to use, write them on a calendar.)

Pull the skin taut; then clean it with an alcohol swab or a cotton ball soaked in alcohol, using a circular motion.

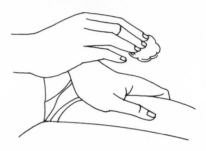

3

Before drawing up the insulin, inject an equal amount of air into the vial. That way you won't create a vacuum in the vial, and it'll be easier to withdraw your insulin.

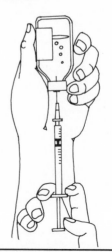

4

If air bubbles appear in the syringe after you fill it with insulin, tap the syringe lightly to remove them. Draw up more insulin, if necessary.

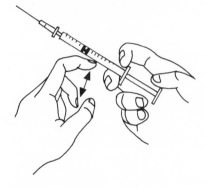

5

Using your thumb and forefinger, pinch the skin at the injection site. Then quickly plunge the needle into the fat fold at a 90-degree angle, up to its hub.

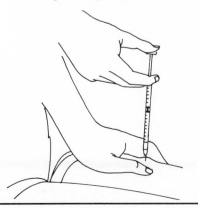

As you hold the syringe with one hand, pull back on the plunger slightly with your other hand to check for a backflow of blood. If blood appears in the syringe, discard everything and start again. If no blood appears, inject the insulin slowly.

6

Place the alcohol swab or cotton ball over the injection site; then press down on it lightly as you withdraw the needle.

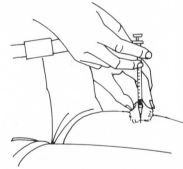

Snap the needle off the syringe, and dispose of both needle and syringe properly.

Important: If you travel, keep a bottle of insulin and a syringe with you at all times. The insulin doesn't need to be refrigerated as long as you keep it away from heat.

control over blood glucose levels.

The most common complications of insulin therapy—hypoglycemia and hyperglycemia—are dose-related. Local allergic reactions may occur at the start of therapy. So can severe allergic reactions, characterized by urticaria, angioedema, lymphadenopathy, bullae, or even anaphylaxis. During therapy, the patient may experience fatty buildup at injection sites if the sites aren't properly rotated. And, over time, insulin resistance may develop. Typically, though, this resistance can be overcome by changing insulins.

Purpose

To regulate blood glucose levels by increasing glucose transport across muscle and fat-cell membranes, by increasing hepatic formation of glycogen from glucose, and by promoting the conversion of glucose into fat.

Preparation

Explain to the patient that subcutaneous insulin injection helps regulate his blood glucose levels. Make sure he understands that insulin treats his illness but doesn't cure it. Emphasize that he needs lifelong medical follow-up and that he should *never* stop taking insulin because of the risk of life-threatening hyperglycemic coma.

Review the patient's medication regimen for possible interactions. For ex-

ample, concurrent use of beta blockers, clofibrate, fenfluramine, monoamine oxidase inhibitors, salicylates, or tetracycline prolongs insulin's hypoglycemic effects. Corticosteroids and thiazide diuretics diminish these effects.

If you'll be giving an insulin injection, gather the necessary equipment and wash your hands. Be sure that the insulin is of the correct type and strength. *Don't* switch the type of insulin.

If you're mixing insulins, follow the doctor's directions for their proportions. If you're mixing NPH or lente insulin in the same syringe with regular insulin, be sure to administer the mixture immediately to avoid binding.

Procedure

Select the appropriate injection site and assess for fatty buildup, which decreases insulin absorption. Make sure the patient hasn't exercised this area or undergone local heat therapy, because these factors promote overly rapid insulin absorption.

Now inject the insulin subcutaneously. Then properly dispose of the needle and syringe.

Monitoring and aftercare

If you're giving insulin to a patient who hasn't received it previously or is switching brands, observe him carefully for allergic reactions. Closely monitor his blood and urine glucose levels, as ordered.

During therapy, be alert for the Somogyi effect—hyperglycemia caused by insulin administration in patients who've received excessive doses of insulin for a prolonged period. Hyperglycemia persists in these patients because the hypoglycemia caused by excess insulin administration stimulates the secretion of large amounts of epinephrine, glucagon, and glucocorticoids. These substances act to elevate blood glucose levels. When insulin levels are lowered, this response decreases and blood glucose levels fall.

Home care instructions

• Explain to the patient that insulin therapy is only part of his care regimen—diet and regular exercise also contribute to good blood glucose control. Tell him that he should consult his doctor if his caloric intake or activity level changes or if he becomes ill, since his insulin requirements may change. Reinforce the importance of good blood glucose control by explaining that this may delay or possibly prevent the vascular and neurologic complications of diabetes.

• Provide instructions for mixing, drawing up, and injecting insulin (see *Giving Yourself a Subcutaneous Insulin Injection*, pages 402 and 403). If the patient's vision is impaired, explain that many devices, such as a magnifying sleeve and the Cornwall syringe, are available to aid him.

• Show the patient how to rotate injection sites, usually among his abdomen, thighs, and upper arms. Explain that he shouldn't use the same site more than once every 2 months, and demonstrate how a site rotation chart can help him to keep track of his injections.

• Tell the patient to store his insulin in a cool, dry place but never to freeze it. (Refrigeration isn't necessary, but it may be convenient.)

• If the patient will be testing his urine for glucose and ketones, show him how to use reagent strips, following the manufacturer's guidelines. If he'll be using a home blood-glucose monitoring system, have him practice obtaining a drop of blood manually or with a blood-letting device. Advise him to test glucose levels before insulin administration or meals.

• Tell him to notify his doctor if he misses an insulin dose or takes the incorrect amount or type.

• Suggest that he wear a Medic Alert bracelet and carry ample supplies of insulin and syringes with him on trips. Also recommend that he carry a fast-acting carbohydrate, such as hard candy or fruit juice, in case of an emergency.

Continuous Subcutaneous Insulin Infusion

One of the most recently developed treatments for Type I (insulin-dependent) diabetes, continuous subcutaneous insulin infusion allows a patient to achieve tight control of blood glucose levels 24 hours a day. In effect, the battery-powered infusion pump mimics the normal pancreatic pattern of insulin secretion. It delivers a basal infusion of regular insulin through tubing to a subcutaneous needle, usually inserted in the patient's abdomen. The pump also enables the patient to trigger delivery of a bolus dose of insulin at mealtimes to counter the blood glucose surge that results from digestion of food.

For many patients, continuous insulin infusion provides dramatically better diabetic control than conventional multiple insulin injections. This, in turn, makes the patient feel more energetic and gives him increasing control over his illness. What's more, continuous infusion can help overcome insulin resistance in peripheral tissues. And it can correct metabolic and hormonal abnormalities—including elevated blood levels of amino acids, lipids, catecholamines, growth hormone, glucagon, and somatomedin C, as well as excessive urinary losses of calcium and phosphorus—that may contribute to complications of diabetes. In fact, research suggests that successful continuous insulin infusion may slow or delay complications of diabetes, such as retinopathy and nephropathy, and may even reverse some already present complications.

Continuous insulin infusion, though, isn't without its drawbacks. The foremost ones are the high cost of equipment and supplies and the potential for

THE INSULIN PUMP:
UNDERSTANDING ITS KEY FEATURES

Most insulin pumps today are smaller, lighter, and easier to use than the models that first appeared on the market in the late 1970s. What's more, they're equipped with sophisticated safety features and alarms that help minimize errors in insulin delivery.

How the pump works

At the heart of most insulin pumps is a syringe. (A few pumps carry the insulin in a special reservoir instead.) It's filled with medication like a regular syringe, attached to the infusion tubing, and simply snapped into the pump. Adjusting the controls on the pump determines the rate of insulin flow from the syringe.

Each insulin pump has a range for the smallest and largest basal rates and bolus doses that it can deliver. Usually, the basal infusion is programmed in units of insulin per hour or day; the bolus is programmed in units alone. A number of pumps can also be programmed to change basal rates automatically at different times of the day. This feature is commonly used to compensate for the "dawn phe-

nomenon"—an early morning rise in blood glucose levels.

All pumps sound an alarm when the battery is running low. Most will also sound an alarm if the infusion tubing is blocked or if the pump has run out of insulin.

A look ahead

Some researchers are currently testing implantable insulin pumps that can be programmed and refilled from the outside. Besides benefiting patients who have frequent skin reactions, implantable pumps allow efficient and reliable insulin delivery directly into the body cavity instead of through the skin. However, they're not readily accessible for repair in case of malfunction.

Perhaps the best hope is an implantable pump that measures blood glucose levels and adjusts insulin delivery automatically. Such a device requires a small, reliable, durable glucose sensor that measures glucose accurately from minute to minute. To date, though, a sensor that meets these qualifications hasn't been approved for widespread use.

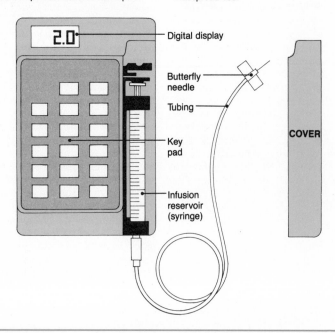

Digital display

Butterfly needle

Tubing

Key pad

COVER

Infusion reservoir (syringe)

rapid onset of hyperglycemia and diabetic ketoacidosis should the insulin flow be interrupted.

Despite these drawbacks, more than 15,000 diabetic patients currently use insulin infusion pumps. What makes someone a good candidate for using this device? First, the patient must be highly motivated and willing to participate in his treatment, since he'll need to check his blood glucose levels at least before and after each meal or snack and before exercise. He must also be emotionally stable so that he won't

COMPLICATIONS

GUARDING AGAINST HAZARDS OF INSULIN INFUSION

Despite the many benefits of continuous subcutaneous insulin infusion, such complications as hypoglycemia, hyperglycemia, or infection can occur. Fortunately, these complications can typically be prevented by careful monitoring and thorough patient teaching.

Heading off hypoglycemia
To help prevent hypoglycemia, stress the importance of testing blood glucose levels several times a day, as ordered. For some patients, such testing may be the only way to detect mild or moderate hypoglycemia. Explain that receiving continuous insulin infusion for a prolonged period can decrease the patient's catecholamine response to hypoglycemia, causing him to be asymptomatic. Make sure he understands how to adjust his diet, exercise, and blood glucose level.

Tell the patient that blood glucose levels drop to their nadir around 3 a.m., thereby creating the potential for excessive insulin delivery at that time. To avoid this nocturnal hypoglycemia, advise the patient to work closely with his doctor to ensure an appropriate basal rate. Also, suggest eating a snack and checking his blood glucose level just before he goes to bed.

Preventing hyperglycemia
If the patient's insulin supply is interrupted because of leakage at the insertion site, loosely connected tubing, a dead battery, or another problem, his blood glucose level can rise abruptly. That's because the insulin pump uses only fast-acting (regular) insulin and is designed to release only as much insulin as he needs at any one moment. So be sure to review the symptoms of hyperglycemia, such as polydipsia and polyuria, with the patient and tell him how to correct them promptly by adjusting his insulin supply.

Alert the patient to causes of equipment malfunction and stress what he can do to prevent them. Typically, the pump itself doesn't malfunction; rather, an obstruction forms between the syringe and the subcutaneous needle. The result of insulin precipitation, this obstruction occurs most commonly in premenstrual women, although its cause is unknown. Insulin precipitation is also often associated with temperature extremes and low basal rates.

If the patient suspects an obstruction, tell him to disconnect the tubing from the needle and to try clearing the obstruction with a bolus of insulin. If this doesn't work, he should change the infusion tubing and needle.

Insulin may also leak from the connection between the syringe and infusion tubing. Unfortunately, the patient can do little to prevent this. However, alert him to check this connection whenever he accidentally bumps or drops the pump.

Tell the patient that he can detect pump malfunction promptly by monitoring his blood glucose levels closely. Tell him to inspect the insulin pump equipment daily and to change the infusion set whenever he detects a loss of diabetic control.

Forestalling infection and local reactions
Minor skin reactions at the needle insertion site, such as small nodules or erythema, may result from allergy to metallic needles or irritation from adhesive tape. To prevent or relieve such reactions, suggest that the patient switch to a Teflon catheter or a different kind of tape. Or suggest that he rotate needle insertion sites more often.

Infection commonly leads to abscess formation at the insertion site. To prevent infection, instruct the patient to keep the site clean and to change the needle daily, using sterile technique. Have him watch for redness and tenderness, early signs of infection.

QUESTIONS PATIENTS ASK ABOUT LIFE-STYLE CHANGES

Since the insulin pump gives me better control of my diabetes, can I eat whatever I want?

No, you'll still need to follow your prescribed diet. The good news is that you'll have more flexibility in scheduling meals. Because the pump uses only fast-acting (regular) insulin, you won't have to time meals to compensate for the peaking action of, say, a morning dose of NPH insulin. Within limits, you can delay or even skip meals by postponing the mealtime bolus.

Can I still participate in sports?

Yes, as long as you have your doctor's approval. In fact, quite a few patients with insulin pumps participate in strenuous sports. Some run daily. Others play tennis. Still others water ski.

When you engage in water sports, you'll probably need to disconnect your pump. Most pumps are not waterproof. (That means you should also disconnect the pump when you're taking a bath or shower.) Ask your doctor how long it's safe for you to remain disconnected from the pump. Once reconnected, you may need to take extra insulin to make up for the amount you've missed. However, if you've removed the pump for strenuous exercise, the exercise itself may make up for the lost insulin.

How can I get a good night's sleep while wearing the pump?

Although this may seem impossible at first, you'll probably soon find that you have little trouble sleeping. Use trial and error to determine what works best for you. For instance, try tucking the pump in a pajama pocket or placing it under your pillow. You might even feel comfortable taking the pump under the covers and learning to shift it as you turn in bed.

harbor unrealistic expectations about therapy; for example, he'll still be vulnerable to fluctuations in blood glucose levels when he becomes ill or emotionally upset. Finally, the patient needs a strong support system to encourage him and to provide a backup in case he's unable to manage the pump himself.

Purpose
To achieve and maintain long-term near-normal glucose levels in the insulin-dependent diabetic patient.

Preparation
Describe to the patient how the insulin pump works: it continuously delivers a small amount of insulin, much like a healthy pancreas does. When the patient needs more insulin for meals or snacks, he can initiate the delivery of extra insulin. Emphasize that the pump doesn't measure his blood glucose levels—he must do that on his own.

Instruct the patient to check his blood glucose levels four times each day for 6 weeks to 3 months, as ordered, before the start of therapy. Stress the importance of meticulously recording each measurement. By studying the patient's glucose levels, the doctor will determine the appropriate basal infusion rate and bolus doses.

Determine the patient's expectations of continuous insulin infusion. To avoid disappointment and depression, he should realize that this therapy will not cure his diabetes and that it will require considerable effort for success.

Procedure
Begin by showing the insulin pump to the patient and describing its operation. Next, review the importance of monitoring blood glucose levels and explain how to adjust his bolus insulin, diet, or exercise regimen in response to changes in blood glucose levels. Also discuss what to do when he's ill and how to troubleshoot for complications of continuous insulin infusion.

After the doctor determines the patient's insulin requirements, gather the insulin pump equipment—the subcutaneous needle, infusion tubing, and pump—and prepare the patient for its setup. Then cleanse the needle insertion site on the patient's abdomen. (Alternative sites include the hip or thigh—or the buttocks if the patient's pregnant. However, the abdomen is favored, mainly because insulin seems to be absorbed most efficiently and predictably there.) Now insert the needle *horizontally* into the skin (the needle is prebent at a 30- to 45-degree angle).

Keep the needle in place by wrapping adhesive tape around the needle hub, crossing the ends, and securing them on either side of the needle. Then loop the infusion tubing and tape it in place to prevent the needle from dislodging. Cover the insertion site with a semipermeable, transparent dressing or gauze. Next, adjust the controls to deliver the appropriate basal infusion rate and check the alarms.

Monitoring and aftercare

Supervise the patient each time he delivers a bolus of insulin. Make sure he delivers the appropriate dose and operates the pump correctly. Then check his blood glucose level.

While the patient's hospitalized (usually for 3 to 7 days after continuous insulin infusion is initiated), help him learn to adjust his daily activities to accommodate the pump. For example, show him how to disconnect the pump before he takes a bath or shower. When he reconnects the pump, have him check his blood glucose level and deliver an insulin bolus, if necessary.

Wake the patient between 3 a.m. and 4 a.m. to check his blood glucose level. If you detect hypoglycemia, notify the doctor so he can adjust the patient's basal infusion rate.

Home care instructions

● Review with the patient how to insert the subcutaneous needle, using sterile technique, and stress the importance of rotating insertion sites every other day to prevent dimpling and minor skin re-

actions. Provide written instructions on how to fill the pump and operate its controls.

● Stress the importance of monitoring blood glucose levels, as ordered, to assess adequacy of insulin dosage.

● Teach the patient how to troubleshoot the equipment. For example, tell him to inspect the pump daily; to check the batteries (rechargeable batteries should be charged daily); to check the infusion tubing for kinks or clogs; and to check the connection site for breaks. Advise him to keep spare parts on hand.

● If problems (such as malfunction) occur with the infusion system, tell the patient to use multiple insulin injections until the problem is resolved and to contact his doctor immediately for dosage instructions. Explain that technical problems with the pump can usually be resolved quickly—most manufacturers have 24-hour technical assistance and part replacement available.

● If the patient expresses concern regarding others' reactions to the pump, encourage him to find ways to make the pump less obvious: by concealing it in a pocket or underneath clothing, by covering it with a coordinated cloth pouch, or by tucking the pump into a large knee pad pulled high on his thigh (see *Questions Patients Ask About Life-Style Changes*).

Sulfonylureas

First introduced in the 1950s, sulfonylureas represent the pharmacologic treatment of choice for Type II (non-insulin-dependent) diabetes mellitus. These oral hypoglycemic drugs work most effectively for patients whose diabetes is mild, nonketotic, uncontrollable by diet alone, and usually associated with obesity. However, they may also prove effective for patients whose diabetes requires dietary modifications and insulin dosages of 40 units or less per day.

Sulfonylureas are classified as first or second generation. First-generation drugs include *tolbutamide, chlorpropamide, acetohexamide,* and *tolazamide*; second-generation drugs include *glyburide* and *glipizide.* (A third generation, the biguanides, is used in Europe. However, phenformin, the biguanide once available in the United States, was removed from distribution because of concerns about lactic acidosis.) Although both first- and second-generation sulfonylureas work equally well, some doctors prefer the second-generation drugs because of their lower incidence of side effects, especially hyponatremia.

Chief side effects of the sulfonylureas include hypoglycemia and hypersensitivity reactions, such as pruritus, rash, and facial flushing. Increased gastric acid secretion may also cause such GI symptoms as heartburn, nausea, vomiting, abdominal pain, or diarrhea. Long-term therapy may increase the risk of death from cardiovascular disease.

Sulfonylureas are contraindicated for patients with Type I (insulin-dependent) diabetes because of the absence of functional beta cells. They're also contraindicated during pregnancy and lactation, and for diabetics undergoing severe stress (such as from surgery or acute infection). They're usually not recommended in hepatic or renal disease.

Purpose and action

Sulfonylureas normalize blood glucose levels by stimulating pancreatic beta cells to produce more insulin; by reducing hepatic glucose output; and by increasing the number of insulin receptors, which improves the insulin sensitivity of extrapancreatic tissues.

Monitoring

Review the patient's medication regimen because many drugs interact with sulfonylureas (see *Hazards of Using Sulfonylureas with Other Agents*). Give sulfonylureas 30 minutes before meals to reduce postprandial blood glucose levels. Dividing the daily dose improves GI tolerance.

If the patient's transferring from insulin therapy to an oral sulfonylurea, check his urine glucose and ketone levels at least three times daily, before meals. Collect a double-voided specimen.

If the patient is taking chlorpropamide, monitor his serum sodium level and be alert for hyponatremia. Notify the doctor if dysuria, anuria, hematuria, or other signs of renal insufficiency occur. Because this drug has a long duration of action (36 hours), monitor the patient for 3 to 5 days to detect hypoglycemia. If it occurs, notify the doctor and, as ordered, give I.V. dextrose.

If your patient is elderly, debilitated, or malnourished, be alert for and report an increased response to sulfonylureas. He may need a lower dosage.

Home care instructions

• Explain to the patient that sulfonylurea therapy represents only part of his diabetes care plan. Emphasize that the drug may be only temporarily effective or even ineffective if he fails to follow his prescribed diet and exercise program.

• Warn the patient not to take other medications without checking with his doctor.

• If the patient is taking chlorpropamide, warn him to avoid alcohol. Even small amounts of alcohol can cause chlorpropamide-alcohol flush, a disulfiram-like reaction that's characterized by extreme discomfort with facial flushing, light-headedness, pounding headache, nausea, vomiting, tachycardia, shortness of breath, and photosensitivity. Explain to the patient that these symptoms can last up to an hour.

• Tell the patient that he'll need continued follow-up care and that he shouldn't discontinue his medication

HAZARDS OF USING SULFONYLUREAS WITH OTHER AGENTS

Alcohol and a wide range of drugs can alter the effectiveness of sulfonylureas. Consequently, you'll need to check the patient's history carefully before you administer sulfonylureas.

Enhanced sulfonylurea action
Alcohol may cause a disulfiram-like reaction that's most severe with chlorpropamide. This reaction, called a chlorpropamide-alcohol flush, may be unpredictable. It can occur with even negligible consumption of alcohol, such as swallowing a mouthful of an alcohol-containing mouthwash.

More than a dozen drugs potentiate the action of sulfonylureas, possibly causing such symptoms of hypoglycemia as headache, nervousness, weakness, irritability, diaphoresis, nausea, and hunger. These drugs include chloramphenicol, clofibrate, dicumarol, guanethidine, methandrostenolone, monoamine oxidase

inhibitors, oxyphenbutazone, oxytetracycline, phenothiazines, phenylbutazone, probenecid, salicylates, sulfisoxazole, sulfonamides, and warfarin.

Similarly, propranolol and other beta blockers may induce hypoglycemia in combination with sulfonylureas. However, these drugs may also *mask* hypoglycemic effects.

Decreased sulfonylurea action
Certain drugs can reduce the effectiveness of sulfonylureas and predispose the patient to hyperglycemia, which is characterized by polyuria, polydipsia, polyphagia, and fatigue. These drugs include acetazolamide, corticosteroids, diazoxide, glucagon, lithium carbonate, oral contraceptives, phenothiazines, phenytoin, rifampin, salicylates, thiazide diuretics, and thyroid hormones.

---

without his doctor's permission. Instruct him to take his medication at the same time each day, as ordered, to help stabilize his blood glucose levels. Tell him to take a missed dose as soon as he remembers, unless it's almost time for his next dose; he should not double-dose.

• Teach the patient how to test his blood or urine glucose levels, as ordered. Explain that if his blood glucose remains uncontrolled after several months of therapy, or if it becomes uncontrolled after successful control by sulfonylureas, he may require insulin therapy. Also tell him he may need insulin if he experiences an acute infection or traumatic injury or if he needs to undergo surgery.

• Tell the patient to wear a Medic Alert bracelet containing information about his condition and his prescribed drug.

• Teach him the symptoms of hypoglycemia. If they occur, he should immediately notify his doctor and ingest a quick-acting sugar, such as hard candy, orange juice, or table sugar.

Thyroid Hormones

Used to treat hypothyroidism, thyroid hormone replacements were first employed in the 1890s. These animal thyroid hormone extracts, such as desiccated thyroid and thyroglobulin, are still in use today despite concerns about variations in their ratio of triiodothyronine (T_3) to thyroxine (T_4) from batch to batch. However, purified synthetic preparations, such as liothyronine, levothyroxine, and liotrix, are used more commonly. In fact, *liothyronine*, a rapidly acting T_3, is the drug of choice for treating myxedema or myxedema coma, mild hypothyroidism, and simple (nontoxic) goiter. However, dosage regulation is difficult and the drug's rapid action may cause cardiotoxic effects or abrupt metabolic changes.

Levothyroxine (synthetic T_4), the drug of choice for long-term therapy, possesses a longer half-life than liothyronine. As a result, it can be administered once daily, making compliance more likely. *Liotrix*, a combination of T_3 and T_4, isn't prescribed frequently, since T_4 is converted to T_3.

Side effects of thyroid hormones are usually dose-related and resolve when the dosage is tapered or the drug discontinued. Thyroid hormones should be used with extreme caution in patients with atherosclerosis and other heart diseases because they can precipitate angina pectoris or even myocardial infarction. They should also be given cautiously to patients with adrenal insufficiency because they can increase tissue demand for adrenal hormones, causing adrenal crisis. These hormones can be given safely to pregnant women but must be used cautiously during lactation because small amounts are excreted in breast milk.

Purpose and action

Exogenous thyroid hormones restore hormonal and metabolic balance in a patient with deficient endogenous thyroid hormones. They accelerate cellular oxidation, stimulate metabolism, enhance carbohydrate and protein synthesis, increase mobilization and use of glucose stores, lower cholesterol levels, and aid normal growth and development.

Monitoring

Before you give thyroid hormones, ask the patient if he has experienced hypersensitivity to aspirin. An aspirin-sensitive patient may be allergic to the dye tartrazine, which is present in some liotrix and levothyroxine preparations. Also check for lactose intolerance, which may forewarn of sensitivity to levothyroxine.

Review the patient's medication regimen for possible interactions. Concurrent use of cholestyramine or colestipol, for example, can impair absorption of thyroid hormones, requiring separation of doses by 4 to 5 hours. Use of cardiac glycosides requires careful monitoring because of the increased risk of glycoside toxicity.

Once the patient begins therapy, closely monitor serum total or free T_4 levels. Expect an improvement in 1 to 3 days if the patient is taking liothyronine; in 1 to 3 weeks if he's taking levothyroxine.

Be alert for symptoms of hyperthyroidism, especially in an elderly patient or one with known cardiac disease. Watch for GI effects, such as diarrhea, abdominal cramps, weight loss, and increased appetite. Check for cardiovascular effects, such as palpitations, chest pain, sweating, tachycardia, increased pulse and blood pressure, angina, and arrhythmias. Also note such other effects as headache, nervousness, heat intolerance, tremors, and insomnia. Report any of these symptoms to the doctor, who may decrease the dosage. He may also order a beta blocker, such as propranolol, to help control palpitations, tachycardia, and angina.

Home care instructions

● Advise the patient that thyroid hormone replacement doesn't cure his disease—it only relieves his symptoms. Stress that, although he'll feel better in a few weeks, he should not stop taking his medication.

● Explain that adherence to his medication schedule is extremely important. He should take his medication at the same time each day to maintain constant hormone levels. Instruct him to take a missed dose as soon as possible unless it's almost time for his next dose; he shouldn't double-dose. Tell him to call his doctor if he misses two or more doses.

● Warn the patient to report symptoms of hypothyroidism or hyperthyroidism immediately. Tell him that such symptoms indicate a need for dosage adjustment.

● Instruct him to keep his medication in its original container and to protect it from light and moisture. Tell him to store it in a cool place (below 40° F., or 4.4° C.).

Thyroid Hormone Antagonists

Thyroid hormone antagonists represent the primary treatment for patients with transient hyperthyroidism (from Graves' disease, multinodular goiter, or thyroiditis), for those who refuse iodine 131 treatment, and for those in whom thyroidectomy is contraindicated. Although these drugs don't permanently affect the thyroid gland, they do curtail hormone production until spontaneous remission of hyperthyroidism occurs. Because they decrease thyroid vascularity, they're also used before thyroid surgery, to prevent hemorrhage and thyroid storm.

Two classes of thyroid hormone antagonists—the stable iodines and the thionamides—are currently used. (A third class, represented by the investigational drug ipodate, has been found to reduce serum triiodothyronine levels rapidly.) The stable iodines, such as *potassium iodide*, were once the only therapy available for hyperthyroidism. These drugs suppress thyroid hormone secretion and reduce the gland's vascularity and size. Although they effectively combat thyrotoxic crisis in adults, they're used less commonly today than the thionamides because they're not as long-acting. With continued use, they may cause reversible iodism, a toxic condition characterized by skin eruptions, swelling and inflammation of the mucous membranes, conjunctivitis, fever, edema, and irritability.

The thionamides, the mainstay of antithyroid drug therapy, inhibit thyroid hormone formation. *Propylthiouracil* (PTU) is the preferred thionamide when rapid action is desired, as with severe hyperthyroidism or thyroid storm. Longer-acting *methimazole* can be given once daily and is preferred for treating mild to moderate hyperthyroidism. (A similar drug, *carbimazole*, is used extensively in Europe but has not yet been approved for use in the United States.) Chief side effects of the thionamides include hypersensitivity reactions (usually pruritus, rash, or fever) developing within the first 3 weeks of therapy. These seem to be dose-related and usually disappear spontaneously. Much more serious is granulocytopenia, which occurs most commonly with doses exceeding 30 mg/ day. This condition usually appears within the first 8 weeks of treatment and, if undetected, may be lethal. Although the patient typically experiences only a sore throat or fever, his white blood cell count may drop precipitously.

Thyroid hormone antagonists should be given cautiously during pregnancy. When they're needed, PTU is usually prescribed because methimazole has been linked with fetal aplasia cutis.

Purpose and action
• To provide temporary euthyroidism in the hyperthyroid patient. The stable iodines achieve this effect by causing high levels of iodine in the thyroid, which reduces the rate of thyroid hormone synthesis. The thionamides block iodine oxidation and thus prevent hormone synthesis; they may also prevent the coupling of monoiodotyrosine and diiodotyrosine.
• To reduce thyroid vascularity and hormone levels before surgery.

Monitoring
If you'll be administering potassium iodide, first check the patient's history for iodine allergies. If none exist, dilute the solution in juice or milk to counteract its metallic taste, and have the patient sip it through a straw to avoid discoloring his teeth. Give this solution after meals to prevent gastric irritation.

If the patient's receiving potassium iodide for a prolonged period, check for signs of iodism—a brassy taste or a burning sensation in his mouth, skin eruptions, conjunctivitis, fever, edema, and irritability. A rare but serious hypersensitivity reaction, marked by angioedema, hemorrhagic skin lesions, and serum sickness, may occur when iodine is given I.V. Call the doctor immediately if this occurs, and keep emergency airway supplies at the patient's bedside.

If the patient's receiving a thionamide, monitor for signs of hypersensitivity and notify the doctor if any occur; he may decrease the dosage. Monitor the patient's CBC periodically to detect leukopenia and granulocytopenia, which may occur 4 to 8 weeks after therapy begins. The doctor may not stop the medication if the patient has only mild leukopenia; however, expect to stop therapy if the patient develops granulocytopenia. Continue to monitor CBC until leukocyte production returns to normal, usually within 1 to 2 weeks after stopping therapy.

Monitor serum thyroid hormone levels to determine how your patient is responding to therapy. If he's taking PTU, expect his hormone levels to return to normal in 14 to 60 days.

Home care instructions

• If the patient is receiving thyroid hormone antagonists in preparation for surgery, explain the intended effects and the importance of maintaining his medication schedule.

• If he's receiving thyroid hormone antagonists as treatment for hyperthyroidism, stress the importance of maintaining his medication schedule to prevent recurrence. Tell him that he may not notice improvement for several weeks, until he exhausts his stores of thyroid hormones. Mention that symptoms related to increased sympathetic activity, such as tachycardia, diaphoresis, and tremors, may disappear rapidly. (If not, the doctor may also order propranolol, a beta blocker.) However, symptoms related to catabolic activity, such as weight loss, hypercalcemia, and myopathy, will take longer to improve.

• If the patient is taking a thionamide, tell him to watch for hypersensitivity

reactions and to report skin eruptions immediately. Emphasize the importance of promptly notifying the doctor if he develops a sore throat, fever, or mouth sores, especially during the 4th to 8th week of therapy.

• Explain that he should not stop taking the prescribed drug without his doctor's permission—abrupt withdrawal may precipitate thyroid storm.

• Tell the patient to take his medication at the same time each day. Depending on GI side effects, advise him to consistently take it either with meals or between them. The reason? Food may alter his response by increasing or decreasing drug absorption.

• Explain dietary restrictions, if ordered. Some doctors may not permit iodine-rich foods during therapy.

• Instruct him to take a missed dose as soon as possible; however, if it's almost time for his next dose, he should take both together. If he misses both doses, he should call his doctor.

• Tell the patient to store his medication in its original light-resistant container. Warn him not to take any over-the-counter drugs (especially decongestants and cough medications, which may contain iodine) without first checking with his doctor.

• Advise him to notify any doctors or dentists of his medication regimen before undergoing any invasive procedures, to minimize the risk of thyrotoxicosis.

DIETARY THERAPY

Diabetic Diet

Dietary therapy serves as a cornerstone of diabetes treatment. Unfortunately, an estimated 50% of diabetic patients don't comply with their diet. One major reason is their failure to understand the rationale behind this diet.

The patient with Type II (non-insulin-dependent) diabetes commonly needs to lose weight to lower his blood glucose levels. If he has mild hyperglycemia, he may only need to restrict calories since weight loss usually reduces both hepatic glucose production and insulin resistance. (This resistance stems primarily from a deficiency of cellular insulin receptors; it diminishes as weight loss reverses this receptor deficiency.) However, if the patient has severe hyperglycemia, he may need to use an exchange system to balance intake of dietary protein, carbohydrate, fat, and calories, distributing them carefully throughout the day.

The patient with Type I (insulin-dependent) diabetes has the additional concern of scheduling his meals and snacks to offset peak insulin action and avoid hypoglycemia. He also needs to follow an exchange system to balance dietary protein, carbohydrate, and fat.

Purpose

To provide a carefully regulated, balanced diet that meets nutritional requirements, achieves weight control, and lowers blood glucose levels without causing hypoglycemia, hyperglycemia, or ketosis.

Preparation

Explain to the patient that he'll require a special diet to help control his blood glucose levels. Take a thorough dietary history, keeping in mind that noncompliance with the diabetic diet may stem from unnecessarily limiting the patient's food preferences and habits. Consider not only *what* the patient eats but also *when* he eats, which will help you set up meal and snack times.

Determine what your patient knows about a diabetic diet. Explain that he needs to keep track of all the foods he eats and to categorize them according to food exchanges. Mention that no foods can be exempted—even so-called dietetic foods. (Dietetic candy, for ex-

ample, may need to be counted as an exchange, depending on its ingredients.)

Now, depending on the patient's type of diabetes, explain the diet's major goals: weight loss with a resulting decrease in blood glucose levels for the Type II diabetic patient; blood glucose control while avoiding hypoglycemia for the Type I diabetic patient.

Procedure

Base the target caloric allowance on the doctor's prescription or calculate it from the patient's ideal body weight. The American Diabetes Association recommends an adult basal caloric need of 10 kcal/lb of ideal body weight, modified for activity according to these formulas:
• ideal body weight muliplied by 3 for a sedentary patient
• ideal weight multiplied by 5 for a patient who exercises moderately
• ideal weight multiplied by 10 for a patient who exercises vigorously.

If weight loss is desired, subtract 500 kcal/day to achieve a weekly decrease of 1 lb.

Once you've determined the patient's daily caloric allowance, divide this between meals and snacks and select foods that meet suggested requirements. Typically, 50% to 60% of his calories should come from carbohydrates, 30% from fat, and the remainder from protein.

Monitoring and aftercare

If your patient is a newly diagnosed diabetic with extremely high blood glucose levels, he'll usually require hospitalization while his blood glucose levels are monitored and his insulin requirements are determined. Monitor him for signs of hypoglycemia, such as nervousness, dizziness, diaphoresis, fatigue, faintness, and possibly seizures or coma. Also watch for signs of hyperglycemia, such as polyuria, polydipsia, and dehydration. Finally, be on guard for signs of ketoacidosis, such as a fruity breath odor, dehydration, weak

HOW EXERCISE AFFECTS CARBOHYDRATE NEEDS

Exercise plays a vital role in treating Type I and Type II diabetes. Prolonged, intensive exercise demands continuous delivery of glucose from the tissues to the muscles, a process that requires insulin. But working muscle is more sensitive to insulin action than resting muscle, so more glucose is assimilated into muscle per unit of insulin during exercise.

What does this mean in practical terms? For the Type II diabetic patient, exercise depletes glucose stores, decreases insulin production, and increases the number of available insulin receptors, making metabolism more efficient. This patient should increase his intake of complex carbohydrates before strenuous exercise to maintain glucose homeostasis. For the Type I diabetic patient, exercise also depletes glucose stores; however, his insulin level (from insulin injection) either remains constant or increases (if he exercises the part of the body into which he's injected insulin), while the sensitivity of his muscles to insulin increases. This increased sensitivity occurs with even mild exercise

INTENSITY OF EXERCISE	CAL/HR	EXAMPLES	DURATION
Mild	50 to 199	Standing Strolling (1 mile/hr) Light housework	Less than 30 min
			More than 30 min
Moderate	200 to 299	Walking (2 miles/hr) Vacuuming Bowling Golf	Less than 30 min
			More than 30 min
Marked	300 to 399	Jogging (3 to 4 miles/hr) Swimming Scrubbing floors	Less than 30 min
			More than 30 min
Vigorous	Over 400	Jogging (5 miles/hr) Skiing Playing tennis	Less than 30 min
			More than 30 min

and rapid pulse, and Kussmaul's respirations.

Home care instructions

● Once you've prepared a diet that takes into account the doctor's prescription, the patient's caloric needs, and the food proportions to be used, work closely with the patient to help him understand it. If he'll be using food exchanges, review these carefully with him. (Teaching materials are readily available from the American Diabetes Association.) Explain to him that foods are broken down into meat exchanges (including high-, medium-, and low-fat groups); fat exchanges; milk exchanges; vegetable exchanges; fruit exchanges; and bread exchanges (including cereal and starchy vegetables). Show the patient how each exchange category lists the foods that fall within that group; the grams of carbohydrate, fat, and protein included in one exchange; and the quantity of food (1

and causes a decreased need for insulin that may last for up to 36 hours after he stops exercising. This patient needs to increase his intake of complex carbohydrates before strenuous exercise, modify his insulin dosage according to his doctor's orders, and, possibly, ingest further carbohydrates during exercise. Instruct him to always carry a source of carbohydrates with him during exercise, to help prevent hypoglycemia. Use this table as a guide to help him determine the type of food he should eat before and during exercise.

DIETARY ADJUSTMENTS

None

None

None

5 g simple carbohydrate every 30 minutes during exercise

15 to 20 g complex carbohydrate plus protein 15 to 30 minutes before exercise

15 to 20 g complex carbohydrate plus protein 15 to 30 minutes before exercise; 10 g simple carbohydrate every 30 minutes during exercise

30 to 40 g complex carbohydrate plus protein 15 to 30 minutes before exercise

30 to 40 g complex carbohydrate plus protein 15 to 30 minutes before exercise; 10 to 20 g simple carbohydrate every 30 minutes during exercise

cup, 1 oz, 1 slice, and so forth) that counts as one exchange.

• Ask the patient to write down the food he normally eats each day and then to use the exchange lists to find the calories and the amount of carbohydrates, fat, and protein that the food contains. Show him how and where his current eating habits veer from his prescribed diet. (For example, he may have been eating 2,400 calories/day rather than the 2,000 he needs, or he may have been getting 50% of his calories from fat rather than the recommended 30%.) Then ask him to use the exchange lists to work out a meal plan that incorporates these same foods but falls within the recommended guidelines. (Remember, working with exchange lists can be extremely confusing at first, so allow the patient to work at his own pace.) The more practice he has in planning enjoyable meals, the more likely he is to comply with his diet. Suggest that he plan meals a few days in advance so that he can secure the correct ingredients and will not be tempted to substitute others.

• Discuss restrictions on sugar intake. Although sugar was formerly forbidden, some doctors now allow their patients to have modest amounts of sucrose (table sugar) if taken with a meal—up to 5% of the daily carbohydrate allowance if spaced throughout the day. However, other doctors prefer that their patients use fructose or sorbitol, which are metabolized more slowly than sucrose, or aspartame, which is sweeter than sugar but low in calories. Explain that aspartame can be used as a "free" food: one that has few or no calories and can be used as often as desired. Fructose and sorbitol, in contrast, have more calories and may need to be counted as exchanges.

• Advise the patient about any alcohol restrictions. Typically, the patient can drink limited amounts of alcohol if his doctor approves and his diabetes is well controlled. The Type II diabetic patient should count alcohol as a fat exchange because the body metabolizes alcohol like fat. In contrast, the Type I diabetic patient should count alcohol as extra calories but should *not* substitute it for an exchange because of the risk of causing hypoglycemia. He should eat all his regular exchanges when he drinks alcohol.

• Encourage the patient to eat foods that contain unrefined carbohydrates and are high in fiber. Daily intake of 10 to 15 g of fiber delays gastric emptying and slows carbohydrate absorp-

tion, which can lower blood glucose levels and reduce insulin requirements.
• If your patient is insulin-dependent (Type I), stress the importance of eating on schedule to balance his insulin therapy. If he has to delay a meal, instruct him to eat hard candy or drink a nondietetic soft drink. Tell him he should always carry hard candy, fruit juice, or another source of simple sugar with him to counteract possible hypoglycemia. Also advise him that he needs to eat even if he becomes sick, to prevent hypoglycemia. Suggest that he substitute soft or liquid foods for his exchanges, as necessary.

SURGERY

Hypophysectomy

New microsurgical methods have dramatically reversed the high mortality once associated with removal of pituitary and sella turcica tumors. Hypophysectomy is now the treatment of choice for pituitary tumors, which can cause acromegaly, gigantism, and Cushing's disease. It can also halt progression of diabetic hemorrhagic retinopathy. And it can be used as a palliative measure for patients with metastatic breast or prostate cancer to relieve pain and reduce the hormonal secretions that spur neoplastic growth.

Hypophysectomy may be performed *transfrontally* (approaching the sella turcica through the cranium) or *transsphenoidally* (entering from the inner aspect of the upper lip through the sphenoid sinus). The transfrontal approach carries a high risk of mortality or of such complications as loss of smell and taste and permanent, severe diabetes insipidus. As a result, this approach is rarely used. The commonly

used transsphenoidal approach uses powerful microscopes and improved radiologic techniques to allow removal of microadenomas. Alternative approaches include laser surgery (still experimental) and cryohypophysectomy (used for growth hormone–secreting adenomas), in which a cryosurgical probe is introduced into the sella turcica through a frontal burr hole.

Contraindications to hypophysectomy include anatomic anomalies barring access to the pituitary, sphenoidal infection, and nasal infection. After surgery, transient diabetes insipidus routinely occurs, requiring careful patient monitoring for 24 to 48 hours. Other potential complications include infection, cerebrospinal fluid (CSF) leakage, hemorrhage, and visual defects. Total removal of the pituitary gland causes a hormonal deficiency that requires close monitoring and replacement therapy; usually, though, the anterior pituitary is preserved.

Purpose
To remove hormone-secreting pituitary tissue.

Preparation
Explain to the patient that this surgery will remove a tumor from his pituitary gland. Tell him that he will receive a general anesthetic and, after surgery, will remain in the intensive care unit for 48 hours to permit careful monitoring. Mention that he'll have a nasal catheter and packing in place for 1 to 2 days after surgery, as well as an indwelling urinary catheter.

Arrange for appropriate tests and examinations, as ordered. For example, if the patient has acromegaly, he'll need a thorough cardiac evaluation since he'll tend to have incipient myocardial ischemia. If the patient has Cushing's disease, he'll need blood pressure checks and serum potassium determinations. For all patients, arrange visual field tests to serve as a baseline.

Review the patient's preoperative medication regimen, if appropriate. If

ADENECTOMY: ALTERNATIVE TO HYPOPHYSECTOMY

Both adenectomy and hypophysectomy can be used to remove pituitary tumors. But how do their indications differ? In hypophysectomy, the doctor removes the tumor and all or part of the pituitary gland. However, if the tumor is confined to the sella turcica, the doctor may be able to perform an adenectomy, in which he removes the lesion while leaving the pituitary intact. Both surgeries employ the transsphenoidal approach shown here.

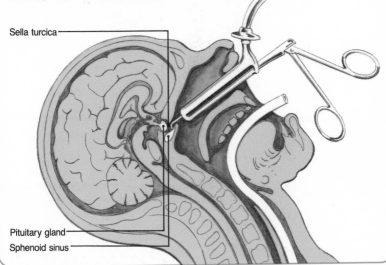

Sella turcica

Pituitary gland

Sphenoid sinus

he's hypothyroid, he may need hormone replacement therapy. If he has a prolactin-secreting tumor, find out if he has been taking ergobromocryptine for 6 weeks before surgery to help shrink and soften the tumor.

Ensure that the patient or a responsible family member has signed a consent form.

Procedure

In transsphenoidal hypophysectomy, the patient is placed under general anesthesia and the doctor makes an incision in the superior gingival tissue of the maxilla. After membrane and tissue dissection, he places a speculum blade in the developed space, slightly anterior to the sphenoid sinus to avoid lateral compression of the opened sinus' anterior walls. (Some doctors prefer the septal passage approach for the speculum.) Then he evaluates the deeper anatomy, using an operating microscope with binocular vision and high-power lighting.

Using a microdrill, the doctor penetrates the sphenoid bone, allowing visualization of the anterior sella floor. He can then resect and aspirate soft tumors downward. Before wound closure, he may apply hemostatic agents, such as Oxycel cotton. Or he may use the patient's own subcutaneous fat or a muscle plug from the thigh as intersellar graft tissue. The sella floor may be sealed off with a small piece of bone or cartilage.

Finally, the doctor inserts nasal catheters with petrolatum gauze packed around them. He closes the initial incision with stitches inside the inner lip.

Monitoring and aftercare

Keep the patient on bed rest for 24 hours after surgery and then encourage ambulation. Keep the head of his bed elevated to avoid placing tension or pressure on the suture line. Tell him not to sneeze, cough, blow his nose, or bend over for several days to avoid disturbing the muscle graft.

Give mild analgesics, as ordered, for headache caused by CSF loss during surgery or for paranasal pain. Paranasal pain typically subsides when the catheters and packing are removed—usually 24 to 48 hours after surgery.

Expect the patient to develop transient diabetes insipidus, usually within 24 hours after surgery. Be alert for increased thirst and increased urinary volume with a low specific gravity. If diabetes insipidus occurs, replace fluids and administer aqueous vasopressin, as ordered. Or give sublingual desmopressin acetate, as ordered. With these measures, diabetes insipidus usually resolves within 72 hours.

Arrange for visual field testing as soon as possible, since visual defects can indicate hemorrhage. Collect a serum sample to measure pituitary hormone levels and evaluate the need for hormone replacement. As ordered, give prophylactic antibiotics.

Home care instructions

• Instruct the patient to report signs of diabetes insipidus immediately. Explain that he may need to limit fluid intake or take prescribed medications.
• If ordered, tell the patient not to brush his teeth for 2 weeks to avoid suture line disruption. Mention that he can use a mouthwash.
• The patient may need hormonal replacement therapy as a result of decreased pituitary secretion of thyroid-stimulating hormone. If he needs cortisol or thyroid hormone replacement, teach him to recognize the signs of excessive or insufficient dosage. Advise him to wear a Medic Alert bracelet.
• Tell the patient with hyperprolactinemia that he'll need follow-up visits for several years because relapse is possible. Explain that he may be placed on bromocriptine if relapse occurs.

Parathyroidectomy

Parathyroidectomy, the surgical removal of one or more of the four parathyroid glands, treats primary hyperparathyroidism. In this disorder, the parathyroids secrete excessive parathyroid hormone (PTH), causing high serum calcium and low serum phosphorus levels.

The number of glands removed depends on the underlying cause of excessive PTH secretion. For example, if the patient has a single adenoma, excision of the affected gland corrects the problem. If more than one gland is enlarged, subtotal parathyroidectomy (removal of the three largest glands and part of the fourth gland) can correct hyperparathyroidism. The remaining glandular segment decreases the risk of postoperative hypoparathyroidism and resulting hypocalcemia since it resumes normal function.

Total parathyroidectomy is necessary when glandular hyperplasia results from malignancy. In this case, the patient will require lifelong treatment for hypoparathyroidism. The doctor may also perform subtotal thyroidectomy along with parathyroidectomy if he's unable to locate the abnormal tissue or adenoma and suspects an intrathyroid lesion.

Serum calcium levels typically decrease within 24 to 48 hours after surgery and become normal within 4 to 5 days. Complications seldom occur but may include hemorrhage, damage to the recurrent laryngeal nerve, and hypoparathyroidism.

Purpose

To remove diseased parathyroid tissue, decreasing circulating levels of PTH and serum calcium.

Preparation

Explain to the patient that this surgery will remove diseased parathyroid tissue. Tell him that he'll be intubated and receive a general anesthetic and that the doctor will make a neck incision, explore the area, and remove parathyroid tissue as necessary. Explain that the doctor may need to perform a subtotal thyroidectomy if he can't find diseased parathyroid tissue. Ensure that the patient or a responsible family member has signed a consent form.

Maintain calcium restrictions, as ordered, before surgery. If the patient's hypercalcemia causes renal calculi, provide plenty of fluids to dilute the excess calcium. If his hypercalcemia is severe, give saline solution with potassium I.V., as ordered, and expect to give a diuretic, such as furosemide. If his calcium level remains elevated once diuresis has begun, you may give I.V. mithramycin (an antihypercalcemic agent), as ordered. As an adjunct, the doctor may also order inorganic phosphates, which appear to lower serum calcium levels by promoting calcium deposition in bone.

Procedure
After the patient's anesthetized, the doctor makes a cervical neck incision and exposes the thyroid gland. Then, he locates the four parathyroids (usually within 2 cm above or below the point where the recurrent laryngeal nerve and the inferior thyroid artery cross) and identifies and tags them. If he can't find one of them, he'll do a cervical thymectomy and thyroid lobectomy on the side where the gland is missing and send a sample for an immediate frozen section. If the missing gland's not found in the removed tissue, the doctor may stop the procedure and order localization studies before a second surgery. Or he may continue surgery by opening the sternum and exploring the mediastinum for the missing gland. Once he has found all four glands, he examines them for hyperplasia and removes the affected ones. Before he sutures the incision, he inserts a Penrose drain or a closed wound drainage device.

Monitoring and aftercare
Keep the patient in high semi-Fowler's position after surgery to promote venous return from the head and neck and to decrease oozing into the incision. As soon as he begins to awaken from anesthesia, check for laryngeal nerve damage by asking him to speak.

Check the patient's dressing and palpate the *back* of his neck, where drainage tends to flow. Expect about 50 ml of drainage in the first 24 hours; if you find no drainage, check for drain kinking or the need to reestablish suction. Expect only scant drainage after 24 hours.

Keep a tracheostomy tray at the patient's bedside for the first 24 hours after surgery, and assess the patient frequently for signs of respiratory distress, such as dyspnea and cyanosis. Upper airway obstruction may result from tracheal collapse, mucus accumulation in the trachea, laryngeal edema, or vocal cord paralysis.

Expect the patient to complain of a sore neck (from hyperextension during surgery), a sore throat (from manipulation), and hoarseness and swallowing difficulty (from anesthesia and intubation). Give mild analgesics, as ordered.

Because transient hypoparathyroidism with resulting hypocalcemia can occur 1 to 4 days after surgery, watch closely for signs of increased neuromuscular excitability. Check for positive Chvostek's and Trousseau's signs, and tell the patient to report numbness and tingling of his fingers and toes or around his mouth (early signs of hypocalcemia) as well as muscle cramps. Keep I.V. calcium on hand in case tetany occurs.

Home care instructions
• Tell the patient to keep his incision site clean and dry, and explain that it will need to be checked in follow-up appointments. Also tell him that he'll need periodic serum calcium determinations to help evaluate the surgery's outcome.

- Advise him not to take any over-the-counter drugs without consulting his doctor. In particular, tell him to avoid magnesium-containing laxatives and antacids, mineral oil, and vitamins A and D.
- If the patient has had a total para-thyroidectomy, instruct him to follow a high-calcium, low-phosphorus diet, as ordered, and to take his calcium medications. (See *Questions Patients Ask About Hypoparathyroid Diet.*) If he'll be receiving dihydrotachysterol and calciferol, tell him not to take vitamins without consulting his doctor. Tell him to call his doctor if he develops signs of hypercalcemia, such as excessive thirst, headache, vertigo, tinnitus, and anorexia.

QUESTIONS PATIENTS ASK ABOUT HYPOPARA-THYROID DIET

Why do I need a special diet?

Because of your parathyroidectomy, your body now lacks parathyroid hormone. This hormone helps maintain a balance between two important minerals: calcium and phosphorus. Without this hormone, your kidneys excrete too much calcium and retain too much phosphorus. Your diet, which is high in calcium and low in phosphorus, tries to make up for this.

Why did my doctor tell me to avoid milk, which is high in calcium?

Because milk is also high in phosphorus, which you need to limit.

Why do I need to take vitamin D supplements with this diet?

This vitamin helps your body absorb calcium faster. Even if you eat lots of high-calcium foods, you may not be getting the full benefit if you don't have enough vitamin D.

How do I know if my diet's working?

Your doctor will order periodic blood tests to check on your calcium and phosphorus levels. Your diet's working if your serum calcium levels are between 8.5 and 10.5 mg/dl and your serum phosphorus levels are between 2 and 4 mg/dl.

Thyroidectomy

The surgical removal of part or all of the thyroid gland, thyroidectomy allows treatment of hyperthyroidism, respiratory obstruction from goiter, and thyroid malignancy. Subtotal thyroidectomy, used to correct hyperthyroidism when drug therapy fails or radiation therapy is contraindicated, reduces secretion of thyroid hormone. It also effectively treats diffuse goiter. After surgery, the remaining thyroid tissue usually supplies enough thyroid hormone for normal function.

Total thyroidectomy is usually performed for extensive malignancy. After this surgery, the patient requires lifelong thyroid hormone replacement therapy.

Most often performed under general anesthesia, thyroidectomy infrequently causes complications if the patient's properly prepared with thyroid hormone antagonists before surgery. Potential complications include thyroid storm; hemorrhage; parathyroid damage, resulting in postoperative hypocalcemia or tetany; and laryngeal nerve damage, causing hoarseness or permanent voice change.

Purpose
- To remove hyperfunctioning or enlarged thyroid tissue, decreasing circulating thyroid hormone levels
- To remove thyroid malignancy.

Preparation

Explain to the patient that thyroidectomy will remove diseased thyroid tissue or, if necessary, the entire gland. Tell him that he'll have an incision in his neck; that he'll have a drain and dressing in place after surgery; and that he may experience some hoarseness and a sore throat from intubation and anesthesia. Reassure him that he'll receive analgesics to relieve his discomfort.

Ensure that the patient has followed his preoperative drug regimen, which will render the gland euthyroid to prevent thyroid storm during surgery. He probably will have received either propylthiouracil or methimazole, usually starting 4 to 6 weeks before surgery. Expect him to be receiving iodine as well for 10 to 14 days before surgery to reduce the gland's vascularity and thus prevent excess bleeding. He may also be receiving propranolol to reduce hypertensive effects. Notify the doctor immediately if the patient has failed to follow his medication regimen.

Collect samples for serum thyroid hormone determinations to check for euthyroidism. If necessary, arrange for an EKG to evaluate cardiac status. Ensure that the patient or a responsible family member has signed a consent form.

Procedure

After the patient's anesthetized, the surgeon extends the neck fully and determines the incision line by measuring bilaterally from each clavicle. Then he cuts through the skin, fascia, and muscle and raises skin flaps from the strap muscles. He separates these muscles midline, revealing the thyroid's isthmus, and ligates the thyroid artery and veins to help prevent bleeding. Next, he locates and visualizes the laryngeal nerves and parathyroid glands and then begins dissection and removal of thyroid tissue, trying not to injure these nearby structures.

Before the surgeon sutures the incision, he inserts a Penrose drain or a closed wound drainage device, such as a Hemovac drain.

Monitoring and aftercare

Keep the patient in high semi-Fowler's position to promote venous return from the head and neck and to decrease oozing into the incision. Check for laryngeal nerve damage by asking the patient to speak as soon as he awakens from anesthesia.

Watch for signs of respiratory distress. Tracheal collapse, tracheal mucus accumulation, laryngeal edema, and vocal cord paralysis can all cause respiratory obstruction, with sudden stridor and restlessness. Keep a tracheostomy tray at the patient's bedside for 24 hours after surgery, and be prepared to assist with emergency tracheostomy, if necessary.

Assess for signs of hemorrhage, which may cause shock, tracheal compression, and respiratory distress. Check the patient's dressing and palpate the *back* of his neck, where drainage tends to flow. Expect about 50 ml of drainage in the first 24 hours; if you find no drainage, check for drain kinking or the need to reestablish suction. Expect only scant drainage after 24 hours.

As ordered, administer a mild analgesic to relieve a sore neck or throat. Reassure the patient that his discomfort should resolve within a few days.

Assess for hypocalcemia, which may occur when bones depleted of calcium from hyperthyroidism begin to heal, rapidly taking up calcium from the blood. Test for Chvostek's and Trousseau's signs, indicators of neuromuscular irritability from hypocalcemia. Keep calcium gluconate available for emergency I.V. administration.

Be alert for signs of thyroid storm, a rare but serious complication (see *Guarding Against Hazards of Thyroidectomy,* page 424).

The doctor will usually remove the drains and half the surgical clips on the second day after surgery; the remaining clips, the following day.

COMPLICATIONS

GUARDING AGAINST HAZARDS
OF THYROIDECTOMY

Thyroidectomy has many benefits and relatively few complications. However, some complications can be life-threatening if not promptly recognized and corrected.

Thyroid storm
This rare but severe form of thyrotoxicosis can occur in a patient who received inadequate preoperative treatment with thyroid hormone antagonists. Its symptoms include high fever; hot, flushed skin; tachycardia and tachyarrhythmias; agitation and restlessness; confusion; and frank psychosis. Without treatment, hypotension, coma, and vascular collapse follow.

If you detect thyroid storm, infuse fluids, apply a hyperthermia blanket, and give acetaminophen. Also give sodium iodide, propranolol, and hydrocortisone I.V. Instill propylthiouracil through a nasogastric tube to block thyroid hormone synthesis and release.

If the patient develops respiratory distress, administer oxygen and ensure a patent airway. Treat extreme restlessness with sedatives as ordered, and monitor vital signs, cardiac rhythm, and serum thyroid hormone levels.

Hypocalcemia
Inadvertent damage to the parathyroids during surgery may cause transient hypoparathyroidism with resulting hypocalcemia. To detect this complication, assess the patient for early signs of hypocalcemia, such as paresthesias in the extremities, every 2 to 4 hours postoperatively. Test for positive Chvostek's and Trousseau's signs. Be alert for later signs of hypocalce-

mia: muscle cramps, tetany, seizures, stridor, dyspnea, diplopia, abdominal pain, and urinary frequency.

If the patient develops acute hypocalcemic tetany, administer I.V. calcium chloride or calcium gluconate. Assist with emergency tracheostomy if stridor and vocal cord paralysis lead to respiratory obstruction.

Hemorrhage
Hemorrhage in the confined space of the deep cervical fascia may appear in the initial hours after surgery, causing acute airway obstruction with increasing respiratory distress and restlessness. If this occurs, maintain airway patency and, if necessary, assist with emergency tracheostomy until the patient can be sent back to surgery to reopen the wound, relieve the pressure, and correct the hemorrhage.

Nerve injury
Inadvertent damage to the recurrent laryngeal nerve can cause temporary or permanent voice change or permanent paralysis. Assess the patient's voice as soon as he awakens from anesthesia, and continue to assess it for 2 days after surgery.

Unilateral nerve damage causes initial hoarseness and a nonexplosive cough, improving until the patient has a normal voice that tires easily. Bilateral injury causes early postoperative stridor and ineffective coughing. The patient may need reintubation for 7 to 10 days and eventually, if no improvement occurs, a tracheostomy. Be prepared to intervene to relieve respiratory distress.

Home care instructions
- If the patient has had a total thyroidectomy, explain the importance of regularly taking his prescribed thyroid hormone replacement. Teach him to recognize and report signs of hypothyroidism and hyperthyroidism.
- If parathyroid damage occurred during surgery, explain to the patient that he'll need to take calcium supplements. Teach him to recognize the warning signs of hypocalcemia.
- Tell the patient to keep the incision

site clean and dry. Help him cope with concerns about its appearance. Suggest loosely buttoned collars, high-necked blouses, jewelry, or scarves, which can hide the incision until it has healed. The doctor may recommend using a mild body lotion to soften the healing scar and improve its appearance.
- Arrange follow-up appointments as necessary and explain to the patient that the doctor needs to check the incision and serum thyroid hormone levels.

Pancreatectomy

Pancreatectomy, which includes various resections, drainage procedures, and anastomoses, may be used to treat pancreatic diseases in which more conservative techniques have failed. It's indicated for palliative treatment of pancreatic cancer and chronic pancreatitis, which often stems from prolonged alcohol abuse. It's also used to treat islet cell tumors (insulinomas).

The type of procedure used depends on the patient's condition, the extent of the disease and its metastasis, and the amount of endocrine and exocrine function the pancreas retains. Often, the procedure is determined only after surgical exploration of the abdomen.

Major complications of pancreatectomy include hemorrhage (during and after surgery), fistulas, abscesses (common with distal pancreatectomy), common bile duct obstruction, and pseudocysts. Subtotal resection sometimes causes insulin dependence, whereas total pancreatectomy always causes permanent and complete insulin dependence.

Purpose
• To remove diseased pancreatic tissue, preserving functioning tissue by providing adequate drainage
• To remove the entire pancreas, preventing metastasis or relieving pain when function can't be preserved.

Preparation
Explain to the patient that the specific procedure will be selected by the surgeon during abdominal exploration. Provide emotional support and encourage the patient to express his feelings. Give analgesics, as ordered.

Arrange for necessary diagnostic studies, as ordered, to help the surgeon determine the existing endocrine and exocrine structure of the pancreas and any anatomic anomalies.

For the patient with chronic pancreatitis or cancer, provide enteral or parenteral nutrition before surgery. As ordered, give low-fat, high-calorie feedings to combat the malnutrition and steatorrhea that result from malabsorption. Give meticulous skin care to prevent tissue breakdown that could complicate postoperative healing. If the patient is hyperglycemic, give oral hypoglycemic agents or insulin, as ordered, and monitor blood and urine glucose levels.

Monitor the patient with a recent history of alcohol abuse for withdrawal symptoms: agitation, tachycardia, tremors, anorexia, and hypertension. Remember that delirium tremens may occur 72 to 96 hours after the patient's last drink and that surgery should be delayed until after this period.

If the patient smokes (many patients with pancreatic cancer are heavy smokers), advise him to stop smoking before surgery. Evaluate his pulmonary status to provide baseline information, and instruct him in deep-breathing and coughing techniques. Explain to the patient that he should turn in bed, perform deep-breathing exercises, and cough every 2 hours for 24 to 72 hours after surgery. If incentive spirometry is indicated, instruct him as appropriate.

Assess the patient for jaundice and increased hematoma formation—signs of liver dysfunction, which commonly accompanies pancreatic disease. As ordered, arrange for liver function and coagulation studies before surgery. If the patient has a prolonged prothrombin time, expect to give vitamin K to prevent postoperative hemorrhage.

Because resection of the transverse colon may be necessary, the doctor may order mechanical and antibiotic bowel preparation as well as prophylactic systemic antibiotics (started 6 hours before surgery and continuing for 72 hours after surgery). Carry out these measures, as directed, and expect to assist with nasogastric tube and indwelling (Foley) catheter insertion.

Ensure that the patient or a respon-

UNDERSTANDING TYPES OF PANCREATECTOMY

SURGERY	INDICATIONS
Pancreaticojejunostomy	• Chronic pancreatitis with extensive pathology • Multiple strictures • Palpable ductal dilatation • Pancreatic ascites
Distal pancreatectomy (subtotal)	• Islet cells tumors (insulinomas) confined to tail of pancreas
Distal pancreatectomy (95%)	• Acute pancreatitis • Chronic pancreatitis with extensive pathology and diffuse calcification • Multiple strictures or obstructions • Intrahepatic cyst formation • Failure of other procedures, such as surgical repair of biliary or pancreatic ducts or the sphincter of Oddi
Total pancreatectomy	• Chronic pancreatitis with marked pancreatic destruction • Multiple intraductal obstructions • Failure of more conservative measures, such as medication and diet, to control severe pain • Malignancy
Fortner regional pancreatectomy	• Pancreatic cancer
Radical pancreaticoduodenectomy (Whipple procedure)	• Malignancy confined to head of pancreas
Partial pancreaticoduodenectomy (Modified Whipple procedure)	• Malignancy confined to head of pancreas

PROCEDURE

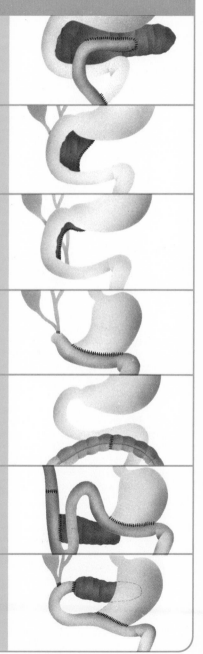

Pancreatic duct, if large enough, is connected to the jejunum, bypassing obstruction; pancreatic tissue is preserved

Removes the neck, body, and tail of the pancreas plus the spleen and splenic vessels; pancreatic duct may be drained into stomach or jejunum; leaves the head and uncinate process of the pancreas to the left of the mesenteric vessels

Removes the neck, body, and tail of the pancreas, as well as a major portion of the head and uncinate process and the entire spleen; leaves only a rim of pancreatic tissue, containing the blood supply to the duodenum and common duct; also includes vagotomy and gastrojejunostomy

Removes the pancreas and spleen completely, leaving the hepatic duct anastomosed to the jejunum; also includes hemigastrectomy and vagotomy or 75% gastrectomy and duodenectomy

Removes the portal vein, entire pancreas, spleen, transverse colon, gallbladder, and common duct

Removes the head of the pancreas along with the duodenum, pylorus and distal half of the stomach, gallbladder, and lower end of the common duct

Preserves the pylorus and stomach by anastomosing the pancreatic remnant to the antrum of the stomach (pancreaticogastrostomy)

sible family member has signed a consent form.

Procedure
After the patient is anesthetized, the surgeon makes an abdominal incision. He selects the procedure based on evaluation of the pancreas, liver, gallbladder, and common duct. If the disease is localized, he may resect a portion of the pancreas and the surrounding organs. If the surgeon detects metastatic disease in the liver or lymph nodes, or tumor invasion of the aorta or superior mesenteric artery, he may decide to bypass the obstruction to lessen the patient's pain.

For further information on the various procedures, see *Understanding Types of Pancreatectomy*, pages 426 and 427.

Monitoring and aftercare
After surgery, the patient usually spends 48 hours in the intensive care unit. Monitor his vital signs closely and administer plasma expanders, as ordered. Use central, arterial, or pulmonary catheter readings to evaluate hemodynamic status; correlate these readings with urinary output and wound drainage. If central venous pressure and urinary output drop, give fluids to avoid hypovolemic shock.

Evaluate nasogastric tube drainage, which should be green-tinged as bile drains from the stomach. A T tube may be placed in the patient's common bile duct; normal bile drainage is 600 to 800 ml daily, decreasing as more bile goes to the intestine. Notify the doctor if bile drainage doesn't decrease, as this may indicate a biliary obstruction leading to possibly fatal peritonitis. Assess Penrose or Shirley sump drainage from the abdomen and inspect the dressing and drainage sites for frank bleeding, which may signal hemorrhage. If a pancreatic drain is in place, prevent skin breakdown from highly excoriating pancreatic enzymes by changing dressings frequently or by using a wound pouching system to contain the drainage.

Monitor the patient's fluid and electrolyte balance closely, evaluate arterial blood gases, and provide I.V. fluid replacements, as ordered. Keep in mind that constant gastric drainage can cause metabolic alkalosis, signaled by apathy, irritability, dehydration, and slow, shallow breathing. Report these signs to the doctor, and expect to administer isotonic fluids. Alternatively, loss of bile and pancreatic secretions can lead to metabolic acidosis, signaled by elevated blood pressure, rapid pulse and respirations, and arrhythmias. Report these signs to the doctor and give I.V. bicarbonate, as ordered.

Have I.V. calcium ready because serum amylase levels commonly rise after pancreatic surgery and amylase can bind to calcium. Evaluate serum calcium levels periodically. Also check urine and blood glucose levels periodically to assess for possible fluctuations. If ordered, give insulin.

Monitor the patient's respiratory status, being alert for shallow breathing, decreased respiratory rate, and respiratory distress. Administer oxygen, if necessary and ordered. Reinforce deep-breathing techniques and encourage the patient to cough.

Be alert for absent bowel sounds, severe abdominal pain, vomiting, or fever—evidence of such complications as fistula development and paralytic ileus. Also check the patient's wound for redness, pain, edema, unusual odor, or suture line separation. Report any of these findings to the doctor.

If no complications develop, expect the patient's GI function to return in 24 to 48 hours. Remove his nasogastric tube, as ordered, and start him on fluids.

Home care instructions
• Teach the patient how to care for his wound, including careful cleansing and dressing each day. Tell him to report any signs of wound infection promptly.
• As needed, teach the patient how to test his urine for glucose and ketones

or how to monitor his blood glucose levels. If he had a total pancreatectomy, provide routine diabetic teaching and show him or a responsible family member how to administer insulin.

• If the patient has chronic pancreatitis, stress that he requires continued follow-up and that he *must* avoid alcohol. As needed, refer him to an outpatient or chemical dependency clinic.

• Because pancreatic exocrine insufficiency leads to malabsorption, provide dietary instructions and inform the patient that he may eventually need pancreatic enzyme replacements.

Adrenalectomy

Adrenalectomy—the resection or removal of one or both adrenal glands—is the treatment of choice for adrenal hyperfunction and hyperaldosteronism. It's also used to treat adrenal tumors, such as adenomas, and has been used to aid treatment of breast and prostate malignancies. The prognosis is good when adrenalectomy's used to treat adrenal adenomas. However, it's less favorable for adrenal carcinomas.

Total bilateral adrenalectomy eliminates the body's reserve of corticosteroids, which the adrenal cortex synthesizes. As these hormones disappear from the circulation, the symptoms produced by their excess also disappear. However, excessive levels of adrenal hormones can also stem from pituitary oversecretion of adrenocorticotropic hormone. In this case, treatment first focuses on removal of a pituitary adenoma by irradiation or surgery. Only if this is impossible will unilateral or bilateral adrenalectomy be considered to prevent excessive secretion of adrenocortical hormones.

Improved use of medications to prepare the patient before surgery has dramatically decreased the risk of postoperative complications. And careful postoperative monitoring further reduces the risk of life-threatening conditions that can arise when hormones that are in excess preoperatively decrease postoperatively.

Purpose
To remove adrenal tissue, reducing adrenal hormone hypersecretion.

Preparation
Explain the procedure to the patient. If he has *hyperaldosteronism*, draw blood, as ordered, for laboratory evaluation. Expect to give oral or I.V. potassium supplements to correct low serum potassium levels. Monitor for muscle twitching and a positive Chvostek's sign (indications of tetany). Keep the patient on a low-sodium, high-potassium diet, as ordered, to help correct hypernatremia. Give aldosterone antagonists, as ordered, for blood pressure control. Explain to the patient that surgery will probably cure his hypertension if it results from an adenoma.

If the patient has a *pheochromocytoma* (a catecholamine-secreting tumor of the adrenal medulla), monitor his blood pressure very carefully. Excess circulating catecholamines may produce paroxysmal attacks of hypertension with severe headache, palpitations or tachycardia, diaphoresis, nausea, vomiting, and visual disturbance. Notify the doctor if these occur, and try to identify the stimulus that triggered the attack. Keep the patient in bed with his head elevated 45 degrees, monitor his vital signs, and document the length of the attack. Before surgery, expect to administer long-acting agents to help control blood pressure. For example, the doctor may order phentolamine to offset the blood pressure effects of excess catecholamines. He may also order phenoxybenzamine for 7 to 10 days before surgery, or he may order metyrosine (which blocks catecholamine synthesis) for 1 to 2 weeks before surgery. He may also order propranolol to control tachycardia. Make sure the patient has taken these medications as directed.

The patient with *adrenal hyperfunction* needs emotional support and a controlled environment to offset his emotional lability. If ordered, give a sedative to help him rest. Expect to administer medications to control his hypertension, edema, diabetes, and cardiovascular symptoms as well as his increased tendency to develop infections. As ordered, give glucocorticoids the morning of surgery to help prevent acute adrenal insufficiency during the surgery.

Ensure that the patient or a responsible family member has signed a consent form.

Procedure

After the patient is anesthetized, the surgeon explores the adrenal glands, using either an anterior (transperitoneal) or a posterior (lumbar) approach. (The anterior approach allows better visualization of both glands.) If he finds a tumor, he either resects it or removes the entire gland, depending on the extent of glandular involvement. If he finds an aldosterone-producing adenoma, he removes the entire gland. If he can find no tumor, he may remove one entire gland and half of the other because of the likelihood of multiple imperceptible adenomas.

In pheochromocytoma removal, the surgeon carefully excises the affected adrenal gland as well as adjacent areolar tissue (often the site of recurring tumors) and palpates abdominal organs for other tumors. To decrease the risk of hypotensive episodes postoperatively, he gives blood or plasma volume expanders, I.V. phentolamine, and I.V. nitroprusside. The patient's blood pressure, pulse, and EKG are monitored carefully. Manipulation of the tumor may cause sudden release of catecholamines with a corresponding rise in blood pressure; removal of the tumor may cause a sudden drop.

Monitoring and aftercare

Monitor vital signs carefully, observing for indications of shock from hemorrhage. Observe the patient's dressing for bleeding, and correlate this with your reading of his vital signs. Report wound drainage or fever immediately. Keep in mind that postoperative hypertension's common, because handling of the adrenal glands stimulates catecholamine release, particularly if surgery was for a pheochromocytoma. Watch for weakness, nausea, and vomiting, which may signal hyponatremia.

Use aseptic technique when changing dressings to minimize the risk of infection. Administer analgesics for pain, and give replacement steroids, as ordered. Remember, glucocorticoids from the adrenal cortex are essential to life and must be replaced to prevent adrenal crisis.

If the patient had primary hyperaldosteronism, he will have had preoperative renin suppression with resulting postoperative hypoaldosteronism. Monitor his serum potassium levels carefully—he may have hyperkalemia if he's receiving spironolactone, a potassium-sparing diuretic for control of postoperative hypertension.

Home care instructions

●Make sure your patient understands the importance of taking his prescribed medications as directed. If he had a unilateral adrenalectomy, explain that he may be able to discontinue his medications in a few months, when his remaining gland resumes function. If he had a bilateral adrenalectomy, explain that he'll need lifelong therapy because his body no longer has a glucocorticoid source.

● Make sure the patient understands that sudden withdrawal of steroids can precipitate adrenal crisis and that he needs continued medical follow-up to adjust his steroid dosage appropriately during stress or illness.

● Describe the signs of adrenal insufficiency and make sure the patient understands how this can progress to adrenal crisis if not treated. Explain that he should consult his doctor if he develops such side effects as weight gain, acne, headaches, fatigue, and increased urinary frequency. Advise him to take his steroids with meals or antacids to minimize gastric irritation.

• If the patient had adrenal hyperfunction, explain that he'll see a reversal of the physical characteristics of his disease over the next few months. However, caution him that his improved physical appearance doesn't mean he can stop his medications.

• If the patient's incision isn't completely healed, provide wound care instructions. Advise him to keep the incision clean, to avoid wearing clothing that may irritate the incision, and to follow his doctor's instructions regarding application of ointments or dressings. Tell him to report fever or any increased drainage, inflammation, or pain at the incision site.

• Advise the patient to wear a Medic Alert bracelet to ensure adequate medical care in an emergency.

RADIATION THERAPY

Iodine 131 Administration

An alternative to thyroidectomy or drug therapy, administration of the isotope iodine 131 (^{131}I) treats hyperthyroidism and is used adjunctively for thyroid cancer. After oral ingestion, ^{131}I is rapidly absorbed and concentrated in the thyroid as if it were normal iodine. The result: acute radiation thyroiditis and gradual thyroid atrophy that eventually reduces thyroid hormone levels.

^{131}I causes symptoms to subside after about 3 weeks and exerts its full effect only after 3 months. A patient with acute hyperthyroidism may require ongoing drug therapy during this period.

Similarly, a patient who also has cardiac disease must be made euthyroid before the start of ^{131}I therapy, to withstand the initial hypermetabolism.

Although one ^{131}I treatment usually suffices, a second or third treatment may be needed several months later if the patient has severe hyperthyroidism or an unusually large gland. Complications include transient or permanent hypothyroidism, requiring administration of thyroid hormone replacements. Rarely, acute exacerbation occurs, resulting in thyroid storm.

^{131}I is the treatment of choice for nonpregnant adults who aren't good candidates for spontaneous remission or who weren't treated successfully with thyroid hormone antagonists. This relatively safe procedure exposes only the thyroid to radiation. However, it's contraindicated during pregnancy and lactation. And, despite the fact that no iatrogenic cancers have been documented in the more than 40 years ^{131}I has been in use, this treatment is used cautiously in children and adolescents because of the potential for cancer or leukemia.

Purpose
To shrink functioning thyroid tissue, decreasing circulating thyroid hormone levels and destroying malignancy.

Preparation
Explain the procedure to the patient and check for any history of allergies to iodine. Ask, for example, about any rashes resulting from eating shellfish.

Unless contraindicated, instruct the patient to stop thyroid hormone antagonists 4 to 7 days before ^{131}I administration because these drugs reduce the sensitivity of thyroid cells to radiation. Also tell the patient to fast overnight, since food may delay ^{131}I absorption. Make sure the patient's not taking lithium carbonate, since this may interact with ^{131}I to cause hypothyroidism.

Inform the patient that ^{131}I won't be administered if he develops severe

432

PRECAUTIONS AFTER RADIOACTIVE IODINE THERAPY

Dear Patient:

You've received a dose of radioactive iodine to help treat your thyroid disease. Although this is a safe treatment, you'll need to follow these instructions to prevent any harm to you or to others.

- All your urine, feces, saliva, and perspiration will be slightly radioactive for 24 hours after therapy. You may use your family bathroom to urinate or defecate but be sure to flush the toilet three times to make certain all waste is discarded. Wash your hands thoroughly afterward.

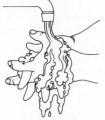

- If you perspire heavily, take a shower and wash your clothes separately.
- Use disposable eating utensils for 48 hours. Resume normal mouth care, but make sure you rinse and drain the sink properly when you've finished.
- If you vomit within 12 hours after therapy, call your doctor immediately. Dispose of your vomitus down the toilet and, if possible, wear gloves while cleaning up. (Discard the gloves in a plastic bag after use.) Discourage other persons from coming in contact with your vomitus. However, if they do, tell them to wash their hands thoroughly afterward.

- Drink plenty of fluids (about 2 quarts, or liters) over the next 24 hours. This will help clear your system and speed elimination of the radioactive iodine from your body.

- Avoid close contact with infants, children, and pregnant women for 48 hours after therapy. For safety's sake, sleep alone and avoid any sexual intimacy for 1 week. After that, you may resume your normal relationship.
- If your neck feels tender, call your doctor. He may want to prescribe medication to make you feel more comfortable.
- If you develop a fever accompanied by restlessness or agitation within 48 hours of therapy, call your doctor immediately.

vomiting or diarrhea because these decrease absorption.

Procedure
In the nuclear medicine or radiation therapy department, the patient receives an oral dose of ^{131}I in solution. The radiation dose delivered to thyroid cells determines the treatment's effectiveness; the effective dose depends on thyroid uptake, the length of time ^{131}I remains within the gland, and the sensitivity of the thyroid cells to radiation.

Monitoring and aftercare
Usually the patient's discharged after ^{131}I administration, with appropriate instructions. However, he may stay in the hospital to be monitored for thyroid storm if he received an unusually large dose or if treatment was for malignancy. In such cases, observe radiation precautions for 3 days. (If you're pregnant, arrange for another nurse to care for this patient.) Encourage the patient to drink plenty of fluids for 48 hours to speed excretion of ^{131}I. Instruct him to urinate into a lead-lined container for 48 hours. Give him disposable eating utensils, and tell him to avoid close contact with young children and pregnant women for 7 days after therapy.

Home care instructions
● Explain to the patient that his urine and saliva will be slightly radioactive for 24 hours and that any vomitus will be highly radioactive for 6 to 8 hours after therapy. Teach him to dispose of these properly (see *Precautions after Radioactive Iodine Therapy*).
● Tell the patient he'll start to see signs of improvement in his condition within several weeks but that maximum effects won't occur for up to 3 months.
● Explain that he should take his prescribed thyroid hormone antagonist, as ordered, starting 3 to 4 days after ^{131}I therapy and continuing until the doctor determines that his thyroid has become atrophic. If the patient's also taking propranolol, tell him that the doctor may have him continue this temporarily to treat tachycardia, diaphoresis, and tremors.
● Inform him that he'll need periodic laboratory tests. If his serum thyroid hormone levels don't fall within 3 months, the doctor may order another dose of ^{131}I.
● Advise the patient that hypothyroidism may occur 2 to 4 months after therapy. If symptoms become severe, the doctor will prescribe a thyroid hormone replacement. If hypothyroidism persists for 6 to 9 months, the patient may require lifelong therapy for permanent hypothyroidism.
● Tell the patient to notify his doctor if he develops pain, swelling, erythema, or fever (from radiation thyroiditis). Reassure him that these symptoms can be treated with anti-inflammatory drugs. Also tell him to notify his doctor if he develops severe exacerbation of hyperthyroidism 3 to 14 days after therapy.
● Advise the female patient of childbearing age to avoid conception for several months after therapy.

Selected References

American Diabetes Association. *The Physician's Guide to Type II Diabetes (NDDM): Diagnosis and Treatment.* New York: American Diabetes Association, 1984.

Atkinson, Lucy, and Kohn, Mary. *Berry and Kohn's Introduction to Operating Room Technique,* 6th ed. New York: McGraw-Hill Book Co., 1986.

Krieger, Dorothy, and Bardin, C., eds. *Current Therapy in Endocrinology 1985-1986.* St. Louis: C.V. Mosby Co., 1985.

Toledo-Pereyra, Luis. *The Pancreas: Principles of Medical and Surgical Practice.* New York: John Wiley & Sons, 1985.

12

Treating Hematologic and Immune Dysfunction

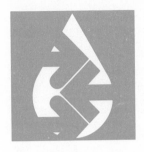

Treating Hematologic and Immune Dysfunction

Introduction

The discovery of the ABO blood groups some 100 years ago was hailed as a milestone in medicine—but only the passage of years has revealed how important it truly was. Its immediate effect was to permit the replacement of blood lost through surgery, trauma, or hemorrhage, but in time it also focused attention on blood's immunologic properties. In doing so, it laid the foundation for two entirely new fields of medicine—hematology and immunology—and led to the discovery of treatments undreamed of by Victorian doctors.

Today, we're learning that a whole range of seemingly unrelated diseases are tied to the immune system. We know that the same forces that fight infection can also attack the body's own tissues, causing such autoimmune disorders as rheumatoid arthritis, lupus erythematosus, and perhaps even multiple sclerosis and diabetes. We've begun to discover how to manipulate the immune system—albeit crudely so far—suppressing it to permit organ transplants, blocking its effects to reverse anaphylaxis, and rebuilding it through bone marrow transplants after it has been destroyed by disease or radiation. We've developed the techniques of transfusion into a sophisticated science, processing blood into a virtual pharmacy of products that can't be duplicated in any laboratory: for example, red cells, which can revive oxygen-starved tissues; leukocytes, which can combat infections that no antibiotic can touch; and clotting factors, plasma, and platelets, which can help patients with hemophilia live virtually normal lives.

But along with all of these benefits come some substantial risks. Mismatched blood can cause death within minutes. Blood-borne hepatitis can also kill if it goes undetected. Immunosuppressants can leave a patient helpless against infection.

Attention to detail

Preventing such problems requires care and diligence on your part. The meticulous procedures you learned in nursing school for administering blood may be cumbersome, but they're still the best way to combat the all-too-human tendency to make mistakes. With immunocompromised patients, such basic nursing tenets as frequent hand washing take on special importance. Patient monitoring must be done with care, to detect the first subtle signs of complications. In other words, the well-being of patients undergoing these new therapies hinges on good old-fashioned nursing care—the kind the first transfusion patient undoubtedly received a century ago.

DRUG THERAPY

Gold Compounds

Gold compounds serve as antirheumatic agents for both juvenile and adult rheumatoid arthritis. Less commonly, they're used to treat psoriatic arthritis. Although they're not curative, they slow the degenerative course of arthritis and may even induce remission.

Three gold compounds are used for treating arthritis: *aurothioglucose* and *gold sodium thiomalate*, which are administered intramuscularly, and *auranofin*, a recently developed oral compound. All three drugs prove equally effective but auranofin appears to be the least toxic. In addition, of course, it obviates the need for an injection—and a trip to the doctor's office to receive it.

Even in the best of cases, gold salts can only *prevent* damage to the bone and cartilage. They can't repair already present damage. Therefore, they're most beneficial when given in the early stages of disease, before irreversible joint changes have occurred.

Gold's therapeutic effects occur slowly. In some patients, improvement occurs after 6 weeks of therapy; in others, it may occur only after 6 months.

Gold's side effects range from mild to potentially life-threatening. Short-term effects include anaphylaxis and arthralgia, whereas long-term ones include stomatitis, dermatitis, and GI upset (especially with auranofin). Rarely, blood dyscrasias, hepatitis, renal impairment, encephalopathy, and pulmonary complications occur.

Gold compounds shouldn't be used in patients with blood dyscrasias, uncontrolled diabetes, compromised cerebral or cardiovascular circulation, colitis, renal or liver disease, urticaria, eczema, or a hypersensitivity to gold or heavy metals.

Purpose and action

Gold compounds reduce inflammation in rheumatoid arthritis. Their anti-inflammatory effects probably result from inhibition of sulfhydryl systems, which alters cellular metabolism. In addition, they alter enzyme function and immune response and suppress phagocytic activity.

Monitoring

Before beginning treatment with gold compounds, obtain a baseline complete blood count and urinalysis. Throughout therapy, monitor these studies to detect blood dyscrasias, proteinuria, or hematuria.

Review the patient's medication regimen for possible interactions. Concurrent use of penicillamine can cause severe hematologic and renal effects.

If the patient will be receiving I.M. injections, record their location so that sites can be rotated. After injection, tell the patient to lie down for 10 to 20 minutes. During this period, observe him for signs of anaphylaxis. Ask the patient if he's experiencing any joint pain. If he is, notify the doctor.

Home care instructions

● Tell the patient to be alert for side effects, which may occur at any time during therapy or even several months after its discontinuation. Tell him to call his doctor immediately if he experiences pruritus (a sign of emerging dermatitis), shortness of breath, a metallic taste (a sign of impending stomatitis), coughing, unusual bleeding or bruising, nausea, vomiting, diarrhea, or abdominal pain.

● Warn the patient that arthralgia may occur a day or two after an injection, but explain that this reaction usually doesn't occur beyond the first few injections.

● Tell him that benefits of therapy may not be apparent for 6 weeks or longer.

Instruct him to record the date that he first notices any relief from stiffness and pain or improvement of joint function.
• Warn the patient that gold compounds may predispose him to mouth ulcers and a sore throat. To help forestall these problems, tell him to brush his teeth and use a mouthwash after every meal.
• Urge the patient to avoid exposure to sunlight, which can worsen gold-induced dermatitis.

Immunosuppressants

The immunosuppressants azathioprine and cyclosporine combat tissue rejection and help control autoimmune disorders. *Azathioprine* treats rheumatoid arthritis when other measures prove ineffective. It's also used preoperatively for renal transplant. *Cyclosporine* helps prevent rejection in various organ transplants, graft-versus-host disease after bone marrow transplant, and chronic rejection in patients receiving other immunosuppressants. When used with corticosteroids, it reduces inflammation in rheumatoid arthritis.

Because azathioprine kills proliferating cells, it can produce severe side effects, such as bone marrow suppression. Cyclosporine, in contrast, minimally suppresses the bone marrow, and patients on this drug have a lower incidence of infection than those on azathioprine. Neither immunosuppressant should be used in patients with recent or existing chicken pox or herpes zoster virus owing to the risk of severe generalized disease. These drugs also shouldn't be used in patients exposed to live virus vaccines and must be used cautiously in patients with hepatic or renal impairment.

Purpose and action
The antimetabolite azathioprine suppresses both humoral and cell-mediated immune responses. It interferes with DNA synthesis by inhibiting purine synthesis.

Cyclosporine's mechanism of action isn't known, but the drug may inhibit production of T-lymphocyte growth factor (interleukin 2). This effect seems more specific for helper T lymphocytes, causing their numbers to diminish during therapy.

Monitoring
Review the patient's drug regimen for possible interactions. Allopurinol, for instance, greatly enhances the action and toxic effects of azathioprine. If these drugs must be given concurrently, the azathioprine dosage should be reduced by two thirds to three quarters.

To monitor bone marrow function, the doctor will usually order a complete blood count (CBC) and platelet count at least every other day at the beginning of therapy or whenever the patient is receiving high doses. In addition, he'll probably order a CBC and platelet count at least weekly for the first 2 months of therapy. Monitor the results of these studies closely, as well as blood urea nitrogen, creatinine, and alkaline phosphatase levels. In addition, watch for any changes in urinary output or signs of jaundice. Report any abnormalities to the doctor immediately.

Be alert for signs of infection, such as fever and sore throat. If any such signs occur, report them to the doctor immediately.

If the patient develops thrombocytopenia, watch for and report any bruises, hematuria, hematochezia, or other signs of bleeding. Avoid giving I.M. injections, if possible, to prevent bleeding.

Home care instructions
• Emphasize the importance of following the prescribed medication schedule. If the patient's taking cyclosporine, tell him to make up a missed dose as soon as possible, unless it's almost time for the next dose—in which case he should simply continue with his reg-

HOW TO AVOID INFECTION

Dear Patient:

You have an increased risk of infection while taking your prescribed drug. Here are some simple steps you can take to protect yourself against it.

Follow your doctor's directions
- Be sure to take all medications exactly as prescribed. Don't discontinue your medication unless your doctor tells you to do so.
- Keep all appointments with your doctor so that he can monitor your progress and the drug's side effects.
- If you need to go to another doctor or to a dentist, be sure to tell him that you're receiving an immunosuppressant drug.

Avoid sources of infection
- To minimize your exposure to infections, avoid crowds and people who are suffering from colds, flu, chicken pox, or other contagious illnesses.
- Don't receive any immunizations, especially with live-virus vaccines, such as poliovirus vaccines. These contain weakened but living viruses, which can cause illness in any person who's taking an immunosuppressant drug. Similarly, avoid contact with any person who has recently received a live-virus vaccine.
- Wash your hands thoroughly before preparing food. Thoroughly cleanse and cook all food before you eat it, to avoid ingesting harmful organisms.
- Examine your mouth daily for lesions.
- Also examine your skin daily for cuts or rashes.

Recognize hazards
- Learn to recognize the early signs and symptoms of infection: sore throat, fever, chills, or malaise. Call your doctor *immediately* if you think you're coming down with an infection.
- Treat minor skin injuries, such as cuts or scrapes, with triple antibiotic ointment. If the injury's a deep one, or if it becomes swollen, red, or tender, call your doctor immediately.

Perform routine hygiene
- Practice good oral and personal hygiene, especially hand washing. Report any mouth sores or ulcerations to your doctor.
- Don't use commercial mouthwashes since their high alcohol and sugar content may irritate your mouth and provide a medium for bacterial growth.

ular schedule. If the patient's taking azathioprine several times a day, he should make up a missed dose as soon as possible. However, if it's time for the next dose, he should take two doses. If a patient misses two consecutive doses of either of these drugs, he should notify his doctor immediately.

• Advise the patient on precautions he can take to prevent infection (see *How to Avoid Infection*).

• Tell him to watch for signs of bleeding, such as melena, hematuria, or easy bruising, and to report them to his doctor. Warn him to avoid aspirin and aspirin-containing compounds, and encourage him to use an electric shaver rather than a razor.

• Caution the patient that immunosuppressants often cause temporary hair loss.

• Inform him that the prescribed drug may cause loss of appetite, nausea, and vomiting. If these GI effects occur, he should take the drug with meals. If they persist, he should notify his doctor, who may order an antiemetic.

• If the patient has refractory arthritis, explain that symptoms may not improve for up to 12 weeks.

• If the patient's taking cyclosporine, instruct him to report symptoms of hypertension, such as frequent headaches or dizziness.

• Also tell him to watch for signs of hepatic impairment, such as clay-colored stools, pruritus, or yellowing of the skin or sclera, and to call the doctor if such signs occur.

Systemic Corticosteroids

Often used for their anti-inflammatory effects, corticosteroids are prescribed for autoimmune disorders, such as rheumatoid arthritis and systemic lupus erythematosus. What's more, they're used adjunctively to help prevent rejection of transplanted organs and as primary therapy for allergic conditions ranging from hay fever to anaphylaxis. They also help treat hematologic disorders, including idiopathic thrombocytopenic purpura, acquired autoimmune hemolytic anemia, and secondary thrombocytopenia in adults.

Corticosteroids are broadly classified as glucocorticoids and mineralocorticoids (see *Comparing Systemic Corticosteroids*, page 440). Glucocorticoids, such as *betamethasone* and *cortisone*, reduce inflammation and affect carbohydrate, fat, and protein metabolism. Mineralocorticoids, by contrast, affect electrolyte and fluid status. Synthetic corticosteroids, such as *prednisone* and *prednisolone*, exert both glucocorticoid and mineralocorticoid effects.

The chief side effects of corticosteroids depend on the duration of therapy and the dosage. Long-term therapy causes cushingoid symptoms, such as moon face, hirsutism, and buffalo hump. In addition, it can cause cataracts, increased intraocular pressure, and peptic ulcers. High corticosteroid doses can cause psychotic behavior.

Corticosteroids should be given with extreme caution to patients with peptic ulcer, heart disease, infection, psychosis, diabetes mellitus, osteoporosis, or glaucoma.

Purpose and action
Corticosteroids are used to produce immunosuppressive and anti-inflammatory actions. How they cause immunosuppression isn't completely understood, but they may prevent or suppress the cell-mediated immune response.

Monitoring
Before beginning therapy, weigh the patient to establish a baseline. During therapy, weigh him regularly to detect any increases caused by corticosteroid-induced appetite stimulation and fluid retention. Check also for edema, thin-

COMPARING DRUGS

COMPARING SYSTEMIC CORTICOSTEROIDS

DRUG	DURATION (HOURS)	ACTION
betamethasone	48 or more	G
cortisone acetate	12 or less	B
dexamethasone	48 or more	G
hydrocortisone	12 or less	B
methylprednisolone	24 to 36	G
paramethasone	48 or more	G
prednisolone	24 to 36	B
prednisone	24 to 36	B
triamcinolone	24 to 36	G

KEY: G indicates that drug acts as a gluco-corticoid. B indicates that drug acts as both a mineralocorticoid and a glucocorticoid.

ning of the extremities, and elevated blood pressure. Notify the doctor if the patient gains weight rapidly or develops edema or hypertension.

Observe the patient's skin for petechiae and bruising, and monitor serum electrolyte and glucose levels to detect hypokalemia, hypernatremia, and hyperglycemia. If ordered, give potassium supplements and place the patient on a salt-restricted diet.

Assess the patient's mental status, especially if he's taking high doses. Report sudden mood swings to the doctor.

If the patient has recently had surgery, monitor the wound for dehiscence and evisceration because corticosteroids may delay healing. Watch for such signs of infection as diminished breath sounds and rhonchi because corticosteroids may mask expected signs.

Review the patient's drug regimen for possible interactions. Concurrent use of indomethacin or aspirin, for example, increases the risk of GI distress and bleeding. Barbiturates, phenytoin,

and rifampin decrease corticosteroid effects.

If the patient complains of GI upset, give antacids, as ordered, to counteract the hyperacidity caused by corticosteroids. Also, give the drug with milk or food.

The corticosteroid dosage must be tapered gradually to prevent adrenal insufficiency. During this period, watch for withdrawal symptoms, such as myalgia, headache, low-grade fever, weight loss, nausea, or vomiting. If such symptoms occur, give aspirin or other nonsteroidal anti-inflammatory drugs to help alleviate them.

Home care instructions

● Tell the patient to take corticosteroids with meals to avoid GI upset and to reduce the risk of developing an ulcer. Explain that the patient should call his doctor if stomach upset, heartburn, or pain persists. Tell the patient to avoid alcohol, which increases the likelihood of an ulcer.

• Provide directions for missed doses. If the patient's on an alternate-day schedule, tell him to take the missed dose later that morning; otherwise, he should take the dose the next morning and then skip the following day, resuming an alternate-day schedule. If he's on a daily schedule, tell him to make up the missed dose as soon as he remembers unless it's almost time for the next dose; tell him *not* to double-dose. If he takes his medication several times daily, tell him to take a missed dose as soon as he remembers and to double-up if it's time for his next dose.
• Tell him that if he vomits within 1 hour of taking his dose, he should take another dose. However, he should call his doctor if vomiting persists.
• Warn him to promptly report signs of adrenal insufficiency: headache, abdominal pain, anorexia, weakness, restlessness, and agitation. Stress that he should *never* abruptly stop taking his medication because this may precipitate adrenal insufficiency or life-threatening adrenal crisis.
• Advise him to report minor stress or illness, such as a cold, or a dental extraction so that the doctor can increase the dosage. Explain that he'll require hospitalization and parenteral steroids if he suffers a major illness or requires an invasive procedure.
• Warn the patient not to take any other drugs, including aspirin, without his doctor's approval.

Antihistamines

Antihistamines can be given orally or by injection to prevent or treat allergic symptoms. These symptoms range in severity from the discomfort caused by hay fever to the distress caused by anaphylaxis. (For information on oral antihistamines, typically used for rhinitis and mild allergies, see "Antihistamines and Decongestants" in Chapter 16.)

Deep I.M. injection of the antihis-tamine *diphenhydramine* 15 to 20 minutes before transfusion helps prevent allergic reactions to blood or blood products in patients with actual or suspected susceptibility. What's more, it can be used with epinephrine for anaphylaxis after acute symptoms have subsided.

Purpose and action
Antihistamines prevent or relieve allergic reactions by blocking the action of histamine.

Monitoring
When giving diphenhydramine to prevent an allergic reaction, monitor its effect by taking the patient's vital signs every 15 minutes until they stabilize. Notify the doctor of any hypertension, tachycardia, or dyspnea.

If you're giving this drug to help combat anaphylaxis, closely monitor the patient's response for signs of an overdose: hallucinations, dyspnea, insomnia, seizures, or facial flushing. Notify the doctor if you suspect an overdose. Typically, he'll order supportive measures, such as oxygen, I.V. fluids, vasopressors, and gastric lavage.

Because antihistamines may cause drowsiness or dizziness, take measures to protect the patient from falls. For example, raise the side rails of his bed.

Home care instructions
Antihistamines are given intramuscularly in the hospital only. As a result, they don't require directions for home use.

Adrenergics
[Sympathomimetics]

Adrenergic drugs stimulate the sympathetic nervous system. One of them, epinephrine, is the drug of choice for treating acute anaphylactic reactions (see *Breaking the Chain of Anaphylaxis*).

Epinephrine may be administered intravenously, subcutaneously, or intramuscularly. I.V. administration of this drug produces an almost immediate response, whereas S.C. or I.M. administration produces effects in 3 to 5 minutes.

Epinephrine can cause severe hypertension when combined with tricyclic antidepressants and certain antihistamines, such as diphenhydramine or chlorpheniramine. Less severe effects include headache, dizziness, palpitations, and anxiety.

Epinephrine should be given with extreme caution to patients with chronic obstructive pulmonary disease who've developed a degenerative cardiac disorder. It should be given cautiously to elderly patients and to those with hyperthyroidism, angina, diabetes mellitus, or hypertension.

BREAKING THE CHAIN OF ANAPHYLAXIS

Anaphylaxis occurs when the body overreacts to an allergic stimulus. If not treated promptly, it can cause death within minutes.

A severe anaphylactic reaction is one of the most frightening conditions you'll encounter in nursing—not only because of its seriousness but also because it's often unexpected. It may start with itching, urticaria, and erythema. Within a few seconds, the patient may start wheezing, coughing, or sneezing as a result of bronchospasm and laryngeal edema. Then, suddenly, his blood pressure drops precipitously, his pulse becomes imperceptible, and the color drains from his skin as a result of peripheral vascular collapse.

What happens in anaphylaxis—and why epinephrine helps

Allergens trigger a massive release of histamine in a previously sensitized patient.

The histamine, in turn, causes extreme vasodilation, and consequently the patient's blood pressure declines sharply. In addition, serum begins to leak through the relaxed walls of the blood vessels, which further lowers the blood pressure and causes edema in adjacent tissues. Laryngeal edema constricts or completely closes the patient's airway, and at the same time his lungs begin to fill with fluid. Meanwhile, the histamines act directly on bronchial tissue, causing bronchospasm.

Epinephrine reverses the effects of histamine on bronchial and vascular tissues. It raises blood pressure by causing vasoconstriction and by acting on the heart's beta-receptors. As blood pressure increases, the edema is reversed. In addition, epinephrine relaxes the smooth muscle of the bronchi, thereby reversing bronchospasm.

WHAT HAPPENS IN ANAPHYLAXIS

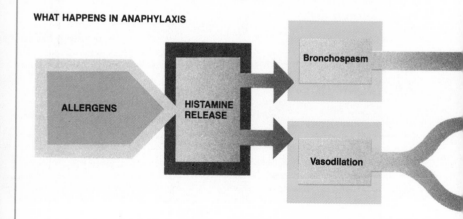

ALLERGENS → HISTAMINE RELEASE → Bronchospasm / Vasodilation

Purpose and action

Epinephrine helps reverse the effects of severe anaphylactic reactions. It stimulates alpha- and beta-adrenergic receptors within the sympathetic nervous system, causing bronchodilation, vasoconstriction, and myocardial stimulation.

Monitoring

Because several concentrations of epinephrine are available, carefully check the label before administering the drug. Use a tuberculin syringe for accuracy. When giving epinephrine subcutaneously or intramuscularly, aspirate the syringe before injection, to prevent inadvertent injection of the drug into a vein.

Monitor the patient's vital signs every 5 minutes and keep resuscitation equipment readily available. Provide oxygen, if necessary. If the patient's blood pressure rises sharply, notify the doctor. He'll probably order rapid-acting vasodilators, such as nitrites, or alpha-adrenergic blocking agents to counteract epinephrine's pressor effects.

Home care instructions

● Explain to the patient that anaphylactic reactions are triggered by certain allergens, including drugs, such as penicillin and local anesthetics; foods, such as eggs and shellfish; and stinging insects, such as bees and wasps.
● Instruct the patient to watch for signs of an allergic reaction, such as flushing, itching, hives, shortness of breath, wheezing, and chest tightness. If the patient has been given an anaphylaxis kit, tell him and a family member to inject epinephrine into the lateral thigh or the deltoid muscle and to massage the injection site to counteract vasoconstriction and increase absorption. Instruct them to rotate sites if more than one injection is given. Tell them to call for help immediately after injecting epinephrine.
● Tell the patient with an anaphylaxis kit to regularly inspect the epinephrine solution for precipitation or discoloration. If the solution isn't clear, tell him to discard it and to ask his doctor for a new prescription. To prevent drug degradation, tell the patient to store epinephrine in a cool, dark place—but to keep it accessible.
● Show family members how to position the patient for optimal oxygenation. Also teach them how to correctly perform cardiopulmonary resuscitation.

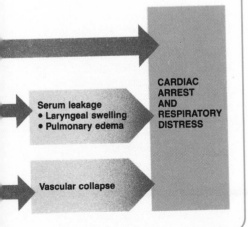

What to do when anaphylaxis strikes

Work quickly, but don't panic. Instead, proceed with the following steps:
● Call for help.
● Insert an oral airway or endotracheal tube, and begin ventilating the patient with a bag and mask.
● Administer aqueous epinephrine—usually 0.2 to 0.5 ml of 1:1,000 dilution subcutaneously.
● If anaphylaxis was triggered by the administration of a parenteral drug or a blood transfusion, apply a tourniquet proximal to the injection or infusion site.
● Insert an I.V. line for drug and fluid administration.
● Provide additional care measures as required: oxygen, antihistamines, aminophylline, volume expanders, or vasopressors.

Serum leakage
● Laryngeal swelling
● Pulmonary edema

Vascular collapse

CARDIAC ARREST AND RESPIRATORY DISTRESS

SURGERY

Splenectomy

Splenectomy, the surgical removal of the spleen, helps treat various hematologic disorders. It's also done as an emergency procedure to stop hemorrhage after traumatic splenic rupture.

The most common reason for splenectomy is hypersplenism—a combination of splenomegaly and cytopenia that occurs in such disorders as hairy cell leukemia, Felty's syndrome, myeloid metaplasia, thalassemia major, and Gaucher's disease. In addition, splenectomy is the treatment of choice for such diseases as hereditary spherocytosis and chronic idiopathic thrombocytopenic purpura. What's more, it may be performed in Hodgkin's disease to establish the stage of the disease and determine the appropriate therapy.

Besides bleeding and infection, splenectomy can cause such complications as pneumonia and atelectasis. The reason: the location of the spleen close to the diaphragm and the need for a high abdominal incision restrict lung expansion after surgery. In addition, splenectomy patients—especially children—are vulnerable to infection because of the spleen's role in the immune response.

Purpose
● To reduce the rate of red blood cell and platelet destruction
● To remove a ruptured spleen
● To stage Hodgkin's disease.

Preparation
Explain to the patient that splenectomy involves removal of his spleen under general anesthesia. Inform him that he'll be able to lead a normal life without it but will be more prone to infection.

Obtain the results of blood studies, including coagulation tests and a complete blood count, and report them to the doctor. If ordered, transfuse blood to correct anemia or hemorrhagic loss. Similarly, give vitamin K to correct clotting factor deficiencies.

Take the patient's vital signs and perform a baseline respiratory assessment. Note especially signs of respiratory infection, such as fever, chills, crackles, rhonchi, and a cough. Notify the doctor if you suspect respiratory infection; he may delay surgery.

Teach the patient coughing and deep-breathing techniques to help prevent postoperative pulmonary complications.

Ensure that the patient or a responsible family member has signed a consent form.

Procedure
After the patient is placed under general anesthesia, the surgeon exposes the peritoneal cavity through a left rectus paramedial or subcostal incision. He ligates the splenic artery and vein and the ligaments that hold the spleen in place. Then he removes the spleen. After carefully checking for any bleeding, he closes the abdomen, often placing a drain in the left subdiaphragmatic space. After the incision site is sutured and dressed, the patient is returned to the recovery room.

Monitoring and aftercare
During the early postoperative period, watch carefully—especially if the patient has a bleeding disorder—for bleeding from the wound or drain and for signs of internal bleeding, such as hematuria or hematochezia.

Leukocytosis and thrombocytosis occur after splenectomy and may persist for years. Because thrombocytosis may predispose the patient to thromboembolism, help the patient exercise and walk as soon as possible after surgery. In addition, encourage him to perform coughing and deep-breathing exercises to reduce the risk of pulmonary complications.

Watch for signs of infection, such as fever and sore throat, and monitor hematologic studies. If infection develops, administer prescribed antibiotics.

Home care instructions

• Inform the patient that he's at an increased risk for infection and urge him to report any of its telltale signs.
• Teach him measures to help prevent infection (see *How to Avoid Infection*, page 438).

TRANSFUSION

Blood Transfusion

Transfusions help treat massive hemorrhage and a range of hematologic disorders. Depending on the disorder, whole blood, packed red cells, platelets, fresh frozen plasma, or granulocytes may be transfused.

Whole blood transfusion replenishes both the volume and oxygen-carrying capacity of the circulatory system. It's typically given only when hemorrhage significantly decreases oxygen-carrying capacity.

Packed red cells consist of blood in which 80% of the plasma has been removed. Like whole blood, packed cells restore the patient's oxygen-carrying capacity, but they don't replenish lost blood volume. They're used to treat symptomatic anemia. However, since red blood cells live for only a short time, they provide only temporary improvement unless the underlying cause of the anemia is corrected.

Transfusion of *platelets*, which are suspended in 30 to 50 ml of plasma, can be administered prophylactically and therapeutically, especially in patients with aplastic anemia or leukemia or those who are receiving antineoplastic chemotherapy. Transfusion usually doesn't increase platelet counts in patients with idiopathic thrombocytopenic purpura, splenomegaly, disseminated intravascular coagulation, or antibody reactions, since these conditions involve platelet destruction. However, such patients may undergo platelet transfusion to treat severe hemorrhage.

Fresh frozen plasma (FFP) is the liquid portion of blood, which is frozen within a few hours of collection. It contains all of the blood's protein coagulation factors and is primarily used to treat clotting factor deficiencies (see "Factor Replacement," page 449). Occasionally, FFP has been used as a volume expander and protein source, but crystalloids, albumin, and plasma protein fraction usually are better choices since they don't carry the risk of transmitting hepatitis or other blood-borne infections.

Granulocytes, the blood cells that help fight bacterial infection, are transfused in granulocytopenic patients who have an infection that doesn't respond to antibiotics. They're usually reserved for patients who have a reasonable likelihood of recovering bone marrow function—for example, neonates, whose immune systems are still undeveloped.

Transfusion, of course, can be lifesaving. Nonetheless, it carries the risk of serious complications, such as an acute hemolytic reaction (see *Managing Transfusion Reactions*, pages 446 and 447). Multiparous women and patients who have been previously transfused are at greatest risk. Patients who've had a previous transfusion reaction stand a 12% chance of having another reaction.

Purpose

• To treat hypovolemic shock by replacing blood lost from hemorrhage

COMPLICATIONS

MANAGING TRANSFUSION REACTIONS

Complications can occur during, immediately after, or up to 4 days after blood transfusion. They result primarily from ABO incompatibility, contaminated blood, or overly rapid

COMPLICATION AND CAUSE	SIGNS AND SYMPTOMS
Acute hemolytic reaction Antibodies in the recipient's plasma react with antigens in donor red blood cells. This leads to donor cell agglutination and capillary occlusion, blocking oxygen and blood flow to vital organs. Eventually, the red blood cells break down and release free hemoglobin into plasma and urine. This free hemoglobin may block the renal tubules, resulting in renal failure.	• Increased pulse and respirations, hypotension • Chills, fever, flushing • Low back or thigh pain • Headache or feeling of fullness in the head • Feeling of chest constriction, pleuritic chest pain, dyspnea • Hemoglobinuria • Abnormal bleeding • Vascular collapse
Febrile reaction Usually due to recipient antibodies directed against donor platelets, lymphocytes, and granulocytes	• Fever with or without chills • Headache, flushing, tachycardia, palpitations • Malaise, myalgia
Mild allergic reaction Etiology unknown, but probably caused by antibodies against plasma proteins	• Pruritus, urticaria, erythema, rash
Anaphylaxis May result from anti-IgA antibodies in patients who are IgA-deficient; occurs within minutes of starting transfusion	• Flushing, dyspnea, wheezing, anxiety, hypotension • Vomiting, cramping, diarrhea • Chest tightness • Pruritus • Cardiac arrest
Hypervolemia Caused by administration of excessive volume or at an excessive rate; most common in children and the elderly, amputees because of decreased vascular space, and those with chronic anemia or compromised cardiac status	• Dry cough, dyspnea, crackles at base of lungs • Distended neck veins • Bounding pulse, increased blood pressure • Chest tightness
Infection Caused by contamination of blood with gram-negative *Pseudomonas*, coliform, or *Achromobacter*	• Chills, fever • Vomiting, diarrhea
Air embolism Caused by air entering blood through tubing	• Cardiac arrest

infusion. Study this chart; you'll learn how to manage these complications and how to prevent their recurrence.

NURSING INTERVENTIONS

- Severest transfusion reaction.
- Stop the transfusion immediately and keep the vein open with normal saline solution. Notify the doctor and the blood bank.
- Monitor vital signs, urine output, and EKG.

- Correct shock by administering oxygen, fluids, and epinephrine, as ordered. Give diuretics to maintain urine flow.
- Send unit, tubing, and filter to the laboratory.
- Collect urine and blood specimens.

- Most common transfusion reaction.
- Can be prevented by giving an antipyretic and an antihistamine before transfusion. However, if a febrile reaction occurs, stop the transfusion and keep the vein open with normal saline solution.

- Assess for signs of an acute hemolytic reaction.
- Give an antipyretic, as ordered. Keep the patient warm and monitor his vital signs.
- If an acute hemolytic reaction has been ruled out, the doctor may simply lower the rate of transfusion.

- Second most common reaction.
- Help prevent this reaction by giving diphenhydramine 15 to 20 minutes before transfusion to patients with allergies.
- If urticaria occurs, stop the transfusion and

keep the vein open with normal saline solution. If no other symptoms develop, resume the transfusion slowly. Administer antihistamines, as ordered.

- Rarely occurs. If it does, stop the transfusion and keep the vein open.
- Maintain intravascular volume, as ordered.

- Give epinephrine and antihistamines, as ordered.
- Monitor vital signs and provide oxygen.

- Monitor venous pressure and lung sounds of patients prone to circulatory overload.
- If hypervolemia occurs, stop the transfusion or slow the rate, and keep the vein open.

- Elevate the head of the bed. Provide oxygen.
- Monitor vital signs and venous pressure.
- Administer diuretics, oxygen, analgesics, vasodilators, and aminophylline, as ordered.

- Uncommon but severe complication. Help prevent it by using anaerobic methods to draw and deliver blood, maintaining strict aseptic techniques, and changing the filter and tubing

every 4 hours and the blood bag at least every 4 hours.
- Treat infection with antibiotics and corticosteroids, as ordered.

- Rare but possibly fatal complication. Can be prevented by expelling air from the tubing before transfusion and not allowing the blood bag to run dry.

- If embolism occurs, treat patient for shock.
- Turn him onto his left side and keep his head down.

• To help treat anemia and other hematologic conditions.

Preparation

Explain the procedure to the patient and ensure that he understands the risks of transfusion. Obtain a blood sample for blood typing and cross-matching and send it to the laboratory. Check to be sure the patient has signed a consent form. If the patient's a Jehovah's Witness, he may refuse the transfusion. (In some circumstances, the patient's or guardian's decision can be legally overridden.)

Review the doctor's orders for any medications that are to be administered before transfusion. If the patient has a history of febrile, nonhemolytic reactions, you may need to give acetaminophen before transfusion. If he'll be receiving granulocytes, you may need to administer meperidine and diphenhydramine.

After ensuring that the ordered blood or blood component is available, begin infusing normal saline solution. (Normal saline is preferred, since solutions containing dextrose can dehydrate and thereby destroy red blood cells and solutions containing calcium, such as lactated Ringer's solution, interfere with the anticoagulant that's used when blood is collected.)

If you'll be transfusing whole blood or packed red cells, prepare a Y-type administration set with an in-line filter (approximately 170 microns) to remove fibrin clots and other aggregates from the blood component. When transfusing products that contain red blood cells, use an 18G catheter, which provides a good flow rate without undue discomfort for the patient. However, if it's difficult to insert an 18G catheter, use the largest size catheter that the patient can tolerate. In such cases, expect a much slower flow rate, so ask the blood bank to send only half the volume ordered, keeping the other half refrigerated until it's needed.

If you'll be transfusing platelets or granulocytes, prepare a straight line set with a 170-micron filter.

If the patient doesn't have an I.V. line in place, perform a venipuncture. Then attach the saline solution to the catheter hub, and start the infusion at a rate just high enough to keep the vein open: about 10 drops/minute. Activate the blood-warming device, if you're using one.

Finally, take the patient's vital signs.

Procedure

After you receive the whole blood or the blood component, check the expiration date on the bag and observe its contents for abnormal color, clumping, gas bubbles, and extraneous materials. Return outdated or abnormal blood to the blood bank.

To prevent a possibly fatal transfusion reaction, carefully check both the amount and the component ordered. Also compare the name and number on the patient's identification band with that on the compatibility slip. Verify ABO and Rh compatibility. And have another nurse double-check each of these steps.

Once you're sure that the blood and patient are compatible, remove the protective cap from the I.V. tubing and insert the connector to an outlet in the blood bag.

To administer whole blood or packed red cells, invert the blood bag and hang it on the I.V. pole. Verify that the tubing contains no air and begin the transfusion. If necessary, adjust the flow rate; the first 10 to 25 ml should be transfused in no less than 15 minutes.

Increase the flow rate so that the transfusion will be completed in 1½ to 2 hours. Under no circumstances should the transfusion take more than 4 hours, since the unrefrigerated blood could become bacterially contaminated.

After the transfusion is complete, flush the filter and tubing with saline solution. Then reconnect the original I.V. solution or remove the I.V. line. Document the site of venous access, the type and quantity of blood component infused, the time of initiation and completion of the transfusion, and the patient's initial and current vital signs. Dispose of the transfusion equipment according to your institution's policy.

Platelets are administered much the same way as red blood cells, but they're transfused at a rate of about one unit every 10 minutes. Granulocytes are also administered in the same fashion as red blood cells. However, severe reactions may occur; monitor the patient especially closely.

Monitoring and aftercare

Keep emergency equipment available for treating a severe hemolytic or anaphylactic reaction (see *Breaking the Chain of Anaphylaxis,* pages 442 and 443). Observe the patient closely for the first 5 minutes to detect signs of an acute reaction. If you note any sign of a reaction, notify the doctor, stop the transfusion, and keep the I.V. line open with normal saline solution.

If no immediate reaction occurs, take the patient's vital signs every 30 minutes during transfusion, noting especially fever or tachycardia. Monitor his intake and output during transfusion and for 8 hours after it. Report any decreased urinary output to the doctor.

During transfusion, assess the needle insertion site often for redness or swelling. If necessary, change the site.

If the infusion rate is too slow, check the patency of the I.V. line and change the administration set (if the filter is clogged). If you're using a gravity-flow infusion, you can raise the height of the bag or apply a pressure bag to increase the flow rate.

If the patient has a mild reaction, administer antipyretics, antihistamines, or corticosteroids, as ordered.

If transfusion is done on an outpatient basis, be sure the patient is observed for at least 2 hours after transfusion before being discharged.

Home care instructions

• Teach the patient and his family the symptoms of a delayed transfusion re-

action and of hepatitis, such as fever, headache, anorexia, nausea, vomiting, or abdominal pain. Warn them that these symptoms may occur 3 weeks to 6 months after transfusion and must be reported immediately.
• Instruct the patient receiving platelets not to use aspirin, since it interferes with platelet function. Instead, recommend acetaminophen for pain relief or fever.

Factor Replacement

Factor replacement—the I.V. infusion of deficient clotting elements—serves as a mainstay of treatment for coagulation disorders. Various blood products are used, depending on the specific disorder being treated. *Fresh frozen plasma* (FFP), for instance, helps treat clotting disorders whose causes aren't known, clotting factor deficiencies resulting from hepatic disease or blood dilution, and deficiencies of clotting factors (such as Factor V) for which no specific replacement product exists.

Cryoprecipitate, which forms when FFP thaws slowly, helps treat von Willebrand's disease, fibrinogen deficiencies, and Factor XIII deficiencies. In addition, it's used for hemophilia patients who are young or whose disease is mild.

Factor VIII (antihemophilic factor) concentrate serves as the long-term treatment of choice for hemophilia A, because the amount of Factor VIII that it contains is less variable than with cryoprecipitate. It's administered intravenously whenever the hemophiliac patient has sustained an injury.

Prothrombin complex, which contains Factors II, VII, IX, and X, can be given to treat hemophilia B, severe liver disease, and acquired deficiencies of the factors it contains. However, it carries a high risk of transmitting hepatitis, since it's collected from large pools of donors.

ADMINISTERING FACTOR REPLACEMENT PRODUCTS

Although all clotting factors are derived from whole blood, they're administered differently. Here's a summary of important pointers for administering these products.

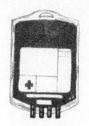

Fresh frozen plasma
• Use fresh frozen plasma within 60 minutes of thawing.
• Administer it only with normal saline solution. Use a blood filter.
• Infuse it as rapidly as the patient will tolerate it—generally, you can give 250 ml over 30 to 45 minutes in patients without symptoms of circulatory overload.
• Watch for side effects and complications. hepatitis, allergic reaction, febrile reaction, and circulatory overload.

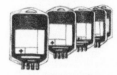

Cryoprecipitate
• Don't refrigerate cryoprecipitate; use it within 6 hours of thawing.
• Administer cryoprecipitate only with normal saline solution. Use a blood filter.
• Infuse it rapidly (10 to 12 units in 30 minutes).
• Watch for symptoms of hepatitis.

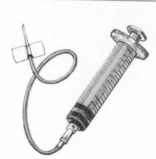

Lyophilized Factor VIII
• Reconstitute vials of Factor VIII according to the manufacturer's directions.
• Administer by slow I.V. push through a butterfly set, at a rate of 1 reconstituted vial every 5 minutes.
• Don't use a glass syringe, since Factor VIII binds to ground glass surfaces.
• Watch for symptoms of hepatitis.

Prothrombin concentrates
• Prothrombin concentrates have a high risk of hepatitis, since they're collected from large donor pools.
• Give via slow I.V. push through a butterfly set, at a rate of 1 vial every 5 minutes.

Purpose
To correct clotting factor deficiencies, thereby stopping or preventing hemorrhage.

Preparation
Explain the procedure and ensure that the patient or a family member has signed a consent form. Gather a standard blood administration set for administering FFP or prothrombin complex, a component syringe or drip set for giving cryoprecipitate, a plastic syringe for I.V. injection of Factor VIII, or a plastic syringe and infusion set for I.V. infusion.

After gathering the equipment, obtain the plasma fraction from the blood bank or pharmacy. Check the expiration date and carefully inspect the plasma fraction for cloudiness and turbidity. If you'll be transfusing FFP, administer it within 4 hours, since it doesn't contain preservatives.

Take the patient's vital signs. If an I.V. line isn't in place, perform a venipuncture and infuse normal saline solution at a keep-vein-open rate.

Procedure
See *Administering Factor Replacement Products* for details.

Monitoring and aftercare

During and after administration of clotting factors, watch for signs of anaphylaxis, other allergic reactions, and fluid overload. Also monitor the patient for bleeding, increased pain or swelling at the transfusion site, and fever. Closely monitor his partial thromboplastin time. Alert the doctor if adverse reactions occur or if you suspect bleeding.

Home care instructions

• Increasingly, factor replacement therapy is being done at home by the patient or his family; in fact, children as young as age 9 can be taught how to do it. If ordered by the doctor, demonstrate correct venipuncture and infusion techniques to the family or patient. Tell them to keep the factor replacement and infusion equipment readily available and to begin treatment immediately if the patient experiences a bleeding episode.

• Tell the patient and his family to watch for signs of anaphylaxis, allergic reactions, or fluid overload. Instruct them to call the doctor immediately if such reactions occur.

• Also tell them to watch for signs of hepatitis, which may appear 3 weeks to 6 months after treatment with blood components.

Exchange Transfusion

Exchange transfusion refers to the methodical replacement of a patient's blood with an equal amount of donor blood. The treatment of choice for erythroblastosis fetalis, exchange transfusion can also be used to treat neonatal sepsis. This treatment replaces red blood cells damaged by anti-Rh-positive antibodies with Rh-negative cells, which aren't harmed by the antibodies. It also removes bilirubin and, to a lesser degree, antibodies from the infant's circulation.

In adults with sickle-cell anemia, exchange transfusion may be used preoperatively to reduce the risks of general anesthesia by lowering hemoglobin S levels. And it's sometimes used during pregnancy in patients with sickle-cell anemia.

Exchange transfusion carries many risks. Necrotizing enterocolitis may result from compromised bowel circulation or a misplaced or clogged catheter, whereas hypoglycemia may result from increased insulin production in response to glucose in the donor blood. What's more, cardiac arrest may result from cardiac overload or decreased output. And hypocalcemia may develop from calcium depletion by sodium citrate in the donor's blood.

Purpose

• To treat erythroblastosis fetalis

• To remove damaged red blood cells and replace them with healthy donor erythrocytes, or to remove damaging toxins from the blood.

Preparation

The steps that follow outline the preparation and procedure for a neonatal exchange transfusion. The steps are similar for adult patients; the major difference is that the umbilical artery or vein is used in infants, whereas the femoral artery is used in adults.

Explain the procedure to the parents, keeping in mind their special needs for information and ongoing emotional support. (See *Questions Parents Ask About Exchange Transfusions*, page 452). Make sure that the parents have signed a consent form.

Once you've prepared the parents, get the infant ready. Typically, he'll have been given nothing by mouth to prevent aspiration of vomitus. If ordered, insert a feeding tube to empty the stomach. Now, swab povidone-iodine over the transfusion site. (Obtain extra blankets for adults, since the transfusion may cause chilling.)

Next, prepare the equipment. Turn on the radiant warmer and set the temperature as prescribed by hospital policy. Place a cardiac monitor at the bedside, along with the transfusion equipment ordered by the doctor. Also check suction and resuscitation equipment and place it at the bedside. Label laboratory tubes for blood samples that will be taken before and after the transfusion.

Next, obtain and verify the ordered blood as prescribed by hospital policy (see "Blood Transfusion," page 444, for recommended identification procedures).

Once you've verified all information, hang the blood bag, insert the spike from the blood tubing, connect the tubing to the blood warmer, and stabilize the temperature at 98.6° F. (37 ° C.). Then run the blood through to the end of the tubing, flushing any air bubbles.

Position the neonate under the radiant warmer to maintain a stable body temperature and provide an accessible working surface. If phototherapy is being used during the procedure to reduce bilirubin levels, place eye pads and shields over the infant's eyes to prevent retinal damage from the phototherapy lights. Turn on the lights.

Restrain the neonate as necessary. Tape a skin or rectal thermometer in place to continuously monitor temperature. Take his baseline vital signs; obtain a blood sample from his finger and test it for glucose. Don't take blood samples from below the infant's waist, to permit accurate detection of a malpositioned catheter, which often causes mottling of the lower extremities.

Remove all of the infant's clothing except his diaper, to allow easy access to the umbilical area. Connect the cardiac monitor to the neonate. Hang the bag for the neonate's discarded blood below the transfusion site.

Next, help the doctor put on a sterile mask, gown, and gloves. The doctor will clean the catheter site and insert a catheter into the umbilical artery, umbilical vein, or both. Then he will attach stopcocks to the catheter.

Procedure

If ordered, inject albumin to bind with and remove bilirubin from the infant's tissues.

As the infant's blood begins to flow through the outflow tubing, draw a blood sample. Place it in the appropriate tube, label it, and send it to the laboratory. Be careful to keep the specimen away from the phototherapy unit to prevent bilirubin decomposition.

The doctor alternately removes and transfuses 10 to 15 portions of blood over 1 to 2 hours, to the desired total volume, to prevent cardiac overload or stress. After the prescribed amount of blood has been exchanged, draw the last blood samples and send them to the laboratory.

After the procedure, the doctor may remove the umbilical catheter; if he anticipates further transfusions, he'll simply flush the catheter with normal saline solution and leave it in place.

Once the exchange transfusion is complete, take the infant's vital signs.

Monitoring and aftercare

Take the infant's vital signs and measure his blood glucose levels every 15 minutes during the procedure. Record the time and amount of collected or transfused blood on the exchange transfusion sheet. Repeat each amount after the doctor specifies it.

Alert the doctor each time 100 ml of blood have been exchanged so he can consider whether to give calcium gluconate to prevent tetany from depletion of serum calcium by sodium citrate in the donor's blood. During administration of calcium gluconate, monitor the infant's heart rate and watch the cardiac monitor for arrhythmias. Document the administration time and amount on the transfusion record.

If the doctor leaves the umbilical catheter in place after the procedure, begin the prescribed I.V. infusion to maintain catheter patency and provide hydration and nourishment. Follow your hospital's policy for cord care while the catheter is in place.

After transfusion, continue to observe the infant for signs of hypoglycemia, hypocalcemia, acidosis, and sepsis. Take his vital signs every 30 minutes for 2 hours, then every hour for 4 hours until he stabilizes, unless hospital policy dictates otherwise.

If the catheter has been removed, check the umbilical area for bleeding.

Home care instructions

• Instruct the parents to keep all follow-up appointments with the doctor.
• Also tell them to call the doctor immediately if the infant develops fever, malaise, or jaundice.

Bone Marrow Transplant

Bone marrow transplant refers to the collection of marrow cells from either the patient or another donor and the subsequent administration of these cells to the patient. It's the treatment of choice for aplastic anemia and severe combined immunodeficiency disease (SCID). It's also used to treat leukemia patients who are at high risk for relapse or who have undergone high-dose chemotherapy and total body irradiation. What's more, bone marrow transplantation is being explored as a treatment for other hematologic disorders and for oncologic disorders, such as multiple myeloma.

There are three types of bone marrow transplants: autologous, syngeneic, and allogeneic. In an *autologous* transplant, marrow tissue is harvested from the patient before he receives chemotherapy and radiation therapy, or while he's in remission, and frozen for later use. Unfortunately, autologous transplantation isn't always possible; for example, the bone marrow may contain malignancies. It can't be used at all for aplastic anemia, since the patient's marrow is already destroyed by the time the disease is diagnosed.

A *syngeneic* transplant refers to the transplantation of marrow between identical twins. Obviously, its use is extremely limited. But when possible, it's the ideal choice, since the twin's

PREPARING THE MARROW DONOR

In syngeneic and allogeneic transplants, be sure not to neglect the donor. Make sure he understands the risks of surgery, and give him the opportunity to ask questions and express his concerns or fears. Tell him what happens during marrow harvesting: it's usually performed in the operating room, under general anesthesia. The doctor repeatedly aspirates blood and marrow from the donor's iliac crest until 500 to 800 ml of material is obtained. This material is mixed with heparin and tissue culture material to prevent coagulation and filtered to remove bone particles and other debris.

Tell the patient that after marrow harvesting, the donor sites will be covered with pressure dressings and he'll be taken to the recovery room. Inform him that he'll probably experience pain when he awakens, but that he'll be given analgesics to relieve it.

marrow is histologically identical to the patient's own tissue, yet is disease-free.

Allogeneic transplantation uses bone marrow tissue from a histocompatible individual, usually a sibling. It's the most common type of bone marrow transplant, but, because the tissues aren't perfectly matched, it requires immunosuppression—and even then, it isn't always successful.

Bone marrow transplantation carries serious risks. During the procedure, a transfusion reaction or respiratory distress may occur. Afterward, hemoglobinuria, infection, or hepatic central vein fibrosis may occur. After an allogeneic transplant, graft-versus-host disease (GVHD), pneumonitis, or rejection may occur.

Purpose

To replace or replenish the bone marrow of patients whose marrow has failed or been suppressed.

Preparation

Begin by reinforcing the doctor's explanation of bone marrow transplant.

Give the patient and his family an opportunity to discuss the procedure with you at length to be sure they understand its risks and benefits. Make sure they know that, if the transplant fails, the patient may die. Then ensure that the patient or a responsible family member has signed a consent form.

Inform the patient that, because his white blood cells will be depleted, he'll be at high risk for infection immediately after the procedure and will be placed in reverse isolation for several weeks. Explain that contact with his family will be limited during this time.

Prepare the patient for the pretransplant regimen. The patient with leukemia, for example, may receive cytotoxic chemotherapy and total body irradiation to eradicate all traces of the leukemia and to prevent rejection of the new bone marrow. The patient with aplastic anemia may also receive cytotoxic drugs for immunosuppression.

During this pretransplant regimen, expect to see side effects, such as parotitis, diarrhea, pancytopenia, fever, cystitis, nausea, vomiting, cardiomyopathy, mucositis, and marrow depression. Administer prophylactic antiemetics, as ordered. Monitor intake and output and administer fluids to prevent fluid and electrolyte imbalances and cystitis.

Before the procedure begins, make sure that diphenhydramine and epinephrine are readily available to manage transfusion reactions. Start an I.V. line for hydration and record vital signs. Obtain an administration set (without a filter, which can trap the marrow cells) and, if ordered, insert a central venous catheter for infusion of the bone marrow.

Procedure

Bone marrow harvesting is performed in the operating room (see *Preparing the Marrow Donor*). In contrast, bone marrow administration is done at bedside using a peripheral I.V. line or a central venous catheter. The bone marrow stem cells circulate in the patient's bloodstream and eventually enter the marrow spaces, where they begin forming new cells. This engraftment period may take as long as 10 to 23 days.

The doctor initiates the transfusion and monitors its progress. The infusion time depends on the amount of marrow to be transfused and the institution's policy; it may range from 30 minutes to 4 hours. If the patient experiences a burning sensation during administration, the doctor can relieve it by slowing the infusion rate and applying warm compresses to the affected area.

Monitoring and aftercare

Once the transfusion has begun, take the patient's vital signs at least every 15 minutes for an hour, every 30 minutes for the next 2 hours, and then every hour for another 4 hours. The patient's vital signs will help you to promptly recognize such reactions as fever, dyspnea, and hypotension.

Monitor the patient for other reactions, such as bronchospasm, urticaria, erythema, chest pain, and back pain. Administer ordered medications to relieve these symptoms.

In addition, assess the patient every 4 hours for any signs of infection, such as fever or chills. Since the patient is pancytopenic, he's at risk for hemorrhage as well as infection. Maintain strict asepsis when caring for him and take measures to protect him from injury. The doctor may also order trans-

fusions of granulocytes or platelets and the patient may be placed in a room with laminar flow to further reduce the possibility of infection.

Draw blood for laboratory analysis, as ordered, and monitor the patient's hematologic status. Notify the doctor immediately of any changes.

Continue to watch for symptoms of GVHD, such as dermatitis, hepatitis, hemolytic anemia, and thrombocytopenia. GVHD usually occurs in the first 90 days after the transplant and may cause transplant failure, lymphatic depletion, infection, or death. GVHD may become chronic. Treatment is symptomatic, although methotrexate has been used in some cases to reduce the occurrence and severity of GVHD.

Home care instructions

• Tell the patient to protect himself from infection—especially if he has chronic GVHD (see *How to Avoid Infection,* page 438). Warn him that he may remain unusually vulnerable to infection for up to a year after the transplant.
• Urge him to keep regular medical appointments so that the doctor can monitor his progress and detect late complications.
• If the patient's a child, explain to the parents that his growth may be impaired by a bone marrow transplant. Tell them to monitor their child's growth; if it lags, he may need hormonal therapy.

Selected References

American Medical Association Council on Scientific Affairs. "Current Status of Therapeutic Plasmapheresis and Related Techniques," *Journal of the American Medical Association* 253(6):819-25, February 8, 1985.

Kasprisin, C.A. "Care of the Patient Receiving Transfusion Therapy," in *Transfusion Therapy: Principles and Procedures,* 2nd ed. Edited by Rutman,

R., and Miller, W. Rockville, Md.: Aspen Systems Corp., 1985.

Kasprisin, C.A. "The Hospitalized Patient: Interactions with the Apheresis Team," in *Therapeutic Hemapheresis.* Edited by Kasprisin, D., and MacPherson, J. Boca Raton, Fla.: CRC Press, 1985.

Stites, D., et al., eds. *Basic and Clinical Immunology,* 5th ed. East Norwalk, Conn.: Appleton & Lange, 1984.

13

Treating Cancer

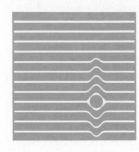

Treating Cancer

Introduction

Not long ago, surgery represented the primary treatment for cancer, with chemotherapy and radiation being used largely as backup measures if cancer recurred. Today, this has changed. Chemotherapy and radiation are full partners with surgery in treating cancer. And joining them are new approaches, such as immunotherapy.

Together these approaches have helped produce lengthy remissions in many patients and cures in others. At the same time, they've radically changed the way we treat cancer patients. Instead of being routinely sent off to surgery, cancer patients are now given individualized courses of treatment. This involves a careful evaluation of the patient's type of malignant tissue, the location and size of the primary tumor and any metastases, and his general health and nutritional status.

Surgery
Cancer surgery can take many forms. For example, it may provide access for other treatments, such as internal radiation implants. More commonly, it's performed for these reasons:
• If the tumor hasn't metastasized, surgery can provide a *cure* by removing the tumor and a margin of normal tissue. Typically, chemotherapy or radiation follows surgery to destroy any undetected cancer cells.
• If a tumor is too large to be removed, *debulking surgery* may be performed. Or preoperative chemotherapy or radiotherapy may be done to shrink it, thereby allowing removal.
• If a tumor depends on hormones for growth and function, *ablative surgery* may be performed to remove the organ responsible for producing the hormone.
• *Emergency surgery* may be necessary to correct hemorrhage caused by chemotherapy, colon perforation, or similar complications.
• When narcotics fail to relieve intractable cancer pain, *palliative surgery* may be necessary to provide relief.
• *Reconstructive surgery*, which ranges from skin grafting to reconstruction of body parts, may be required after radical surgery or radiation therapy.
• After radical surgery or radiation, *rehabilitative surgery* can help restore function.

To locate specific cancer surgeries, such as radical neck dissection or cordotomy, consult the appropriate body system chapters in this reference.

Chemotherapy
Chemotherapy aims to destroy cancer cells or suppress their growth. When a single drug is used, response is usually limited. When two or more drugs are used, long remissions or cures can

occur. Unfortunately, remissions and cures aren't commonplace since many cancers develop resistance to chemotherapeutic drugs over time. Also, these drugs' toxic effects contraindicate dosages high enough to be effective. Perhaps in the future, though, autologous bone marrow transplants may help overcome the life-threatening myelosuppression commonly seen in high-dose regimens, making more aggressive chemotherapy possible.

To increase the effectiveness of chemotherapy today, smaller doses of several drugs may be administered in complementary combinations, producing a cumulative effect similar to large doses of a single drug but causing less toxicity. Also, because different drugs work at different stages of the cell cycle or use different mechanisms to kill cancer cells, using several drugs decreases the likelihood of tumor resistance.

Hormones are also used to fight cancer. For example, diethylstilbestrol is given to create an unfavorable environment for neoplastic growth. And hormone antagonists, such as tamoxifen, are given to slow neoplastic growth by suppressing the action of hormones that nourish tumor cells.

Radiation
About half of all cancer patients receive radiation therapy to destroy malignant cells or inhibit their growth. Delivered externally or internally, radiation can be used as a primary treatment or as an adjunctive procedure intended to kill cancer cells that may have survived other treatments.

New treatments
Several emerging areas of cancer treatment hold promise for the future. New surgical treatments, using lasers and intraoperative radiation, can effectively remove tumors or reduce their size at the time of initial surgery and staging. Biological response modifiers, such as interferon and interleukin, may alter the immune response to interfere with tumor growth.

DRUG THERAPY

Nitrogen Mustards

The oldest anticancer drugs, the nitrogen mustards include the alkylating agents *cyclophosphamide, chlorambucil, mechlorethamine,* and *melphalan.* Cyclophosphamide, the most widely used alkylating agent, helps treat breast, lung, and ovarian cancer and hematologic malignancies, such as lymphomas, chronic leukemia, and Hodgkin's disease. (See *Comparing Nitrogen Mustards* for information on the other, less commonly used alkylating agents.)

Like the other nitrogen mustards, cyclophosphamide causes severe side effects, such as bone marrow depression. It should be used cautiously in leukopenia, thrombocytopenia, and metastasis to the bone or after recent chemotherapy or radiation therapy.

Hemorrhagic cystitis may develop several weeks after the start of cyclophosphamide therapy. Severe nausea and vomiting may also occur along with reversible alopecia (most common with high doses) and irreversible amenorrhea.

Purpose and action
Cyclophosphamide inhibits cellular growth, leading to cell death. The drug achieves this effect by cross-linking strands of DNA and RNA and interfering with protein synthesis.

Monitoring
Before the start of therapy, establish baseline white blood cell and platelet counts, hemoglobin level, and hematocrit. During therapy, monitor these studies to detect leukopenia or thrombocytopenia. Typically, leukopenia

COMPARING NITROGEN MUSTARDS

Although cyclophosphamide is most commonly prescribed, the nitrogen mustards chlorambucil, mechlorethamine, and melphalan have a place in chemotherapeutic regimens. Because these drugs suppress the bone marrow and cause atrophy of lymphoid tissue, they were initially used to treat lymphomas and leukemia. However, their severe side effects and frequent complications have resulted in their replacement, whenever feasible, by less toxic drugs.

When administering nitrogen mustards, be alert for side effects that commonly occur with most antineoplastic drugs, such as anorexia, nausea and vomiting, diarrhea, stomatitis, and bone marrow depression. Also be alert for other severe reactions, such as those discussed below.

Chlorambucil: Skin care crucial
Used to treat chronic lymphocytic leukemia, lymphomas, and Hodgkin's disease, chlorambucil can cause exfoliative dermatitis and hyperuricemia. If the patient develops exfoliative dermatitis, provide meticulous skin care to combat further breakdown and infection. To prevent hyperuricemia, monitor serum uric acid levels, keep the patient well hydrated, and administer allopurinol, as ordered. Also screen the patient's urine for calculi.

Mechlorethamine: Extravasation hazard
The treatment of choice for Hodgkin's disease, mechlorethamine can also be used to treat solid tumors. When preparing mechlorethamine solution, wear gloves and don't let the solution spill onto your skin. Because this drug is unstable in solution, prepare it immediately before infusion, use within 5 minutes, and discard any remaining solution.

When giving the drug, take measures to prevent extravasation and thrombophlebitis, such as injecting the drug into a free-flowing I.V. line. However, if the drug extravasates, apply cold compresses and infiltrate the area with isotonic sodium thiosulfate.

Melphalan: Hydration important
Melphalan is used to treat nonresectable ovarian cancer and is currently the drug of choice for multiple myeloma. Besides causing the side effects that are common to chemotherapeutic agents, the drug also causes hyperuricemia, pneumonitis, and pulmonary fibrosis.

To combat these effects, monitor the patient's serum uric acid levels and promote intake of fluids. Also be sure to watch for and report any signs of pulmonary infection, such as coughing, dyspnea, and fever.

---

reaches its nadir 9 to 14 days after administration.

Review the patient's drug regimen for possible interactions. For instance, use of cyclophosphamide with succinylcholine can lead to apnea. Use of corticosteroids or chloramphenicol can impair cyclophosphamide's effectiveness. However, stopping corticosteroids may produce cyclophosphamide toxicity.

During therapy, be alert for cardiotoxicity, which may occur with high doses of cyclophosphamide or concurrent use of doxorubicin. Also watch for fever, chills, dyspnea, and tachycardia. Report these symptoms to the doctor; he may need to reduce the dosage.

Assess for dysuria and hematuria,

which may signal hemorrhagic cystitis. Check the patient's serum uric acid level and renal function tests regularly. What's more, avoid giving this drug at night, when infrequent voiding may promote cystitis. If signs of cystitis occur, report them immediately. The doctor may discontinue the drug.

If the patient experiences vomiting, record his intake and output and keep him well hydrated. If ordered, administer antiemetics prophylactically.

Home care instructions
● Stress the importance of taking cyclophosphamide as ordered even though side effects may be severe. If the patient vomits shortly after taking the drug, he should contact the doctor.

MANAGING COMMON SIDE EFFECTS OF CHEMOTHERAPY

SIDE EFFECT	NURSING ACTIONS
Bone marrow depression (leukopenia, thrombocytopenia, anemia)	• Establish baseline white blood cell (WBC) and platelet counts, hemoglobin levels, and hematocrit before therapy begins. Monitor these studies during therapy. • If WBC count drops suddenly or falls below 2,000/mm³, stop the drug and notify the doctor. The drug may be discontinued or the dosage reduced. Initiate reverse isolation if WBC count falls below 1,500/mm³. Report a platelet count below 100,000/mm³. If necessary, assist with transfusion. • Monitor temperature orally every 4 hours, and regularly inspect the skin and body orifices for signs of infection. Observe for petechiae, easy bruising, and bleeding. Check for hematuria and monitor the patient's blood pressure. Be alert for signs of anemia. • Limit S.C. and I.M. injections. If these are necessary, apply pressure for 3 to 5 minutes after injection to prevent leakage or hematoma. Report unusual bleeding after injection. • Take precautions to prevent bleeding. Use extra care with razors, nail trimmers, dental floss, toothbrushes, and other sharp or abrasive objects. • Administer vitamin and iron supplements, as ordered. Provide a diet high in iron.
Anorexia	• Assess the patient's nutritional status before and during chemotherapy. Weigh him weekly or as ordered. • Explain the need for adequate nutrition despite loss of appetite.
Nausea and vomiting	• Before chemotherapy begins, administer antiemetics, as ordered, to reduce the severity of these reactions. • Monitor and record the frequency, character, and amount of vomitus. • Monitor serum electrolyte levels and provide I.V. hyperalimentation, if necessary.
Diarrhea and abdominal cramps	• Assess the frequency, color, consistency, and amount of diarrhea. Give antidiarrheals, as ordered. • Assess the severity of cramps, and observe for signs of dehydration (poor skin turgor, oliguria, irritability) and acidosis (confusion, nausea, vomiting, decreased level of consciousness), which may indicate electrolyte imbalance. • Encourage fluids and, if ordered, give I.V. fluids and potassium supplements. • Provide good skin care, especially to the perianal area.
Stomatitis	• Before drug administration, observe for dry mouth, erythema, and white patchy areas on the oral mucosa. Be alert for bleeding gums or complaints of a burning sensation when drinking acidic liquids. • Emphasize the principles of good mouth care with the patient and his family. • Provide mouth care every 4 to 6 hours with normal saline solution or half-strength hydrogen peroxide. Coat the oral mucosa with milk of magnesia. Avoid lemon or glycerin swabs because they tend to reduce saliva and change mouth pH. • To make eating more comfortable, apply a topical viscous anesthetic, such as lidocaine, before meals. Administer special mouthwashes, as ordered. • Consult the dietitian to provide bland foods at medium temperatures. • Treat cracked or burning lips with petrolatum.
Alopecia	• Reassure the patient that alopecia is usually temporary. • Inform him that he may experience discomfort before hair loss starts.

HOME CARE INSTRUCTIONS

• Instruct the patient to immediately report fever, chills, sore throat, lethargy, unusual fatigue, or pallor.
• Warn him to avoid exposure to persons with infections during chemotherapy and for several months after it.
• Explain that the patient and his family shouldn't receive immunizations during or shortly after chemotherapy since an exagger-

ated reaction may occur.
• Tell the patient to avoid activities that could cause traumatic injury and bleeding. Advise him to report any episodes of bleeding or bruising to the doctor.
• Tell him to eat high-iron foods, such as liver and spinach.
• Stress the importance of follow-up blood studies after completion of treatment.

• Encourage the patient's family to supply favorite foods to help him maintain adequate nutrition.

• Suggest that the patient eat small meals frequently.

• Teach the patient and his family how to insert antiemetic suppositories.
• Tell the patient to take the drug whenever it's least likely to cause nausea and vomiting: on an empty stomach, with meals, or at bedtime.

Reassure him that GI upset indicates that the drug is working.
• Instruct him to report any vomiting to the doctor, who may change the drug regimen.
• Tell the patient to follow a high-protein diet.

• Teach the patient how to use antidiarrheals and instruct him to report diarrhea to the doctor.
• Encourage him to maintain adequate fluid in-

take and to follow a bland, low-fiber diet.
• Explain that good perianal hygiene can help prevent tissue breakdown and infection.

• Teach the patient good mouth care. Instruct him to rinse his mouth with 1 tsp of salt dissolved in 8 oz of warm water or hydrogen peroxide diluted to half strength with water.

• Advise him to avoid acidic, spicy, or extremely hot or cold foods.
• Instruct the patient to report stomatitis to the doctor, who may order a change in medication.

• Suggest to the patient that he have his hair cut short to make thinning hair less noticeable.
• Advise washing his hair with a mild shampoo

and avoiding frequent brushing or combing.
• Suggest wearing a hat or scarf, or a toupee or wig.

• Stress the importance of returning for follow-up examinations and laboratory studies to help prevent or treat complications of therapy. Teach the patient how to deal with the common side effects of chemotherapy. (See *Managing Common Side Effects of Chemotherapy*, pages 460 and 461.)

• If the patient is using the tablet form, advise him to take the drug with water on an empty stomach to improve absorption. However, if GI upset occurs, he should take it with meals.

• Inform him to notify the doctor if he misses a dose. He should never double-dose.

• Instruct him to drink 3 qt (or liters) of fluid daily to help prevent cystitis. Caution him to report painful, bloody urination.

• Tell him to report fever, chills, or sore throat; these symptoms may indicate leukopenia.

• Because cyclophosphamide has teratogenic effects, advise both male and female patients to use contraceptive measures during treatment and for 4 months afterward. Ask the female patient to report any menstrual irregularities, such as amenorrhea.

Cisplatin
[Cis-platinum]

The only heavy metal compound commonly used as an antineoplastic agent, cisplatin effectively treats testicular, ovarian, head and neck, and bladder cancer and squamous cell neoplasms. In testicular cancer, cisplatin is often used with bleomycin and vinblastine. In ovarian cancer, it's most often combined with doxorubicin and cyclophosphamide.

Because cisplatin can cause nephrotoxicity, it's generally given I.V. only after hydration and mannitol diuresis. These pretreatment measures may also curtail ototoxic and neurotoxic effects.

To reduce the risk of cumulative toxicity, courses of cisplatin should be scheduled at least 3 weeks apart.

Cisplatin should be given cautiously to patients with renal or auditory impairment or myelosuppression. It shouldn't be given with other nephrotoxic drugs.

Purpose and action
Cisplatin cross-links strands of cellular DNA. This causes an imbalance of growth and leads to destruction of cancer cells.

Monitoring
Before the start of therapy, ensure that baseline audiometric tests have been performed. Also ensure that blood urea nitrogen, creatinine clearance, and serum creatinine tests have been done to provide a baseline for renal function. Similarly, check that hematologic studies—hemoglobin level, hematocrit, and platelet and white blood cell counts—have been performed.

If ordered, give corticosteroids and an antiemetic, to help prevent nausea and vomiting. Hydrate the patient with normal saline solution, establishing a urine output of 100 ml/hour for 4 consecutive hours before giving cisplatin. As ordered, give an I.V. bolus of mannitol and, during and for up to 24 hours after cisplatin infusion, follow with an infusion of mannitol to maintain urine output.

At the start of cisplatin infusion, be alert for signs of anaphylaxis: warm, moist skin; edema; light-headedness; paresthesias; and diffuse erythema or urticaria. If these signs occur, stop the infusion, ensure adequate ventilation, and notify the doctor immediately. As ordered, administer epinephrine, corticosteroids, or antihistamines.

Pay special attention to complaints of loss of taste or tingling in the fingers, toes, or face. These symptoms, which may occur after a single dose or after prolonged therapy, may be irreversible. Report such symptoms immediately; the doctor may discontinue the drug.

After the patient receives the initial dose, monitor intake and output for 24 hours and infuse 1 to 2 qt (or liters) of fluid over 8 to 12 hours or until the patient can tolerate adequate oral fluids. If oliguria occurs, notify the doctor; he may stop the drug until renal function is restored. If severe, protracted vomiting occurs, also notify the doctor. Nausea and vomiting may develop 1 to 4 hours after the start of therapy and persist for up to 24 hours.

During therapy, continue to monitor renal function and hematologic tests. Be alert for signs of infection, which may indicate leukopenia, and for unusual bruising or bleeding, which may indicate thrombocytopenia. These hematologic effects are more pronounced at high doses. Circulating platelets and leukocytes reach their nadir on days 18 to 23, with recovery by day 39.

Ask the patient about tinnitus and review audiometric tests for a high-frequency hearing loss. If you detect either, notify the doctor. He'll discontinue the drug or reduce its dosage to prevent permanent hearing loss.

Home care instructions

● Explain that harmful effects of cisplatin therapy can occur even after treatment ends. Instruct the patient to report symptoms of ototoxicity (hearing loss, ringing in the ears), bone marrow depression (easy bruising, unusual bleeding), nephrotoxicity (burning on urination, fever), or peripheral neuropathy (loss of taste, tingling in the fingers, toes, or face).

● Tell the patient to return for follow-up examinations and for blood and audiometric tests.

Nitrosureas

The most commonly used nitrosureas, I.V. *carmustine (BCNU)* and oral *lomustine (CCNU)*, readily cross the blood-brain barrier, making them useful in treating CNS malignancies. Both drugs can be used to treat colon and lung cancer, Hodgkin's disease, malignant melanoma, and multiple myeloma. Carmustine also helps treat stomach and liver cancer, whereas lomustine is effective against hematologic malignancies, renal cell carcinoma, and lymphomas.

Myelosuppression, a major side effect, commonly reaches its nadir 4 to 6 weeks after administration. As a result, the nitrosureas should be used cautiously in preexisting myelosuppression. Carmustine shouldn't be used with cimetidine, since heightened bone marrow toxicity could result.

Because carmustine and lomustine are detoxified in the liver and excreted through the kidneys, they should be used carefully in patients with impaired hepatic or renal function.

Purpose and action

Carmustine and lomustine exert their cytotoxic effects by cross-linking strands of DNA, causing an imbalance of growth and leading to cell death.

Monitoring

Before beginning therapy, establish baseline white blood cell (WBC) and platelet counts. During treatment, monitor them weekly and report a WBC count below 2,000/mm^3 or a platelet count below 25,000/mm^3.

Before administering a nitrosurea, give an antiemetic, if ordered, to reduce the severity of GI effects. Severe nausea and vomiting may begin 2 to 6 hours after administration and may last 4 to 6 hours with carmustine and up to 24 hours with lomustine.

If you'll be giving carmustine, dissolve 100 mg of the drug in 3 ml absolute alcohol and dilute this solution with 17 ml of sterile water. (This will give you a solution containing 5 mg carmustine/ml in 10% alcohol.) Now dilute this in normal saline solution or dextrose 5% in water, and infuse at least 250 ml over 1 to 2 hours. During infusion, assess for pain or burning at the site, which may indicate venospasm caused by the drug's alcohol base. To reduce pain, decrease the infusion rate. Also be alert for extravasation; if it occurs, notify the doctor immediately. (See *Combating Chemotherapeutic Drug Extravasation*, page 470.)

Home care instructions
• Explain to the patient that bone marrow suppression reaches its nadir 4 to 6 weeks after drug administration. Warn him to watch for and report signs of infection and bone marrow toxicity, including easy bruising, nose or gum bleeding, and melena. Tell him to take his temperature daily.
• If the patient's receiving carmustine, tell him to report a hacking cough or dyspnea. These symptoms may indicate pneumonitis or pulmonary fibrosis.
• Emphasize the importance of weekly WBC and platelet counts to monitor the extent of myelosuppression.
• Teach the patient how to deal with other side effects of chemotherapy. (See *Managing Common Side Effects of Chemotherapy*, pages 460 and 461.)

Folic Acid Antagonist

The folic acid antagonist *methotrexate* exerts a palliative effect in breast, head and neck, and lung cancer and induces remission of some leukemias, lymphosarcoma, and disseminated neoplasms in children. What's more, the drug can cure uterine choriocarcinoma.

Methotrexate can be given orally, intramuscularly, intravenously, or intrathecally. It doesn't cross the blood-brain barrier unless given intrathecally or in extremely high doses. With high doses, leucovorin calcium is given within 4 hours of methotrexate to block its systemic effects and protect healthy cells while allowing malignant cells to absorb methotrexate.

Like most chemotherapeutic drugs, methotrexate causes severe side effects,

including GI upset, myelosuppression, stomatitis, CNS disturbances, and renal and hepatic toxicity. The drug should be given cautiously to patients with infection, peptic ulcer, ulcerative colitis, or impaired hepatorenal function and to young, elderly, or debilitated patients. In patients with preexisting bone marrow depression, the drug should be given with extreme caution, if at all.

Purpose and action
Methotrexate destroys cancer cells by inhibiting DNA synthesis and cell reproduction. It achieves these effects by binding to dehydrofolate reductase, thus preventing the reduction of folic acid to tetrahydrofolate. (See *How Chemotherapeutic Drugs Disrupt the Cell Cycle*.)

Monitoring
Before starting therapy, assess the patient's vital signs, skin and oral mucosa, and nutritional status. Collect samples for a complete blood count and creatinine clearance test. These data will help detect thrombocytopenia, leukopenia, anemia, or agranulocytosis. During therapy, report any drop in white blood cell (WBC) or platelet count. An abnormal creatinine clearance test may signal renal dysfunction.

Check the drug regimen to anticipate possible interactions. For example, probenecid, phenylbutazone, salicylates, and sulfonamides enhance methotrexate's toxic effects and shouldn't be used concurrently with the drug.

Use care in the preparation, administration, and disposal of methotrexate; it's absorbed through the skin and, like other antineoplastic agents, has mutagenic, teratogenic, and carcinogenic potential.

Once therapy begins, be alert for side effects, which can occur within the first 12 hours and may extend over 2 weeks. Diarrhea can indicate GI toxicity, which may require a change in dosage.

If you're giving methotrexate intrathecally, watch for symptoms of

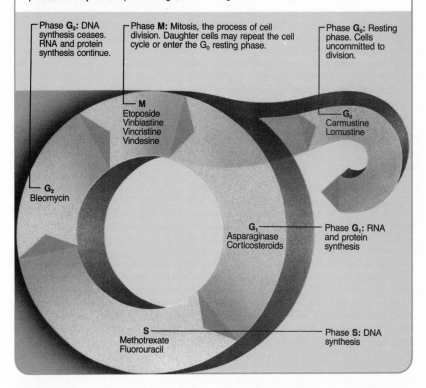

HOW CHEMOTHERAPEUTIC DRUGS DISRUPT THE CELL CYCLE

Chemotherapeutic drugs may be either cell-cycle-specific or cell-cycle-nonspecific. Cell-cycle-specific drugs, such as methotrexate, act at one or more cell-cycle phases. Cell-cycle-nonspecific drugs, such as busulfan, can act on both replicating and resting cells.

Note: The drugs listed in this diagram are only examples of cell-cycle-specific agents.

Phase G_2: DNA synthesis ceases. RNA and protein synthesis continue.

Phase **M**: Mitosis, the process of cell division. Daughter cells may repeat the cell cycle or enter the G_0 resting phase.

Phase G_0: Resting phase. Cells uncommitted to division.

M
Etoposide
Vinblastine
Vincristine
Vindesine

G_0
Carmustine
Lomustine

G_2
Bleomycin

G_1
Asparaginase
Corticosteroids

Phase G_1: RNA and protein synthesis

S
Methotrexate
Fluorouracil

Phase **S**: DNA synthesis

arachnoiditis within hours of administration. Report such symptoms as paresthesias, decreased hand strength, loss of coordination, and foot or wrist drop to the doctor. A change in medication or a decreased dosage may be indicated to prevent further neurotoxicity and irreversible loss of function.

Observe for stomatitis, which can occur 48 to 72 hours after administration. Be alert for signs of infection, which could indicate leukopenia. To detect thrombocytopenia, carefully monitor the patient's platelet count, since a count below 150,000/mm³ can lead to irreversible bone marrow depression. To detect anemia, watch for pallor, lethargy, or increased fatigue.

Monitor SGOT, SGPT, and alkaline phosphatase levels; increased levels indicate hepatotoxicity. Report any pulmonary effects to the doctor and give corticosteroids, if ordered.

Home care instructions

● Explain to the patient that continued monitoring is essential because the side effects may be cumulative, with myelosuppression occurring weeks after the start of therapy.

• Warn him to avoid alcohol, which increases the risk of hepatotoxicity.

• Inform him that certain over-the-counter drugs contain salicylates, which can increase methotrexate's toxicity. Urge him to read all labels on products and to consult the doctor before taking such medications.

• Since methotrexate may increase photosensitivity, caution the patient to avoid overexposure to the sun. Stress that a sunscreen should be used during even minimal exposure to sunlight.

• Instruct the female patient of child-bearing age to practice birth control during and immediately after methotrexate therapy because of the risk of abortion or congenital anomalies.

• Teach the patient how to deal with other side effects of chemotherapy (see *Managing Common Side Effects of Chemotherapy,* pages 460 and 461).

Pyrimidine Antagonists

The antimetabolites fluorouracil (5-fluorouracil) and cytarabine (ARA-C or cytosine arabinoside) interfere with pyrimidine synthesis.

Fluorouracil relieves pain and reduces the size of tumors of the GI tract, breast, liver, pancreas, ovaries, or bladder. It's used topically for premalignant skin lesions and superficial basal cell carcinoma. And it has a palliative effect in any carcinoma that can't be cured by surgery or radiation.

Most commonly used for acute myelocytic leukemia, *cytarabine* is also used for acute lymphocytic leukemia, chronic myelocytic leukemia, erythroleukemia, and meningeal leukemia. When given with other chemotherapeutic drugs, it helps treat non-Hodgkin's lymphoma in children.

The side effects of pyrimidine antagonists include leukopenia, thrombocytopenia, stomatitis, anorexia, nausea, vomiting, and diarrhea. Stomatitis commonly occurs with fluorouracil. Megaloblastosis, an uncommon but potentially life-threatening reaction, can occur with cytarabine.

Cytarabine is usually given in combination with other drugs, thereby affecting the incidence and intensity of side effects. For example, when given with methotrexate, a synergistic cytotoxic effect may occur, requiring a change in dosage.

Both fluorouracil and cytarabine are administered parenterally, since they aren't absorbed orally. Fluorouracil, which is primarily given intravenously, can also be administered via intraarterial infusion for treatment of hepatic metastasis. I.V. infusion extending over 2 to 8 hours appears to reduce toxic effects, but I.V. injection over 1 to 2 minutes proves more effective.

Cytarabine may also be given by continuous infusion or I.V. injection. In maintenance doses, it may be given subcutaneously. This drug may be given intrathecally for acute leukemia and, with other agents, such as methotrexate, for CNS metastasis or recurrent CNS neoplasms. Leukopenia and thrombocytopenia are more common when cytarabine is given by continuous I.V. infusion; nausea and vomiting are more severe with rapid I.V. injection.

Since cytarabine and fluorouracil are metabolized in the liver and excreted through the kidneys, they should be used cautiously in renal or hepatic disease. Both drugs are contraindicated if the patient has chicken pox or herpes zoster or has recently been exposed to these diseases. Fluorouracil should be avoided in any patient with poor nutrition, bone marrow depression, or potentially serious infections.

Purpose and action

Fluorouracil and cytarabine destroy neoplastic cells by inhibiting the enzyme thymidylate synthetase, thereby blocking DNA and RNA synthesis. As cell-cycle-specific drugs, they act in the S phase of cell division. (See *How Chemotherapeutic Drugs Disrupt the Cell Cycle,* page 465.)

Monitoring

Before chemotherapy begins, establish baseline vital signs, complete blood count, and renal and hepatic studies as well as skin condition and nutritional status. Before beginning cytarabine therapy, assess the patient's joints, since pain and swelling occur in leukemia as well as from drug toxicity.

Since fluorouracil causes tissue inflammation, use caution when handling the drug. Wear gloves and avoid contact with the eyes, nose, and mouth. Wash your hands thoroughly after use.

Observe for the common side effects of pyrimidine antagonists, such as ecchymosis, easy bruising, petechiae, anorexia, diarrhea, nausea, and vomiting. (When high doses of cytarabine are given by rapid I.V. injection, projectile vomiting, a frightening side effect, may occur. Reassure the patient that this is an anticipated reaction and will subside.)

Be alert for symptoms of cytarabine syndrome, which may occur 6 to 12 hours after the drug is given. These include bone pain, fever, maculopapular rash, conjunctivitis, chest pain, or malaise. If these symptoms develop, give corticosteroids, as ordered.

If the patient receiving fluorouracil has intractable vomiting, stomatitis, or diarrhea, notify the doctor. He may modify the dosage or stop the drug.

Monitor white blood cell (WBC) and platelet counts, blood urea nitrogen levels, and hematocrit frequently. A WBC count below 3,500/mm³ or a platelet count below 100,000/mm³ may require interruption of fluorouracil therapy. Similarly, a WBC count below 1,000/mm³ or a platelet count below 50,000/mm³ may require interruption of cytarabine therapy.

Monitor uric acid level for signs of hyperuricemia. Maintain high fluid intake and administer allopurinol, if ordered, to prevent urate nephropathy. Have the patient report dysuria and maintain good perineal care to prevent excoriation from acidic urine.

Closely monitor the patient's skin for breakdown and maculopapular rash, especially if he's receiving fluorouracil. If rash or another skin problem develops, provide meticulous care to help prevent infection. However, if you detect infection, report this immediately to the doctor since a local infection may rapidly become systemic because of a lack of granulocytes.

Home care instructions

- Teach the patient how to deal with chemotherapy's side effects (see *Managing Common Side Effects of Chemotherapy*, pages 460 and 461).
- Warn the patient on fluorouracil that it may cause photosensitivity. Advise him to wear protective clothing and use a sun blocker when outdoors to prevent inflammatory erythematous dermatitis. Explain that this reaction will subside when fluorouracil is stopped.

Antibiotic Antineoplastics

Doxorubicin, one of the most versatile and effective chemotherapeutic agents, belongs to the family of cancer-fighting drugs known as antibiotic antineoplastics. (See *Comparing Antibiotic Antineoplastics*, pages 468 and 469, for information on the drugs bleomycin, dactinomycin, daunorubicin, plicamycin, and procarbazine.) These drugs are derived from naturally occurring microorganisms but differ from other antibiotics in their ability to affect host cells as well as bacterial cells.

Doxorubicin treats a wide range of cancers, including breast, lung, ovarian, and gastric cancers as well as sarcomas, lymphomas, and acute leukemias. Like most antineoplastics, it can cause severe side effects, sometimes weeks or months after administration. Cardiotoxic effects can lead to congestive heart failure, and some-

COMPARING ANTIBIOTIC ANTINEOPLASTICS

DRUG AND ACTION	INDICATIONS	MAJOR SIDE EFFECTS
Bleomycin Inhibits DNA synthesis and causes scission of single- and double-stranded DNA	Squamous cell carcinomas, lymphomas, Hodgkin's disease, and esophageal, head and neck, cervical, and testicular cancer	*GI:* stomatitis, anorexia, nausea, vomiting, diarrhea *Skin:* erythema, hyperpigmentation, vesiculation *Other:* reversible alopecia, anaphylaxis, fever, chills, pulmonary reactions (basilar crackles, dyspnea, tachypnea, nonproductive cough)
Dactinomycin A cell-cycle-specific drug that links to DNA, blocking DNA-dependent RNA synthesis	Uterine and testicular tumors, osteogenic sarcoma, Ewing's sarcoma, melanoma, and rhabdomyosarcoma; used in combination with surgery or radiation for Wilms' tumor	*Blood:* leukopenia, thrombocytopenia, pancytopenia *GI:* anorexia, nausea, vomiting, stomatitis *Skin:* erythema, hyperpigmentation (especially in previously irradiated areas), reversible acne *Other:* reversible alopecia, severe damage to soft tissue
Daunorubicin Interferes with DNA-dependent RNA synthesis by intercalation	Acute nonlymphocytic leukemia in adults and acute lymphocytic leukemia in children; often combined with cytarabine or vincristine and prednisone for increased effectiveness	*CV:* potentially fatal congestive heart failure (CHF), arrhythmias *Blood:* bone marrow depression *GI:* stomatitis, esophagitis, nausea, severe vomiting (lasting 24 to 48 hours) *GU:* transient red urine, hyperuricemia *Other:* reversible alopecia, severe tissue necrosis
Plicamycin (Mithramycin) Interferes with DNA-dependent RNA synthesis by intercalation. This drug also inhibits osteocytic activity, blocking calcium and phosphorus resorption from the bone.	Testicular cancer and hypercalcemia and hypercalciuria in advanced malignancy	*Blood:* thrombocytopenia, bleeding (from epistaxis to generalized hemorrhage), facial flushing *GI:* nausea, vomiting *Metabolic:* decreased serum calcium level, which could lead to tetany (carpopedal spasm, Chvostek's sign, and muscle cramps) *Local:* irritation and cellulitis, if extravasation occurs
Procarbazine Inhibits synthesis of DNA, RNA, and protein	Hodgkin's disease, lymphomas, and brain and lung cancer	*Blood:* thrombocytopenia, leukopenia, anemia *CNS:* hallucinations *GI:* anorexia, nausea, vomiting *Skin:* photosensitivity

NURSING CONSIDERATIONS

• Contraindicated in renal and pulmonary disease.
• Auscultate the lungs and obtain baseline chest X-rays. Monitor pulmonary function during treatment and report any abnormalities.
• To observe for anaphylaxis, administer I.V. slowly (over 10 minutes). If an anaphylactic reaction occurs, stop the drug immediately, notify the doctor, and provide emergency care. Also observe for delayed (up to several hours) allergic reaction.
• Provide supportive care if GI side effects occur. (See *Managing Common Side Effects of Chemotherapy,* pages 460 and 461.)
• If skin reactions occur, provide meticulous care to prevent tissue breakdown. Observe for signs of extravasation.
• Administer antipyretics for fever.

• Contraindicated in renal, hepatic, or bone marrow impairment, chicken pox or herpes zoster, pregnancy, and lactation.
• Monitor white blood cell (WBC) count daily and platelet count every 3 days. Report low levels to the doctor.
• Monitor renal and hepatic function and report any abnormalities to the doctor.
• Use only sterile water (without preservatives) as diluent.
• Because of dactinomycin's strong vesicant action, infuse cautiously through a running I.V. line to avoid infiltration.
• Provide supportive care if GI effects occur.
• Report erythema, which can be severe, especially in previously irradiated areas. Desquamation and sloughing may occur if this condition isn't treated.

• Use cautiously in pregnancy, heart disease, renal or hepatic failure, or bone marrow depression.
• Perform EKG before and during treatment. Be alert for symptoms of CHF, including edema, dyspnea, and cyanosis. Also monitor resting pulse—a high rate indicates cardiac side effects. Keep digitalis and diuretics on hand. Report signs of CHF to the doctor and stop the drug immediately.
• Monitor complete blood count and hepatic function, and encourage fluids to avoid hyperuricemia.
• Provide supportive care if GI effects occur.
• To avoid extravasation, inject the drug into a free-flowing I.V. line. Never give I.M. or S.C.
• Inform the patient that urine discoloration is harmless.

• Contraindicated in children under age 15 and in patients with thrombocytopenia or coagulation disorders. Use cautiously in renal, hepatic, or bone marrow impairment.
• Monitor platelet count, WBC count, and prothrombin time before and during therapy. Discontinue therapy if WBC count falls below 3,000/mm^3 or if prothrombin time increases 4 seconds over baseline. Also monitor liver and renal function tests.
• Give slowly to reduce nausea that develops with I.V. push. To prevent extravasation, inject drug into the tubing of a free-flowing I.V. line. Never give I.M. or S.C.
• Report early signs of bleeding, such as facial flushing, and immediately stop therapy.
• Check for signs of tetany: carpopedal spasm, Chvostek's sign, or muscle cramps.
• Monitor serum calcium for decreased levels. Report any abnormalities to the doctor.
• Avoid contact with skin or mucous membranes.

• Use cautiously in bone marrow depression or impaired renal or hepatic function.
• Since procarbazine inhibits monoamine oxidase (MAO), use cautiously with other MAO inhibitors and with tricyclic antidepressants.
• Evaluate WBC and platelet counts before and during treatment.
• Instruct the patient to avoid alcoholic beverages and foods with high tyramine content (such as beer, caffeine, and some cheeses) while taking this drug. Their combination may cause throbbing headache, chest pain, and palpitations.
• Provide supportive care if GI effects occur.
• Warn the patient that this drug heightens photosensitivity. Instruct him to avoid exposure to the sun and to use a sunscreen when exposure is unavoidable.

COMBATING CHEMOTHERA-PEUTIC DRUG EXTRAVASATION

Doxorubicin and other chemotherapeutic drugs, especially the vinca alkaloids, cause extensive cell damage if they infiltrate surrounding tissues during I.V. infusion.

Extravasation may result from vein fragility, the use of improper technique or equipment, poor selection of the injection site, or accidental dislodgment of the needle or catheter. Signs and symptoms of extravasation include pain, erythema, edema, leakage of I.V. solution, phlebitis, and tissue necrosis.

Preventing extravasation
Follow these tips to help you prevent extravasation:
- Choose a large vein for the infusion.
- Initially infuse normal saline or dextrose solution to assess vein patency and correct needle placement.
- Inject the solution into the tubing of a free-flowing I.V. line.
- Assess the I.V. site continuously. If stinging or burning occurs, stop the infusion immediately and notify the doctor.

Treating extravasation
If extravasation *does* occur, notify the doctor and discontinue the infusion immediately. Then follow these measures:
- Elevate the affected arm.
- Apply ice for 24 hours followed by warm compresses for 24 to 72 hours.
- Give steroids topically or subcutaneously, as ordered.
- Observe for extensive tissue necrosis. If present, early excision of the area and plastic surgery may be necessary.

times bone marrow depression forces dosage reductions or interruptions in therapy. Severe stomatitis and nausea and vomiting are also common.

Because the drug is metabolized in the liver and excreted in bile, it should be used cautiously in hepatic impairment. Because of its cardiotoxic potential, it's contraindicated in patients with heart disease.

Purpose and action
Doxorubicin destroys cancer cells by binding to DNA, thereby blocking DNA and RNA synthesis. A cell-cycle-specific drug, doxorubicin acts at the S phase of cell division.

Monitoring
Before chemotherapy begins, collect serum samples for complete blood count, platelet count, and liver function studies. Also perform an EKG and, if ordered, assist with coronary angiography to determine the patient's ejection fraction. Check the patient's drug regimen to anticipate any interactions. For example, concurrent use of doxorubicin and streptozocin can cause increased and prolonged drug blood levels, requiring a dosage adjustment.

Handle and dispose of this drug cautiously. Avoid inhaling any of its particles. If it touches the skin—yours or the patient's—flood the area with water and cleanse thoroughly with soap.

Avoid mixing doxorubicin with heparin, since a precipitate will form. Monitor I.V. administration carefully. If extravasation occurs, stop administration and choose another injection site. (See *Combating Chemotherapeutic Drug Extravasation.*) To minimize the risk of extravasation, never give this drug I.M. or S.C.

Be alert for facial flushing, which indicates overly rapid injection. If this reaction occurs, decrease the administration rate.

Watch for signs of cardiotoxicity—dyspnea, swelling of the legs, or an unusually rapid or irregular heartbeat—occurring within minutes of a single I.V. dose. If any of these signs occur, slow the infusion rate. Then, if any still persist, withhold the drug and notify the doctor immediately.

During the initial course of therapy, monitor for hyperuricemia and urine discoloration. Typically, the urine is red for 1 or 2 days when treatment begins. Encourage fluids and, if ordered, give allopurinol to alkalinize the urine.

If the patient has previously had radiation therapy, monitor for erythema, edema, and desquamation since they can recur with doxorubicin. Reassure the patient that these effects will sub-side after 7 days.

Home care instructions
• Teach the patient how to deal with chemotherapy's side effects (see *Managing Common Side Effects of Chemotherapy,* pages 460 and 461).
• Warn the patient that cardiotoxicity can occur 1 to 6 months after completion of therapy and must be reported promptly. Emphasize the importance of early detection to prevent severe and potentially fatal complications.

• Instruct the patient to return for follow-up EKGs and blood studies.

Vinca and Related Alkaloids

The vinca alkaloids *vinblastine, vincristine,* and *vindesine* provide palliative treatment for lymphomas, leukemias, sarcomas, and some car-

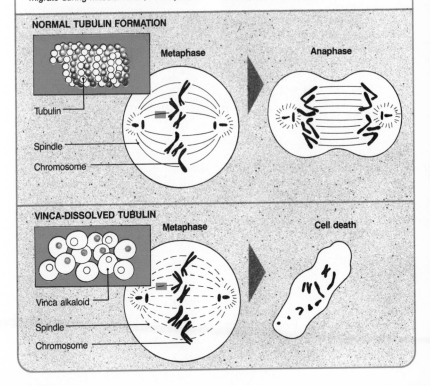

HOW VINCA ALKALOIDS AFFECT MITOSIS

The vinca alkaloids arrest cells in metaphase, the second phase of mitosis.
As cell-cycle-specific drugs, they stop mitosis by binding to tubulin, a protein found in the cytoplasm of all cells.
Normally, tubulin molecules stack to form the spindles along which chromosomes migrate during mitosis. Then, in anaphase

(the third phase of mitosis), the spindle fibers pull the chromosome pairs apart toward opposite poles of the cell as the process of cell division continues.
However, by binding to tubulin, the vinca alkaloids interrupt this process, causing dissolution of the mitotic spindle and subsequent cell death.

NORMAL TUBULIN FORMATION

Tubulin
Spindle
Chromosome

Metaphase

Anaphase

VINCA-DISSOLVED TUBULIN

Vinca alkaloid
Spindle
Chromosome

Metaphase

Cell death

cinomas. In addition, vinblastine is often used with cisplatin and bleomycin to treat disseminated, nonseminomatous testicular cancer. Vincristine, when used with corticosteroids, proves highly effective against childhood leukemias. *Etoposide*, a podophyllin derivative, has the same mechanism of action and major uses as the vinca alkaloids. This drug has produced complete remissions in testicular cancer and small-cell carcinoma of the lung.

The chief side effects of the vinca alkaloids include acute bronchospasm, myelosuppression, neurotoxicity, and GI upset. And because these drugs are painful vesicants, they cause severe tissue damage if extravasation occurs. (See *Combating Chemotherapeutic Drug Extravasation*, page 470.)

The vinca alkaloids are contraindicated in severe leukopenia, bacterial infection, neuromuscular disease, or concurrent use of other neurotoxic drugs. They should be used cautiously in hepatic disease.

Purpose and action
The vinca alkaloids and etoposide damage cancer cells by arresting mitosis in metaphase. (See *How Vinca Alkaloids Affect Mitosis*, page 471.)

Monitoring
Before therapy, ensure that a complete blood count and liver function tests have been performed. During therapy, monitor these tests to detect myelosuppression and hepatotoxicity.

If you're administering etoposide, take the patient's blood pressure readings before infusion and every 30 minutes during it. If systolic pressure drops below 90 mm Hg, stop the infusion and notify the doctor. Also monitor for anaphylaxis, a rare but life-threatening reaction.

If you're administering a vinca alkaloid, be alert for and report acute bronchospasm, a life-threatening reaction most common in the patient who's also receiving mitomycin. Assess for signs of neurotoxicity, including paresthesias in the extremities or a change in bowel habits, especially constipation. Be sure to report constipation that lasts longer than 24 hours since paralytic ileus could also occur.

Observe the oral mucosa for stomatitis. If it occurs, inform the doctor; he may discontinue the drug.

Home care instructions
- Explain to the patient that the therapeutic response to vinca alkaloids isn't immediate.
- Inform him that he'll need periodic blood tests to monitor his hematologic status. Instruct him to promptly report fever, sore throat, easy bruising or bleeding, pallor, or unusual fatigue.
- Also instruct him to report neurotoxic symptoms, such as paresthesias in his fingers or toes or jaw pain.
- To prevent constipation, tell the patient to eat high-fiber foods, drink plenty of fluids, and take a stool softener, if prescribed.
- Teach the patient how to deal with the side effects of chemotherapy. (See *Managing Common Side Effects of Chemotherapy*, pages 460 and 461.)

Antiestrogens

The antiestrogens include estrogen antagonists, such as tamoxifen, and androgens. (See *Comparing Androgens: Hormones for Cancer Therapy* for information on the androgens.) Tamoxifen, the most commonly used antiestrogen, currently serves as the treatment of choice for metastatic breast cancer in postmenopausal women, replacing hormonal treatments, adrenalectomy, and hypophysectomy. This drug is most effective in women with positive estrogen receptors, which indicates that estrogens are binding to normal tissue—and to cancer cells. Tamoxifen also proves effective against ovarian cancer and breast cancer in men.

COMPARING ANDROGENS: HORMONES FOR CANCER THERAPY

The androgens *fluoxymesterone, methyltestosterone, and testolactone* have been used since 1950 to treat advanced breast cancer in postmenopausal women. Today, they've been largely replaced by tamoxifen, a safer and more effective drug.

The androgens provide palliative treatment for inoperable breast cancer with metastasis to the bone. They exert their cytotoxic effect by changing the tumor's hormonal environment and altering the neoplastic process.

If you're administering any of these androgens, you'll need to understand some key differences in their side effects, administration, and onset of effectiveness.

Side effects: Sometimes severe
Hypercalcemia commonly occurs with all three drugs but may also indicate bone metastasis. However, if a bone scan reveals no metastasis, exercise and increased fluids can aid calcium excretion and may prevent hypercalcemia.

Use of fluoxymesterone or methyltestos-

terone may cause possibly irreversible virilization, characterized by deepening of the voice, oily skin, acne, clitoral enlargement, and amenorrhea. The degree of virilization is usually dose-dependent. In contrast, the synthetic testolactone doesn't cause virilization.

Route varies
Fluoxymesterone is given orally in tablet form, whereas methyltestosterone comes in two tablet forms: one for swallowing and the other for buccal absorption. Testolactone can be given orally or by deep I.M. injection.

Response time delayed
After taking fluoxymesterone, the patient may notice improvement in about 1 month, with objective changes noted by blood tests and a bone scan in about 3 months. With methyltestosterone and testolactone, the therapeutic response takes about 3 months.

Tamoxifen's side effects rarely prove severe enough to interrupt treatment. The most common ones include hot flashes, nausea, vomiting, vaginal discharge, menstrual irregularities, and rash. Hypercalcemia, headaches, lightheadedness, and anorexia may also occur. In the early stages of treatment, increased bone and tumor pain may occur, signaling destruction of the malignancy.

Because tamoxifen causes mild to moderate myelosuppression, it should be used cautiously in patients with preexisting thrombocytopenia or leukopenia.

Purpose and action
Tamoxifen destroys cancer cells by competing with estrogens for binding sites in the cells of certain tissues, including breast tissue. The drug can also reduce metastatic lesions in the bone and other sites.

Monitoring
Before therapy begins, establish a baseline for white blood cell and platelet counts and calcium level. Continue to monitor hematologic studies during therapy to detect leukopenia and thrombocytopenia. Also monitor serum calcium levels to detect hypercalcemia; keep the patient well hydrated to minimize the effects of this condition.

If the patient complains of increased bone pain, adjust the dosage of the analgesic, as ordered. Explain that tamoxifen may initially worsen pain, but reassure the patient that this usually indicates a good therapeutic response.

Home care instructions
• Inform the patient that tamoxifen usually produces a therapeutic response in 4 to 10 weeks. If the cancer has metastasized to the bone, this response may take several months.
• Stress the importance of following the

LEUPROLIDE: ALTERNATIVE TO ESTROGENS

Leuprolide, a drug with antiandrogenic properties, provides an effective alternative to estrogen therapy in advanced prostatic cancer. What's more, it produces fewer side effects than estrogens do.

How leuprolide works
Leuprolide is a synthetic analog of gonadotropin-releasing hormone. Given by S.C. injection, this drug initially raises levels of luteinizing hormone and follicle-stimulating hormone, leading to a brief increase in testosterone levels. However, these effects quickly reverse, leading to sharply reduced testosterone levels within 4 weeks. Because most prostate tumors depend on testosterone for growth and function, leuprolide can arrest their development.

Fewer side effects
Compared to estrogens, leuprolide has markedly fewer side effects. For example, thrombophlebitis, MI, and pulmonary embolism rarely occur with leuprolide. Gynecomastia, nausea, and vomiting occur less commonly, too. However, sudden hot flashes and increased bone or tumor pain may occur soon after the start of therapy. Symptoms of prostatic cancer may also worsen temporarily. This exacerbation of symptoms coincides with the transient elevation of testosterone levels early in the course of therapy and subsides once levels decline.

medication schedule closely. Instruct the patient to continue taking tamoxifen even if GI upset occurs. However, if she vomits soon after taking a dose, she should contact the doctor.
• If the patient misses a dose, explain that she shouldn't increase the next dose. Instead, she should contact the doctor and ask for instructions.
• Warn the patient to avoid taking antacids within 1 or 2 hours of taking enteric-coated tamoxifen tablets since this can worsen GI upset.
• Tell the patient to report sudden confusion, dizziness, or headaches.
• Since tamoxifen induces ovulation in premenopausal women, advise the pa-

tient to use mechanical contraception during therapy.
• Remind the patient to keep appointments for scheduled blood tests.

Estrogens

The estrogens *chlorotrianisene* and *estrone* effectively treat prostatic cancer. *Diethylstilbestrol, estradiol, ethinyl estradiol,* and the *esterified estrogens* help treat prostatic cancer as well as male metastatic breast cancer and postmenopausal breast cancer. Estrogens may be given to women in whom antiestrogen therapy was initially effective but subsequently unsuccessful.

These drugs can cause potentially life-threatening complications, such as thromboembolism, MI, cerebrovascular accident, and severe hypercalcemia. Other effects include nausea and vomiting, thrombophlebitis, and edema. In women, menstrual changes may accompany a loss of libido. In men, gynecomastia, testicular atrophy, and impotence may occur.

Estrogens are contraindicated in preexisting thrombophlebitis. They should be used cautiously in hypertension, depression, heart failure, diabetes mellitus, and hepatic or renal dysfunction.

Purpose and action
Estrogens are thought to inhibit the reproduction of cancer cells by causing changes in the stroma of the tissue. In breast and prostatic cancer, they may stimulate the body's immune defenses (and may account for some remissions in breast cancer). They inhibit prostatic tissue growth and compete with androgens for the same receptor sites in prostatic cancer cells. Estrogens reduce secretion of testosterone by the testes and adrenal glands by inhibiting the hypothalamic secretion of gonadotropin-releasing hormone, leading to reduced pituitary secretion of follicle-

stimulating hormone and luteinizing hormone.

Monitoring

Because estrogens can cause fatal cardiovascular complications, you'll need to evaluate the patient's cardiovascular status before therapy. You'll also need to establish a baseline for renal and hepatic function. During therapy, you'll need to monitor these as well as the patient's blood pressure.

Home care instructions

• Instruct the patient to follow the prescribed dosage schedule. Explain that if he misses a dose, he should take it as soon as he remembers. However, if it's almost time for the next dose, he should skip the missed dose and resume his regular schedule. He should never double-dose.

• Advise the patient to immediately report abdominal pain, numbness or stiffness in his legs or buttocks, chest pain or pressure, shortness of breath, severe headaches, and visual disturbances—any of which may indicate blood clots. Also have him report yellow sclera or skin, dark urine, or light-colored stools, which could indicate hepatitis or gallbladder dysfunction.

• Tell the patient to be alert for sudden weight gain and swelling of his hands and feet, which could indicate sodium and fluid retention.

• Reassure the male patient that gynecomastia and impotence will subside once therapy is completed.

• Advise taking estrogens with food or immediately after meals to reduce nausea.

• Warn that cigarette smoking increases the risk of side effects.

Interferons

One of the newer forms of biological response modifiers, interferons are being widely investigated for cancer

HOW DO INTERFERONS WORK?

How interferons destroy cancer cells isn't fully understood. One theory holds that interferons change the physical structure of cancer cells, strengthening and stiffening the cell membrane. In turn, the stronger cell membrane may inhibit tumor masses from forming and metastasizing throughout the body. Interferons may also inhibit the action of oncogenes—the normal human genes that, when activated in certain tumors, apparently contribute to the development of malignancies within cells.

It's also thought that interferons may strip away the cancer cell membranes, exposing the antigens. The weak antigens on the surface of cancer cells may go unnoticed by the immune system, so the cells continue to replicate. But when stronger interior antigens are exposed, the body may more easily identify them as foreign and develop antibodies to destroy them.

therapy. Currently two interferons, alfa-2a and alfa-2b, are commercially available, for treatment of hairy-cell leukemia. In clinical trials, the gamma interferons show promise in treating non-Hodgkin's lymphoma, renal cell carcinoma, multiple myeloma, chronic myelogenous leukemia, and Kaposi's sarcoma.

Interferons produce primarily mild side effects, such as flulike symptoms, that subside after 2 to 4 weeks of treatment. Uncommon effects of these drugs include bone marrow depression, hypotension, neurotoxicity, nausea, vomiting, and anorexia. Mild, transient hypertension and alopecia are also possible.

Because interferons have cardiotoxic potential, they should be administered cautiously to patients with heart disease.

Purpose and action

Interferons inhibit tumor growth possibly by a direct cytotoxic effect against the tumor cell or by altering the immune response. (See *How Do Interferons Work?*)

Monitoring

Make sure the patient realizes that interferon therapy is investigational before he gives his consent. If he doesn't clearly understand this, he may harbor unrealistic expectations about the drug's therapeutic capabilities.

Before therapy begins, establish white blood cell and platelet counts. Monitor these studies during therapy to detect leukopenia and thrombocytopenia, which, in interferon therapy, are seldom symptomatic.

During therapy, observe for hypotension by monitoring blood pressure before treatment and at 30-minute intervals during initial therapy. Reduce the risk of hypotension by providing adequate hydration. Also be alert for chest pain or an irregular heartbeat, which may indicate cardiotoxicity, especially in an elderly patient. Report these symptoms immediately.

Observe for fatigue, depression, insomnia, reduced attention span, and memory deficits, which may indicate neurotoxicity. Treat headache, fever, and chills with acetaminophen. However, if the patient has persistent headaches, notify the doctor; he may need to reduce the dosage.

Home care instructions

• Since many patients receive interferon at home, teach the patient to perform self-injection. If he'll be using undiluted interferon, show him how to reconstitute the drug.

• Help the patient design a medication schedule so that he can record daily injections and any side effects. These notes will help the doctor monitor for toxicity.

• Tell the patient he'll need periodic blood tests during treatment. Discuss the signs of myelosuppression and have him report their occurrence.

• Advise the patient to avoid alcohol because of its CNS-depressant effects.

• Instruct the patient to notify his doctor if he misses a drug dose. Warn him against routinely increasing the next dose.

RADIOTHERAPY

Radiation Treatments

About half of all cancer patients require radiation treatments to destroy neoplastic cells or curtail their growth. In curative applications, radiation is commonly used preoperatively to shrink a tumor, thus allowing total excision, and postoperatively to eradicate any neoplastic cells that may have gone undetected during surgery. In other curative applications, preliminary surgery may be performed to provide access for radiation treatment and chemotherapy. Radiation treatments can also be used to relieve cancer pain and enhance the patient's quality of life when hope for a cure no longer exists.

Radiation can be delivered by an external source or administered internally (see *Understanding Types of Radiation*). Because radiation doesn't distinguish between malignant and normal cells, healthy cells can experience damaging effects. These effects are generally related to the radiation dosage, the number of treatments, the type of body tissue, and the area of the body treated. For example, in the GI tract and bone marrow, where cells divide rapidly, side effects may develop quickly. In endothelial and connective tissue, where cells divide slowly, side effects may only occur several months after cessation of therapy.

Purpose

Radiation deters the proliferation of malignant cells by decreasing the rate of mitosis or impairing the synthesis of DNA and RNA.

Preparation

Since the patient may misinterpret radiation therapy as terminal care, be

UNDERSTANDING TYPES OF RADIATION

Radiation may be delivered externally or internally, depending on the patient's condition and medical history, the location and size of the tumor, its type and radiosensitivity, the presence of metastases, and the expected outcome.

External radiation
The most common form of radiation, external radiation is delivered via *X-rays* that emit a beam of electrons into the target area. The dosage and rate are based on the desired outcome—for example, treatment of the tumor and metastasis or treatment of just the tumor.

Another form uses a stream of *gamma rays* to deliver radiation. The most common source of gamma rays is cobalt 60, but radium and cesium 127 are used as well. When this form is used, the dosage, rate, and penetration depth are predetermined by the radiation source.

The machines used for external radiation are classified by their energy-producing capabilities. Adapted from diagnostic X-ray machines, the *orthovoltage machine* produces 100,000 to 500,000 volts of energy. Once the predominant device for delivering radiation, this machine is seldom used today because it doesn't penetrate deeper tissue. Instead, it deposits the maximum radiation dose on the skin and in the subcutaneous tissue.

Today, the mainstay of radiation therapy is the *megavoltage or supervoltage machine*. It produces energy of 1 million or more volts, thus improving the penetrating ability of the radiation beam. With this machine, the maximum dose penetrates deeper tissue with minimal skin damage. Two types of machines are used: units containing cobalt or cesium as radioactive sources for gamma rays and linear accelerators that use electricity to produce X-rays. Linear accelerators are capable of producing high energy with great penetrating ability. Some also produce electron beams with a shorter range of penetration. These are often used for superficial tumors.

Indications for external radiation include cancer of the lungs, head and neck, breast, abdomen, and pelvis; Hodgkin's disease; and superficial tumors.

Internal radiation
Internal radiation is delivered locally or systemically. If delivered locally, it places radioactive substances permanently or temporarily into tissues surrounding the tumor or into the tumor itself, using the *interstitial* approach. Or it may involve delivery of radioactive substances into a hollow body cavity, using the *intracavitary* approach. For the interstitial approach, radioactive sources (radium, radon, iridium, cesium, cobalt, or iodine 125) are sealed in applicators, such as needles, beads, seeds, or ribbons, and implanted directly in the tissues. Radioactive sources may also be implanted in previously inserted applicators in interstitial tissue or body cavities. Unsealed sources, such as radioactive phosphorus or gold 198, are used for intracavitary applications.

Indications for interstitial implantation include cancer of the buccal mucosa, head, tongue, neck, and chest. This approach may also be used for cancer of the prostate, uterus, and cervix. Intracavitary applications treat metastatic breast and bone cancer; malignant pleural effusions; cancer of the bladder, head and neck, and prostate; and cervical and uterine cancer.

Internal radiation can be delivered systemically, using radioactive materials in solutions or colloidal suspensions that are given orally, intravenously, or by instillation. Systemic applications are used for primary and metastatic thyroid carcinoma, chronic myelocytic leukemia, and chronic lymphocytic leukemia.

sure to stress its purpose. Point out the potentially curative effects of radiation and its ability to improve the patient's quality of life. Before treatment begins, explain the type of therapy to be performed. Take the patient on a tour of the radiation facilities and encourage him to ask questions.

Obtain baseline white blood cell (WBC) and platelet counts. Also obtain a thorough patient history, including any previous radiation treatments and side effects. Because radiation therapy can reduce the production of sperm, tell the male patient about sperm banking if he intends to start a family later on. Tell the female patient undergoing pelvic irradiation that this treatment can decrease hormone levels, which may lead to infertility and amenorrhea.

If the patient will be receiving external radiation, tell him that the radiation therapist may mark the exact areas of treatment on his skin with a pen or dye. Instruct the patient not to remove these markings until after the completion of therapy.

If the patient will be receiving internal radiation, explain the need for temporary isolation after implantation. If the patient will be immobilized during internal radiation owing to the lo-

MANAGING SIDE EFFECTS OF RADIATION THERAPY

Radiation therapy can cause both local and systemic effects. Local effects, such as headaches from cranial tissue irradiation and erythema, are discussed in the chart below. Systemic effects, which are similar for both radiation therapy and chemotherapy, are discussed in *Managing Common Side Effects of Chemotherapy,* pages 460 and 461. These effects include GI upset, stomatitis, alopecia, and bone marrow depression.

SIDE EFFECT	NURSING CONSIDERATIONS
Headaches, caused by cerebral edema	• Assess for pain. Administer corticosteroids or analgesics, as ordered.
Pneumonitis, pericarditis, or myocarditis caused by irradiation of lung or heart areas	• Auscultate the patient's heart and lungs daily. Monitor his vital signs, as ordered. • Watch for and report coughing, dyspnea, weakness, or pain on inspiration.
Mucositis, pharyngitis, decreased salivation and taste sensation (caused by irradiation of the head and neck area)	• Inspect the oral cavity and evaluate the patient's nutritional status. Tell him to maintain optimal nutrition, emphasizing protein and carbohydrates. • Administer analgesics, such as lidocaine solution or ointment, before meals. • Tell the patient to avoid dry or thick foods, to use artificial saliva, and to drink plenty of fluids with meals. • Instruct the patient to rinse his mouth before meals with equal parts of hydrogen peroxide and water to prevent accumulation of debris and to improve his appetite. • Suggest use of sugarless lemon drops or mints to increase salivation.
Erythema	• Observe reddened areas daily and record any changes. Keep the skin dry and exposed to air.
Desquamation	• If dead surface cells peel off, apply cornstarch to prevent pruritus and irritation from clothing and bed linens. • If desquamation is moist, apply lanolin to relieve dryness and pruritus, if ordered. Use dressings (nonadherent pads, gauze, and nonallergenic tape) to absorb drainage and prevent irritation from clothing. Keep the skin exposed whenever possible.
Epilation (usually temporary but may be permanent with high doses of radiation)	• If hair loss occurs in the treatment area, be supportive and encourage the use of cosmetic replacements, such as false eyelashes.
Sweat gland destruction	• To maintain skin integrity, instruct the patient to avoid exposure to intense sunlight, wind, or cold. • Apply emollient-based lotions. • Observe for ulceration, telangiectasia, and poor healing after trauma.

cation of applicators, such as needles, be sure to explain this. Assess for possible problems in positioning, range of motion, and comfort. Prepare the patient for a temporary change in appearance if the implant's placed in a visible area, such as the neck or breast.

Finally, make sure the patient or a responsible family member has signed a consent form.

Procedure

For external radiation, the patient lies immobile on a treatment table in the X-ray department while a large machine, usually overhead, directs radiation at the target site for the prescribed period. Afterward, the patient can return to his room or go home.

For internal radiation, the patient may be taken to the operating room—or the procedure may be performed in his room. If he's having an interstitial application, the doctor may place special radioactive needles or guides within the tumor mass. Or the doctor may surgically place radioactive gold grains into cancerous tissue.

If the patient is having intracavitary radiation, the doctor places the radioactive source in a special apparatus (such as a nasogastric tube) and inserts it into a body cavity near the tumor. The patient may also have a type of internal radiation involving I.V. or oral administration of a radioactive solution or suspension. Or he may undergo intracavitary instillation of a suspension, usually by paracentesis or thoracentesis. This suspension is distributed by rotating the patient every 15 minutes for 2 or 3 hours while he lies on a flat surface.

Monitoring and aftercare

Monitor the patient's WBC and platelet counts to help evaluate myelosuppressive effects. Also monitor for other common side effects of radiation treatment, such as erythema and nausea and vomiting. (See *Managing Side Effects of Radiation Therapy* for details.)

If the patient has had internal radiation, take precautions against radioactive contamination. Be sure to spend no more time than necessary with the patient. And when you're in his room, stay as far away from him as possible. (If you're pregnant, don't go into his room at all. Ask your supervisor to assign another nurse to the patient.) If your hospital provides radiation badges, be sure to wear one.

Home care instructions

● Explain that the full benefit of radiation treatment may not occur for up to several months. Instruct the patient to report any long-term side effects.
● Stress the importance of keeping appointments with the doctor.
● Refer the patient to a support group, such as a local chapter of the American Cancer Society.

Selected References

Clinical Oncology: A Multidisciplinary Approach, 6th ed. American Cancer Society, 1983.

DeVita, Vincent, et al. *Principles and Practice of Oncology*, 2nd ed. Philadelphia: J.B. Lippincott Co., 1985.

Groenwald, S.L. *Cancer Nursing: Principles and Practice*. Boston: Jones & Bartlett, 1987.

Krachoff, Irvin A. "Cancer Chemotherapy—March/April 1987," in *Cancer: A Journal for Clinicians*. American Cancer Society, 1987.

Nursing88 Drug Handbook. Springhouse, Pa.: Springhouse Corp., 1988.

Yasko, Joyce M. *Nursing Management of Symptoms Associated with Chemotherapy*. Adria Laboratories, 1986.

14

Treating Infection

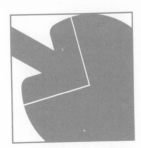

Treating Infection

Introduction

Infections. Because they're so prevalent, they may sometimes seem like a tiresome topic. After all, despite the development of new penicillins and cephalosporins, treatment protocols for most infections remain the same. However, there's much you can do to improve the chances of treatment's success. For example, by rigorously following infection control policies, you can help prevent an infection from worsening—and from causing contagion. What's more, you can help speed a patient's recovery and guard against complications through timely collection of culture specimens and careful monitoring of his drug regimen.

Providing a healthful environment

Within the hospital, the risk of nosocomial infection always remains great. Urinary catheters and I.V.s, for example, provide portals for pathogens to enter the body. And any surgical procedure always carries the risk of infection.

Fortunately, though, you can reduce the risk of nosocomial infection. Hand washing, for instance, is the single most important measure you can take to prevent contagion. Other measures include isolation procedures, proper sterilization of equipment, and the use of disinfectants and antiseptics.

Advice about antibiotic therapy

Before giving antibiotics, you'll need to ensure timely collection of specimens for culture and sensitivity studies. (These specimens have no value *after* therapy begins.) Choice of antibiotic depends on these studies, which are especially important in gram-negative infections because of the high incidence of drug-resistant organisms. You'll also need to obtain an accurate history, including the patient's weight and height, current drug use, previous adverse effects, and hepatorenal status.

Although most patients respond well to antibiotic therapy, you'll need to be alert for side effects, such as hypersensitivity. Most common with penicillins, hypersensitivity may show itself as a slight rash or as life-threatening anaphylaxis occurring within minutes of administration. Serum sickness, another severe effect, may occur a week or more after therapy begins.

Monitoring recovery

You'll usually be responsible for monitoring the patient's progress. In local infection, expect to see decreased redness, edema, and heat or pain, usually within 48 hours. In systemic infection, look for decreased fever and white blood cell count. And, in respiratory infection, anticipate decreased dyspnea, coughing, and secretions.

DRUG THERAPY

Penicillins

Because of their effectiveness, low incidence of toxicity, and minimal cost, penicillins are one of the most widely used antimicrobial classes. This class consists of extracts from several strains of *Penicillium* mold and semisynthetic derivatives. Penicillin derivatives differ in their spectrum of antimicrobial activity, gastric acid stability, degree of protein binding, and resistance to inactivation by penicillinase.

Penicillins effectively treat bacterial infections, such as streptococcal pharyngitis, pneumococcal pneumonia, gas gangrene, gonorrhea, syphilis, tetanus, and cellulitis. (See *Comparing Penicillins*.) They're also used prophylacti-

COMPARING DRUGS

COMPARING PENICILLINS

DRUG AND ROUTE	MAJOR INDICATIONS	SPECIAL CONSIDERATIONS
Natural penicillins		
penicillin G benzathine P.O. **penicillin G potassium** I.V., I.M., P.O. **penicillin G procaine** I.M. **penicillin G sodium** I.V., I.M. **penicillin V** P.O.	Infections caused by various organisms, including gram-negative bacteria and clostridia; meningococcal meningitis	• Contraindicated in patients with a history of severe hypersensitivity reactions. Use cautiously in patients with allergies, colitis (penicillins can cause pseudomembranous colitis), or renal impairment. • Notify the doctor if a hypersensitivity reaction develops. • Expect false-positive reactions on copper sulfate urine glucose tests. • Oral form can cause nausea, vomiting, and diarrhea. Tell the patient to take it on an empty stomach. He should avoid taking it with fruit juice, because acidic fluids inactivate the drug.
Aminopenicillins		
amoxicillin P.O. **ampicillin** I.V., I.M., P.O. **bacampicillin** P.O. **cyclacillin** P.O.	Infections caused by gram-positive and gram-negative bacteria (*H. influenzae, Proteus mirabilis, Salmonella, Shigella,* and most strains of *E. coli*); especially useful in treating urinary tract infections	• Contraindicated in patients with a history of severe hypersensitivity reactions. Use cautiously in patients with allergies, colitis, infectious mononucleosis, or renal impairment. • Report any hypersensitivity reaction. • Oral form can cause GI upset. Tell the patient to take drug on an empty stomach. • Expect false-positive reactions on copper sulfate urine glucose tests. • Reassure the patient that the darkened tongue this drug can cause is harmless. • Concurrent use of allopurinol increases the incidence of rashes. Probenecid raises blood levels of ampicillin and amoxicillin.

cally before dental surgery or other invasive procedures in patients with a history of streptococcal rheumatic fever or bacterial endocarditis.

Choice of a specific penicillin can be complicated since a previously susceptible organism sometimes develops resistance. For example, staphylococci have become resistant to penicillin G even though other bacteria, such as streptococci, remain susceptible to it.

Hypersensitivity, the major side effect, occurs with both natural extracts and derivatives and most commonly af-

fects patients with asthma or a history of allergies. This reaction ranges in severity from a rash and pruritus to serum sickness and anaphylaxis.

Penicillins are contraindicated in any patient with a previous anaphylactic response to penicillin or a cephalosporin (possible cross-allergenicity). Unfortunately, a negative history doesn't rule out a future allergy.

Purpose and action

• To combat bacterial infection by interfering with the reproduction of mi-

DRUG AND ROUTE	MAJOR INDICATIONS	SPECIAL CONSIDERATIONS
Penicillinase-resistant penicillins		
cloxacillin P.O. **dicloxacillin** P.O. **methicillin** I.V., I.M. **nafcillin** I.V., I.M., P.O. **oxacillin** I.V., I.M., P.O.	Systemic infections caused by penicillinase-producing staphylococci	• Contraindicated in patients with a history of severe hypersensitivity reactions. Use cautiously in patients with allergies or colitis. • Notify the doctor if a hypersensitivity reaction develops. • Give oral form of the drug on an empty stomach. • If you're giving oxacillin, monitor hepatic enzyme levels. If you're giving methicillin, monitor renal function. • Probenecid increases penicillin blood levels. It's often used for this purpose.
Extended-spectrum penicillins		
azlocillin I.V. **carbenicillin disodium** I.V., I.M. **carbenicillin indanyl sodium** P.O. **mezlocillin** I.V., I.M. **piperacillin** I.V., I.M. **ticarcillin** I.V., I.M.	Systemic infections caused by gram-positive and gram-negative organisms (*Pseudomonas* and some strains of *Proteus* and *Enterobacter* are resistant to ampicillin.)	• Contraindicated in patients with a history of severe hypersensitivity reactions. Use cautiously in patients with allergies or colitis, or on sodium-restricted diets. • Reduce dosage for patients with renal impairment to prevent nephrotoxicity. • Monitor intake and output. • Monitor complete blood count since these drugs may cause thrombocytopenia. • Contact the doctor if a hypersensitivity reaction develops. • Carbenicillin disodium contains large amounts of sodium. Monitor serum potassium levels, which may fall because of increased sodium. • Give carbenicillin indanyl sodium on an empty stomach to prevent GI upset and promote absorption.

crobial enzymes, causing lysis and cell death. Although usually bactericidal, penicillins exert a bacteriostatic effect in inadequate concentrations.
• To provide prophylaxis before invasive procedures.

Monitoring
Always keep epinephrine and other emergency resuscitation supplies available when giving penicillins. Watch for signs of hypersensitivity, such as rash or pruritus, which may develop within 20 minutes (or sometimes only after several days). Be especially alert for signs of anaphylaxis, such as dyspnea, choking, fulminating hypotension, thready pulse, anxiety, weakness, sweating, and dizziness. If the patient develops these signs, notify the doctor immediately. Check the patient's blood pressure regularly and prepare to give I.V. fluids for hypotension.

Besides monitoring the patient for hypersensitivity, you'll need to review his medication regimen for possible interactions. Concurrent use of antacids reduces penicillin's effectiveness by decreasing its absorption from the GI tract. Erythromycins and tetracyclines also reduce its effectiveness. Acidifying drugs, such as ammonium chloride, and acidic foods reduce oral penicillin's effectiveness. In contrast, aspirin and phenylbutazone raise serum levels of penicillin by reducing plasma protein binding. Probenecid, too, raises serum penicillin levels. In fact, it's commonly used for this purpose.

If the patient receives penicillin for a prolonged period, observe for superinfection. This occurs most commonly in elderly, debilitated, or immunosuppressed patients.

Home care instructions
• Instruct the patient to call the doctor if he experiences a rash, hives, itching, or wheezing. If he's had a severe penicillin reaction, stress the importance of wearing a Medic Alert bracelet or necklace. If he carries an anaphylaxis kit, review the instructions with him.

• Emphasize the importance of completing the full course of penicillin, even if he feels better. Explain that residual organisms can cause a relapse.
• If the patient misses a dose, instruct him to take it as soon as possible. Then he should space the remaining daily doses closer together to make up for the missed dose. Penicillins are most effective if a constant serum concentration is maintained.
• Tell the patient to avoid orange juice, other acidic juices, and vitamin C supplements while taking oral penicillin; they reduce the drug's effectiveness.
• If diarrhea occurs, tell the patient to check with his doctor or pharmacist before taking his medication. Antiperistaltic antidiarrheals aren't recommended because they can delay elimination of toxins.
• Tell the patient to call his doctor if symptoms don't improve within a few days.

Cephalosporins

Chemically related to penicillin, cephalosporins are a group of semisynthetic broad-spectrum antibiotics. Although effective against gram-positive bacteria, they're most important for their role in treating gram-negative infection. Specifically, they combat infections of the skin, soft tissues, bones, joints, and urinary and respiratory tracts caused by staphylococci, streptococci, *E. coli*, *Proteus mirabilis*, and *Shigella*. They may also be used prophylactically before cardiac, orthopedic, gynecologic, or bowel surgery.

Differences among individual cephalosporins relate to their bacterial sensitivity, duration of action, and routes of administration and excretion. The first-generation cephalosporins include such drugs as *cefadroxil* and *cefazolin*. The second-generation drugs, such as *cefamandole* and *cefoxitin*, have expanded antibacterial activity

HOW CEPHALOSPORINS ATTACK BACTERIA

The antibacterial action of cephalosporins depends on their ability to penetrate the bacterial cell wall and bind with proteins in the cytoplasmic membrane. Once the drug damages the cell wall, the body's natural defense mechanisms destroy the bacteria.

To understand how cephalosporins work, you'll need to understand the structure of a bacterial cell. Outside the *cytoplasmic membrane* lies a chemically complex, rigid cell wall that protects the cell against osmotic pressure and the outside environment. This cell wall contains a *mucocomplex layer*, which forms a sac around the bacterium. Acting as a filter, this layer prevents large molecules from passing through it. Gram-positive bacteria have a thick mucocomplex layer extending from the cytoplasmic membrane to the *teichoic acid layer* that coats the cell's exterior. In contrast, the mucocomplex layer in gram-negative cells is thin and supported by a complex outer cell wall composed of polysaccharides, lipids, and proteins. The gram-negative cell also contains *periplasmic space*, which lies between the cytoplasmic membrane and the cell wall.

Both gram-positive and gram-negative bacterial cell walls contain chemically similar *peptidoglycans,* which are necessary for cell wall strength and rigidity. Cephalosporins inhibit the synthesis of these walls apparently by interfering with enzymatic action and preventing cross-linkage of these peptidoglycan chains.

BACTERIAL CELL

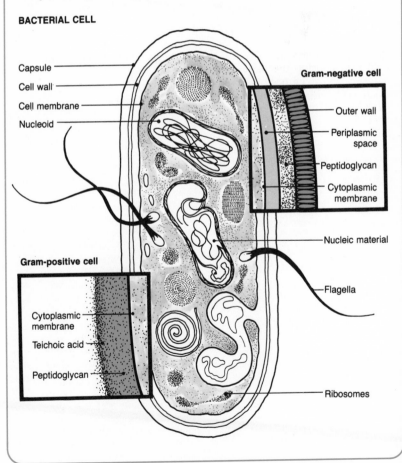

Capsule
Cell wall
Cell membrane
Nucleoid

Gram-negative cell
Outer wall
Periplasmic space
Peptidoglycan
Cytoplasmic membrane

Nucleic material

Gram-positive cell

Cytoplasmic membrane
Teichoic acid
Peptidoglycan

Flagella

Ribosomes

against some gram-negative organisms, such as *Bacteroides fragilis*, which is resistant to other antibiotics. Third-generation drugs, such as *cefotaxime, ceftazidime,* and *moxalactam,* further expand the spectrum of antibacterial activity. This generation proves effective against *Pseudomonas aeruginosa,* an organism resistant to all other cephalosporins.

INQUIRY

QUESTIONS PATIENTS ASK ABOUT CEPHALOSPORINS

I'm allergic to penicillin. Is it safe for me to take Keflex?

Usually, Keflex and similar cephalosporin drugs are safe for most people who are allergic to penicillin. But some of these people may also be allergic to Keflex. So watch for signs of a Keflex allergy: itching, redness, or hives. If you notice any of these signs, call your doctor and don't take any additional doses.

I've had diarrhea and vaginal itching since I've been taking Keflex. Should I stop taking it?

No. You're getting these symptoms because Keflex disrupts the normal bacteria in your intestinal tract and vaginal lining. You can relieve them by including 8 ounces of yogurt or buttermilk in your daily diet.

Since I've been taking Keflex, I've been testing positive for glucose in my urine. Do I need more insulin?

You probably don't need more insulin, but you may have to change the type of urine test you're using. If you're using Clinitest tablets, you're getting unreliable results because Keflex chemically interferes with the test. Ask your doctor if you should use a glucose oxidase reagent, such as Clinistix or Tes-Tape, as an alternative. Keflex won't affect them.

The third-generation drugs also penetrate cerebrospinal fluid.

Cephalosporins are contraindicated in patients with a previous anaphylactic reaction to cephalosporins or penicillins (possible cross-allergenicity). They shouldn't be used concurrently with other nephrotoxic drugs. In patients with renal impairment, they should be used cautiously.

Purpose and action

• To treat infection caused by gram-negative and, to a lesser extent, gram-positive organisms by interfering with the final stage of bacterial cell wall formation, resulting in unstable cell membranes. Eventually, autolysis causes cell death. (See *How Cephalosporins Attack Bacteria,* page 485.)

• To provide prophylaxis before surgery.

Monitoring

Be alert for signs of cephalosporin hypersensitivity. Similar to penicillin hypersensitivity, it's characterized by a maculopapular rash with possible fever, lymphadenopathy, urticaria, and eosinophilia. Also be alert for signs of pseudomembranous colitis (copious watery or bloody diarrhea, abdominal pain, and fever). If such signs occur, stop the drug and give fluid, electrolyte, and protein replacements.

If you're giving a cephalosporin I.V., infuse it over at least 30 minutes; overly rapid infusion causes pain, vein irritation, and phlebitis. If you're giving it I.M., apply ice packs to the site before and after injection. If you're giving it orally, watch for nausea, vomiting, or diarrhea; to relieve these, give the drug with food. Some experts believe that regular intake of yogurt or buttermilk can prevent these GI effects by replenishing normal flora in the digestive tract.

Check for signs of superinfection, a common complication of oral administration marked by diarrhea, vaginal itching, or sore mouth. Also monitor prothrombin time because some cephalosporins, such as moxalactam, can cause hypoprothrombinemia.

If your patient's undergoing dialysis, administer cephalosporins *after* a treatment to prevent reduced drug effectiveness. If he's receiving probenecid, expect increased cephalosporin blood levels. Notify the doctor.

Home care instructions

• Instruct the patient to immediately report signs of an allergic reaction (rash, hives, and possibly fever) or decreased urine output to his doctor.

• Tell him to take oral cephalosporins on an empty stomach unless they cause GI upset. Suggest that he have yogurt or buttermilk with a meal to help replace normal GI flora.

• Advise the patient to avoid alcohol. Some cephalosporins interact with it, causing flushing, nausea, and palpitations.

Aminoglycosides

These broad-spectrum antibiotics are used primarily to treat severe gram-negative infections caused by *Pseudomonas*, *E. coli*, *Proteus*, *Klebsiella*, and *Enterobacter*. Because the aminoglycosides can cause ototoxicity and nephrotoxicity at therapeutic levels, their systemic use is characteristically reserved for infections that are unresponsive to less toxic drugs.

The aminoglycosides are given intramuscularly or intravenously for severe urinary tract, bone, joint, and pleural infections. They can be given intrathecally for CNS infections. What's more, they can be applied topically or nebulized and given by inhalation.

The aminoglycosides include amikacin, gentamicin, neomycin, kanamycin, netilmicin, streptomycin, and tobramycin. *Amikacin*, a semisynthetic derivative, combats urinary tract infections resistant to other aminoglycosides. *Gentamicin* is the drug of choice for gram-negative sepsis. Given intrathecally for meningitis, it's also used with carbenicillin for severe *Pseudomonas aeruginosa* infections. *Neomycin*, the most toxic aminoglycoside, can be given orally for profuse diarrhea caused by *E. coli*, for preoperative bowel antisepsis, and for urinary tract infections. Topically, it's used in eye, ear, and skin infections. However, because of its potential toxicity, it isn't used parenterally. Closely resembling neomycin, *kanamycin* effectively combats many gram-negative infections. It's used for intestinal infections, for preoperative bowel antisepsis, and for intraperitoneal and wound irrigation. It may be given as an aerosol for respiratory infections. Another semisynthetic derivative, *netilmicin* is used parenterally in severe staphylococcal and gram-negative infections. *Streptomycin*, a primary treatment for tuberculosis, may be administered with other antituberculars, although the emergence of resistant organisms has diminished its efficacy. It's also used to treat bacterial endocarditis (resulting from *H. influenzae*), tularemia, bubonic plague, and cholera. Closely related to gentamicin but causing less nephrotoxicity, *tobramycin* treats meningitis and neonatal sepsis. It may also be used with carbenicillin to combat *Pseudomonas*.

Although oral aminoglycosides are used for preoperative bowel sterilization, they shouldn't be given to patients with intestinal obstructions. Also, aminoglycosides shouldn't be used with other ototoxic, neurotoxic, or nephrotoxic drugs, general anesthetics, muscle relaxants, or diuretics.

Purpose and action

To treat severe gram-negative infections caused by susceptible organisms. Aminoglycosides act directly on the ribosomes of pathogens: by binding directly to the 30S ribosomal subunit, they inhibit protein synthesis. They're bactericidal in high concentrations and bacteriostatic in low concentrations.

COMPLICATIONS

GUARDING AGAINST AMINOGLYCOSIDE TOXICITY

Because aminoglycosides can seriously damage auditory and renal function, you'll need to take precautions before, during, and after therapy. And, if the patient's taking a muscle relaxant, you'll need to promptly recognize any neurotoxic effects.
Be especially alert for aminoglycoside toxicity when treatment lasts longer than 7 days.

BEFORE THERAPY

• Assess the patient's renal function. Check urinalysis findings, blood urea nitrogen (BUN) and serum creatinine levels, and creatinine clearance.
• Evaluate the patient's hearing, using the results from audiometric tests.
• Before and during therapy, keep the patient well hydrated to avoid renal irritation.

DURING THERAPY

• Keep in mind that ototoxicity can occur even with therapeutic aminoglycoside levels. Notify the doctor if the patient complains of tinnitus or vertigo. This indicates vestibular injury, which occurs most commonly with gentamicin and streptomycin. Also notify him if you suspect a hearing loss or if audiometric tests reveal a high-frequency loss; this occurs most commonly with kanamycin and neomycin. If the pa-

tient develops ototoxic effects, the doctor will probably discontinue the drug.
• Be alert for early signs of nephrotoxicity, such as decreased urine output. Supporting laboratory findings include casts, albumin, or red or white blood cells in the urine; changes in creatinine clearance (decreased or increased); and elevated BUN levels. Report any of these changes immediately. They signal a need for dosage reduction or drug discontinuation.
• If the patient's taking a muscle relaxant, monitor for signs of neurotoxicity, such as apnea or depressed respirations. Stop the drug and contact the doctor immediately if any of these signs occur.

AFTER THERAPY

Continue to monitor auditory and vestibular function for 4 weeks after stopping the drug; the onset of hearing loss may be delayed.

Monitoring

To ensure adequate blood levels and avoid toxicity, monitor serum aminoglycoside levels frequently. Draw trough levels just before giving a dose and peak levels 30 to 60 minutes after giving it.

Recognize that prolonged administration of aminoglycosides can cause ototoxicity and nephrotoxicity. (See *Guarding Against Aminoglycoside Toxicity*.) Be alert for other side effects: optic neuritis, blurred vision, joint pain, nausea, and rash. Also watch for signs of superinfection.

Is the patient also taking ethacrynic acid or furosemide? They increase the risk of ototoxicity. And keep in mind that aminoglycosides act synergistically with antipseudomonal penicillins.

Home care instructions

• Stress the importance of immediately reporting ototoxic or nephrotoxic signs.
• If not contraindicated, encourage the patient to drink plenty of fluids to reduce the risk of nephrotoxicity.

Erythromycins

Effective against more gram-positive organisms than gram-negative ones, erythromycins treat mild to severe streptococcal infections, especially if penicillin is contraindicated. They're also used in diphtheria, pneumonia caused by *Mycoplasma pneumoniae*, and Legionnaire's disease. Prophylactically, these antibiotics are used for pertussis and rheumatic fever. In neonates, the ophthalmic form prevents conjunctivitis caused by *Chlamydia trachomatis* and gonococcal ophthalmia. The topical form effectively treats acne and superficial skin infections.

Erythromycins should be avoided in patients with hepatic impairment and used cautiously in those with biliary disease. Because they're irritating to the tissues, they shouldn't be given rectally or intramuscularly.

Purpose and action
• To treat and prevent susceptible gram-positive and gram-negative infections. Erythromycins inhibit bacterial protein synthesis by binding to the 50S ribosomal subunit. They're bacteriostatic.
• To provide prophylaxis against pertussis and rheumatic fever.

Monitoring
When giving erythromycin intravenously, dilute it in at least 100 ml of fluid and administer it over 15 to 20 minutes to reduce the risk of phlebitis.

If the patient's receiving erythromycin orally, ask him to report any nausea or abdominal pain. If stomatitis or perianal irritation occurs, provide frequent topical care.

If the patient's receiving erythromycin estolate in high doses or for a prolonged period, you'll need to monitor liver function tests to detect any hepatotoxic effects.

Home care instructions
• Is the patient allergic to penicillin? If so, instruct him to watch for signs of hypersensitivity to erythromycin.
• Tell him to complete the full course of therapy even if symptoms disappear.
• Advise him to take the drug on an empty stomach with a full glass of water. However, he can take enteric-coated erythromycin on an empty stomach or with meals.
• If he misses a dose, tell him to take it as soon as possible and to take the day's remaining doses closer together.

• Advise him to contact his doctor if he experiences nausea, vomiting, fever, jaundice, abdominal cramps, or diarrhea; all occur commonly.

Tetracyclines

Used for severe infections that prove resistant to other antibiotics, tetracyclines treat infections caused by sensitive gram-positive and gram-negative organisms, *Rickettsia* (Rocky Mountain spotted fever, Q fever), mycoplasmal pneumonia, and *Chlamydia* (lymphogranuloma venereum, psittacosis, trachoma). However, because of widespread microbial resistance (by *Proteus* and *Pseudomonas*, for example), tetracyclines serve as the drugs of choice in relatively few situations.

The tetracycline family includes the drugs demeclocycline, doxycycline, minocycline, oxytetracycline, and tetracycline hydrochloride. *Demeclocycline* treats gonorrhea and infections caused by gram-negative and gram-positive organisms, rickettsiae, and *Chlamydia*. *Doxycycline*, which can be used safely in renal impairment, treats infections caused by gram-positive and gram-negative organisms, *Rickettsia*, *Mycoplasma*, and *Chlamydia*. *Minocycline* proves effective for asymptomatic carriers of *Neisseria meningitidis* (but it's not recommended for meningococcal infections), gonorrhea, syphilis, or chlamydial infections. A naturally derived tetracycline, *oxytetracycline* treats urinary tract infections. As a substitute for penicillin, it may be used in brucellosis, syphilis, and gonorrhea. *Tetracycline hydrochloride*, the most widely used and least expensive tetracycline, is commonly used for acne, gonorrhea, syphilis, and chlamydial infections. This drug is available as an ophthalmic and topical preparation.

These drugs should be avoided in patients with renal impairment since they

INTERACTIONS

PREVENTING TETRACYCLINE MALABSORPTION

If your patient experiences GI upset during tetracycline therapy, his natural inclination might be to drink a glass of milk. Or he might take some stomach-soothing product, such as an antacid.

Unfortunately, taking milk or an antacid with tetracyclines significantly reduces blood levels of these drugs. The calcium, magnesium, or aluminum in these products forms insoluble tetracycline complexes that are poorly absorbed by the body.

What should your patient do to ward off his GI upset while still promoting proper drug absorption? He can take each dose with a full glass of water on an empty stomach. And you can review his diet for foods or drugs that interfere with tetracycline absorption:

• calcium-containing foods, such as cheese and ice cream
• calcium supplements
• antacids that contain calcium, magnesium, or aluminum
• iron preparations, such as vitamins containing iron
• other products that contain magnesium, including sodium bicarbonate and Milk of Magnesia
• colestipol, which blocks absorption of tetracyclines.

Advise the patient to take any of these products at least 1 hour before or 2 hours after taking tetracycline.

Monitoring

Watch for overgrowth of nonsusceptible organisms, evidenced by mycotic infections of the mouth, throat, and vagina. The patient may experience a sore mouth, black hairy tongue, oral thrush, and itching in the rectal and perineal areas. To help relieve these symptoms, provide meticulous skin care in the affected areas two to three times daily.

If the patient has diarrhea, you'll need to carefully evaluate it to rule out enteritis resulting from superinfection; this can be life-threatening and usually requires stopping the drug.

If the patient's receiving a tetracycline I.V., infuse it slowly in a well-diluted solution. With long-term administration, monitor complete blood counts and blood urea nitrogen levels for evidence of blood dyscrasias. Watch for signs of diabetes insipidus, such as polyuria and polydipsia.

Oral tetracyclines irritate the GI mucosa, causing nausea, vomiting, and flatulence. Giving the drug with water minimizes gastric irritation. If the patient still reports discomfort, give the drug with a light snack, such as crackers, although absorption may be slightly reduced. Or the doctor may lower the dose and increase the frequency of administration.

Avoid giving oral tetracyclines close together with dairy products, antacids, or laxatives. (See *Preventing Tetracycline Malabsorption*.) If oral tetracycline and an iron preparation are ordered, space doses as far apart as possible, because iron combines with tetracyclines (as do other metallic ions) to inhibit absorption.

Home care instructions

• Instruct the patient to take tetracycline at least 1 hour before or 2 hours after ingesting dairy products, antacids, or laxatives. To prevent GI upset, advise taking it with a glass of water.
• Warn him to avoid intense or prolonged exposure to sunlight. If exposure is unavoidable, advise him to wear protective clothing and use a sunscreen

increase tissue breakdown and, therefore, waste products in the blood. They're also contraindicated during pregnancy because they may permanently discolor the teeth of the fetus. In children under age 8, they may cause permanent tooth discoloration, enamel defects, and impeded bone growth.

Because tetracyclines irritate the tissues, they're rarely given by I.M. injection.

Purpose and action

To treat infection caused by susceptible organisms by binding to the 30S ribosomal subunit, thereby inhibiting protein synthesis and cell multiplication.

to prevent photosensitivity.
• Explain to the patient that his stools may be looser than usual during therapy. However, emphasize that he should report diarrhea and abdominal cramps immediately.

Sulfonamides

Developed in the mid-1930s, sulfonamides were the first systemic antibacterial drugs used in people. They're effective against both gram-positive and gram-negative organisms, and although increased microbial resistance has since limited their usefulness, they're still the drugs of choice for treating urinary tract infections. For other conditions, such as trachoma and toxoplasmosis, they're used as secondary drugs.

Short-acting systemic sulfonamides, such as *sulfisoxazole*, are quickly absorbed and rapidly eliminated. In contrast, intermediate-acting drugs, such as *sulfamethoxazole*, are absorbed and excreted more slowly.

Systemic sulfonamides are usually given orally, since they can precipitate out of I.V. solutions and irritate tissues. Topical sulfonamides prevent burn infections and treat ocular, vaginal, and other soft-tissue infections.

Sulfonamides should be avoided during late pregnancy and lactation and in premature infants and newborns. They easily cross the placenta and are excreted in breast milk, possibly causing kernicterus by displacing bilirubin from binding sites on albumin. The drugs should be used cautiously and the dosage reduced in patients with impaired renal or hepatic function, porphyria, intestinal or urinary obstruction, blood dyscrasias, allergies, or asthma.

Purpose and action
To treat infection caused by susceptible gram-positive and gram-negative organisms. Sulfonamides curb cell multiplication by inhibiting folic acid production.

Monitoring
Give the drug on an empty stomach. To prevent crystalluria, encourage the patient to drink plenty of fluids throughout therapy.

Be sure to test the patient's urine for excessive acidity before long-term administration of sulfonamides. If his urine pH is low, you'll need to administer sodium bicarbonate to ensure drug solubility.

Sulfonamides can cause blood dyscrasias and renal impairment, especially with prolonged therapy. Consequently, you'll need to monitor the patient's complete blood count, urinalysis, and intake and output. Also watch for signs of erythema multiforme; if they occur, discontinue the drug and notify the doctor.

Review the patient's medication regimen for possible interactions. For example, methenamine compounds, urinary acidifiers, and paraldehyde may cause precipitation of sulfonamides, leading to renal damage. Also watch for hypoglycemia (caused by pancreatic stimulation) and suppressed thyroid function.

Home care instructions
• Stress the need to complete the full course of therapy, even if symptoms disappear.
• Instruct the patient to watch for signs of blood dyscrasias, such as sore throat, fever, mucosal ulcers, or jaundice. If these signs occur, the patient should stop the drug and contact his doctor immediately.
• If appropriate, encourage the patient to drink at least 3 quarts of fluid daily to prevent formation of urine crystals. If necessary, have him record intake and output to monitor hydration.
• If the patient's using a topical sulfonamide, tell him to stop the drug if he notices local irritation or other allergic signs.

UNDERSTANDING OTHER IMPORTANT ANTI-INFECTIVES

Besides the drugs discussed on the preceding 10 pages, numerous other drugs help combat or prevent infections. This table highlights some of them: the important antiviral, antifungal, and antitubercular drugs.

DRUG AND MAJOR USES	MECHANISM OF ACTION	SIDE EFFECTS
acyclovir Treatment for severe genital herpes and recurrent mucocutaneous herpes simplex virus	Suppresses viral replication by inhibiting DNA polypeptide synthesis.	Burning and stinging (with topical form only); confusion; erythema, pain, and phlebitis at injection site; lethargy; tremors
amantadine Prophylaxis or symptomatic treatment of respiratory tract infections caused by the influenza A virus; also used for symptomatic treatment of parkinsonism	Interferes with penetration of influenza A virus into susceptible cells, probably by inhibiting the uncoating of the RNA virus. In parkinsonism, the drug may enhance dopamine release from presynaptic nerve endings.	Anxiety, confusion, constipation, decreased coordination, depression, dizziness, drowsiness, dry mouth, dyspnea, edema, inability to concentrate, insomnia, irritability, orthostatic hypotension, slurred speech, urinary frequency, urinary retention, visual disturbances
amphotericin B Treatment for aspergillosis, coccidioidomycosis, histoplasmosis, leishmaniasis, disseminated candidiasis, blastomycosis, and amebic meningoencephalitis	Binds with the sterols in the fungal cell membrane to increase cellular permeability. This allows leakage of cell contents, such as potassium, causing the organism's death.	Anorexia, blurred vision, bone marrow depression, chills, confusion, dizziness, drowsiness, fever, hallucinations, headache, hearing loss, hepatic impairment, irritability, joint and muscle pain, malaise, nausea, numbness and tingling in extremities, phlebitis and pain at injection site, renal impairment, seizures, tinnitus, vertigo, weakness

SPECIAL CONSIDERATIONS

• Use cautiously in patients with renal impairment or neurologic disorders. Risk of renal toxicity rises with I.V. form or if patient is dehydrated. During infusion, ensure adequate hydration. Give the infusion over 1 hour to prevent renal tubular damage. Avoid infiltration.
• Patients with life-threatening herpes virus infection require increasingly higher doses.

Drug concentration shouldn't exceed 6 mg/ml.
• The topical form decreases healing time and the duration of viral shedding in genital herpes.
• Instruct the patient to wear a finger cot or glove when applying ointment. Tell him to dispose of the finger cot or glove in a sealed plastic bag to prevent spreading infection.

• Amantadine is contraindicated in seizure disorders, uncontrolled psychoses, or severe neuroses because of the drug's CNS effects. It's also contraindicated in congestive heart failure.
• Use cautiously in hepatic disease because the drug may accumulate. Reduce dosage in renal impairment.
• To prevent orthostatic hypotension, instruct the patient to rise slowly from a recumbent position and to lie down if he feels dizzy or weak.
• To reduce CNS symptoms, give amantadine in two divided doses rather than in a single dose. If insomnia occurs, give the second daily dose at least 6 hours before bedtime.
• Advise the patient to avoid driving or operating machinery; this drug can affect his vision, coordination, and concentration.
• Instruct him to report any anticholinergic reactions, such as dry mouth, constipation, or urinary retention. He should also inform the doctor if he's taking other medications; amantadine's effects increase when combined

with other anticholinergics.
• If the patient misses a dose, tell him to take it as soon as possible. However, he shouldn't take two doses within 4 hours. And he shouldn't double-dose.
• In an outbreak of influenza A, prophylaxis should begin before exposure, or as soon as possible after it, and continue for at least 10 days. If influenza develops, treatment should continue for 2 days after symptoms disappear.
  Candidates for prophylactic treatment include all unimmunized residents and care-givers in a chronic care facility where exposure has occurred; patients with chronic or debilitating diseases who were immunized too late to develop an antibody response (takes about 2 weeks) as well as their caregivers; immunodeficient patients, who may have a poor response to the influenza vaccine; and persons for whom the influenza vaccine is contraindicated, such as those with a hypersensitivity to eggs.

• Because this drug causes severe side effects, it should be used only in patients with a confirmed diagnosis of life-threatening fungal infection. Patients may become more ill after therapy is initiated.
• Concomitant use of aminoglycosides increases the risk of renal toxicity.
• When administering the drug I.V., institute seizure precautions and watch closely for allergic reactions and hepatorenal impairment. Keep the patient well hydrated to help prevent renal damage. Monitor blood urea nitrogen, nonprotein nitrogen, and creatinine levels every other day. Assess daily for signs of CNS involvement, such as blurred

vision, confusion, irritability, or seizures. Check for signs of hypokalemia, such as EKG changes, weakness, and numbness and tingling in the extremities. Encourage the patient to eat potassium-rich foods, such as bananas, oranges, and apricots, to combat hypokalemia. Potassium supplements may be ordered.
• To prevent phlebitis at the I.V. site, add heparin to the infusion, if ordered.
• Provide supportive care, such as giving antipyretics, antiemetics, antihistamines, and corticosteroids, to relieve side effects.
• Report signs of ototoxicity, such as hearing loss, tinnitus, or vertigo.

(continued)

UNDERSTANDING OTHER IMPORTANT ANTI-INFECTIVES *(continued)*

DRUG AND MAJOR USES	MECHANISM OF ACTION	SIDE EFFECTS
isoniazid (INH) Primary drug for treatment and prevention of tuberculosis; in treating tuberculosis, administered orally or intramuscularly, usually with another antitubercular drug, to inhibit the emergence of drug-resistant organisms	Interferes with bacterial metabolism, resulting in alteration of the bacterial cell wall. INH may have a bacteriostatic or bactericidal effect, depending on its concentration and the susceptibility of the pathogens.	GI upset, hepatic impairment (marked by anorexia, fatigue, weakness), optic neuritis (decreased vision or color discrimination), numbness or tingling in extremities, syndromes resembling systemic lupus erythematosus and rheumatic arthritis, urinary retention
metronidazole Treatment for amebiasis, giardiasis, trichomoniasis, and anaerobic bacterial infections; also used to prevent anaerobic infections in patients undergoing intestinal surgery	Inhibits the growth of bacteria, trichomonads, and amoebas, probably by disrupting DNA and inhibiting nucleic acid synthesis.	Diarrhea, dizziness, epigastric distress, nausea, numbness, peripheral neuropathy, reddish brown urine, tremors, vertigo
miconazole Treatment for severe fungal infections, including meningitis. Also used as a bladder irrigant or instillation to treat bladder mycoses. Topically, the drug is used to treat various forms of candidiasis.	Increases cell wall permeability, causing leakage of cell contents. The drug is fungicidal or fungistatic, depending on the dosage.	Anorexia, chills, diarrhea, fever, itching or burning (with topical form), nausea, phlebitis at infusion site, pruritic rash, vomiting
rifampin Along with other drugs, treatment for INH-resistant tuberculosis. Also used as prophylaxis for asymptomatic carriers of *Neisseria meningitidis*. Used with dapsone to treat leprosy and to prevent meningitis due to *H. influenzae*.	Suppresses RNA synthesis, thereby interfering with bacterial replication. Rifampin has a bactericidal or bacteriostatic effect, depending on its concentration and the susceptibility of the pathogens.	Anorexia; decreased urine output; fatigue; fever; flulike symptoms (joint pain, malaise); hematuria; jaundice; numbness or tingling in extremities; orange urine, feces, saliva, sputum, and tears; pale stools; renal impairment; weakness

SPECIAL CONSIDERATIONS

• Use cautiously in seizure disorders (and only if controlled by anticonvulsants), renal or hepatic impairment, or alcoholism.
• Tell the patient to complete full course of therapy. Relapse can occur if treatment is stopped early, and drug-resistant strains may appear with inadequate dosage. Treatment can last for months or years.
• Monitor liver function tests since INH can cause hepatic impairment.
• Check for paresthesias in extremities, which may signal pyridoxine deficiency. This occurs most commonly in malnourished, alcoholic, or diabetic patients.
• Monitor vision. INH can lower serum levels of vitamin D, producing optic neuritis.
• Tell the patient to immediately report decreased urine output or any symptoms of hepatic impairment or optic neuritis.
• Instruct him to avoid antacids, which may decrease drug absorption, and alcohol, which increases the risk of hepatotoxicity.
• INH should be given to family members and other close contacts of patients with recently diagnosed tuberculosis; patients with a significant reaction to the Mantoux test, a chest X-ray revealing fibrotic lesions, negative bacteriologic findings, and no past antitubercular treatment; newly infected patients with a tuberculin skin test conversion within the last 2 years; and patients with a significant reaction to the Mantoux test who are receiving immunosuppressive therapy or have a chronic or debilitating disease.

• Metronidazole is contraindicated during the first trimester of pregnancy because it may cause teratogenic effects. It's also contraindicated for alcoholics taking disulfiram because of toxic reaction.
• Use cautiously in patients with blood dyscrasia, hepatic disease, or alcoholism because the drug and its metabolites can accumulate in the blood. Also use cautiously in patients with CNS disorders or retinal or visual field changes.
• Give drug with meals to reduce GI upset.
• Instruct the patient to report tremors, dizziness, or numbness. Inform him that his urine may turn a reddish brown.
• Advise him to avoid alcohol because abdominal cramps, flushing, and headache may occur.
• Inform the patient with trichomoniasis that sexual partners should be treated simultaneously to avoid reinfection. Advise him to avoid sexual relations until the infection disappears.

• Use cautiously in patients with hepatic impairment because this drug is metabolized by the liver.
• Inform the patient that topical miconazole can cause itching or burning. Advise him to keep the drug away from his eyes.
• Therapeutic levels are reached most reliably with I.V. infusion. When the drug is given I.V., monitor for changes in hemoglobin, hematocrit, electrolyte, and lipid levels.
• When used vaginally, only small amounts of the drug are absorbed.

• Use cautiously in patients with hepatic disease because the drug is metabolized by the liver.
• Instruct the patient to complete the prescribed course of therapy. Remind him to take every dose. Treatment for tuberculosis may continue for months or years.
• Contact the doctor promptly if you detect signs of hepatotoxicity (anorexia, dark urine, fever, jaundice, malaise, or pale stools).
• Instruct the patient to report fatigue, weakness, numbness or tingling in the extremities, or decreased urine output.
• Suggest an alternate form of contraception if the patient is taking an oral contraceptive.
• Patients who intermittently receive high doses of this drug may experience flulike symptoms. Also, hypersensitivity reactions (hematuria, renal impairment) may occur with intermittent therapy, indicating that the drug should be discontinued.
• Tell the patient to avoid alcohol, which increases the risk of hepatotoxicity.

SURGERY

Incision and Drainage

Called an I & D, this common procedure drains accumulated pus from an infected area through a surgically created incision. It's indicated when an infection fails to resolve spontaneously. For example, in a furuncle or carbuncle, inflammation traps bacteria within a small, localized area. Because antibiotics can't reach this area, an I & D is required to drain it.

The timing of an I & D is critical. If induration is just beginning, more pus is likely to form, so the procedure should be postponed. In that case, the area should be treated with moist heat until the pus consolidates, thereby allowing an I & D to be most effective.

Purpose
To treat suppurative infections.

Preparation
Explain to the patient that the surgeon will make an incision in the infected area to drain pus. Inform him that he'll receive a local anesthetic before the procedure and that he'll receive analgesics afterward to relieve pain.

Now assemble sterile equipment to perform the procedure and specimen tubes to collect culture samples. Prepare the skin with antiseptic solution and cover the area with sterile drapes.

Procedure
The surgeon begins by anesthetizing the area. If the infected area is superficial and nearly ready to rupture, he may simply aspirate the pus with needle and syringe. If the area's large, he may make an incision directly over the suppurative area, spreading its edges to allow drainage of pus. Now immediately collect culture specimens.

After the pus drains, the surgeon leaves the cavity open to promote healing. If the cavity is large, he may pack it with gauze to provide further drainage and to assist debridement. Finally, he applies a sterile dressing.

Monitoring and aftercare
Frequently change the patient's dressings, using sterile technique. Record the appearance and amount of drainage and check for signs of infection.

Give analgesics, as ordered, and assess any complaints of excessive pain. Typically, local pain should wane soon after the I & D. Be alert for signs of systemic infection: fever, malaise, and chills. Check culture results.

Home care instructions
• Tell the patient to report inflammation, warmth, swelling, excessive pain, or changed appearance of drainage.
• Warn him not to pierce any lesions. Doing so could spread the infection.
• If the doctor orders warm soaks to promote further drainage, teach the patient to perform this procedure.
• If the patient must change the dressings at home, stress the importance of maintaining sterile technique and correctly disposing of soiled dressings.

MOIST HEAT

Warm Soaks

Immersion of a body part in warm water causes peripheral vasodilation, helping to relieve pain and promote healing. With the application of heat, leukocytes speed to the infection site, where they rapidly remove toxins and accelerate pus formation. This consolidated pus may then open a tract and drain to the outside of the body.

Moist heat achieves its full effect in 20 to 30 minutes. In fact, after an hour, it does more harm than good because vasoconstriction occurs. Warm soaks shouldn't be used in malignancy because heat promotes tissue growth.

Purpose
To promote healing by increasing local circulation.

Preparation
Examine the skin for abrasions, bleeding, or impaired circulation. Does the patient complain of paresthesias or cool sensations? Does the area look mottled?

Evaluate the patient's ability to determine when heat is injurious. Body areas with impaired circulation have a lower tolerance for heat. Assess the size and appearance of the wound or skin. (Most soaks are applied with clean tap water and clean technique, but broken skin requires sterile solution and equipment.)

Assemble a basin, bath thermometer, plastic sheet, hot tap water or sterile solution, towels, and dressing materials, if needed. To warm a sterile solution, place it in a basin of hot water for 15 minutes; the prescribed temperature is between 105° and 110° F. (40.6° and 43.3° C.).

Explain the procedure and position the patient in bed or in a chair. Cover bedding with a plastic sheet.

Procedure
If necessary, remove the soiled dressing, place it in a nonpermeable, disposable bag, and seal the bag. (If the dressing sticks to the wound, leave it in place.) Fill the basin half full with the warmed liquid. Slowly submerge the body part into the basin, covering the entire treatment area.

Using a bath thermometer, check the temperature every 5 minutes. If it drops below the prescribed range, remove some of the cooled water with a cup, and ask the patient to remove the body part from the basin while you add more hot water. Mix and check temperature. To prevent chilling and vasoconstriction, wrap the affected part in a towel while you change the liquid. Leave the body part immersed for 20 minutes, or as ordered, and then dry gently.

Monitoring and aftercare
Watch for excessive redness, drainage, bleeding, or maceration. If pain or any such signs occur, stop treatment and tell the doctor. After treatment, wrap the body part with towels to prevent vasoconstriction. If prescribed, apply medication or a dressing. Discard the water and dispose of soiled materials properly. Clean and disinfect the basin.

Home care instructions
• Teach the patient to perform the procedure. Advise him to use a clean basin and a cooking thermometer if he doesn't have a bath thermometer.
• Instruct him to report increased pain, bleeding, or skin changes.

Selected References

Advice for the Patient, vol. 2, 7th ed. Rockville, Md.: United States Pharmacopeial Convention, 1985.

Benenson, Abram, ed. *Control of Communicable Diseases in Man,* 14th ed. Washington, D.C.: American Public Health Association, 1985.

Brunner, Lillian, and Suddarth, Doris.

The Lippincott Manual of Nursing Practice, 4th ed. Philadelphia: J.B. Lippincott Co., 1986.

Drug Information for the Health Care Provider, vol. 1, 7th ed. Rockville Md.: United States Pharmacopeial Convention, 1985.

15

Treating Visual Dysfunction

Treating Visual Dysfunction

Introduction

It goes without saying that you give your patients the best nursing care you can possibly provide. However, the patient with a visual problem deserves an extra measure of understanding and support because failing eyesight can affect every aspect of his daily life.

Cause for concern
The patient with a visual problem faces an especially difficult situation. Because of his impairment, he may feel increasingly isolated from his family and friends. Ultimately, he may fear blindness.

These special fears require a caring and compassionate nursing response. Consider the patient with a detached retina: he may find himself suddenly admitted to the hospital, placed on complete bed rest, and having both eyes patched. Besides preparing him for surgery, you'll need to orient him to his surroundings and relieve his anxieties.

You're also responsible for monitoring and helping to correct complications that can result from treatment. Consider the patient who has had a corneal transplant. For this patient, you'll need to examine the eye regularly for cloudiness, excessive redness, or other signs of graft rejection. What's more, you'll need to impress upon the patient the importance of daily observation for early signs of rejection—per-

haps for the rest of his life.

In other eye surgeries, such as scleral buckling, you'll need to monitor for infection and teach the patient ways to avoid activities that elevate intraocular pressure.

Cause for optimism
Despite the patient's apprehensions and the risk of complications, the future is far from bleak. Over the past 15 years, technological advances have revolutionized the treatment of many eye disorders. Lasers, for instance, once gleamed only from the pages of science fiction stories and comic books. Today, their finely focused beams are being used to repair detached retinas, to perform trabeculoplasties and iridectomies, and to accomplish other surgical goals. And these devices offer marked advantages over previous methods: they shorten recovery time, cause little or no discomfort, and prove less taxing for elderly or debilitated patients. What's more, they avert the common complications of most surgical techniques—hemorrhage and infection.

Still, despite the undeniable impact of technology, you mustn't forget that patients with visual disorders require a sensitive human response. The caring and counsel you provide can make a significant difference in the effectiveness of any treatment.

DRUG THERAPY

Miotics

Miotics refer to two groups: cholinergics, which directly stimulate parasympathetic cells, and anticholinesterase drugs, which inhibit cholinesterase. The first group, which includes *acetylcholine*, *carbachol*, and *pilocarpine*, causes the sphincter muscle of the iris to contract, resulting in miosis. The second group, which includes *demecarium*, *echothiophate*, *isoflurophate*, and *physostigmine*, inhibits the enzymatic destruction of acetylcholine by inactivating cholinesterase. This leaves acetylcholine free to act on the iridic sphincter, causing pupillary constriction.

Miotics (especially pilocarpine) are used in the treatment of acute angle-closure glaucoma, but they have been largely replaced by beta-adrenergic blockers in the initial treatment of chronic open-angle glaucoma. They're also therapeutic in iridectomy, anterior segment surgery, and other eye surgery. When used with mydriatics, they prevent adhesions after ocular surgery.

The side effects of miotic drugs usually occur as a result of their local action on eye structures. Common effects include poor night vision, myopia, eyelid twitching, brow pain, headache, eye pain, lacrimation, and eye irritation. The longer-acting miotics, such as demecarium and echothiophate, cause severer reactions. For instance, in patients over age 60, these drugs can hasten cataract development. In children, they can cause cysts on the iris, which may interfere with vision. What's more, they can cause detachment of the retina in predisposed patients, resulting from the spasm of accommodation that causes the lens and vitreous to move forward, creating a retinal tear.

Systemic effects of miotics are uncommon. However, if they do occur, they're more likely to occur with the anticholinesterase group. In fact, toxic doses may affect the central nervous system and cause respiratory failure. Patients with bronchial asthma, bradycardia, or hypotension are especially susceptible.

Because miotics worsen inflammation, they're contraindicated in iritis and corneal abrasions. They should be used cautiously in acute heart failure, bronchial asthma, peptic ulcer, hyperthyroidism, and Parkinson's disease.

Purpose and action

Miotics may reduce intraocular pressure in two ways. In chronic open-angle glaucoma, they cause contraction of the ciliary muscle, which widens the spaces of the trabecular meshwork. This reduces outflow resistance, thus lowering intraocular pressure. In acute angle-closure glaucoma, miotics pull the peripheral iris away from the trabecular meshwork, again by constricting the pupil.

Monitoring

Before giving miotics, check the drug history for possible interactions. Concurrent use of anticholinergics may have additive effects. After administration, observe for signs of local allergy, such as redness or itching. Don't use echothiophate or isoflurophate in patients who are exposed to organophosphate insecticides.

Watch for retinal detachment, which can occur from 1 hour to several weeks after therapy begins. Also pay special attention to complaints of acute, severe eye pain, headache, and visual problems. Evaluate the patient's vision in dim light. If his night vision is poor, make sure he can ambulate safely.

Monitor the patient on anticholinesterase drugs for signs of an overdose. Telltale signs include weakness, hypersalivation, sweating, nausea, vomiting, abdominal pain, urinary incontinence, diarrhea, bradycardia, severe hypotension, and bronchospasms. If any of these signs occur, stop the drug and notify the doctor.

Home care instructions
• Teach the patient how to instill the eye drops. Warn him not to touch the tip of the dropper to the eye or surrounding tissue. Instruct him to apply light finger pressure to the lacrimal sac for 1 minute after instillation to reduce systemic absorption.
• Instruct the patient to stop the drug immediately and contact the doctor if he develops excessive salivation, diarrhea, weakness, or other signs of toxicity.
• Reassure the patient that the blurred vision caused by these drugs usually diminishes with continued use. However, if these drugs cause poor night vision, caution against driving or operating machinery after dark.
• Explain that close medical supervision is vital during miotic therapy to monitor intraocular pressure.

Carbonic Anhydrase Inhibitors

The carbonic anhydrase inhibitors *acetazolamide*, *dichlorphenamide*, and *methazolamide* treat chronic open-angle, acute angle-closure, and secondary glaucoma. These drugs reduce intraocular pressure by diminishing the production of aqueous humor up to 60%. They also produce systemic acidosis, which adds to their ocular hypotensive effect.

Carbonic anhydrase inhibitors are commonly used with other antiglaucoma drugs, such as the miotics and mydriatics, in ophthalmic emergencies. They may also be given with osmotic drugs. (See *Osmotic Drugs: Emergency Prevention of Blindness*,

page 502.) Although carbonic anhydrase inhibitors are administered orally, acetazolamide, the most widely used drug in this class, may also be given parenterally.

This class of drugs commonly causes malaise, anorexia, weight loss, fatigue, weakness, drowsiness, and, in infants, a failure to thrive. Other common effects include nausea, vomiting, and diarrhea. Diuresis may occur initially but commonly subsides with continued therapy or a change in dosage. With prolonged therapy, renal calculi may form.

Carbonic anhydrase inhibitors should be used cautiously in diabetes mellitus (because they may raise glucose levels) and in obstructive pulmonary disease (because they may precipitate acute respiratory failure).

Purpose and action
Carbonic anhydrase inhibitors reduce aqueous humor production, thus lowering intraocular pressure.

Monitoring
Because GI symptoms commonly occur with carbonic anhydrase inhibitors, give the drug with food. Assess for signs of CNS toxicity, such as incoordination, seizures, cardiac abnormalities, or confusion. As ordered, monitor the patient's intake and output, weight, and serum electrolyte levels.

Home care instructions
• Advise the patient to schedule doses at mealtimes, if possible, to lessen GI distress. To prevent nocturnal diuresis, tell him to take the last dose no later than 6 p.m.
• Tell the patient to take a missed dose as soon as he remembers, unless it's within 2 hours of the next scheduled dose. In that case he should omit the missed dose and maintain his regular schedule. He should never double-dose.
• Warn him to report signs of hypokalemia, such as fatigue, muscle cramps, and increased thirst. If appropriate, tell him to eat high-potassium

OSMOTIC DRUGS: EMERGENCY PREVENTION OF BLINDNESS

In acute angle-closure glaucoma, hyperosmotic solutions, such as *glycerin, isosorbide, urea, and mannitol,* effectively control sharply rising intraocular pressure. Without prompt treatment, this ophthalmic emergency could result in blindness.

How osmotics work

Hyperosmotic solutions rapidly reduce intraocular pressure and vitreous volume while the patient is prepared for surgery or laser treatment. These drugs draw fluid from the eyeball by osmosis to increase blood osmolarity; at the same time, they decrease corneal edema. Their effectiveness hinges on an intact blood-aqueous vascular system and on the absence of inflammatory disease.

Comparing osmotics

In an emergency, mannitol and urea are equally effective in reducing intraocular pressure and vitreous volume. They reduce intraocular pressure in 30 to 60 minutes and remain effective for 6 to 8 hours. Both are given I.V., but mannitol is more convenient to administer and less toxic. Urea irritates the tissues, causing pain at the infusion site. And if this drug is infused into a leg vein, it can also precipitate thrombosis.

In contrast, glycerin and isosorbide are given orally. They work more slowly than the other osmotics, but they're safer and more convenient to use. Glycerin reduces intraocular pressure in about 1 hour and its effects subside after 5 hours. Isosorbide has a similar duration of action. However, it's preferred over glycerin in diabetic patients because it doesn't alter their blood glucose levels.

---

foods, such as bananas and avocados.
• Tell him to contact the doctor if he experiences depression, difficult or painful urination, or lower back pain.
• Inform him that this drug may make him drowsy. If it does, he should avoid driving or other activities that require alertness.
• Advise the patient not to store capsule or tablet forms of the drug in the bathroom since heat and moisture will cause them to decompose.

Beta-Adrenergic Blockers

Ophthalmic beta-adrenergic blockers, such as *timolol, betaxolol,* and *levobunolol,* are used to treat chronic open-angle glaucoma and suspected glaucoma. Because these drugs may be absorbed systemically, the choice of a specific drug requires careful consideration. Nonselective beta blockers, such as timolol and levobunolol, can cause bradycardia, heart block, ventricular ectopy, congestive heart failure, and exacerbation of asthma. In contrast, the cardioselective beta blocker betaxolol doesn't significantly affect the heart rate and exerts relatively mild pulmonary effects.

Beta blockers should be used cautiously in diabetes mellitus since they mask symptoms of hypoglycemia.

Purpose and action

Ophthalmic beta blockers reduce intraocular pressure by decreasing the production and increasing the outflow of aqueous humor. They may achieve this effect by blocking the response of the eye to sympathetic nerve stimulation and circulating catecholamines.

Monitoring

Before giving an ophthalmic beta blocker, review the patient's drug regimen for possible interactions. Concurrent use of timolol or levobunolol with other beta blockers, such as propranolol or metoprolol, can potentiate the systemic and ocular effects of these drugs. In such patients, betaxolol should be substituted.

Be alert for toxic signs, especially in children, the elderly, or patients with hepatic disease. Toxic effects may include bradycardia, premature ventricular contractions, hypotension, seizures, confusion, depression, unusual fatigue, or weakness.

If the patient is diabetic, monitor his serum glucose levels, as ordered.

Home care instructions

• Show the patient how to instill the drug. Explain that he should use his middle finger to apply light pressure to the inside corner of the eye during administration and for 1 minute after it.
• Warn the patient to avoid touching the applicator tip to any surface (including the eye) to prevent contamination of the eye drops.
• Tell him to keep the medication container tightly closed and to store it away from heat and direct sunlight. He should discard outdated medicine as instructed.
• Instruct the patient to notify the doctor if he experiences photophobia, confusion, depression, fatigue, or wheezing.
• Inform him that if he misses a dose he should administer it as soon as possible, unless it's within 2 hours of the next scheduled dose. If that happens, he should skip the missed dose and return to his regular schedule.
• Stress the importance of keeping follow-up appointments to have intraocular pressure checked.

Mydriatics

Topical mydriatics include a group of anticholinergic drugs: *atropine*, *cyclopentolate*, *homatropine*, *scopolamine*, and *tropicamide*. They also include a group of adrenergic drugs: *epinephrine*, *epinephryl*, *hydroxyamphetamine*, and *phenylephrine*.

Atropine, homatropine, and scopolamine help relieve acute inflammation of the iris (iritis), ciliary body, or choroid (uveitis). Cyclopentolate, hydroxyamphetamine, phenylephrine, and tropicamide are used in diagnostic procedures, whereas the epinephrine salts help treat chronic open-angle glaucoma.

Mydriatics, especially the anticholinergic ones, may cause systemic effects, such as tachycardia and dry mouth. Because mydriatics increase intraocular pressure, they're contraindicated in acute angle-closure glaucoma.

Purpose and action

The anticholinergic mydriatics cause pupillary dilation and paralysis of accommodation by blocking the action of acetylcholine. The adrenergics constrict the dilator muscle of the pupil. (See *Understanding Mydriatic Action*, page 504.)

Monitoring

In a patient with anatomically narrow ocular angles, be alert for symptoms of acute angle-closure glaucoma, such as pain, blurred vision, and headache, when the pupil becomes dilated from these drugs.

In children and the elderly especially, check for systemic effects, including tachycardia, flushing, and dry skin. Also ask about photophobia and blurred vision.

If the patient's taking an adrenergic mydriatic, tell him to report brow pain, headache, blurred vision, pain, or tearing. Also check for pigment granules (aqueous floaters) in the anterior chamber. These should disappear 12 to 24 hours after drug instillation.

Home care instructions

• Teach the correct technique for instilling the medication; caution the patient not to touch the tip of the dropper or tube to the eye or the surrounding tissue.
• Show the patient how to reduce the drug's systemic effects by applying light finger pressure on the lacrimal sac for 1 minute after instillation.
• Stress the importance of immediately reporting signs of increasing intraocular pressure, such as pain and persistent blurred vision.
• Because mydriatics will temporarily blur vision, caution the patient against

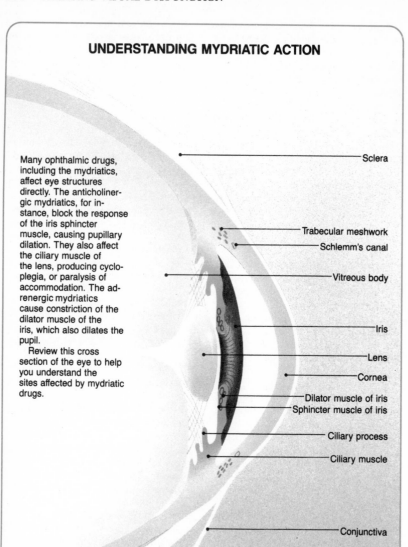

UNDERSTANDING MYDRIATIC ACTION

Many ophthalmic drugs, including the mydriatics, affect eye structures directly. The anticholinergic mydriatics, for instance, block the response of the iris sphincter muscle, causing pupillary dilation. They also affect the ciliary muscle of the lens, producing cycloplegia, or paralysis of accommodation. The adrenergic mydriatics cause constriction of the dilator muscle of the iris, which also dilates the pupil.

Review this cross section of the eye to help you understand the sites affected by mydriatic drugs.

Sclera

Trabecular meshwork
Schlemm's canal

Vitreous body

Iris

Lens

Cornea

Dilator muscle of iris
Sphincter muscle of iris

Ciliary process

Ciliary muscle

Conjunctiva

driving or operating machinery until his vision clears.
• If photophobia occurs, suggest that the patient wear dark glasses when he's outdoors in the sunlight.
• Instruct him to keep the medication container tightly sealed and to store it away from heat and light. Mention that he shouldn't use the mydriatic if it becomes discolored or cloudy.

Vasoconstrictors

Typically sold as over-the-counter eye drops, vasoconstrictors relieve the itching and redness associated with eye irritation and inflammation caused by pollen-related allergies, colds, dust, smog, swimming, and contact lenses. They also provide relief from eye strain caused by reading or driving.

The most commonly used ophthalmic vasoconstrictors include *naphazoline, phenylephrine, ephedrine, tetrahydrozoline,* and *zinc sulfate.* These agents are available in varying strengths and may be found in combination products.

Vasoconstrictors should be used with extreme caution, if at all, in infants and children, since they may produce severe CNS depression. Also, their variable systemic absorption may cause a severe drop in body temperature. However, zinc sulfate is an exception; it produces only a local effect.

Contraindicated in acute angle-closure glaucoma, vasoconstrictors should be used cautiously in hyperthyroidism, heart disease, hypertension, or diabetes mellitus because toxic reactions are possible.

Purpose and action
Ophthalmic vasoconstrictors temporarily relieve eye itching and redness. Naphazoline, phenylephrine, and tetrahydrozoline act directly on the conjunctival arterioles to produce constriction. Zinc sulfate acts as an astringent on the conjunctiva.

Monitoring
Review the patient's drug regimen for possible interactions. Concurrent use of ophthalmic vasoconstrictors and monoamine oxidase inhibitors, for instance, may trigger a hypertensive crisis. Use of tricyclic antidepressants can cause toxic effects.

During therapy, monitor the patient's vital signs and mental status. Report symptoms of toxicity, such as tachycardia, headache, and excessive drowsiness.

Home care instructions
• Instruct the patient to report symptoms of toxicity, including headache, dizziness, irregular heartbeat, or excessive drowsiness.

• If the patient is administering his own eye drops, teach him the proper technique. Emphasize that he shouldn't touch the tip of the dropper to the eye or surrounding tissue. Tell him to apply gentle pressure to the inside corner of the eye during administration and for 1 minute after it to prevent drug absorption through the tear duct.

• Emphasize that the drug usually shouldn't be used for more than 4 days. Longer use may actually worsen eye irritation as well as increase the risk of side effects.

• Warn against exceeding the recommended dose since rebound irritation and inflammation can occur.

• Tell the patient not to use the solution if it changes color, becomes cloudy, or develops a precipitate.

Corticosteroids

Because of their anti-inflammatory properties, corticosteroids reduce scarring and prevent vision loss that may result from inflammatory disorders of the eyelids, conjunctiva, cornea, and anterior segment of the globe. They're also used in eye allergies (such as contact dermatitis), corneal injury from chemical or thermal burns, and injuries caused by ocular penetration by foreign bodies.

The ophthalmic corticosteroids include *betamethasone, dexamethasone, fluorometholone, hydrocortisone, medrysone,* and *prednisone.* The choice of a specific corticosteroid depends on the underlying disorder and the patient's response. In ocular infections, corticosteroids are normally administered with an antibiotic drug to eradicate the causative organism.

Commonly available as drops or ointment, corticosteroids also come in a solution or suspension, allowing subcutaneous injection to enhance topical therapy. The chief side effects of topical corticosteroids include burning and

COMBINATION PRODUCTS: USE WITH CAUTION

Fixed-dose corticosteroids may be combined with one or more antibacterial agents to treat keratitis secondary to staphylococcal infection, allergic conjunctivitis secondary to chronic bacterial conjunctivitis, and certain types of postoperative inflammation. However, the corticosteroid and antibacterial must be used together carefully.

Think twice

The reason? The corticosteroid in these combination products may actually weaken ocular defense mechanisms, thus lowering resistance to fungal and bacterial infections. For example, using a corticosteroid with an antibacterial to treat corneal abrasion may cause an increased susceptibility to fungal infections.

These combination products may also mask signs of worsening infection, such as fever, pain, and inflammation. What's more, if the causative organism is resistant to the antibacterial, scarring and nerve damage (leading to blindness) can occur before the antibacterial's ineffectiveness is noted. As a result, if a combination product is to be used at all, it should be used with caution and only after identification of the causative organism.

Purpose and action

Ophthalmic corticosteroids relieve redness, irritation, and ophthalmic pain while preventing scarring. They do this by restoring the normal permeability of the inflamed capillaries, thereby decreasing leukocyte infiltration.

Monitoring

During therapy, assess the patient for any increase in eye redness, drainage, or pain. These signs may indicate exacerbation of a preexisting infection or the onset of a secondary infection of the cornea.

Carefully monitor the duration of therapy and the results of intraocular pressure measurements, which are usually ordered every 2 months. Be especially alert for increased intraocular pressure in the glaucoma patient. If it occurs, notify the doctor.

Home care instructions

• Tell the patient to stop the drug and notify the doctor immediately if he notices a change in his vision.

• Teach the patient the correct technique for administering the drug. If the drug is in suspension form, instruct him to shake the bottle thoroughly before application. If he's using drops, warn him not to touch the dropper to his eye and explain that he must apply light finger pressure to the lacrimal sac during instillation and for 1 minute after it. If he's using an ointment, tell him to apply it with a pad and to exert slight pressure on the eye to enhance drug absorption.

• Explain that if he misses a dose he should apply it as soon as possible, unless the next scheduled dose is less than 1 hour away. Then he should skip the missed dose and return to his regular schedule.

• Tell the patient to store the medication in a tightly covered, light-resistant container.

• Instruct him to schedule regular ophthalmologic examinations to check intraocular pressure.

stinging, making their instillation uncomfortable, especially for young children. Repeated administration, especially of dexamethasone or prednisone, can increase intraocular pressure and damage the optic nerve. Such damage is reversible with drug discontinuation after an initial course of therapy, but permanent damage may occur with repeated courses.

Corticosteroids are contraindicated in acute superficial herpes simplex (dendritic keratitis), vaccinia, varicella, and other fungal or viral diseases of the cornea and conjunctiva. Their use should also be avoided in diabetes mellitus, ocular tuberculosis, or any acute, purulent, untreated eye infection. Corticosteroids should be used cautiously in corneal abrasions with possible infection (especially herpes) and in glaucoma.

SURGERY

Radial Keratotomy

This investigational treatment for myopia involves surgical creation of small radial incisions in the cornea. These incisions flatten the cornea to help properly focus light on the retina. This procedure is used for patients whose vision with glasses or contact lenses is unsatisfactory. Cosmetic reasons alone, however, should not be the motivating factor. Results are unpredictable.

Because keratotomy has been widely used only since the 1970s, its long-term effects aren't known. Complications include overcorrection or undercorrection, corneal perforation (usually self-healing), fluctuating vision (lasting for 1 to 4 years), and temporary photophobia and night glare.

Purpose
To correct myopia by flattening the cornea, thereby reducing the corneal curvature.

Preparation
The patient will already have had an ophthalmologic examination to evaluate visual acuity and refraction, the thickness and curvature of the cornea, endothelial cell count, and intraocular pressure. Explain the keratotomy procedure, and answer any questions he may have. During this question-and-answer session, form an impression of the patient's motivation for surgery to ensure that better vision is the desired result and not just freedom from wearing glasses.

Tell the patient that his face will be cleansed with an antiseptic and a sedative will be given to help him relax. He'll also have a drape placed over his

---

INVESTIGATIONAL REFRACTIVE SURGERY

Radial keratotomy is just one of several investigational surgeries that attempt to correct refractive corneal problems. In *epikeratophakia*, a piece of precarved, freeze-dried, reconstituted tissue from a donor cornea is attached to the patient's cornea. Another investigational procedure called *keratomileusis* involves the removal of part of the patient's own cornea, which is then reshaped and replaced.

Pros and cons
Proponents of refractive corneal surgery argue that these procedures are no different than surgery performed to eliminate the need for a leg brace or a hearing aid. Opponents counter that a healthy eye shouldn't be tampered with, especially if vision can be corrected by glasses or contact lenses. Both groups agree that these procedures require careful screening and education about their risks and the expected extent of improvement.

---

face, supplemental oxygen provided, and a local anesthetic instilled in the affected eye. Explain that the procedure takes 3 to 8 minutes and that he must remain still until it's over. Inform him that the doctor may cover the eye with a dressing after surgery.

Ensure that the patient has signed a consent form.

Procedure
After the patient has been prepared, the surgeon marks the visual axis to determine the proper placement of the incisions. He then measures the corneal thickness by pachymeter and sets a diamond knife by micrometer to the exact depth for the cut. Next, the surgeon makes 8 to 16 incisions into the cornea in a radial pattern, irrigating them with balanced salt solution. Finally, he instills antibiotic drops, such as gentamicin, and may patch the eye.

Monitoring and aftercare
After the patient recovers from the local anesthetic, he may experience some

discomfort. Warn him not to rub the eye—this may damage the cornea.

If the patient's eye isn't patched, lower the lights since brightness may aggravate his discomfort.

Home care instructions

• If the doctor prescribes eye drops, review their use with the patient. Emphasize the importance of instilling them as prescribed.

• Explain that photophobia commonly occurs after keratotomy but usually subsides in a month or two. Suggest that the patient wear dark sunglasses or glasses with polarizing lenses when he's in bright sunlight. Warn him to avoid night driving if he's bothered by glare from oncoming lights.

• Because the patient's vision may fluctuate, advise him to avoid any activity that requires clear vision until symptoms subside.

• Instruct the patient to protect the affected eye from soap and water when showering and bathing and to avoid contact and water sports until the doctor gives permission. Also advise the female patient to refrain from wearing eye makeup temporarily.

Cataract Removal

Lens opacities, called cataracts, can be removed by one of two techniques. In the first technique, *intracapsular cataract extraction* (ICCE), the entire lens is removed, most commonly with a cryoprobe.

In the other technique, *extracapsular cataract extraction* (ECCE), the patient's anterior capsule, cortex, and nucleus are removed, leaving the pos-

---

COMPARING METHODS OF CATARACT REMOVAL

Cataracts can be removed by intracapsular or extracapsular techniques.

Intracapsular cataract extraction
In this technique, the surgeon makes a partial incision at the superior limbus arc. He then removes the lens, using specially designed forceps or a cryoprobe, which freezes and adheres to the lens, facilitating its removal.

Extracapsular cataract extraction
In this technique, the surgeon may use *irrigation and aspiration* or *phacoemulsification.* In the former approach, the surgeon makes an incision at the limbus, opens the anterior lens capsule with a cystotome, and exerts pressure from below to express the lens. He then irrigates and suctions the remaining lens cortex.

In phacoemulsification, he uses an ultrasonic probe to break the lens into minute particles, which are aspirated by the probe.

INTRACAPSULAR EXTRACTION

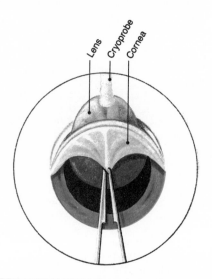

Lens Cryoprobe Cornea

terior capsule intact. This technique may be carried out using manual extraction, irrigation and aspiration, or phacoemulsification. ECCE represents the primary treatment for congenital and traumatic cataracts. It's characteristically used to treat children and young adults because the posterior capsule adheres to the vitreous until about age 20. By leaving the posterior capsule undisturbed, ECCE avoids disruption and loss of vitreous.

Immediately after removal of the natural lens, many patients receive an intraocular lens implant. An implant is especially well suited for elderly patients who are unable to use eyeglasses or contact lenses (because of arthritis or tremors, for example).

Cataract removal can cause numerous complications. Fortunately, most can be corrected. Complications include pupillary block, corneal decom-

pensation, vitreous loss, hemorrhage, cystoid macular edema, lens dislocation, secondary membrane opacification, and retinal detachment.

Purpose
● To remove a cloudy, cataractal lens that prevents light rays from reaching the retina
● To correct aphakia by implanting an intraocular lens.

Preparation
Explain the planned surgical technique to the patient. Tell him that he'll receive mydriatics and cycloplegics to dilate the eye and facilitate cataract removal, that he'll receive osmotics and antibiotics to reduce the risk of infection, and that he may receive a sedative to help him relax.

Inform the patient that after surgery he'll have to wear an eye patch tem-

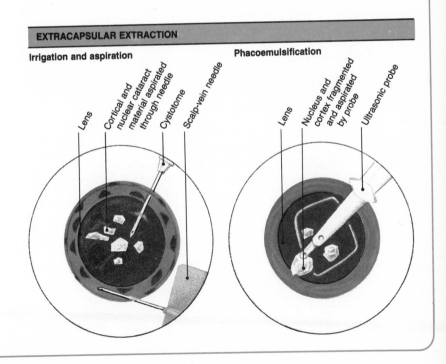

EXTRACAPSULAR EXTRACTION

Irrigation and aspiration

- Lens
- Cortical and nuclear cataract material aspirated through needle
- Cystotome
- Scalp-vein needle

Phacoemulsification

- Lens
- Nucleus and cortex fragmented and aspirated by probe
- Ultrasonic probe

porarily to prevent traumatic injury and infection. Instruct him to call for help when getting out of bed, and tell him that he should sleep on the unaffected side to reduce ocular pressure. Explain to the patient that he'll temporarily experience loss of depth perception and decreased peripheral vision on the operative side.

If ordered, perform an antiseptic facial scrub to reduce the risk of infection. Ensure that the patient has signed a consent form.

Procedure

The patient may receive a local or general anesthetic.

For a review of cataract removal procedures, see *Comparing Methods of Cataract Removal*, pages 508 and 509. After cataract removal, the surgeon may insert a lens implant. After enlarging the incision, he'll implant the lens into the capsular sac. If he implants the lens without sutures, he'll administer miotic agents, such as pilocarpine, to prevent the iris from dilating too widely and causing the lens to slip.

In both ICCE and ECCE, the surgeon may also perform a peripheral iridectomy to reduce intraocular pressure, and he may briefly instill alpha-chymotrypsin, a proteolytic enzyme, in the anterior chamber to dissolve resistant zonular fibers. After the procedure, the surgeon may administer miotics to constrict the pupil. Then he'll close the sutures, instill antibiotic drops or ointment, and patch and shield the eye.

Monitoring and aftercare

After the patient returns to his room, notify the doctor if severe pain, bleeding, increased drainage, or fever occurs. Also report any increased intraocular pressure.

Because of the change in the patient's depth perception, keep the side rails of his bed raised, assist him with ambulation, and observe other safety precautions.

Maintain the eye patch and have the patient wear an eye shield, especially when sleeping. Tell him to continue wearing the shield during sleep for several weeks, as ordered.

Home care instructions

● Warn the patient to immediately contact the doctor if sudden eye pain, red or watery eyes, photophobia, or sudden visual changes occur.
● Instruct the patient to avoid activities that raise intraocular pressure, including heavy lifting, bending, straining during defecation, or vigorous coughing and sneezing. Tell him not to exercise strenuously for 6 to 10 weeks.
● Explain that follow-up appointments are necessary to monitor the results of the surgery and to detect any complications.
● Teach the patient or a family member how to instill eye drops and ointments and how to change the eye patch.
● Suggest that the patient wear dark glasses to relieve the glare that he might experience.
● If the patient will be wearing eyeglasses, explain that changes in his vision can present safety hazards. To compensate for loss of depth perception, show him how to use up-and-down head movements to judge distances. To overcome the loss of peripheral vision on the operative side, teach him to turn his head fully in that direction to view objects to his side.
● If the patient will be wearing contact lenses, teach him how to insert, remove, and care for his lenses, or have him arrange to visit a doctor routinely for removal, cleansing, and reinsertion of extended-wear lenses.

Corneal Transplant

[Keratoplasty]

In a corneal transplant, healthy corneal tissue from a human donor replaces a damaged part of the cornea. Corneal

COMPARING CORNEAL TRANSPLANTS

A corneal transplant may involve replacement of the entire cornea or simply a thin layer of corneal tissue. In a full-thickness transplant, the surgeon removes the corneal disk, which measures 7 to 8 mm, and replaces it with a matching "button" from a donor. In a lamellar, or partial-thickness, transplant, the surgeon removes the superficial corneal tissue only and replaces it with donor tissue. By using this procedure, he spares the stroma and the entire endothelium.

FULL-THICKNESS TRANSPLANT

Removal of cornea

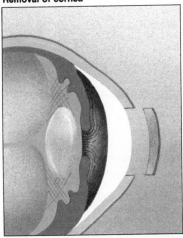

Insertion of donor cornea

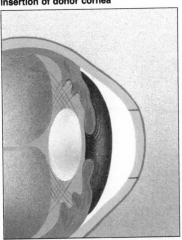

LAMELLAR TRANSPLANT

Removal of lamellae

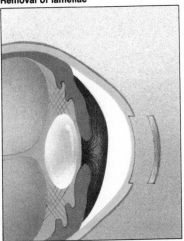

Insertion of donor lamellae

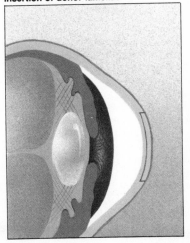

QUESTIONS PATIENTS ASK ABOUT CORNEAL TRANSPLANT

Will I be able to see better right after surgery?

Probably, but your vision should continue to improve. It will be best after the doctor removes the sutures when your eye has healed—in about 6 months to 1 year.

Will I feel the sutures?

Yes, they'll probably feel uncomfortable, but you *mustn't rub your eye.* Instead, take aspirin or acetaminophen. If that doesn't help relieve your symptoms, contact your ophthalmologist.

How will I know if my eye is rejecting the graft?

If your eye begins to reject the graft, the cornea becomes cloudy and opaque, and your vision will become extremely poor. Remember that rejection can occur at any time during the rest of your life. So be sure to check your eye every morning for persistent redness or discharge or a change in your vision. If you notice any changes and they last for at least 24 hours, contact your ophthalmologist *immediately.* If rejection is just starting, he may treat it with medication.

transplants help restore corneal clarity lost through injury, inflammation, ulceration, or chemical burns. They may also correct corneal dystrophies, such as keratoconus, the abnormal thinning and bulging of the central portion of the cornea.

A corneal transplant can take one of two forms: a full-thickness penetrating keratoplasty, involving excision and replacement of the entire cornea, or a lamellar keratoplasty, which removes and replaces a superficial layer of corneal tissue. The full-thickness procedure, the more common of the two, produces a high degree of clarity and restores vision in 95% of patients.

A lamellar transplant is used if damage is limited to the anterior stroma or if the patient is uncooperative and may be expected to exert pressure on the eye after surgery. The degree of clarity produced by a lamellar transplant rarely matches that of a full-thickness graft. As a treatment for dystrophies, its success depends on the type and extent of the abnormality.

Because the cornea is avascular and doesn't recover as rapidly as other parts of the body, healing may take up to a year. Usually, sutures remain in place and vision isn't completely functional until healing occurs.

Graft rejection may occur in about 15% of patients; it may happen at any time during the patient's life. Uncommon complications include wound leakage, loosening of the sutures, dehiscence, and infection.

Purpose
To replace damaged or opaque corneal tissue with a clear, healthy corneal graft.

Preparation
Explain the transplant procedure to the patient and answer any questions he may have (see *Questions Patients Ask About Corneal Transplant*). Advise him that healing will be slow and that his vision may not be completely restored until the sutures are removed, which may be in about a year.

Tell the patient that most corneal transplants are performed under local anesthesia and that he can expect momentary burning during injection of the anesthetic. Explain to him that the procedure will last for about an hour and that he must remain still until it has been completed.

Tell the patient that analgesics will be available after surgery, since he may experience a dull aching. Inform him that a bandage and protective shield will be placed over the eye.

As ordered, administer a sedative or an osmotic agent to reduce intraocular pressure. Ensure that the patient has signed a consent form.

Procedure

In a *full-thickness keratoplasty*, the surgeon cuts a "button" from the donor cornea and a button from the host cornea, sized to remove the abnormality. Next, he anchors the donor button in place with extremely fine sutures. To end the procedure, he patches the eye and tapes a shield in place over it.

In a *lamellar*, or *partial-thickness*, *keratoplasty*, the surgeon excises a shallower layer of corneal tissue in both the donor and host corneas. He then peels away the excised layers of tissue and sutures the donor graft in place. As in the full-thickness procedure, he patches the eye and applies a rigid shield.

Monitoring and aftercare

After the patient recovers from the anesthetic, assess for and immediately report sudden, sharp, or excessive pain; bloody, purulent, or clear viscous drainage; or fever. As ordered, instill corticosteroid eye drops or topical antibiotics to prevent inflammation and graft rejection.

Instruct the patient to lie on his back or on his unaffected side, with the bed flat or slightly elevated, as ordered. Also have him avoid rapid head movements, hard coughing or sneezing, bending over, and other activities that could increase intraocular pressure; likewise, he shouldn't squint or rub his eyes.

Remind the patient to ask for help in standing or walking until he adjusts to changes in his vision. And make sure that all his personal items are within his field of vision.

Home care instructions

• Teach the patient and his family to recognize the signs of graft rejection (inflammation, cloudiness, drainage,

and pain at the graft site.) Instruct them to immediately notify the doctor if any of these signs occur. Emphasize that rejection can occur many years after surgery; stress the need for assessing the graft *daily* for the rest of the patient's life. Also remind the patient to keep regular appointments with his doctor.

• Tell the patient to avoid activities that increase intraocular pressure, including extreme exertion, sudden, jerky movements, lifting or pushing heavy objects, or straining during defecation.

• Explain that photophobia, a common side effect, gradually decreases as healing progresses. Suggest wearing dark glasses in bright light.

• Teach the patient how to correctly instill prescribed eye drops.

• Remind the patient to wear an eye shield when sleeping.

Iridectomy

Performed by laser or standard surgery, an iridectomy reduces intraocular pressure by facilitating the drainage of aqueous humor. This procedure removes part of the iris, creating an opening through which the aqueous humor can flow to bypass the pupil.

Iridectomy is commonly used to treat acute angle-closure glaucoma. In this disorder, the iris occludes the angle between itself and the cornea, inhibiting normal drainage and causing a buildup of intraocular pressure. If not relieved, this emergency condition can result in nerve damage and permanent vision loss.

Because glaucoma is a bilateral disorder, preventive iridectomy is often performed on the unaffected eye. It may also be indicated for a patient with an anatomically narrow angle between the cornea and iris. Iridectomy is also used in chronic angle-closure glaucoma, in excision of tissue for biopsy or treatment, and sometimes with other eye surgeries, such as cataract removal, keratoplasty, and glaucoma-filtering procedures.

Most iridectomies are performed in the superior peripheral area of the iris because the eyelid will cover the iridectomy. Occasionally, spontaneous hemorrhage may occur in the anterior chamber (hyphema), causing increased pressure and injuring the eye.

Purpose
• To lower intraocular pressure
• To prevent increased intraocular pressure.

Preparation
Make it clear to the patient that an iridectomy can't restore vision loss caused by glaucoma but that it may prevent further loss. Explain that most iridectomies are performed under local anesthesia. As a result, he may have dimmed or blurred vision for several hours afterward. Instruct him to remain still throughout the procedure, which should last for about 30 minutes.

Before iridectomy, administer miotics, topical beta blockers, and oral or I.V. osmotic agents, as ordered, to reduce intraocular pressure.

Procedure
If the patient's having an iridectomy performed by laser, see "Laser Surgery," page 528. If the surgeon is using a conventional approach, he performs the iridectomy under a conjunctival flap at the limbus or through the clear cornea.

In the limbal approach, the surgeon applies slight pressure to the globe, causing the iris to prolapse. He then excises part of the iris and redeposits it in the chamber.

In the corneal approach, the surgeon tents the iris through an incision in the anterior chamber, incises part of the iris, and redeposits it in the chamber. If the chamber hasn't reformed, the surgeon does so with a balanced salt solution or air. He then closes the scleral or corneal incision and the conjunctival flap. He administers pilocarpine to constrict the pupil and ensure that none of the iris remains in the wound.

The surgeon then applies an antibiotic-corticosteroid ointment and patches the eye.

Monitoring and aftercare
After an iridectomy, be alert for hyphema with sudden, sharp eye pain (mild or aching pain is common and not a concern) or the presence of a small half-moon–shaped blood speck in the anterior chamber. (Check with a flashlight.) If either occurs, have the patient rest quietly in bed with his head elevated, and notify the doctor.

To prevent adhesions between the lens and the iris, administer topical corticosteroids and medication to dilate the pupil. And if the patient received osmotic therapy before iridectomy, encourage him to increase his fluid intake to restore normal hydration and electrolyte balance.

To prevent elevated intraocular pressure from increased venous pressure in the head, neck, and eyes, administer stool softeners to prevent constipation and straining during bowel movements. Also, keep the head of the bed elevated 15 to 20 degrees and advise the patient to refrain from coughing, sneezing, vigorous nose blowing, or rubbing and squeezing his eyes.

Home care instructions
• Instruct the patient to immediately report any sudden, sharp eye pain, since this may indicate bleeding.
• Explain that increased venous pressure in the head, neck, and eyes can strain the suture line or the blood vessels in the affected area. Instruct the patient to prevent this by avoiding constipation or straining during bowel movements. Also have him refrain from strenuous activity and sexual intercourse for 3 weeks, and explain how coughing, sneezing, or vigorous blowing of his nose all raise venous pressure. Finally, tell the patient to move

slowly, keep his head raised, and sleep on two pillows.

● Tell him to make an appointment with the ophthalmologist, and inform him that he'll need periodic tests to determine if visual loss has ceased.

Trabeculectomy

A surgical filtering procedure, trabeculectomy removes part of the trabecular meshwork to allow aqueous humor to bypass blocked outflow channels and flow safely away from the eye. This procedure creates a filtering bleb or opening under the conjunctiva. Then an iridectomy is performed to prevent the iris from prolapsing into the new opening and obstructing the flow of aqueous humor.

A trabeculectomy helps treat glaucoma that doesn't respond to drug therapy. Possible complications of this procedure include a temporary rise in intraocular pressure, collapse of the filtering bleb, collapse of the flat anterior chamber, a severe inflammatory reaction, infection, and hyphema.

Purpose
To create a new path for aqueous outflow, preventing the buildup of intraocular pressure that can further damage the optic nerve and cause vision loss.

Preparation
Inform the patient that this procedure will probably prevent further visual impairment but that it can't restore vision that's already lost. Explain that it will temporarily affect his depth perception and peripheral vision on the affected side.

Continue to administer prescribed antiglaucoma drugs until the patient leaves for the operating room. Warn him to avoid any activities that could increase intraocular pressure, such as bending, vigorous coughing or sneezing, or straining during defecation.

Explain that he'll receive a local anesthetic, which may cause a temporary burning sensation. Tell him that during surgery he should lie still and that afterward the doctor will periodically perform tonometry measurements to detect any increase in intraocular pressure. (Make sure the necessary equipment is available.)

Tell the patient to expect a dressing or patch on the eye after surgery. If he doesn't have a patch, he'll experience blurred vision until the effects of the eye drops wear off, which could take several days or even longer. Also, tell him not to be alarmed by the bleb in his eye.

Before a trabeculectomy, ensure that the patient has signed a consent form.

Procedure
The surgeon begins by making a conjunctival flap at the limbus in the upper part of the globe. Then he dissects a flap of sclera and removes a portion of the trabecular meshwork, providing an entrance into the anterior chamber. After tenting the iris upward into the opening, he excises a small part of the iris to prevent it from plugging the opening for aqueous outflow. The surgeon ends the procedure by suturing the scleral and conjunctival flaps back into place. Aqueous fluid quickly fills the conjunctival flap, forming a bleb. After the procedure, the surgeon applies antibiotic ointment and may patch the eye.

Monitoring and aftercare
After a trabeculectomy, report any excessive bleeding from the affected area. Also observe for nausea and administer antiemetics, since vomiting can raise intraocular pressure.

Administer eye drops, as ordered: miotics, such as pilocarpine, immediately after surgery and mydriatics, such as atropine, after 3 or 4 days. Also if ordered, give corticosteroids to reduce iritis, analgesics to relieve pain, and antiglaucoma drugs to reduce

QUESTIONS PATIENTS ASK ABOUT TRABECULECTOMY

Now that I've had surgery for glaucoma, can I stop using eye drops?

No, you shouldn't stop using them unless your ophthalmologist says so. In fact, you may need to continue your medication indefinitely because surgery only relieves the buildup of intraocular pressure. And if you've been using drops in your opposite eye, you'll need to continue using them in that eye, too, because glaucoma often affects both eyes.

Will my vision get better after surgery?

Unfortunately, it won't. Damage to the optic nerve from high intraocular pressure is permanent. The surgery prevents further vision loss.

Why does the doctor keep ordering vision tests?

Visual field tests keep track of glaucoma, a disease that robs vision like "a thief in the night." That means you may not be aware of any further vision loss until the progression is pronounced. Visual field studies are sensitive to even minute losses. The ophthalmologist will monitor these studies so he can adjust your glaucoma medication when necessary to prevent further vision loss.

Home care instructions

• Instruct the patient to immediately report sudden onset of severe eye pain, photophobia, excessive lacrimation, inflammation, or vision loss.

• Explain that glaucoma isn't curable but can be controlled. Stress that he can take prescribed drugs regularly to treat this condition.

• Warn him to avoid wearing constrictive clothing around his neck or torso since it can increase intraocular pressure.

• Remind the patient that changes in his vision can present safety hazards. To compensate for loss of depth perception, show him how to use up-and-down head movements to judge distance. To overcome the loss of peripheral vision, teach him to turn his head fully to view objects on his side.

• Stress the importance of regular appointments with the doctor, who will periodically monitor peripheral vision and intraocular pressure. Urge family members to have regular eye examinations, too, since glaucoma is often a familial disease.

Vitrectomy

This microsurgical procedure removes part or all of the vitreous humor—the transparent gelatinous substance that fills the cavity behind the lens. A vitrectomy helps treat vitreous hemorrhage and other opacities, traction retinal detachment, and retinal detachment with vitreous contraction. It's also used for removal of foreign bodies. Vitrectomy yields varying results; depending on the patient's condition, the quality of his resulting vision may range from poor to good.

Complications of vitrectomy include endophthalmitis (requiring intravitreous and systemic antibiotics and possibly a second vitrectomy), iatrogenic cataracts (requiring removal later), vitreous hemorrhage (which

pressure in the unoperated eye.

Remind the patient to avoid activities that increase intraocular pressure, and instruct him not to sleep on the affected side until the doctor gives permission. Because the patient's depth perception may be affected after the surgery, remind him to ask for help when rising from bed or walking.

UNDERSTANDING VITRECTOMY

In vitrectomy, the surgeon first performs a peritomy and recession of the conjunctiva. He sutures the rectus muscle for traction and makes two incisions in the sclera, one for the insertion of vitrectomy instruments and the other to provide an opening for a fiberoptic light. He also places a contact lens over the cornea to enhance the view of the posterior segment.

Next, the surgeon cuts and aspirates the membranes and vitreous. At the same time, he infuses saline solution into the vitreous cavity to maintain intraocular pressure. He may then inject air or sulfur hexafluoride gas to hold the retina in place until a firm adhesion develops. Finally, he administers antibiotics and usually patches both eyes.

HORIZONTAL VIEW OF EYE

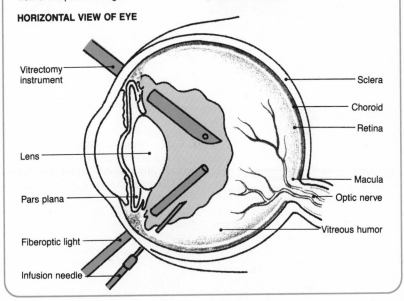

may clear by itself or may require laser photocoagulation), and retinal detachment (which may require scleral buckling).

Purpose
● To remove vitreous opacities
● To allow access to the retina for treatment of detachment and tears
● To allow removal of foreign bodies.

Preparation
Orient the visually handicapped patient to his surroundings to help relieve his anxieties. Tell him that before the procedure he'll receive mydriatic and cycloplegic drugs to dilate the pupil and perhaps antibiotics to prevent infection. Explain that most vitrectomies are

performed under general anesthesia and that the procedure should last for 2 to 3 hours. Tell him to expect patches on both eyes after surgery and that he'll go home in about 5 to 7 days.

Ensure that the patient has signed a consent form.

Procedure
Once the patient is draped and the microscope positioned, the surgeon performs the vitrectomy. See *Understanding Vitrectomy* for details of the procedure.

Monitoring and aftercare
After vitrectomy, closely monitor the patient's blood pressure, since prolonged hypotension could affect retinal

artery circulation. Administer antiemetics to prevent vomiting. Tell the patient to avoid coughing and straining during defecation to prevent elevating intraocular pressure, thereby compromising the sclerotomy incision.

If the patient received injections of air or gas during surgery, inform him that he'll need to assume a certain position, usually face down, to keep the gas bubble in place over the retina. Explain that he must maintain this position for several days, although he'll be allowed to sit upright when eating meals or stand so he can use the bathroom. Suggest to the patient that he listen to a radio or have a family member read to him to help pass the time in this uncomfortable position.

If the patient has continued bleeding or hemorrhage, notify the doctor. If the patient doesn't have a gas bubble, place him in semi-Fowler's position to allow the blood to pool inferiorly and to keep the visual axis clear.

As ordered, administer I.M. or oral analgesics and instill mydriatic and cycloplegic drops to maintain the patient's pupil dilation and antibiotic and corticosteroid drops to prevent infection and control edema. Apply cold compresses to manage eyelid and conjunctival edema.

Expect a moderate amount of drainage for 48 hours, but be sure to report any unusual color or large amounts of discharge.

Home care instructions
• Tell the patient who's had a gas bubble injected into his eye to avoid air travel until the bubble is completely absorbed, usually about 4 to 6 days after surgery.
• Instruct the patient not to stoop, lift heavy objects, or exercise strenuously. However, he may engage in reading, watching TV, going up and down stairs, and taking walks.
• Suggest wearing dark glasses if photosensitivity develops.
• Emphasize the importance of instilling eye drops as prescribed for up to 6 weeks to prevent infection and inflammation.
• Remind the patient to schedule a follow-up appointment for 1 week after discharge.

Scleral Buckling

Used to repair retinal detachment, scleral buckling involves application of external pressure to the separated retinal layers, bringing the choroid into contact with the retina. Indenting (or buckling) brings the layers together so that an adhesion can form. It also prevents vitreous fluid from seeping between the detached layers of the retina and leading to further detachment and possible blindness. When the break or tear is small enough, laser therapy, diathermy, or cryotherapy may be used to seal the retina.

Scleral buckling is successful in about 95% of patients. Its effectiveness depends on the cause, location, and duration of detachment. If the retinal macula is detached, visual acuity may still be poor after surgery.

The two most common complications of scleral buckling are glaucoma and infection. In about 20% of patients, the retina fails to reattach, possibly requiring repeat surgery.

Purpose
To seal retinal breaks and reattach the retina.

Preparation
You'll need to provide ongoing support for the patient with a detached retina. He'll be apprehensive about vision loss, impending surgery, and activity restrictions. Usually, the patient is immediately admitted to the hospital, both of his eyes are patched, and he's placed on complete bed rest. Despite his anxiety, you'll need to stress the importance of remaining still to prevent further detachment of the retina.

Explain that scleral buckling aims to reattach the retina. Depending on the patient's age and the surgeon's preference, advise him whether he'll receive a local or general anesthetic. Tell him to expect postoperative bruises around the affected eye but reassure him that these will disappear in a few weeks. Inform him that he'll be walking within 48 hours after surgery and will probably go home in 3 to 7 days.

Have the patient wash his face with an antiseptic solution to prevent infection. Administer mydriatic and cycloplegic drugs, as ordered, to dilate the pupils and relax the focusing muscles of the eye. Also, as ordered, administer a sedative.

If you'll be assisting with the procedure, you'll need to familiarize yourself with the operating room and the location of equipment to prevent accidents during the lights-out period. You'll repeatedly be required to adjust the surgeon's light and viewing apparatus and to darken the room to facilitate examination of the detachment.

After scrubbing, gowning, and gloving, rinse the silicone material to be used—first in saline solution and then in antibiotic solution. Keep the material readily available.

Procedure

The surgeon begins by making an incision in the conjunctiva, exposing the sclera, and tagging the rectus muscles with sutures to aid in positioning the eye. Using a drawing that shows the location of landmarks and the retinal tear, the surgeon locates the retinal break and marks its position on the sclera by diathermy or cryotherapy. This forms an adhesive, exudative choroiditis at the site of the retinal hole. (As this heals, the scar should keep the retina in place.)

For an *explant* procedure, the surgeon sutures a scleral silicone sponge over the retinal hole. For an *implant* procedure, he'll dissect the scleral bed. Then he may drain the subretinal fluid to allow the retina to contact the cho-

roid. He does this by perforating the choroid and, if necessary, indenting the globe to drain the fluid. The surgeon then places the silicone sponge in the prepared site and sutures the scleral flaps over the sponge. He may also place a band around the entire globe and suture it in place.

After scleral buckling, the surgeon may inject gas or air into the posterior cavity to create a bubble that pushes the retina into place against the choroid. Finally, he'll instill antibiotic ointment or drops and patch the eye.

Monitoring and aftercare

After scleral buckling, place the patient in the ordered position. Notify the doctor immediately if you observe any eye discharge or if the patient experiences fever or sudden, sharp, or severe pain.

Because the patient will probably have binocular patches in place for several days, institute safety precautions. Raise the side rails of his bed and help him when he walks.

Advise him to avoid activities that increase intraocular pressure, such as hard coughing or sneezing, bending, or straining during defecation. Is the patient nauseated? If he is, administer ordered antiemetics, since vomiting increases intraocular pressure.

Emphasize that the patient mustn't squint, or rub or squeeze his eyes. This can rupture the suture line or cause retinal detachment.

As ordered, administer mydriatic and cycloplegic eye drops to keep the pupil dilated and antibiotics and corticosteroids to reduce inflammation and infection. If the patient's eyelid or conjunctiva swells, apply ice packs.

Home care instructions

• Instruct the patient to notify the doctor of any signs of recurring detachment, including floating spots, flashing lights, and progressive shadow. He should also report any fever or eye pain or drainage.
• Stress the importance of avoiding strenuous activity or situations (such

SCLERAL BUCKLING PROCEDURES

For an *explant*, the surgeon may mark the site over the retinal tear with cryotherapy or diathermy. He then sutures a silicone explant sponge over the retinal tear. For an *implant*, the surgeon may likewise use diathermy or cryotherapy to identify the retinal tear. He then dissects partial-thickness scleral flaps, sutures the implant in the prepared scleral bed, and sutures the scleral flaps over the implant.

For either procedure, he may apply a band around the globe to hold the implant or, as shown here, the explant in place.

EXPLANT WITH BAND

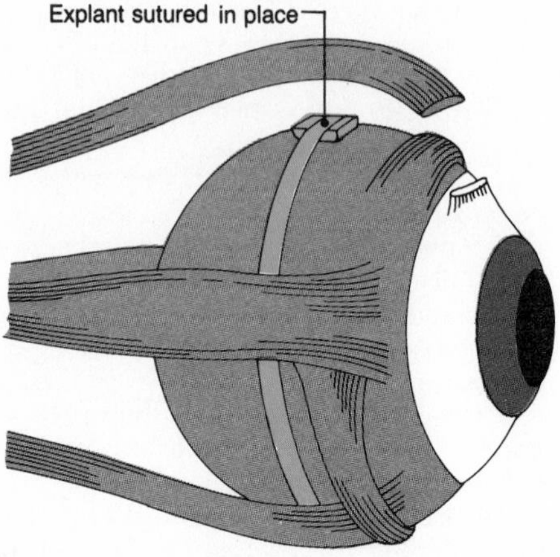

Explant sutured in place

---

as crowds) in which jostling or eye injury could occur. Warn against heavy lifting, straining, or any strenuous activity that increases intraocular pressure.

• Tell the patient to avoid rapid eye movement, as in reading, until the doctor gives permission.

• Show him how to use prescribed dilating, antibiotic, or corticosteroid drops. Stress the importance of meticulous cleanliness to avoid infection.

• Explain the importance of keeping follow-up appointments with the doctor to check for further retinal detachment, glaucoma, and other complications.

Dacryocystectomy and Dacryocystorhinostomy

These surgical procedures treat disorders of the lacrimal system. Dacryocystectomy is the surgery of choice for

removing a lacrimal gland tumor, whereas dacryocystorhinostomy establishes a new drainage path for tears. However, before either of these surgeries can be performed, any dacryocystitis must be controlled with hot packs, antibiotics, and incision and drainage of an abscess.

The complications of dacryocystectomy and dacryocystorhinostomy include excessive bleeding and infection.

Purpose
• *For dacryocystectomy*: To excise a neoplasm of the lacrimal sac and duct tissue.
• *For dacryocystorhinostomy*: To establish a new passage for tears to drain into the nose.

Preparation
For 2 weeks before either procedure, instruct the patient to avoid aspirin since bleeding may occur postoperatively. Also instruct him to take prescribed antibiotics. If the patient's taking anticoagulants, make sure he closely follows the doctor's directions.

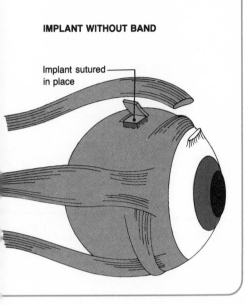

IMPLANT WITHOUT BAND

Implant sutured in place

then removes the lacrimal sac and tumor. In *dacryocystorhinostomy*, he retracts the sac and makes an opening through the bone into the nasal mucosa. He then sutures tissue from the lacrimal sac to the nasal mucosa, forming a new drainage channel into the nose.

To complete either procedure, the surgeon closes the incision, packs the nose with gauze, and applies antibiotic ointment to the incision site and the conjunctival sac. Finally, he applies a dressing.

Monitoring and aftercare

In the immediate postoperative period, notify the doctor if you discover excessive bleeding or signs of infection, such as fever, increased pain, or redness at the surgical site. Administer analgesics, as ordered, and apply cold compresses to the surgical site for 24 hours to reduce swelling, bleeding, and pain.

Besides monitoring the patient for complications, check the nasal packs for proper positioning. (The surgeon may suture the nasal packs to the external nares to prevent slippage.) Leave the nasal packs undisturbed for at least 48 hours.

Home care instructions

• Instruct the patient to immediately contact the doctor if fever occurs or if discharge, redness, or swelling develops at the surgical site. Also have him report bleeding or increased bruising around his nose and eyes.
• Tell the patient to use hot compresses at home, as ordered by the doctor, for 48 to 72 hours after surgery to relieve pain and promote healing.
• Advise the patient to avoid forcibly blowing his nose since this could exert excessive pressure on the surgical site.
• Remind the patient to make an appointment to have the sutures removed 5 to 7 days after surgery.
• If the patient has had dacryocystectomy, tell him to keep follow-up appointments to monitor and treat any metastasis.

Check prothrombin time and report any abnormalities.

Explain to the patient that he'll receive a local anesthetic. Tell him that he'll have postoperative bruising and swelling around his eyes and nose. He'll also have nasal packs in place. Assure him that the doctor will prescribe analgesics to relieve any postsurgical pain.

If the patient's having a dacryocystorhinostomy, explain that he'll probably be discharged after 1 day. The dacryocystectomy patient may require longer hospitalization for the treatment of metastasis.

Ensure that the patient has signed a consent form.

Procedure

For either procedure, the patient is placed in the reverse Trendelenburg position to reduce venous pressure at the surgical site. The surgeon packs the nose with cotton soaked in a 5% cocaine solution, then makes an incision along the side of the nose, exposing the lacrimal sac. In *dacryocystectomy*, he

Eye Muscle Surgery

This surgery corrects defects in the strength or placement of the eye muscles. These defects cause misalignment of the eye, disrupting the visual axis, and, possibly, diplopia. Eye muscle surgery adjusts the pull that the muscles exert on the affected eye, thereby realigning the visual axis and restoring binocular vision.

Two types of eye muscle surgery may be performed. *Resection*, the most common procedure, shortens and strengthens eye muscles; *recessive surgery* weakens the muscles by repositioning them. One or both techniques may be used to carefully position the eye back into proper alignment.

Although eye muscle surgery is most commonly performed in children, it may also be therapeutic for adults. It's usually successful in restoring binocular vision, but a few years after the surgery, the operated eye may drift out of alignment again, necessitating repeat surgery.

Complications rarely occur but may include minor infection and a small amount of bleeding.

Purpose
To correct strabismus.

Preparation
Inform the patient that the surgery will be performed under general anesthesia. (Deep general anesthesia allows the eyes to return to their primary position before surgery begins.) Explain that if the operation is performed in the same day surgery area, he'll come in early in the morning and leave the same day; if he requires hospitalization for eye muscle surgery, he'll be admitted for a day or two.

If the patient is a child, take special measures to reduce his anxiety about the procedure. Take him on a tour of the surgical area, and if possible, introduce him to the nurse who will care for him. Assure him that his parents will be with him when he awakens after surgery. Also let him know if he should expect an eye patch after surgery. (Many doctors no longer use patches on children's eyes after the surgery.)

Explain that the patient shouldn't eat or drink anything after midnight of the night before surgery. If the patient is a child, be sure his parents understand how to administer any preoperative medications.

Tell the patient that after surgery the doctor may order orthoptic exercises to help train the eyes to work together and enhance restoration of binocular vision.

Before the procedure, ensure that the patient or a responsible family member has signed a consent form.

Procedure
If the patient's having medial rectus recessive surgery, the surgeon opens the conjunctiva at the limbal base of the corneal-scleral junction or adjacent to the muscle insertion site. He then isolates the muscle with a hook and places sutures just posterior to the insertion point. He severs the muscle, moves it to the new insertion point, and sutures it in place. He ends the procedure by closing the conjunctiva and instilling antibiotic ointment in the conjunctival sac.

In resective surgery, the surgeon isolates the muscle as for recessive surgery, then clamps it, and places sutures at the site to be resutured. He then cuts the muscle anterior to the clamp and the sutures and trims the muscle tissue remaining at the insertion site. He reinserts the muscle from the clamped site to the insertion point. Then he closes the conjunctiva and applies antibiotic ointment.

Monitoring and aftercare
If the patient's a child, make sure that he doesn't pull at the eye patch or scratch the eye after surgery. Apply an

arm splint, if necessary, to prevent disruption of the surgical site.

Watch for and report excessive amounts of eye discharge.

Home care instructions
• If appropriate, teach the patient or his parents to instill antibiotic or corticosteroid eye drops.
• Tell the patient or his parents that the conjunctiva will be red for 1 or 2 weeks. Emphasize the importance of notifying the doctor if increased redness, fever, or eye discharge occurs.
• Advise the patient to shield his eyes from light to prevent tearing, burning, and excessive redness.
• Explain that double vision may persist for several months. Stress the importance of keeping appointments with the doctor to monitor this condition.
• Review the prescribed orthoptic techniques, and make sure the patient or his parents understand the importance of practicing them as ordered.
• Caution the patient to avoid vigorous sports until the doctor gives permission.

Tarsorrhaphy

Tarsorrhaphy refers to the intermarginal closing of the eyelids by sutures. This surgery protects the cornea exposed by exophthalmos, neuroparalytic lids, exposure keratitis, superficial ulcerative keratitis, wounds, burns with scarring, or entropion. It's also performed for a disfigured or blind eye that doesn't require enucleation.

Tarsorrhaphy may be permanent or temporary. In this procedure, small portions of the palpebral fissure (the space between the upper and lower lids) remain open for secretion drainage. Typically, at least one of the spaces is in the medial corner of the lids.

Complications of tarsorrhaphy are few and minor. They include superficial infection and lid edema.

Purpose
• To protect the eye from exposure
• To correct an eyelid deformity.

Preparation
Explain the procedure to the patient. Tell him that he'll receive a local anesthetic and supplemental oxygen and that he'll have surgical drapes placed over his face during surgery. Emphasize that he must remain still during the procedure.

Explain that if the entire lid is closed with sutures he'll have monocular vision, reduced depth perception, and partial loss of peripheral vision on the affected side. As a result, he'll need to move about cautiously until he adjusts to his visual limitations.

Ensure that the patient has signed a consent form.

Procedure
For a *temporary closure*, the surgeon inserts a suture through the skin above the center of the upper eyelid border and in front of the tarsus. The suture emerges from the center of the eyelid border, and then passes through the lower lid border and the skin on the outside of the lid. The surgeon then ties the suture over a plastic peg or rubber strip.

For a *permanent closure*, the surgeon marks the upper and lower lid margins in two or three corresponding positions. He then strips the lid margins of the mucosa at those points and passes sutures through the plastic pegs or rubber strips and then through the opposing upper and lower lids at the denuded points. He then ties them, bringing the raw edges together into firm apposition. In either procedure, he finishes by applying antibiotic ointment (such as bacitracin, neomycin, or sulfacetamide sodium) and patching the eye.

Monitoring and aftercare
To ensure the patient's stability, help him get up and walk around until he adjusts to his altered vision.

HOW TO INSTILL EYE DROPS AFTER TARSORRHAPHY

Before giving eye drops, verify the contents of the bottle and the strength of the medication. Also check the expiration date. Then follow these directions:
• Wash your hands.
• Have the patient lie down and turn his head sideways to allow gravity to pull the drops down and into the eye. (If you're putting drops in the right eye, turn his head to the right; if you're putting them in the left eye, turn it to the left.) Or the patient can sit and *tilt* his head sideways.
• Identify the small medial opening, and pull the lower lid down to make an opening. If necessary, wrap a gauze square around your finger to hold the lid firmly.
• Next, squeeze the prescribed number of drops into the opening, taking care not to touch the eyelid with the dropper.
• Have the patient remain in position for 60 seconds after instillation so that the drops will flow inside the opening.
• Now, using a tissue, gently remove excess medication. Wash your hands again.

Home care instructions
• For mild discomfort after tarsorrhaphy, instruct the patient to take an analgesic, such as acetaminophen. For severe or persistent pain, he should contact the doctor.
• If the patient has had a temporary tarsorrhaphy, inform him that the doctor will remove the sutures in 2 weeks. If he's to use drops or ointments after discharge, teach him how to apply them properly (see *How to Instill Eye Drops after Tarsorrhaphy*).
• Warn the patient to avoid rubbing the affected eye, and instruct the female patient to avoid wearing eye makeup until approved by the doctor. If tearing occurs, tell the patient to dab, rather than wipe, the tears.
• Explain that if the affected eye becomes irritated or if a foreign particle becomes lodged there, he should notify the doctor and not try to treat these conditions himself.
• Give the patient and family members

instructions for accommodating visual limitations in daily activities. Suggest, for instance, placing dishes and beverages on the unaffected side because loss of peripheral vision may interfere with eating. To avoid spills when pouring liquids, advise the patient to touch the pouring container to the receiving container. And when setting objects down, he should release them only when they've contacted the surface.
• Caution family members to make sure pathways are clear of obstacles and to inform the patient before rearranging furniture.
• Instruct the patient to exercise caution in assessing the height of curbs or stairs. Reduced depth perception may impair his judgment.
• Because peripheral vision is decreased, instruct the patient to turn his head fully when crossing the street, to see any traffic.
• If the patient drives, advise him to compensate for changes in his vision by turning his head farther or relying more heavily on his mirrors.

Enucleation

When no other options exist, enucleation—the surgical removal of the eyeball—is indicated for intractable pain in a blind eye, intraocular malignant tumors, or marked intraocular inflammation following a penetrating injury. Occasionally, it's used for cosmetic reasons when the eye is both blind and disfigured.

Complications seldom occur after enucleation, but they may include extrusion of the implanted ball from the socket, hemorrhage, and infection, which can occasionally result in abscess, thrombosis, or meningitis.

The nurse plays a critical role in supporting the patient before and after this procedure. The patient's eye may be blind and painful or disfigured, but losing it will nonetheless be a traumatic experience. She assesses the patient's emotional state and listens to his concerns. She also provides information concerning the procedure's effect on his pain and appearance and instructs him in wearing the prosthesis and caring for it.

Purpose

To remove a severely degenerated, painful, blind eye and to replace it with a cosmetically acceptable prosthesis.

Preparation

Before the patient undergoes the traumatic experience of losing an eye, be sure to address his emotional concerns. Explain that temporary depression is a common reaction, and reassure him that his appearance will be normal with the artificial eye.

Remember to positively identify the eye to be removed, fully describing it on the patient's chart.

Inform the patient that enucleation is usually performed under general anesthesia. Tell him to expect only mild pain and that he'll receive analgesics for any discomfort. He can also expect a large pressure bandage over the operative site for several days to prevent swelling and bleeding.

Make sure the patient understands that the temporary prosthesis will be white or clear, unlike the permanent prosthesis, which he'll wear later. Advise him that the permanent prosthesis probably won't achieve parallel movement with the unaffected eye. But reassure him that although this may be quite disconcerting at first, his appearance will be normal.

Ensure that the patient has signed a consent form.

Procedure

The surgeon begins by incising the conjunctiva in a 360-degree pattern at the limbal base of the cornea and sclera. He tags the lateral, medial, superior, and inferior rectus muscles with sutures and severs them at their insertion site at the sclera. He then cuts the two oblique muscles so that the globe floats freely in the socket. He turns and lifts the globe slightly to allow a hemostat to be clamped over the optic nerve. Using the hemostat, he crushes the blood vessels in the optic nerve, then severs the nerve behind the hemostat, and lifts the globe from the socket. The surgeon immediately places saline packs in the cavity to staunch the flow of blood. (Electrocautery may also be used.)

Next, he places a plastic or silicone ball into the cavity and attaches the rectus muscles across the ball. He then closes Tenon's capsule over the muscles and sutures the conjunctiva in a separate layer, completely covering the implanted ball. The surgeon applies antibiotic ointment in the conjunctival lid sac, inserts a temporary prosthesis, and applies a pressure bandage to complete the procedure.

Monitoring and aftercare

When the patient returns to his room, be alert for oozing or bleeding at the dressing site; if either occurs, notify the doctor immediately. Also promptly report any signs of infection, such as fever or pain and headache on the side of the enucleation.

Make sure the pressure dressing remains in position for 24 to 48 hours after surgery or until the doctor orders its removal. Warn the patient not to remove the bandage, since it's an important safeguard against hemorrhage.

Because the patient may not realize the finality of enucleation until after the surgery, you'll need to be especially supportive in discussing his fears and concerns.

Home care instructions

• Instruct the patient to schedule a follow-up examination for 7 to 10 days after discharge from the hospital. Also tell him to make an appointment with an ocularist (a professional who makes ocular prostheses) in 6 to 8 weeks to begin the fitting process for a permanent prosthesis.

• Explain that his prosthesis will be

526

HOW TO REMOVE AND INSERT A PROSTHESIS

Dear Patient:

Your prosthesis has been custom-designed just for you. Learning how to properly remove and insert it will ensure a comfortable, pleasing appearance.

Removing the prosthesis
Always wash your hands first and place a towel on the hard surface you will be working over to protect the polished surface of the prosthesis.

1

To begin, tilt your head slightly downward. Using your fingertip, gently depress the lower lid backward and downward toward your cheekbone. This will break the suction that holds the prosthesis in place.

2

Now cup your other hand under the prosthesis to catch it when it slips out. Don't let the prosthesis fall on a hard surface.

    If you can't remove the prosthesis, contact the doctor or an ocularist to obtain a specially designed suction cup to help you.

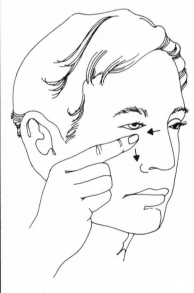

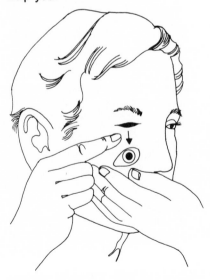

Inserting the prosthesis

Stand in front of a mirror and place a towel on any hard surface you're working over. Moisten the prosthesis with lukewarm water. (Don't insert a dry prosthesis since friction makes insertion difficult.)

1

Hold the prosthesis with the painted side facing out and the narrow end toward your nose.

3

Now pull the lower lid downward and then push slightly upward to enclose the lower edge of the prosthesis.

2

Use the index finger on your opposite hand to secure the upper lid against the bony surface above the socket. At the same time, slide the prosthesis upward into the socket under the upper lid until it's seated at the top of the socket.

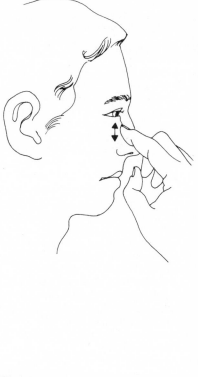

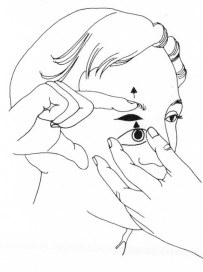

custom-made to closely match his healthy eye. Give him written instructions for removing, cleaning, and inserting the prosthesis. (See *How to Remove and Insert a Prosthesis*, pages 526 and 527.) He should clean it every day and check it every 4 to 6 weeks for surface deposits of tears or mucus that could irritate the conjunctival sac. Explain that the ocularist should check and polish the prosthesis once a year. The doctor should check the socket once a year to be sure the prosthesis is correctly placed and the socket covering has maintained its integrity.

• Instruct the patient to contact the doctor if the socket becomes painful or if excessive discharge occurs.

• Urge him to protect the healthy eye from injury—for example, by wearing shatterproof glasses.

Laser Surgery

The treatment of choice for a wide variety of ophthalmic disorders, laser surgery is relatively painless and especially useful for elderly patients, who may be poor surgical risks.

How do these former science fiction wonders work? To begin, a laser generates focused, or monochromatic, light waves. Then it magnifies their power by deflecting them off a series of mirrors. The result: a finely focused, high-energy beam. Depending on the type of laser, this beam shines at a specific wavelength and color. An argon laser, for example, produces a blue-green beam with a short wavelength that's highly absorbed by the colors red and orange, making it ideal for surgery on the highly vascular retina.

Laser treatment may employ thermal or nonthermal effects to achieve its desired results. The thermal lasers—xenon arc, pulsed ruby, carbon dioxide, krypton, and argon—cause photocoagulation or photovaporization. These lasers are used primarily in retinal detachments and tears, diabetic retinopathy, cystoid macular edema, and glaucoma procedures, such as trabeculoplasty and iridectomy.

The nonthermal, or cutting, lasers—Q-switched ruby, Q-switched neodymium-YAG, and the mode-locked neodymium-YAG—use photodisruptive beams to perforate tissue. When used following cataract surgery, these lasers permit microsurgical incision of the posterior lens capsule, thereby avoiding the more invasive techniques of conventional surgery.

Another laser technology combines the action of the thermal and nonthermal lasers. Using this type of laser in an iridectomy, for example, allows the surgeon to cut through tissue while simultaneously controlling bleeding. Yet another laser, the tunable dye device, has recently shown effectiveness in treating choroidol melanomas. In this procedure, a photosensitive dye, given 72 hours before treatment, increases the susceptibility of the tumor cells to the laser's effects.

Laser treatment avoids the common complications of more invasive surgeries—for example, hemorrhage and infection. However, laser treatments do pose certain risks, including increased intraocular pressure, iritis, bleeding, pitting of the intraocular lenses, and, in rare cases, cataract formation.

Purpose
To repair retinal detachment, open the anterior capsule preceding cataract removal or open the posterior capsule following cataract removal, and perform other ophthalmic procedures.

Preparation
Explain the goals and risks of laser treatment to the patient. Assure him that he should feel little pain.

Inform the patient that he'll have anesthetic eye drops instilled before treatment and a special contact lens inserted to prevent him from closing his eye during the procedure. Tell him that the lens also absorbs some of the thermal en-

SAFETY PRECAUTIONS DURING LASER SURGERY

Despite their many advantages, lasers present safety hazards for health care workers and patients alike. Such hazards include possible laser-produced eye damage, skin burns, and fire. As a result, lasers must be used in accordance with established regulations, manufacturers' recommendations, and hospital policy.

Some important safety precautions for laser use include:

• direct supervision by a person knowledgeable in laser technology and safety
• safety latches or locks on doors to prevent unauthorized personnel from entering areas of laser use
• warning labels in laser use areas and on all laser equipment, specifying: "Danger: Laser Radiation. Avoid eye or skin exposure to direct or scattered radiation."
• coverings on all windows to reduce laser radiation to levels at or below the maximum permissible exposure to the eye. (The eye is the most susceptible organ to laser injury.)
• eye protection for everyone in the room, including the patient—either safety goggles or moistened gauze sponges in place—while the laser is being used. A lack of protection may result in permanent damage to the eye's anterior portion, the corneal epithelium, and the retina, causing a blind spot (scotoma).
• skin protection from laser burns by avoiding exposure to direct or reflected laser energy
• fire protection by avoiding unnecessary reflection from the laser beam. Dull-surfaced instruments prevent reflection. If metal instruments are used, reflection of the beam from a smooth surface, such as a refractor, to an alternate area, such as a disposable drape, can cause a fire.

---

ergy generated by the laser.

Explain that during the treatment, he'll sit facing the doctor with his chin supported on a rest, while he focuses on a particular object. Stress the importance of sitting still throughout the procedure. Agree with the patient on a signal for movement, such as raising the right hand. Tell him that he'll see periodic flashes of light from the laser but that he mustn't look away or move. A few hours after treatment he may return home.

Inform the patient that after treatment his eye may be bloodshot, and his eyelid may turn black and blue. Explain that he may experience blurred vision and decreased night vision and may see spots before his eyes. Also, the bright laser light may cause a headache. Assure him that these are temporary effects.

Ensure that the patient has signed a consent form. Keep in mind that some lasers are considered investigational and require special consent forms.

Procedure

The patient is comfortably seated in front of the slit lamp of the laser, the goniolens is positioned with a methylcellulose bridge to protect the cornea, and the treatment sites are identified. Then the surgeon directs the laser beam at the sites, allowing the laser to work for the appropriate time.

In a *trabeculoplasty*, the surgeon directs the beam at the trabecular meshwork. The beam creates multiple burns around the meshwork to reduce intraocular pressure.

In an *iridectomy*, the surgeon creates a series of mild laser burns, causing a localized area of the midperipheral iris to bulge forward. He then uses a beam of much higher energy to perforate the central portion of the iris, thereby creating an opening between the anterior and posterior chambers to allow for aqueous outflow.

The surgeon may also use the laser beam to prevent *retinal detachment* by repairing peripheral retinal thinning, holes, or tears. Or he can surround an existing localized detachment with laser burn scars to limit its size and prevent further damage.

When the treatment is complete, the surgeon turns off the laser and the patient is taken to the recovery room.

Monitoring and aftercare
Notify the doctor immediately if you observe signs of bleeding, such as an extremely red eye. Keep in mind that slight redness occurs normally and may persist for 48 hours.

Observe for slight localized corneal edema and perilimbal congestion, which commonly develops during laser treatment. To reduce edema and resultant discomfort, apply ice packs to the site for 20 minutes. Ask the patient if he has a headache, which can result from the laser beam's brightness. If he does report a headache, administer acetaminophen, if ordered.

Take the patient's vital signs and observe his overall appearance. Be alert for decreased pulse and blood pressure, pallor, and sweating, which could point to a vasovagal attack. If these signs occur, provide symptomatic treatment.

Home care instructions
• Teach the patient how to instill the prescribed eye drops.
• Emphasize the importance of immediately notifying the doctor if he experiences bleeding or any extreme blurring of vision.
• Warn the patient to avoid activities, such as straining during defecation, that increase venous pressure in the head, neck, and eyes. Instruct him to keep his head up, to move slowly, and to avoid bending over or moving suddenly. If necessary, suggest using a stool softener to avoid constipation. And advise the patient to sleep with several pillows under his head to reduce intraocular pressure.
• Instruct the patient to avoid strenuous exercise for about 3 weeks. But encourage mild forms of exercise, such as walking, to promote circulation and a sense of well-being.
• Warn him to avoid using epinephrine-containing nose drops or sprays since these may raise his blood pressure.
• If the patient received treatment with a tunable dye laser, tell him that he may experience photosensitivity for about 30 days. Advise him to wear sunglasses when he's outdoors during daylight hours.
• Remind the patient to return for a checkup 24 hours after treatment and at scheduled intervals thereafter.

MISCELLANEOUS TREATMENT

Foreign Body Removal

Typically, removal of a foreign body from the eye is a first-aid measure. However, if the object is embedded in the cornea, medical assistance is required for removal and a local anesthetic and an antibiotic need to be applied.

The nurse may remove a foreign body in the conjunctiva. She'll also help the doctor remove foreign bodies from the cornea.

Purpose
To remove a foreign body from the eye, thereby decreasing pain, preventing further damage by abrasion, and reducing the risk of infection.

Preparation
Before removing a foreign body, try to calm the patient's fears about having his eye manipulated. Tell him what to expect, and if you'll need to evert the patient's eyelid to remove the particle, review how this is done. If the foreign body is lodged in the cornea, tell him that an anesthetic will be placed in his eye to reduce discomfort.

Caution the patient not to rub his eye because this will cause further damage, making removal more difficult. Consider placing a protective shield over the eye to prevent the patient from rubbing it.

Procedure

If a foreign particle is lying on the surface of the conjunctiva, instruct the patient to tilt his head back and move his eyes away from the site of the particle. Hold the patient's eyelids open to prevent blinking. Then gently touch the particle with the tip of a cotton swab and lift it from the eye, taking care not to drag the swab across the surface of the cornea.

If the particle is embedded in the conjunctiva in a place that requires better visualization or stabilization during removal (such as the upper fornix), you may need to evert the eyelid. To do so, have the patient look downward, then hold the upper eyelashes, and push down on the upper tarsal border with a small stick or tongue blade, exerting pressure to evert the lid. Once you've done this, appose the fingers, applying pressure on both the upper and lower lid lashes to widen the area of inspection. Now remove the particle with the tip of a cotton swab.

If the patient has a corneal injury, the doctor will examine the eye, using a slit lamp to determine the particle's location and depth. He'll administer a topical anesthetic and remove the foreign particle in the cornea with an appropriate instrument. Then he'll apply an antibiotic ointment and an eye patch.

Monitoring and aftercare

Before the doctor removes a particle from the cornea, ask the patient if the anesthetic has taken effect.

After an embedded particle has been removed, instruct the patient to sit quietly for a few minutes with his eyes closed. Warn him not to rub the eye because this will aggravate the abraded area.

Home care instructions

• Teach the patient how to correctly apply the antibiotic ointment by pulling down the lower lid and applying the ointment along the entire length of the conjunctival sac. Caution him to avoid touching the tip of the tube to the eye or lid.
• Show the patient how to apply an eye patch. Explain that the patch is a comfort measure and will only be necessary for 24 hours.
• Tell the patient to be sure to contact the doctor if his eye pain doesn't decrease in 24 hours or if his vision deteriorates.

Selected References

Belcher, C., et al. *Photocoagulation for Glaucoma and Anterior Segment Disease.* Baltimore: Williams & Wilkins Co., 1984.

Boyd-Monk, H. "A Fortunate Accident: Radial Keratotomy," *Today's OR Nurse* 6(3):25-26, 31, March 1984.

Marta, M. "A Guide to the Posterior Vitrectomy," *Today's OR Nurse* 5(1):26-29, 69, March 1983.

Nursing88 Drug Handbook. Springhouse, Pa.: Springhouse Corp., 1988.

Sliney, D.H. *YAG Laser Ophthalmic Microsurgery.* East Norwalk, Conn.: Appleton-Century-Crofts, 1985.

Smith, J. "The Patient Having Laser Trabeculoplasty," *Journal of Ophthalmic Nursing Technology* 3(5):207-08, September/October 1984.

Smith, S. *Standards of Ophthalmic Nursing Practice,* AAO, 1985.

Spaeth, G. *Ophthalmic Surgery: Principles and Practice.* Philadelphia: W.B. Saunders Co., 1982.

Whitton, S. "Penetrating Keratoplasty: The Gift of Sight," *Today's OR Nurse* 5(1):20-22, 24, March 1983.

Zack, P., and Smirnow, I. "Intraocular Lens Implantation," *Today's OR Nurse* 5(1):12-16, 18, 68-69, March 1983.

16

Treating Dysfunction of the Ears, Nose, and Throat

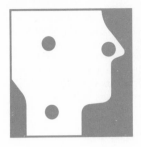

Treating Dysfunction of the Ears, Nose, and Throat

Introduction

Ear, nose, and throat disorders are as common as they are troublesome. And the care you give may be as simple as warning the patient who's taking antihistamines to avoid drinking alcohol because of increased CNS sedation. Or it may be as complex and emotionally taxing as helping the patient with laryngeal cancer cope with major changes in his life-style and self-image.

Treating ear problems
Ear problems affect the young and old alike. In fact, they're especially prevalent among the young and the old.

Chronic otitis media, for example, most commonly affects children. If antibiotics fail to curb the infection, myringotomy may be performed. Before and after this surgery, you'll need to provide thorough teaching, especially for the patient's parents. For example, they'll need to learn about myringotomy tube care and restrictions on bathing and swimming.

Hearing loss, a common problem in the elderly, may also challenge your skills. After all, some patients may have grown accustomed to being unable to hear. Others may fail to realize the marked improvement a hearing aid could give them. And those who do try a hearing aid may fail to use it correctly because of problems adjusting the controls or caring for the device. It's up to you to detect problems like these—and to help patients overcome them.

Treating nasal problems
Treatments for nasal problems range from cosmetic correction of a hook nose to emergency insertion of nasal packing to halt severe epistaxis. On the surface, these treatments seem to require widely different nursing skills. But keep in mind that cosmetic measures may be as important to some patients as therapeutic measures are to others.

Treating throat conditions
Perhaps no disease conjures up images of death, disability, or disfigurement more than cancer. And laryngeal cancer is no exception. Even though survival rates remain high for most patients, the prospect of having a permanent tracheostomy can prove especially frightening. The patient may ask himself, "What will I look like after surgery?" "Will I be able to talk?" "How can I possibly take care of myself?"

There's much you can do to help the patient address his concerns. For example, you can introduce him to a laryngectomee who has adapted well to his condition. You can arrange a preoperative visit with a speech therapist. And you can point out that there are only a few activities, such as swimming, that he won't be able to do.

Antihistamines and Decongestants

Antihistamines and decongestants relieve sneezing, rhinorrhea, and nasal congestion associated with colds and allergies. Antihistamines include such drugs as *azatadine, brompheniramine, carbinoxamine, chlorpheniramine, clemastine, cyproheptadine, methdilazine, promethazine, terfenadine, trimeprazine, tripelennamine,* and *triprolidine.*

Although most antihistamines are given orally, brompheniramine, chlorpheniramine, and promethazine can also be given by deep I.M. injection. Such injection brings rapid relief but may cause local stinging and burning, sweating, and transient hypotension.

Decongestants, including *ephedrine, pseudoephedrine,* and *phenylpropanolamine,* relieve nasal stuffiness. They're available for oral use in tablets and extended-release capsules.

Antihistamines and decongestants are often combined in cold and allergy medications to relieve a wide range of symptoms. For example, chlorpheniramine and phenylpropanolamine are combined to relieve rhinorrhea and nasal stuffiness.

Although both prescription and over-the-counter antihistamines and decongestants are generally well tolerated, they may produce many systemic effects. Antihistamines, for instance, affect the cardiovascular and central nervous systems and also cause dry mouth. Decongestants, which affect the same systems, may cause restlessness, irritability, insomnia, and palpitations. Neither are recommended for use in newborns, premature infants, or the elderly. Antihistamines should be avoided in patients with acute asthma because they increase the viscosity of tracheobronchial secretions. They should also be avoided in patients with urinary retention or prostatic hypertrophy.

Purpose and action

Antihistamines decrease rhinorrhea and dry nasal passages by competing with histamine for receptor sites on effector cells. Decongestants decrease nasal stuffiness by acting on the respiratory tract's alpha-adrenergic receptors to produce vasoconstriction.

Monitoring

Before giving an antihistamine or a decongestant, check the patient's drug regimen for possible interactions. For instance, concurrent use of antihistamines with CNS depressants may cause increased sedation. Use of decongestants with monoamine oxidase inhibitors can cause life-threatening hypertensive crisis.

If you're giving antihistamines by deep I.M. injection, monitor the patient's vital signs, noting hypotension, irregular pulse, or other untoward effects. Be alert for signs of overdose: hypotension, seizures, flushing, palpitations, restlessness, and chest tightness.

Watch for changes in the patient's mental status. If the patient is taking an antihistamine and experiences drowsiness, raise the side rails of his bed and assist him with ambulation, if necessary. If he's taking a decongestant, watch for increased restlessness and insomnia. Give the last dose 2 to 3 hours before bedtime, and caution the patient not to crush or chew the tablets or capsules (especially if they're extended-release).

Home care instructions

• Tell the patient to take his drug exactly as directed. Explain that he may develop a tolerance to it; however he shouldn't alter the dosage on his own, but rather should contact the doctor.

• Instruct the patient to take a missed dose as soon as possible, unless it's within 2 hours of his next dose (or within 12 hours if he's taking an extended-release product). Warn him not to double-dose.

• If the patient is taking an antihistamine, explain that drowsiness commonly occurs. Instruct him to avoid driving and operating machinery until his response is clear. Tell him that caffeinated beverages may combat drowsiness and that he should avoid drinking alcohol or taking sedatives unless directed otherwise by the doctor. Suggest relieving dry mouth with ice chips, sugarless gum, or hard candy. If he develops GI irritation, advise him to take the drug with soup or milk.

• If the patient is taking a decongestant, tell him to avoid excessive intake of caffeinated beverages because these potentiate CNS stimulation. Instruct him to notify the doctor if his cold symptoms don't improve in a week or if fever persists.

REPAIRING A PERFORATED EARDRUM

A ruptured tympanic membrane can result from excessive fluid buildup in acute otitis media or from traumatic injury. Such injury most commonly results from overly deep insertion of a cotton-tipped applicator when a patient cleans his ear. Perforation may be quite dangerous in the posterior-superior quadrant, leading to disruption of the ossicles or cholesteatoma formation.

To repair a ruptured tympanic membrane, the doctor may perform a myringoplasty. In this surgery, he approximates the edges of the membrane or applies a graft taken from the fascia of the temporalis muscle.

After myringoplasty, give the patient antibiotic eardrops, as ordered, to reduce the risk of infection. If the patient has a graft, instruct him to avoid strenuous activity for 2 weeks to prevent its dislodgment. Also tell him to avoid blowing his nose vigorously for at least 2 weeks. If the patient perforated his eardrum with a cotton-tipped applicator, warn him to use such applicators only for cleaning the outer ear. He should never probe deeply to dislodge earwax. Instead, he should call his doctor, who will irrigate the ear or order medicated eardrops.

SURGERY

Myringotomy

The surgical incision of the tympanic membrane, myringotomy relieves pain and prevents membrane rupture by allowing drainage of pus or fluid from the middle ear. It's most commonly performed on children with acute otitis media. Typically, it's employed when antibiotics and decongestants or antihistamines fail to correct the causative infection or when the infection itself damages the middle ear mucosa or causes such severe pressure that the tympanic membrane may rupture. If the tympanic membrane does rupture, though, the doctor may perform a myringoplasty (see *Repairing a Perforated Eardrum*).

Myringotomy may be performed on one or both ears. After myringotomy, a pressure-equalizing tube may be inserted through the incision to allow fluid drainage. Usually, myringotomy provides almost instant symptomatic relief, and the incision typically heals in 2 to 3 weeks. (If tubes have been inserted, they're generally expelled spontaneously after 6 to 12 months.)

Myringotomy can cause minor complications, such as bleeding during tube insertion if the ear canal's inadvertently scratched, and scars or sclerotic patches on the tympanic membrane. When tubes are inserted, ear discharge can become chronic.

Purpose
To relieve pain and drain fluid from the middle ear.

Preparation

Explain to the patient or his parents that myringotomy removes fluid or pus from the middle ear and relieves ear pain. Inform the patient or his parents whether the surgery will be performed on one or both ears and whether a local or general anesthetic will be used. Mention that the doctor may insert a tube through the incision to allow drainage until the inflammation subsides. Then he may either remove the tube or allow it to drop out naturally.

Before the procedure, make sure the patient or a responsible family member has signed a consent form.

Procedure

Typically, an adult or older child receives a local anesthetic. However, if the patient is a young child, uncooperative, or beset with severe otitis media, he may receive a light general anesthetic. (An infant, though, may receive no anesthetic.)

After the anesthetic takes effect, the doctor visualizes the tympanic membrane and makes a radial or circumferential incision. A radial incision, used when serous fluid is present, involves a small slit in the membrane. After making this incision, the doctor inserts a plastic tube or a Teflon grommet. A circumferential incision, used when pus or thick drainage is present, involves a larger U-shaped incision that permits more drainage. After making this incision, the doctor may irrigate the middle ear or apply gentle suction to remove tenacious drainage. If drainage is copious, the doctor may apply a dressing over the ear.

If the patient's having a bilateral myringotomy, the doctor also performs the procedure on the opposite ear.

Monitoring and aftercare

Assess the condition of the patient's ear. Is fluid draining from it? If so, note the amount, type, color, and odor. If you see bright red blood in the drainage, notify the doctor immediately; this may indicate injury to the ear canal.

If needed, cover the ear with a gauze pad or lay cotton fluff gently over the ear's orifice to absorb drainage. Apply petrolatum or zinc oxide to the external ear to protect it from excoriation by drainage, and change dressings as needed. If exudate cakes on the outer ear, remove it by gently swabbing with a cotton-tipped applicator dipped in hydrogen peroxide. Don't attempt to clean the ear canal or allow peroxide to run into the ear.

Home care instructions

• If the patient has a dressing in place to absorb ear drainage, tell him or his parents to wash their hands before and after changing it and to dispose of old dressings by placing them in a small paper or plastic bag before throwing them in the trash. Emphasize the need to notify the doctor if drainage lasts more than 1 week or changes in color or character, for example, from serous to purulent. Advise reporting any ear pain or fever, which may signal blocked tubing or reinfection.
• Explain the importance of not allowing water to enter the ear canal until the tympanic membrane is intact. Show the patient or his parents how to roll absorbent cotton in petrolatum to form a plug and then how to insert the plug in the outer part of the ear before showering or washing hair. If the doctor permits swimming, advise inserting ear plugs first and avoid ducking beneath the water.
• Tell the patient or his parents to expect considerable drainage through the tubes.
• Emphasize the need to return for follow-up examinations and to notify the doctor if the tubes are expelled.

Stapedectomy

The surgical removal of all or part of the stapes, stapedectomy is the treatment of choice for otosclerosis, a hereditary condition in which new bone grows around the ear's oval window, limiting movement of the stapes and causing a conductive hearing loss. Because otosclerosis is usually bilateral, stapedectomy is usually performed twice: first in the ear with the greatest hearing loss and then, a year or so later, in the second ear.

A *total stapedectomy* involves removal of both the suprastructure and the footplate of the stapes followed by the insertion of a graft and prosthesis to bridge the gap between the incus and the inner ear. A *partial stapedectomy* can involve severing and removing the anterior crus and the anterior portion of the footplate. Or it can entail removing the entire suprastructure while leaving the footplate in place, drilling it, and fitting it with a piston. *Laser stapedectomy*, a relatively new technique, is easier to perform but carries some risk of the laser beam's penetrating the bone.

Stapedectomy is contraindicated in external otitis media and inner ear disease. It should be performed cautiously, if at all, in patients with complete hearing loss in the opposite ear because of the risk of complications. These may include sudden sensorineural hearing loss if the prosthesis slips into the vestibule or if fibrosis develops at the site. Other possible complications include transient vertigo, nausea, and vomiting. Facial nerve paralysis can result from the surgery or the local anesthetic.

Purpose
To remove otosclerotic growths from the stapes and restore hearing.

Preparation
Explain to the patient that stapedectomy involves the removal of bone growth from the stapes. Also explain that the stapes' footplate and the entire stapes may also be removed. Tell him whether he'll be receiving a local or general anesthetic. Mention that improved hearing may not be evident for

several weeks after surgery since ear packing and edema may mask any initial improvement. Tell him that the doctor usually removes the packing after a week.

Tell the patient that he may experience vertigo, nausea, and vomiting after surgery but that he'll receive medication for these symptoms and for pain. Explain that he can minimize these symptoms by changing position slowly. Mention that the doctor may restrict his activity after surgery and ask him to lie in one position to keep the prosthesis from dislodging.

As ordered, prepare the patient for surgery, which may include washing his hair or shaving around the auricle. Give eardrops, ointments, irrigations, and hot or cold compresses to decrease any inflammation or relieve discomfort. Also insert ear wicks loosely into the external meatus to remove any drainage by capillary action. Before the procedure, make sure the patient has signed a consent form.

Procedure
After the patient is given a local or general anesthetic, the surgeon uses a binocular microscope to visualize the area and makes a curved incision near the eardrum. He raises the tympanomeatal flap to visualize the stapes, confirms that the stapes is immobile, and determines which procedure he'll use.

In a *total stapedectomy*, the surgeon removes the suprastructure and footplate. Then he attaches a prosthesis to the incus and covers the oval window with a graft. (See *Understanding Types of Stapedectomy*, pages 538 and 539.)

In a *partial stapedectomy*, the surgeon removes the anterior crus and anterior portion of the footplate. Or he removes the entire suprastructure, drills a hole through the footplate, and attaches a piston between the footplate and the incus.

If the surgeon is using a laser, he approaches the middle ear as for conventional stapedectomy, but then uses a laser to vaporize the tendon and pos-

UNDERSTANDING TYPES OF STAPEDECTOMY

Stapedectomy may be total or partial, depending on the extent of otosclerotic growth. It may also be performed using a variety of techniques, as shown below.

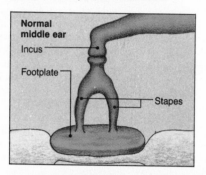

Normal middle ear

Incus

Footplate

Stapes

PARTIAL STAPEDECTOMY

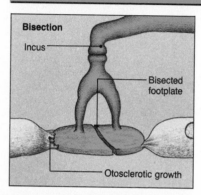

Bisection

Incus

Bisected footplate

Otosclerotic growth

TOTAL STAPEDECTOMY

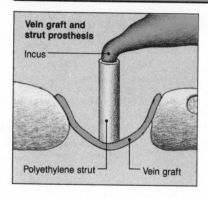

Vein graft and strut prosthesis

Incus

Polyethylene strut

Vein graft

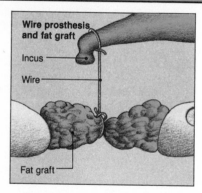

Wire prosthesis and fat graft

Incus

Wire

Fat graft

terior crus. Next, he severs the incudostapedial joint, removes the stapes, and inserts the piston with a vein graft.

After completing the surgery, the surgeon applies a dressing over the ear.

Monitoring and aftercare

After surgery, position the patient as ordered. The doctor may prefer that the patient lie on his operated ear to facilitate drainage; on his opposite ear to avoid graft displacement; or simply in the most comfortable position. Advise the patient to move slowly without bending when he changes position, to

help prevent vertigo and nausea. If he develops these symptoms anyway, administer antiemetic drugs, as ordered, and keep the bed's side rails up at all times. Help the patient when he first tries to walk, because he may feel dizzy. Keep in mind that vertigo may also indicate labyrinthitis or an inner ear reaction. Provide pain medication, as ordered.

Monitor the patient for other signs of complications, such as fever, headache, ear pain, or persistent facial nerve paralysis. If facial paralysis results from the surgery, facial nerve decompres-

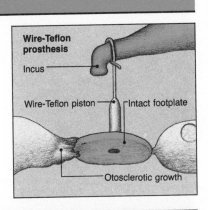

Wire-Teflon prosthesis

Incus

Wire-Teflon piston

Intact footplate

Otosclerotic growth

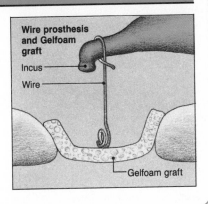

Wire prosthesis and Gelfoam graft

Incus

Wire

Gelfoam graft

sion or corticosteroid therapy may be necessary.

When you change the patient's dressings, use aseptic technique. Replace soiled or bloody pledgets in the ear canal as needed, and be sure to keep the ear dry. Tell the patient to refrain from coughing, sneezing, or blowing his nose because these actions could dislodge his prosthesis and graft.

Home care instructions
● Instruct the patient to call the doctor immediately if he develops fever, pain, changes in taste, prolonged vertigo, or a "sloshing" feeling in his ear. These signs may indicate infection or displacement of the prosthesis.
● Tell him to protect his ear from cold drafts for 1 week and to avoid contact with people who have colds, influenza, or other contagious illnesses. Explain that he should take his prescribed antibiotics and report any respiratory infection to his doctor immediately.
● Advise him to postpone washing his hair for 2 weeks. Then, for the next 4 weeks, he should avoid getting water in his ears when washing his hair.
● Instruct him not to swim for 6 weeks, unless the doctor specifically allows it.
● To avoid prosthesis dislodgment, warn him to avoid blowing his nose for at least 1 week after surgery and not to travel by airplane for 6 months.

Ethmoidectomy

The only effective treatment for chronic nasal polyps, ethmoidectomy surgically removes nasal polyps and diseased tissue from the ethmoid sinuses. It may be used when polyps recur after more conservative surgery. Typically, these polyps recur and obstruct breathing as they enlarge and prolapse into the nose.

Ethmoidectomy may also be done to treat chronic infection of the ethmoid sinus, which occurs most commonly in children and, if untreated, can lead to vision loss. As with any nasal surgery, ethmoidectomy's most common complication is bleeding.

Purpose
● To remove nasal polyps and prevent their recurrence
● To treat chronic infection of the ethmoid sinuses.

Preparation
Explain to the patient that ethmoidectomy removes nasal polyps and ethmoid tissue. If the surgery will be done

using a local anesthetic, explain to the patient that he'll hear and feel scraping and pulling during the procedure but that he won't feel any pain.

Inform the patient that nasal packing will be inserted directly after surgery to help reduce bleeding and swelling. Explain that the packing will cause him to breathe through his mouth and may give him a sensation of facial fullness but that he'll receive analgesics to reduce his discomfort. Warn him not to pull or otherwise move the packing.

Before the procedure, ensure that the patient or a responsible family member has signed a consent form.

Procedure

Depending on the patient's condition and cooperativeness, he'll receive a local or general anesthetic. Then the surgeon performs the procedure, using an external, frontal, or intranasal approach, as needed.

In an *external ethmoidectomy*, the surgeon makes a curved incision around the inner canthus of the eye, exposing the bony wall of the ethmoid area. Then he removes the ethmoid cells, diseased tissue, and the lateral wall of the nose medial to the ethmoid area. If the sphenoid sinuses are involved, he may also remove some of the sphenoidal mucosal lining.

In a *frontoethmoidectomy*, the surgeon makes a similar incision but extends it to the eyebrow, exposing portions of the frontal sinus. Then he removes the ethmoid cells and the mucosal lining of the frontal sinus. He may also remove some of the bony floor of the frontal sinus to create a pathway for drainage into the nose.

In an *intranasal ethmoidectomy*, which is typically performed under local and topical anesthesia, the surgeon fractures the middle turbinate medially toward the nasal septum, or partially removes it, to gain access to the ethmoid sinus. Then he removes the ethmoid cells and diseased tissue through the nose. Depending on the extent of disease, he may also remove the medial wall of the orbit or the floor of the frontal sinus to promote drainage into the nose.

After any of these procedures, the surgeon inserts nasal packing.

Monitoring and aftercare

After surgery, closely monitor the patient for airway obstruction because the nasal packing may become dislodged and fall into the nasal pharynx. If he begins to choke on the dislodged packing, remove it gently and promptly notify the doctor. Also be sure to watch for bleeding from his nose or in vomitus.

As ordered, administer analgesics to help relieve the patient's discomfort from the nasal packing. And because his mouth may be uncomfortably dry from mouth breathing, perform oral care every 2 hours after the anesthetic's effects wear off. Assist with gentle rinses, using tepid water and dilute mouthwash. Offer ice chips and fluids unless the patient's nauseated.

When the doctor removes the nasal packing (usually within 24 hours after surgery), encourage the patient to take regular deep breaths through his mouth. Also provide him with a basin, so he can expectorate any blood. Explain that his eyes may tear when the doctor removes the packing but that this is normal.

Home care instructions

● Tell the patient to expect some oozing of blood-tinged fluid from his nose for a day or two after surgery. However, he should report any frank, heavy bleeding or any discharge that persists for more than 3 days.
● Warn the patient to engage in quiet activities and not to blow his nose or sneeze for 10 days. If he needs to clear his nostrils, he should sniff gently. However, if he can't avoid sneezing, he should keep his mouth open.
● Advise the patient to use a laxative if he becomes constipated because straining during defecation may trigger nasal bleeding.

Caldwell-Luc Procedure

A surgical approach to the maxillary sinus, the Caldwell-Luc procedure permits visualization of the antrum, facilitates sinus drainage, and allows access to infected sinuses when an intranasal approach isn't possible because of suppuration or inflammation. It's most commonly performed to treat chronic sinusitis that's unresponsive to other treatments. In maxillary sinusitis, the most common sinus infection, the procedure includes stripping the maxillary sinus of infected mucosa to facilitate drainage. When multiple sinuses are involved, this procedure may resolve infection by draining the upper sinuses.

This procedure may also be performed to halt persistent epistaxis, to obtain a tissue sample for histologic analysis, and in conjunction with other treatments, such as ethmoidectomy. Most often performed under local anesthesia, it is usually well tolerated and causes little bleeding.

Purpose
• To treat chronic sinusitis
• To ligate the maxillary artery in persistent epistaxis
• To close an oroantral fistula resulting from dental extraction or maxillary carcinoma
• To remove nasal polyps in the ethmoid sinuses
• To obtain a tissue sample from the antrum.

Preparation
Explain the procedure to the patient, telling him that it involves a sublabial incision. Instruct him not to touch the area beneath his upper lip postoperatively. Warn him to expect considerable swelling of his cheek and numbness and tingling on his upper lip. If he wears dentures, inform him that he won't be able to wear his upper plate until the incision heals.

Explain to the patient that he may have a gauze dressing placed under his nose to absorb any drainage. If he has severe sinusitis, he may have a plastic drainage tube inserted into the antral opening for irrigation. Inform him that bleeding sometimes occurs after surgery. If it does, the doctor will lightly pack the maxillary sinus, extending the packing through the patient's nose.

Make sure the patient has signed a consent form.

Procedure
After the patient receives an anesthetic, the surgeon incises the mouth at the junction of the buccal and alveolar mucosa. He retracts the periosteum to expose the fossa above the upper canine teeth. Then he incises the antrum wall. If the patient has sinusitis, he'll strip the diseased sinus lining and make an opening between the nose and the antrum to improve drainage (an intranasal antrostomy). If the patient has an antral lesion, the surgeon will take a tissue sample for histologic analysis and leave the maxillary mucosa intact.

If the patient has persistent epistaxis, the surgeon will remove part of the posterior sinus wall, exposing the internal maxillary artery. Then he'll ligate the artery.

The surgeon may suture the incision loosely; however, it's usually left to heal by itself. If bleeding occurs, he may pack the maxillary sinus.

Monitoring and aftercare
Right after surgery, check for facial edema and advise the patient to report any untoward symptoms, such as paresthesias of his upper lip. Explain that these symptoms usually resolve in a few days. (Occasionally, upper lip sensation may be permanently diminished.) If the patient has packing in place, explain that the doctor will remove it within 48 hours. If he has a drainage tube in place for irrigation, assist with

ANTRAL PUNCTURE AND LAVAGE: ALTERNATIVE TREATMENT FOR SINUS INFECTION

Used as an alternative to the Caldwell-Luc procedure, antral puncture and lavage is a conservative treatment for sinus infection. After the patient receives local and topical anesthetics, the doctor inserts a trochar and a cannula through the patient's nostril under the inferior turbinate, passing through the nose's thin lateral wall into the antrum. Then he irrigates the sinus through the cannula with about 500 ml of normal saline solution. As the patient sits with his head bent over a basin, the irrigation washes out infectious material, soothing inflamed mucosa and facilitating drainage.

Calming the patient's fears

Before antral puncture and lavage, you'll need to reassure the patient by explaining the procedure and describing the brief sound he'll hear and the pressure he'll feel as his nasal wall is punctured. Be sure to emphasize that he'll feel no pain. During the procedure, as the patient hangs his head over the basin, advise him to breathe slowly through his mouth. If he needs bilateral irrigation, provide emotional support before the doctor repeats the procedure on the opposite side. When the irrigation is complete, give the patient a mouthwash and ask him to gently rinse his mouth.

irrigation and tell him that the tube will be removed in 3 to 4 days.

Assess the patient's mouth frequently. Although bleeding doesn't normally occur after the procedure, check anyway for bright red blood at the back of the throat and in any drainage or emesis. Remind the patient not to touch the incision with his tongue or finger. If he wears dentures, instruct him not to insert his upper plate. Also caution him not to brush his teeth, but rather to rinse his mouth gently with tepid saline solution or dilute mouthwash.

Start the patient on fluids 4 hours after surgery, unless he's nauseated. Progress to a full soft diet, as ordered. Until the incision heals, avoid giving foods that require thorough chewing.

Home care instructions

• Tell the patient to expect some drainage from his nose for a few days after surgery. Instruct him to monitor its amount, color, and odor. Advise him to call the doctor if he notices any bleeding or foul smell or if drainage persists for more than 5 days.
• Instruct the patient to cleanse his teeth with gauze pads wrapped around his finger, supplemented by gentle mouthwashes.
• Warn him not to rub or bump his incision. Explain that he should plan menus for the next 2 weeks that don't require much chewing, to avoid injuring the incision. If he wears dentures, he shouldn't insert the upper plate for 2 weeks.
• Tell the patient not to engage in vigorous activity or blow his nose forcefully for 2 weeks. If he needs to clear his nostrils, he should sniff gently.

Rhinoplasty and Septoplasty

Whether performed independently or together, these surgical procedures treat deformities of the nose. Rhinoplasty changes the nose's external appearance, correcting congenital or traumatic deformity. Septoplasty corrects a deviated septum, preventing nasal obstruction, thick discharge, and secondary pharyngeal, sinus, and ear problems. Usually, they're performed using local and topical anesthetics. Although they're generally well tolerated, they may cause swelling, nasal bleeding and hemorrhage, and septal hematoma. Other possible complications include nasal skin necrosis, infection, and septal perforation.

Purpose
- *For rhinoplasty:* to correct deformity and enhance the nose's appearance
- *For septoplasty:* to correct a deviated septum and restore easy breathing.

Preparation
Reinforce the surgeon's explanation of the planned procedure. In rhinoplasty, the surgeon will explain the extent of the procedure and how the nose should look postoperatively. Emphasize that changes may not be evident for up to several months. Point out that the facial swelling accompanying this surgery should subside in 3 to 4 weeks. Also tell the patient that he'll be awake during the surgery but will feel no pain.

For both rhinoplasty and septoplasty, tell the patient to expect nasal packing after surgery and that this, along with swelling, may give him an uncomfortable sensation of facial fullness. Warn him against trying to relieve this by manipulating the packing.

Ensure that the patient has signed a consent form.

Procedure
In both procedures, the patient receives topical and local anesthetics. In *rhinoplasty*, the surgeon fractures the nasal bones, removes excess tissue, and then repositions the bones. He makes an incision in the groove between the upper and lower nasal cartilages and trims the soft tissue to reshape the tip of the nose. He may also insert a cartilage implant to bolster a saddle-bridge or retracted columella.

In *septoplasty*, the surgeon makes an incision inside the nose past the mucocutaneous junction. He separates the perichondrium from the cartilage and septal bone and cuts the deviated cartilage into pieces or incises and repositions it midline. Alternatively, in a procedure known as submucous resection, he removes the cartilage entirely except for a small wedge that supports the nose.

After either procedure, the doctor may insert nasal packing.

Monitoring and aftercare
If the patient has nasal packing in place, watch closely to make sure the packing doesn't slip and obstruct the airway. At first, assess airway patency every hour and frequently check the nasal pack's position. If the patient becomes restless or starts to choke, notify the doctor—the nasal pack may have slipped. If needed, provide analgesics, as ordered, to relieve headache. Tell the patient that the doctor will remove the packing 24 to 48 hours after surgery.

Monitor vital signs and observe for hemorrhage, which may be immediate or delayed. Keep the patient on his side to prevent inhalation of blood, and periodically examine the back of his throat for fresh blood. Also check any sputum or emesis for bleeding.

Watch for signs of infection, especially if the patient is debilitated or has had an implant. Also watch for and report signs of septal perforation: crusting and bleeding from the edge of the perforation and a whistling sound when the patient breathes. The doctor may treat the perforation by enlarging the opening or by placing a Silastic septal button in the perforation.

Help the patient rinse his mouth every 2 to 4 hours, and give him ice chips as needed. Offer fluids 4 hours after surgery and expect the patient to be able to resume his normal diet the next day.

Home care instructions
- After the nasal packing is removed, instruct the patient not to blow his nose for at least 10 days because this may precipitate bleeding. If he needs to clear his nose, tell him to sniff gently.
- If the patient has a bandage or an external splint in place, tell him not to manipulate it because he may cause misalignment or stimulate bleeding.
- If the doctor prescribes inhalation treatments to reduce swelling and prevent crusting, instruct the patient to place a bowl of hot water before him and to drape a towel over his head, creating a type of tent. Then he should

breathe in the warmed air.

• If the doctor prescribes nose drops, tell the patient how to administer them: he should lie flat on his back, instill the drops, and remain supine for 5 minutes to facilitate absorption by swollen tissues. Then he should turn his head from side to side for 30 seconds to distribute the drops inside his nose.

Tonsillectomy and Adenoidectomy

Tonsillectomy—the surgical removal of the palatine tonsils—and adenoidectomy—the surgical removal of the pharyngeal tonsils—were once routinely performed for enlarged tonsils and adenoids. Often combined and performed as an adenotonsillectomy, these procedures aren't as commonly used today. Instead, antibiotics are prescribed to treat tonsils and adenoids enlarged by bacterial infection. However, either or both of these surgeries may be indicated when tonsillar tissue enlarges sufficiently to obstruct the upper airway, causing hypoxia or sleep apnea. Tonsillectomy is also the preferred treatment for peritonsillar abscess. What's more, it may be indicated in chronic tonsillitis that results in more than seven acute attacks within 2 years. Adenoidectomy may be performed to prevent recurrent otitis media, although some experts dispute its effectiveness.

Tonsillectomy is most commonly performed in children, but it isn't advised for those under age 3. Adenoidectomy is performed almost exclusively in children because adenoid tissue usually atrophies after adolescence. The most serious complication of these surgeries is hemorrhage, which may occur within 24 hours after surgery or up to 7 to 10 days later, when the membrane formed at the operative site begins to slough off.

Adenoidectomy is contraindicated in cleft palate because the procedure allows air to escape through the nose, creating severe speech problems. Both procedures are contraindicated in recent upper respiratory infections and in bleeding disorders.

Purpose
To remove the palatine or pharyngeal tonsils, preventing hypoxia, sleep apnea, or chronic tonsillitis.

Preparation
Determine if the patient has a bleeding disorder or any recent upper respiratory tract infection. Both of these conditions may contraindicate surgery.

Explain the planned surgery to the child and his parents, and answer any questions they may have. If the child is scheduled for an adenoidectomy, evaluate whether he has nasal speech or difficulty articulating. If you note these, arrange for an evaluation by a speech therapist.

For either procedure, make sure the parents have signed a consent form.

Procedure
In a *tonsillectomy*, a child typically receives a general anesthetic. (An adult patient may receive a local anesthetic.) After the anesthetic takes effect, the surgeon removes tonsillar tissue by dissection and snare.

In an *adenoidectomy* or *adenotonsillectomy*, the child receives a general anesthetic. Adenoidectomy is usually performed before tonsillectomy. With the child in Rose's position (his head tilted far back), the surgeon removes adenoidal tissue with a gentle, sweeping motion. If necessary, he then removes tonsillar tissue.

Monitoring and aftercare
While the child is recovering from the effects of anesthesia, place him on his side to prevent aspiration of blood and slightly elevate the head of his bed. Monitor vital signs closely for 24 hours and watch for hemorrhage. Use a flash-

light to check the throat and assess for bleeding—remember, blood can seep down the back of his throat. Pay special attention to frequent swallowing; it may indicate excessive bleeding.

As the child becomes more alert, offer fluids. Start with ice chips, progressing to tepid water, clear liquids, and eventually full liquids. Take care not to dislodge clots: make sure the child doesn't place straws or other utensils in his mouth. When ordered, start the child on soft foods.

To help prevent excessive bleeding, don't give aspirin or aspirin-containing products. Instead, give mild analgesics, such as acetaminophen, as ordered. Expect some vomiting; even coffee-ground emesis is normal—the result of swallowed blood. However, notify the doctor if you see bright red blood; this indicates that vomiting has induced bleeding at the operative site.

If the child complains of a sore throat, provide cool compresses or an ice collar.

Home care instructions

• Instruct the parents to report any bleeding immediately. Mention that the child's especially at risk 7 to 10 days after surgery, when the membrane formed at the operative site begins to slough off. Ensure that they understand to feed him only liquids and soft foods for 1 to 2 weeks to avoid dislodging clots or precipitating bleeding.
• Inform the parents that the child will have some minor discomfort, such as ear pain (especially on swallowing), a sore throat, and voice changes for 1 to 2 weeks after surgery. Advise giving him at least 1 to 2 quarts of soothing fluids daily, avoiding such liquids as carbonated beverages.
• Tell the parents that the child can brush his teeth gently. However, he should avoid vigorous brushing, gargling, and irritating mouthwashes for several weeks.
• Warn them to avoid giving the child aspirin or aspirin-containing preparations because these may precipitate

bleeding. Advise them to treat any fever with acetaminophen and to notify the doctor if fever doesn't resolve within 24 hours.
• Instruct the parents to have the child avoid vigorous activity for 3 days after discharge. A child may usually return to school after 10 to 14 days. Also stress that he should avoid exposure to persons with colds or other contagious illnesses for at least 2 weeks.

Laryngectomy

The removal of all or part of the larynx, laryngectomy is most commonly performed to treat laryngeal cancer. The type and site of the tumor, the extent and location of metastases, and vocal cord mobility determine the specific procedure used. (Laryngoscopy, which requires no incision, may be used to remove a localized glottic tumor. It doesn't affect the voice and usually causes no other complications.)

Laryngofissure may be used to remove a glottic tumor limited to one vocal cord. However, radiation is now replacing this procedure since both treatments have similar survival rates but radiation leaves the patient with a better voice. More widespread tumors may require a *vertical hemilaryngectomy* or a *horizontal supraglottic laryngectomy*. For a large glottic or supraglottic tumor with vocal cord fixation, a *total laryngectomy* may be needed.

The prognosis after laryngectomy, though generally good, reflects the extent of the disease at the time of surgery. After laryngectomy and radiation treatments, the 5-year survival rate is 80% to 90% for lesions without vocal cord fixation; 75% for tumors with cord fixation; and 50% for tumors with metastases to the cervical lymph nodes.

Many complications can result from laryngectomy. Immediately after surgery, respiratory distress or, rarely,

UNDERSTANDING TYPES OF LARYNGECTOMY

Although laryngoscopic surgery may be used to remove an early localized glottic tumor, other techniques must be used to excise more widespread tumors. These include total laryngectomy, horizontal supraglottic laryngectomy, vertical hemilaryngectomy, and laryngofissure.

Total laryngectomy

Used to excise a large glottic or supraglottic tumor with vocal cord fixation, this procedure involves removal of the true vocal cords, false vocal cords, epiglottis, hyoid bone, cricoid cartilage, and two or three rings of the trachea. Neighboring areas may also be removed, depending on the extent of the tumor. A permanent tracheostomy is performed, creating a laryngeal stoma that leaves the patient without speech.

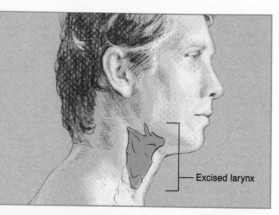

Excised larynx

Horizontal supraglottic laryngectomy

Performed to remove a large supraglottic tumor, this procedure excises the top of the larynx (the epiglottis, the hyoid bone, and the false vocal cords), leaving the true vocal cords intact. Although there's no laryngectomy stoma, a temporary tracheostomy may be performed to ensure a patent airway until edema subsides. The patient's voice is unaffected, but removal of the epiglottis may cause swallowing difficulty.

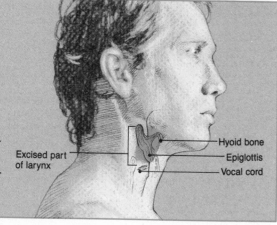

Excised part of larynx

Hyoid bone
Epiglottis
Vocal cord

bleeding into the wound or hematoma formation may occur. Later complications include pneumonia, atelectasis, and pharyngeal fistula.

Purpose

To remove a laryngeal tumor.

Preparation

Not only will you have to prepare the patient for surgery but you'll also have to prepare him and his family for the dramatic impact laryngectomy will have on their life-style. Begin by describing the surgery and its aftercare in detail, and answer any questions they may have. Explain the expected voice quality and extent of speech.

If the patient will be having a total laryngectomy, explain that he'll breathe through an opening in his neck after surgery. Inform him that he won't be

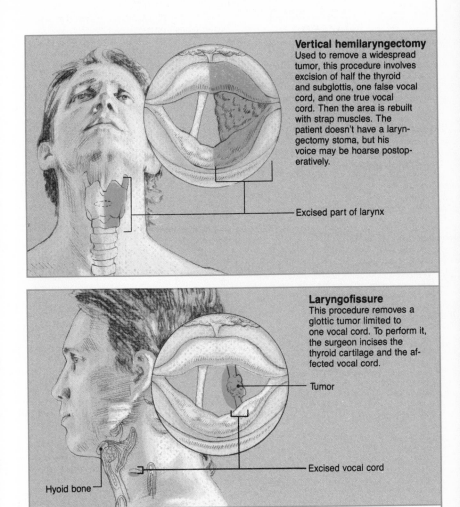

Vertical hemilaryngectomy
Used to remove a widespread tumor, this procedure involves excision of half the thyroid and subglottis, one false vocal cord, and one true vocal cord. Then the area is rebuilt with strap muscles. The patient doesn't have a laryngectomy stoma, but his voice may be hoarse postoperatively.

Excised part of larynx

Laryngofissure
This procedure removes a glottic tumor limited to one vocal cord. To perform it, the surgeon incises the thyroid cartilage and the affected vocal cord.

Tumor

Excised vocal cord

Hyoid bone

able to smell, blow his nose, whistle, gargle, sip, or suck on a straw after surgery. Describe the laryngectomy stoma and show him pictures. Explain that he'll expectorate secretions through his stoma; they'll need suctioning periodically. Emphasize that he'll be able to perform stoma care and suction himself. If possible, arrange a meeting with a laryngectomee who has adjusted well to having a stoma.

If the patient will be unable to speak after surgery, suggest a communication system, such as flash cards, paper and pencil, or a magic slate. Also coordinate visits by a speech pathologist, who will evaluate the patient, reinforce earlier information, and answer questions about reestablishing speech.

Inform the patient that he may have a laryngectomy tube after surgery (shorter and thicker than a tracheos-

COMPLICATIONS

RECOGNIZING HAZARDS OF LARYNGECTOMY

Immediately after a laryngectomy, you'll need to monitor the patient closely for bleeding and signs of respiratory distress. But you'll also need to be alert for later complications.

Pneumonia and atelectasis

To detect these respiratory complications, monitor the patient's breath sounds and temperature. Stress the importance of frequent turning, coughing, and deep breathing. If the patient has a tracheostomy, suction regularly until he can do it himself.

Wound infection

Watch for tissue necrosis and drainage, and monitor the patient's temperature. Report signs of infection to the doctor, who may order additional drains and antibiotics.

Pharyngeal fistula

Suspect this major complication if you note secretions leaking from the wound about 10 days after surgery. Notify the doctor immediately and discontinue oral feedings, administer antibiotics, and assist with drain insertion.

Hemorrhage

The carotid artery may rupture 8 to 20 days after a wound infection begins or sooner as a result of surgical injury or weakening from preoperative radiation. Watch for a bright red stain on the wound's margin or for signs of bleeding in necrotic tissue. If you detect bleeding, notify the doctor immediately, apply pressure, and call for help. Don't leave the patient unattended.

tomy tube but requiring the same care) and that it's usually removed after 7 to 10 days. Explain that he'll also have a nasogastric tube in place for 7 to 10 days; this will provide a route for nourishment until his suture line heals. Mention that he'll begin receiving oral feedings (thick, easy-to-swallow fluids,

such as Jell-O or ice cream) about 10 days after his surgery.

Before a laryngectomy, make sure the patient has signed a consent form.

Procedure

After the patient receives a general anesthetic, the surgeon removes the diseased vocal cord, a part of the larynx, or the entire vocal cords, larynx, and thyroid cartilage. (See *Understanding Types of Laryngectomy*, pages 546 and 547.)

Monitoring and aftercare

After surgery, keep emergency resuscitation equipment readily available. Elevate the head of the bed 30 degrees to prevent tension on the incision line, decrease neck edema, and prevent aspiration during feeding. Be sure to support the patient's head, neck, and back for 24 to 48 hours.

Periodically auscultate the patient's lungs to detect any pulmonary congestion. Also check the rate and depth of his respirations and observe for accessory muscle use. If the patient has a tracheostomy tube, suction it gently, as ordered, using sterile technique. Provide humidification. If the patient experiences respiratory difficulty, notify the doctor immediately.

For 8 hours after surgery, check the incision site hourly for bleeding or signs of hematoma formation (swelling or bulging of the stoma under the skin flap). Report any abnormalities. Perform tracheostomy care every 8 hours or as needed, and check the site for signs of infection. If neck drains are in place, ensure their patency.

As ordered, give I.V. fluids and nasogastric tube feedings, and monitor intake and output. If the patient experiences discomfort, give analgesics and sedatives, as ordered, through the nasogastric tube or I.V. line. Keep in mind, though, that narcotics depress respirations and inhibit coughing.

To help relieve the patient's anxiety, use the communication system you developed before surgery. If he has had a partial laryngectomy, tell him not to use his voice until the doctor gives permission. Reassure him that speech rehabilitation will enable him to speak again.

Home care instructions
• Begin patient teaching as soon as possible, since the patient must know how to care for himself before discharge. Call the visiting nurse association to arrange help for the patient at home and, if possible, have one of the nurses attend the teaching sessions. If the patient has had a total laryngectomy, explain that a speech pathologist will work closely with him.
• If appropriate, teach the patient how to perform tracheostomy care using clean technique. Instruct him to clean the inner cannula of his tube with hydrogen peroxide and water daily to help maintain a patent airway and prevent infection. Explain that he must suction the outer cannula to keep his airway patent when he feels congested, when his breathing sounds raspy or wheezy, or when excess mucus forms. Also, tell him to watch for bloody secretions, which may indicate local trauma. Finally, have him demonstrate correct cleaning and suctioning techniques.
• Emphasize the importance of daily stoma care, using warm water, to maintain a patent airway, promote healing, and prevent infection. Warn him not to use tissues, loose cotton, or soap during cleaning because these may get in his airway. Tell him to wear a bib or dressing over his stoma to act as a filter and to warm incoming air. Also instruct him to avoid swimming and getting water in his stoma. Mention that he'll need to humidify his home, especially during the winter.
• Instruct him to notify the doctor if he develops symptoms of a respiratory infection, such as fever, cough, yellow or green drainage from the stoma, or erythema around the stoma.
• Stress the importance of keeping follow-up medical appointments to monitor for recurrence of cancer.

• Provide emotional support and help the patient adjust to his new self-image. Suggest that he contact the International Association of Laryngectomees.

Radical Neck Dissection

Performed alone or with other major head and neck surgery, radical neck dissection removes the cervical chain of lymph nodes, the sternomastoid muscle, the fascia, and the internal jugular vein. Because many head and neck tumors eventually metastasize to the cervical lymph nodes, this treatment is indicated if the cervical lymph nodes are palpable or if metastasis to the nodes is suspected. This surgery is also indicated if a primary lesion appears in the neck or in an area with a high incidence of neck metastasis or if metastasis occurs on one or both sides of the neck after laryngectomy.

Radical neck dissection can cause disfigurement as well as severe complications, such as shoulder weakness and drop and carotid artery rupture. Shoulder weakness and drop may result from severing of the spinal accessory nerve that innervates the trapezius muscle and from removal of the sternomastoid muscle. Life-threatening carotid artery rupture may result from removal of the muscle and fascia that previously covered and protected the artery. Although a dermal graft or muscle pedicle graft may be used to protect this area, the carotid artery may rupture anyway if a pharyngeal fistula, an infection, or necrosis develops.

Purpose
To prevent or treat metastasis to the cervical lymph nodes.

Preparation
If the patient is scheduled for a total laryngectomy along with a radical neck

dissection, discuss the procedure with him and tell him that he'll have a stoma after surgery. (See "Laryngectomy," page 545.) Explain that he'll also have neck drains in place after surgery and that he won't be able to speak while his tracheostomy tube's in place. Establish a communication system with him, using flash cards, paper and pencil, or a magic slate. If surgery will leave him without speech, arrange a consultation with a speech therapist.

Encourage the patient to express his fears about cancer, the surgery, and his prognosis, and answer any questions he may have. Because radical neck dissection causes major disfigurement, you'll need to provide strong emotional support. And you'll need to help mobilize the resources—family members, rehabilitation services, and support groups—that will provide sustenance and care for the patient after his discharge.

Before the surgery, make sure the patient has signed a consent form.

Procedure

After the patient receives a general anesthetic, the surgeon makes large incisions in the neck, unfolding skin flaps that allow access to the involved area. He then removes muscle and fascia anterior to the prevertebral fascia, including the cervical chain of lymph nodes, the internal jugular vein, and the sternomastoid muscle. He also severs the spinal accessory nerve but spares the carotid artery and the vagus nerve. If necessary, he performs a laryngectomy.

Next, the surgeon inserts drains, carefully positions the skin flaps over the dissected area, and sutures them to ensure a good blood supply. Finally, he applies a dressing to the patient's neck.

Monitoring and aftercare

When the patient returns to his room, elevate the head of his bed 30 to 45 degrees to reduce tension on the suture line and decrease edema. Also, monitor respiratory rate and depth, and check for accessory muscle use. Report dyspnea or increasing edema to the doctor.

If the patient has a tracheostomy tube, provide tracheostomy care every 4 hours. Also, observe skin flap color and report any hematoma formation at the suture line. Make sure the patient's neck drains are patent. (Usually, they're connected to a closed drainage system.) Monitor the amount and character of the drainage.

Report any pulmonary congestion and suction the patient orally or through his tracheostomy tube, as ordered. To avoid disrupting the incision line, suction gently. When the patient changes position, support his head and neck because removal of the sternomastoid muscle renders him unable to support his head on his own. To find out how the patient feels, use the communication system you've established. If he needs analgesics, give them as ordered, but remember that narcotics depress respirations and inhibit coughing.

Assess the patient's incision for redness, swelling, drainage, and other signs of infection. Monitor for skin flap necrosis, which may occur if the surgeon was unable to save enough blood vessels to adequately nourish the flap. Keep in mind that if necrosis affects the carotid artery wall, massive hemorrhage can result. A hemorrhage can also occur 8 to 20 days after a wound infection begins or sooner as the result of surgical injury or weakening of the artery from preoperative radiation. Watch for a bright red stain on the wound's margin or for signs of bleeding in necrotic tissue. If hemorrhage occurs, apply pressure, stay with the patient, and call for help.

Home care instructions
● Inform the patient that he may experience shoulder discomfort for months after the surgery. Instruct him to use heat and massage to relieve discomfort.
● Explain that surgery severed the nerve in one of his shoulder muscles

STRENGTHENING EXERCISES FOR YOUR NECK AND SHOULDER

Dear Patient:

After your neck incision is sufficiently healed and your doctor has given permission, you can start doing the exercises described below. Perform them each morning and evening. At first, do each exercise once. Then, as your strength increases, repeat each exercise one at a time until you can do each one 10 times. If an exercise tires you, rest before beginning the next one.

Exercising your neck
Do these exercises to help you regain maximum neck function.

1
Turn your head as far to the right as possible and then as far to the left as possible.

2
Tilt your head to the right and then to the left; to the front and then to the back.

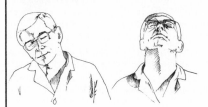

Exercising your shoulder
These exercises will help restore muscle function in your shoulder.

1
Place the hand of your unaffected arm on a flat surface, such as a stool, for support. Let your affected (free) arm hang loosely. Gradually swing your affected arm up and back as far as possible without discomfort. Work toward executing a complete circle—each day, try to move your arm a little more.

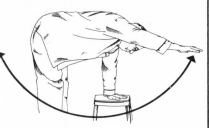

2
Stand facing a wall, and place the fingertips of the hand on your affected side on the wall. Then climb the wall with your fingertips as high as possible without discomfort—each day, try to climb a little higher.

and removed some muscle, causing weakness. Caution him not to lie on the affected side and not to lift more than 2 lb with that arm. Teach him exercises that will allow him to regain mobility. (See *Strengthening Exercises for Your Neck and Shoulder*, page 551.) However, caution him not to perform these exercises until his neck incision has healed and his doctor has given permission.

• If the patient has also had a laryngectomy, teach him stoma and tracheostomy care and arrange for visits by a speech therapist.

• Emphasize the importance of keeping follow-up doctor's appointments to monitor for possible recurrence of cancer.

• Provide the patient and his family with information about counseling and membership in a support group.

MISCELLANEOUS TREATMENTS

Hearing Aids

Powered by a replaceable battery, a hearing aid consists of a microphone, an amplifier, a receiver, and an ear mold. The microphone picks up sound and converts it to electrical energy. The amplifier magnifies this energy electronically and the receiver converts it back to sound waves, which the ear mold directs into the patient's ear.

Four types of hearing aid are commonly available: behind-the-ear, eyeglass, in-the-ear, and body aids. A *behind-the-ear aid*, the most commonly used type, consists of a short curved plastic tube that connects the unit (which rests behind the ear) to an acrylic ear mold. In an *eyeglass aid*, a similar unit, the components are contained in an eyeglass temple. An *in-the-ear aid*, the most compact device, consists of one piece fashioned like an ear mold, which houses the microphone, amplifier, and receiver. A *body aid*, most suitable for the patient with severe or profound hearing loss or with limited manual dexterity, has a larger microphone, amplifier, and power supply than the other types of aid and produces less distortion. It's built into a case that can be clipped to the patient's pocket or worn on his body. A long wire connects the unit to an ear mold.

A bone-conduction aid, which delivers sound waves to the mastoid process, may be used when an acrylic mold can't be inserted into the patient's ear. This aid comes in all styles, including the eyeglass type.

Although largely beneficial, hearing aids have a few disadvantages. For example, body aids pick up the sound of the patient's clothing rubbing against his body. Behind-the-ear aids eliminate this problem, but they're less durable and more prone to acoustic feedback. What's more, any hearing aid requires a period of adjustment since the patient may hear background noises that he hasn't heard in years.

Purpose
To amplify sound for the hearing-impaired patient.

Preparation
After an audiologist describes the hearing aid and its operation to the patient, reinforce this explanation to the patient. Point out that the device will improve his hearing but that he'll need time to adjust to amplification. Initially, he may find background noise, such as traffic or the chirping of birds, annoying. Encourage him to wear the hearing aid, to keep it turned on, and to use the prescribed setting.

Procedure
Typically, an audiologist administers hearing tests, such as pure tone and speech audiometry, to determine the type and extent of the patient's hearing

loss. Then, based on these results and on the patient's age, dexterity, preference, and prospect of compliance, the audiologist selects a hearing aid. Next, the audiologist or hearing aid dealer makes an ear mold and fits the patient with the appropriate aid.

Monitoring and aftercare
After the patient is fitted with a hearing aid, explain that adjustment to it may take up to 6 months. Encourage him to wear the aid every day and to gradually increase the degree of amplification, if necessary.

Home care instructions
• Teach the patient's family to help him adjust to his hearing aid. Instruct them to be patient, to speak in a normal voice, and not to equate hearing impairment with feeblemindedness. They should get the patient's attention before speaking and, if possible, eliminate background noise, such as TV or radio noise. They should repeat messages, if necessary, and reword them.
• Tell the patient how to use the hearing aid's on/off switch and volume control and how to change the battery.
• Instruct him to store the aid in a dry place when he's not using it and to avoid getting it wet. Have him inspect the unit daily for a cracked case, corroded battery contacts, frayed wires, or an occluded ear mold. Unless he has an in-the-ear aid, tell him that he can clean the ear mold with warm, soapy water after he has disconnected it from the unit. Warn against using hairspray when wearing the aid because this may damage the microphone. Also warn him not to stick sharp objects, such as a needle or pencil point, into the unit. If he suspects that the unit's malfunctioning, he should contact the audiologist or hearing aid dealer.
• Tell the patient about organizations that offer help for the hearing-impaired, such as the Alexander Graham Bell Association for the Deaf. Also help him obtain additional devices, such as a loop system to allow him to hear television more clearly, a coupler for his telephone to improve clarity, and a battery tester.

Nasal Packing

When direct pressure or cautery fails to stop severe epistaxis, nasal packing may be used. An anterior pack consists of a strip of petrolatum or iodoform gauze layered horizontally in the anterior nostrils, usually near the turbinates. A posterior pack consists of a rolled gauze pack secured with strong silk sutures and inserted into the nasopharynx. The loose ends of the sutures, brought through the nostrils, provide traction against the bleeding vessels. Insertion of a posterior pack requires sedation and hospitalization. Alternative methods to control posterior epistaxis include insertion of Foley or nasal balloon catheters. (See *Understanding Nasal Balloon Catheters*, page 554.)

Possible complications of nasal packing include hypoxia and shock from blood loss and respiratory compromise. In the sedated patient with posterior packing, aspiration and airway obstruction may also occur. Less frequent complications include sinusitis, otitis media, and pressure necrosis.

Purpose
To control severe epistaxis that's uncontrolled by other treatments.

Preparation
Explain the procedure to the patient, and inform him that he'll have the pack in place for several days. If he's to have a posterior pack, inform him that he'll have to cooperate with the doctor to ease the passage of the catheter. Also explain that he'll have to breathe through his mouth, which will make his mouth dry, but that you'll provide mouthwashes to relieve this. Mention that pain medication will be available

UNDERSTANDING NASAL BALLOON CATHETERS

To control posterior epistaxis, the doctor may use a nasal balloon catheter instead of posterior nasal packing. These catheters are self-retaining and disposable and can be either single- or double-cuffed. The single-cuffed catheter consists of a cuff that, when inflated, compresses the blood vessels and a soft, collapsible outside bulb that prevents the catheter from slipping out of place posteriorly.

The double-cuffed catheter consists of a posterior cuff that, when inflated, secures the catheter in the nasopharynx; an anterior cuff that, when inflated, compresses the blood vessels; and a central airway that helps the patient breathe more comfortably. Each cuff is inflated independently.

Before insertion, the doctor lubricates the catheter with an antibiotic ointment and inserts it through the patient's nostril. He then inflates the balloon by inserting

sterile saline solution into the appropriate valve. (If a double-cuffed catheter is used, the doctor will inflate the posterior cuff first.) He may secure the catheter by taping its anterior tip to the outside of the patient's nose.

To remove the catheter, the doctor deflates the balloon by inserting the hub of a syringe deeply into the valve and withdrawing the solution. He then gently withdraws the catheter from the nostril.

Check the placement of these catheters routinely. With a double-cuffed catheter, you may clean the central airway with a small-gauge suction catheter to remove clots or secretions. The doctor may want to deflate the cuff for 10 minutes every 24 hours to prevent damage to the patient's nasal mucosa. Expect to find a small amount of discharge around the catheter each day.

**SINGLE-CUFFED CATHETER
INFLATED IN PLACE**

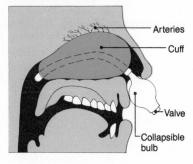

Arteries
Cuff
Valve
Collapsible bulb

**DOUBLE-CUFFED CATHETER
INFLATED IN PLACE**

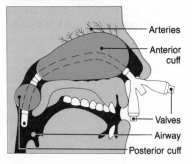

Arteries
Anterior cuff
Valves
Airway
Posterior cuff

to relieve the headache that often accompanies nasal packing. If the patient will be sedated, explain the routine preoperative and postoperative procedures.

Prepare to assist the doctor as directed. Gather the necessary equipment and prepare the patient as ordered. If he's to be sedated, administer the ordered sedative or tranquilizer.

Procedure

To begin, have the patient lean forward to prevent blood from draining into his throat. Monitor his vital signs and watch for impending hypovolemic

shock from blood loss. The doctor anesthetizes the patient's nasal passages with a vasoconstrictive agent, which may help control the bleeding. Then, as soon as the anesthetic takes effect, he suctions the patient's nose to remove any clots and locate the bleeding site.

If bleeding is from the anterior nose, the doctor uses forceps to layer petrolatum or iodoform gauze strips horizontally in the nose. Horizontal layers ensure uniform packing and prevent displacement of the pack into the patient's throat. The doctor leaves one end of the gauze at the tip of the nostril to allow easy removal of the packing.

If bleeding is from the posterior nose, the doctor inserts a lubricated catheter into the nose and advances it into the nasopharynx. To minimize gagging, tell the patient to pant during this procedure. When the catheter appears in the nasopharynx, the doctor pulls it out through the mouth and secures it to the sutures of the posterior pack. Then he withdraws the catheter through the nose, pulling the pack into its proper position behind the soft palate and against the posterior part of the septum. He checks to make sure the uvula is free of the packing and then detaches the catheter from the packing, securing the pack with tape and dental rolls.

Monitoring and aftercare

After nasal packing, watch for signs and symptoms of hypoxia, such as tachycardia, confusion, and restlessness. Check arterial blood gases, as ordered, and monitor the patient's pulse and blood pressure. Keep emergency equipment (flashlight, scissors, and hemostat) at the patient's bedside, and place a call bell within his reach. If he has a posterior pack, check its placement frequently, and remove it immediately if it's visible at the back of his throat and he appears to be choking. Avoid tension on the sutures taped in place, because this may dislodge the posterior pack.

Monitor blood loss to help detect impending hypovolemia. Note the amount of bleeding on the dental rolls, and have the patient report any fresh blood in the back of his throat or blood he spits out. Also monitor fluid status. Note the patient's intake and output, and maintain an I.V. line if one is in place. Check the oral mucosa and skin turgor for signs of dehydration, and instruct the patient to report any nausea and vomiting.

Offer mouthwashes or ice chips to keep the patient's mouth moist, and provide sedation as ordered. If he develops a headache, provide analgesics as ordered. Also monitor his temperature—fever may indicate infection.

Home care instructions

● When the nasal packs have been removed and the patient is ready for discharge, instruct him to avoid blowing his nose for 2 to 3 days, because this may precipitate bleeding. Inform him that he can expect slight oozing of blood-stained fluid from his nose for the next few days but that he should report any frank bleeding.

● Teach the patient how to use a steam inhaler at home to help prevent crusting inside the nose. Suggest using menthol and eucalyptus in the steam inhaler for a more soothing effect. Explain that he can start using the inhaler 6 hours after the packing is removed.

Selected References

Farb, S. *Otorhinolaryngology*, 3rd ed. New Hyde Park, N.Y.: Medical Examination Pub. Co., 1983.

Fujita, Shiro. "UPPP for Sleep Apnea and Snoring," *Ear, Nose and Throat Journal* 63(5):227-35, May 1984.

Holt, R., et al. *Decision Making in Otolaryngology: Head and Neck Surgery*. St. Louis: C.V. Mosby Co., 1983.

Innes, A., and Gates, N., *ENT Surgery and Disorders with Notes on Nursing Care and Clinical Management*. London: Faber & Faber, 1985.

Katz, A., ed. *Manual of Otolaryngology: Head and Neck Therapeutics*. Philadelphia: Lea & Febiger, 1986.

Raymond C.A. "Popular, Yes, But Jury Still Out on Apnea Surgery," *JAMA* 256(4):439-41, July 25, 1986.

Saunders W., et al. *Nursing Care in Eye, Ear, Nose and Throat Disorders*, 4th ed. St Louis: C.V. Mosby Co., 1979.

Yanagisawa, E., et al. *The Surgical Atlas of Otology and Neuro-Otology*. Edited by Lee, K. New York: Grune & Stratton, 1983.

17

Treating Skin Dysfunction

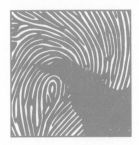

Treating Skin Dysfunction

Introduction

The skin is the largest organ of the body—and, in many ways, it's the most abused. It bears the brunt of contact with the world, making it prone to a host of ailments: burns, infections, irritation, ulcers, trauma, and cancer.

Fortunately, skin possesses some impressive qualities. It's tough yet flexible. It regenerates quickly. It can be stretched, if necessary, to cover a defect or harvested from one part of the body and grafted to another.

Hands-on health care
In addition, it's accessible. That means the treatment of skin disorders is usually a quite literal example of hands-on health care. Most medications are applied topically; surgery is usually performed with only a local anesthetic; monitoring depends less on laboratory tests than on simple observation.

Not that skin treatments are unsophisticated. Consider laser surgery—which has at last made it possible to treat disfiguring port wine stains—and Moh's surgery, a meticulous technique for removing tumors while preserving virtually all of the surrounding skin. With these new skin treatments, as well as with the traditional ones, you play a key role. For example, you're responsible for carrying out or directly assisting with many dermatologic treatments. And because

therapy often depends on the patient's compliance with home care regimens that can last for months or even years, your patient teaching and monitoring are vitally important.

In fact, one of the most difficult aspects of treating skin disorders falls squarely within your domain. Even minor skin disorders are often painfully obvious to both the patient and the world, and the scars they leave on the patient's psyche can be much greater than the physical ones.

It's easy to overlook these psychological problems, especially when the disorder seems minor and you're seeing the patient only occasionally to monitor his progress. What's more, the patient may be reluctant to bring up these matters with you—either because he's embarrassed or simply because he doesn't think you can help him. So gently explore these areas with him. Help him to express his concerns, and point out ways of improving his appearance—for example, with cosmetics or new clothes. Encourage him when his spirits flag. Cheer his successes and offer support when he suffers setbacks.

And above all, show that you accept him, both by your words and your actions. The patient may feel cut off from humanity because of his disease, and the best care you can offer him may well be the simple touch of your hand.

DRUG THERAPY

Topical Corticosteroids

Topical corticosteroids are the mainstay of treatment for inflammatory, pruritic, hyperplastic, or infiltrative skin disorders. Although mainly used for symptomatic relief, they sometimes cure these conditions.

Besides being easy to apply and fast-acting, topical corticosteroids effectively treat a wide variety of common eruptions, such as psoriasis, pemphigus, eczema, contact dermatitis, cutaneous sarcoid, and lichen planus. They're also unlikely to cause sensitivity reactions or other side effects; the few side effects that do occur are usually related to the vehicle rather than to the corticosteroid itself. What's more, these corticosteroids are compatible with almost all other topical medications, and they have a long shelf life.

Three factors determine the effectiveness of a topical corticosteroid: its potency, the type of vehicle, and the depth of penetration. Potency varies according to the specific corticosteroid, with Class I corticosteroids being the most potent and Class VII being the least potent. (See *Comparing Topical Corticosteroids* for details on the potency and nursing concerns for these drugs.)

Topical corticosteroids come in cream, ointment, and gel forms. Cream-based medications (oil-in-water emulsions) permit easy application and lubricate the skin, but they don't penetrate deeply and are removed with perspiration. Ointments (water-in-oil emulsions) are indicated when marked lubrication and enhanced penetration are required, as in extremely hyperkeratotic skin. However, they may cause folliculitis, stain clothing, and produce an unacceptable cosmetic effect unless they're properly applied. Gels—semisolid mixtures with a consistency between those of creams and ointments—are easily applied and greaseless. However, they wear off easily and, because they contain alcohol, they tend to dehydrate the skin and may burn if they're applied to broken skin.

Typically, chronic skin disorders are treated with the lowest-potency corticosteroid capable of producing the desired results, thereby reducing the risk of systemic side effects. Sometimes chronic conditions become recalcitrant, requiring brief cessation of therapy. When potent corticosteroids are discontinued, the patient may experience a rebound phenomenon; such patients may be switched to another corticosteroid or may gradually be weaned to less potent corticosteroids.

Topical corticosteroids are usually contraindicated in bacterial or fungal infections, herpes simplex virus, varicella, and viral exanthematous diseases since they inhibit the body's immune reponse and can actually worsen these infections. Nonetheless, they're sometimes combined with antibiotic or antifungal preparations, to reduce inflammation and pruritus while the underlying disease is treated.

Purpose and action
Corticosteroids are potent anti-inflammatory agents. They decrease the number of circulating lymphocytes, monocytes, eosinophils, and basophils. And they interfere with prostaglandin synthesis. Their vasoconstrictive effect controls erythema and pruritus, whereas their antiproliferative effect helps control psoriasis, which is characterized by epidermal proliferation.

Monitoring
During therapy, observe the lesions under treatment and note any apparent results of treatment or side effects. Keep

COMPARING TOPICAL CORTICOSTEROIDS

DRUG	NURSING CONSIDERATIONS
Class I betamethasone dipropionate ointment 0.05%	• Highest potency of all topical steroids. Should be used only for short periods. • Don't apply to broken skin, to areas where skin is normally thin, or to face, groin, or axillae. Don't cover with occlusive dressing. • Watch for side effects. If patient's condition worsens, stop drug and notify doctor.
Class II amcinonide ointment 0.1% desoximetasone cream 0.25%, gel 0.05%, ointment 0.25% diflorasone diacetate ointment 0.05% fluocinonide cream 0.05%, gel 0.05%, ointment 0.05% halcinonide cream 0.1%	• Don't apply to compromised skin or to areas where skin is normally thin. • Apply sparingly and only to areas specified. Unless ordered, don't cover with an occlusive dressing. • Observe for side effects. If patient's condition worsens, stop drug and notify doctor.
Class III betamethasone dipropionate cream 0.05% betamethasone valerate ointment 0.1% diflorasone diacetate cream 0.05% triamcinolone acetonide cream 0.5%	• See information for Class II.
Class IV betamethasone benzoate ointment 0.025% desoximetasone cream 0.05% fluocinolone acetonide cream 0.2%, ointment 0.025% flurandrenolide ointment 0.05% hydrocortisone valerate ointment 0.2% triamcinolone acetonide ointment 0.1%	• See information for Class II. However, note that these steroids may be occluded for up to 2 hours.
Class V betamethasone benzoate cream 0.025% betamethasone dipropionate lotion 0.02% betamethasone valerate cream 0.1%, lotion 0.1% fluocinolone acetonide cream 0.025% flurandrenolide cream 0.05% hydrocortisone butyrate cream 0.1% hydrocortisone valerate cream 0.2% triamcinolone acetonide cream 0.1%, lotion 0.1%	• See information for Class II. However, note that these steroids may be occluded for up to 2 hours.
Class VI desonide cream 0.05% fluocinolone acetonide solution 0.01% flumethasone pivalate cream 0.03%	• See information for Class II. However, note that these steroids may be occluded for extended periods. • Can be used on the face, groin, axillae.
Class VII topicals with hydrocortisone, dexamethasone, flumethasone, prednisolone, or methylprednisolone	• Lowest potency of all topical steroids. • May be used on any area of the body and occluded for extended periods. • Observe for side effects. If patient's condition worsens, stop drug and notify doctor.

in mind that contact dermatitis may result from the vehicle; suspect it if the patient's condition worsens in spite of adequate topical treatment. Local side effects caused by the corticosteroid itself may include thinning of skin, striae, acne-like eruptions, and telangiectasia. The risk of these side effects increases when corticosteroids are applied to areas where the skin is thin, such as the eyelids.

Observe the patient for cushingoid symptoms, such as moon face or truncal obesity, since topical corticosteroids may suppress adrenal function. Such suppression, though rare, is most likely to occur when potent corticosteroids are used or when less potent drugs are occluded, used for an extended period, or applied to areas of thin or denuded skin.

Home care instructions
• Explain the possible side effects to the patient, such as contact dermatitis and telangiectasia. Tell him that, if side effects occur, he should stop the medication and notify his doctor.
• To ensure the full benefit of therapy, teach the patient proper application techniques. Tell him first to place a small amount of medication (between a teaspoonful and a tablespoonful) on his palm and then to soften it by briskly rubbing his hands together. Then tell him to apply it evenly, using long strokes and following the direction of hair growth to avoid irritating the hair follicles. When he's done, his skin should feel lubricated but not greasy. If possible, have him apply the medication in your presence so that you can be sure he's doing it correctly.
• Encourage strict compliance with the treatment regimen. Tell the patient that using a large amount of medication won't work any better than using the correct amount; it's simply messier and more costly. Warn him to use the medication only on areas specified, to prevent exacerbation of an infection and unintended side effects.
• Instruct the patient to apply topical

preparations after a bath or shower, when the blood vessels are dilated and absorption is increased.
• If the patient's using a potent corticosteroid, tell him not to rub it on his face, axillae, perianal region, or genitalia unless the doctor has specifically ordered him to do so. Instruct him not to use an occlusive dressing unless the doctor has ordered one.

Antihistamine Antipruritics

The antihistamine antipruritics include *tripelennamine, diphenhydramine, chlorpheniramine, methdilazine, trimeprazine, meclizine,* and *cyproheptadine.* These systemic antihistamines offer symptomatic relief of pruritic dermatoses. Although they don't cure the underlying disorder, they help break the scratch-itch cycle and thus promote healing.

Sedation and drowsiness, the major side effects of systemic antihistamines, are magnified when these drugs are combined with CNS depressants, such as barbiturates, alcohol, anticonvulsants, or muscle relaxants. When used with monoamine oxidase (MAO) inhibitors, the antihistamines can cause anticholinergic effects, such as tachycardia, constipation, and urinary retention. Increased cholinergic effects may occur when antihistamines are used with tricyclic antidepressants.

In children and the elderly, antihistamines may cause paradoxical restlessness and hyperactivity. Children are especially prone to toxicity.

Contraindications to therapy include known hypersensitivity to antihistamines, stenosing peptic ulcer, and bladder neck obstruction. Although these drugs seem to be safe during pregnancy, they should be used cautiously in the first trimester. They shouldn't be used during lactation.

Purpose and action

Antihistamines block the action of histamines by occupying the same receptor sites on target tissue.

Monitoring

Before administering antihistamines, check the patient's drug regimen to see if he's taking CNS depressants, MAO inhibitors, or tricyclic antidepressants. If he is, ask the doctor whether the dosage should be adjusted or whether the drug should be withheld.

Watch children for signs of toxicity, such as hallucinations, incoordination, tonic-clonic seizures, flushing, and fever. Notify the doctor of such signs immediately; toxicity can cause cerebral edema, deepening coma, and respiratory collapse in 2 to 18 hours.

For most patients taking systemic antihistamines, expect to see some degree of sedation. Ask the patient or his parents if these effects are bothersome or interfering with his daily activities; if they are, the doctor may adjust the dosage or try another antihistamine. (See *Questions Patients Ask About Antihistamines.*)

Assess the patient taking antihistamines for excessive dryness of the mouth, nose, and throat. Continuing mouth dryness may lead to tooth decay, gum disease, or thrush. Dehydration of the nose and throat may predispose him to upper respiratory tract infections. If the patient reports excessive dryness, notify the doctor.

Home care instructions

• Emphasize the importance of adhering to the prescribed drug regimen.
• Tell the patient to check with his doctor before taking any over-the-counter drug.
• Alert parents to side effects that may occur in children taking systemic antihistamines, such as nightmares and hyperactivity. For all patients, briefly describe other possible side effects, such as sedation, blurred vision, painful or difficult urination, dizziness, rash, sore throat, or fever. Tell the pa-

tient that, if such reactions occur, he should stop the drug and notify the doctor immediately.
• To prevent excessive sedation, tell the patient not to make up any missed doses.
• Instruct him to take the drug with food or a glass of water or milk to minimize GI upset.
• Recommend sugarless candy or gum to relieve mouth dryness.
• If the patient is using a topical antihistamine, warn him not to apply it to denuded skin.

INQUIRY

QUESTIONS PATIENTS ASK ABOUT ANTIHISTAMINES

How will I be able to work if this drug is going to make me sleepy?

First try taking the drug when you're at home and see how you react. Then take it at work. If drowsiness begins to interfere with your job, tell the doctor. He may be able to change the amount you take or switch you to another antihistamine that won't make you as tired. Sometimes people who take antihistamines for a long time begin to adapt to the medicine and don't feel quite so sleepy.

Can I become addicted to antihistamines?

No. Antihistamines aren't physically addictive. But since they have a mild calming effect, it's possible that someone might want to take them whenever he feels nervous.

Can I drink alcohol while I'm taking antihistamines?

Avoid drinking alcohol, since the combination will make you tired and slow your reflexes.

Topical Antifungals

Topical antifungal agents are effective against dermatophytoses, such as tinea capitis, tinea corporis, tinea cruris, tinea pedis, and tinea versicolor. These antifungals may be formulated as aerosol powders or solutions, topical powders, creams, gels, or spray solutions. They may contain a number of agents, such as *acrisorcin, carbolfuchsin solution, clotrimazole, haloprogin, miconazole nitrate,* and *nystatin.*

Antifungal preparations have similar effects, and the choice of drug and vehicle is largely a matter of preference. The powder form offers some advantages for treating moist skin areas, where its drying effect can help promote healing. When bacterial overgrowth complicates the infection, the doctor may choose a combination product.

Topical antifungals have low toxicity and are unlikely to cause hypersensitivity reactions. Percutaneous absorption is virtually nonexistent unless the preparation is applied to compromised skin. Side effects occur rarely and are usually mild. They include overgrowth of nonsusceptible organisms, skin irritation, photosensitivity, edema, erythematous vesicular eruptions, hives, pruritus, stinging, peeling, blistering, maceration, and angioedema.

Purpose and action
Antifungal agents inhibit or destroy dermatophytes by interfering with their metabolic activity.

Monitoring
Because these drugs are safe, effective, and usually prescribed for outpatients, monitoring is minimal. However, you'll need to watch for signs of hypersensitivity, such as skin irritation that wasn't present before therapy.

Assess the patient's response to therapy. In severe fungal infection, you may not see improvement for up to 3 weeks. However, if the patient's condition appears to be *worsening* with treatment, notify the doctor so that he can reevaluate the patient and confirm the diagnosis.

Home care instructions
● Show the patient how to apply the medication. The specific procedure will depend on the type of medication prescribed; in general, a half-inch ribbon of cream is used for every 4 square inches of body surface; aerosols are sprayed onto the affected area from a distance of 6″ to 10″; spray solutions are released from a distance of 4″ to 6″; and topical powders are dusted lightly onto the affected area and gently rubbed in.
● Tell the patient to keep the affected areas clean and dry to promote maximum drug effectiveness. Instruct him to cleanse crusted or oozing lesions before applying the drug and to treat these areas frequently.
● Warn the patient not to expect immediate improvement. However, tell him that he should call the doctor if the infection worsens or if he notes any evidence of new blistering, burning, peeling, or swelling.
● Emphasize the need to continue with the full course of treatment even if symptoms have cleared within a few days. Explain that the infection will still be present and that symptoms will reappear if the drug is discontinued prematurely.
● Tell the patient to return for a culture after completion of therapy to check for any remaining infection or overgrowth of new fungi.

Pediculicides

The topical drugs *lindane, pyrethrins,* and *permethrin* eradicate infestations of head, body, or pubic lice. These drugs come in various forms: lindane in a shampoo, cream, or lotion; pyrethrins in a gel or solution shampoo or in a topical solution; and permethrin in a lotion. Typically, two applications are required; the first eradicates adult lice and the second, given about 10 days later, kills newly hatched lice.

Pediculicides are generally safe, causing only local stinging and burning. Rarely, they cause a severe rash. However, they should be applied cautiously, especially in children, because systemic absorption can cause CNS effects. In fact, permethrin shouldn't be used on children under age 2. Pyrethrins, though poorly absorbed through the skin, can cause sneezing, sinusitis, wheezing, vomiting, respiratory distress, and even paralysis if inhaled.

Purpose and action

Pediculicides attack the central nervous system of lice, paralyzing them or causing seizures and death.

Monitoring

When treating patients for lice infestation, watch for local and systemic reactions and assess the effectiveness of therapy. Although the patient's skin may be irritated by the lice infestation itself, be on guard for any new rashes that occur after treatment. Report them to the doctor; he may order treatment with topical steroids. Check the patient's skin and scalp for lice and nits. Also check other family members since transmission is common.

When using preparations containing lindane, watch for signs of systemic absorption and CNS toxicity, especially in young patients. Dizziness, muscle cramps, irritability, tachycardia, vomiting, and seizures are common signs of CNS toxicity. With pyrethrins, watch for signs of respiratory distress caused by inadvertent inhalation of the drug.

Home care instructions

• Because pediculicides are usually applied at home, provide thorough directions for their use. Keep in mind that the method of application depends on

the product that's used. If the patient's using lindane shampoo, tell him to apply it to dry hair, to rub it in thoroughly, and to leave it in place for 4 minutes. Then he should apply a little water, work the shampoo into a lather, and rinse his hair thoroughly. Afterward, he should use a fine-tooth comb to remove nits and nit shells.

Pyrethrins administration is similar. Depending on the type of infestation, pyrethrins may be applied to the scalp, body, or pubic area. If the patient's using a gel or solution form, he should first wash the affected area with warm water and soap or regular shampoo; if he's using a shampoo, he should apply it to dry hair and work it into a lather, using a small amount of water. With all forms of pyrethrins, he should leave the medication on the affected area for 10 minutes and then rinse thoroughly. Afterward, he should comb his hair with a fine-tooth comb.

• No matter which pediculicide is used, instruct the patient to apply it again after 7 to 10 days to kill any newly hatched lice.

• Tell him never to apply pediculicides to broken skin and to keep them away from the face (especially the eyes), mucous membranes, and urethral meatus. Briefly describe the signs of CNS toxicity, and advise him to notify the doctor immediately if any occur. Explain that lindane shouldn't be used during or immediately after a bath or shower and that pyrethrins should be applied in a well-ventilated area.

• Tell the patient that, if a rash or an irritation develops during application, he should wash off the medication and notify his doctor. Pruritus may persist for several weeks after successful treatment and may be treated with topical corticosteroids.

• Instruct the patient on how to prevent reinfestation. Tell him to clean the house thoroughly, vacuuming upholstered furniture, rugs, and floors; to wash all recently worn clothing, bed linens, and towels in hot water or to have them dry-cleaned; and to wash

hair brushes and combs in hot, soapy water for 5 to 10 minutes. Explain that hats, combs, and brushes should never be shared.
• If the patient's undergoing treatment for pubic lice, explain that the toilet seat should be scrubbed frequently and that sexual partners must receive concurrent treatment.

Retinoids

Etretinate and *isotretinoin*, two synthetic derivatives of vitamin A, often yield excellent results and prolonged remissions in skin disorders. Etretinate is indicated for severe recalcitrant psoriasis; isotretinoin's greatest value is in treating severe nodulocystic or inflammatory papulopustular acne that's unresponsive to other drugs. Both retinoids are sometimes used to treat other skin disorders, such as ichthyosis and Darier's disease, and research suggests that etretinate may prove useful for treating some carcinomas.

Retinoid therapy usually lasts 15 to 20 weeks, continuing until about two thirds of the lesions clear. Often the patient's condition will worsen before it improves.

Both etretinate and isotretinoin have numerous side effects. Mucocutaneous and dermatologic effects include dryness and peeling of lips, skin, and mucous membranes; alopecia; dry eyes; and photosensitivity. Some patients also experience muscle, bone, or joint pain and GI disturbances. These drugs may also contribute to the development of pseudomotor cerebri, hyperuricemia, regional ileitis, and corneal opacities. And they may cause effects similar to those seen with vitamin A toxicity, such as increased cerebrospinal fluid pressure, papillary edema, diplopia, hepatomegaly, splenomegaly, hemorrhage, and hypoprothrombinemia.

In addition, retinoids can have additive photosensitizing effects when they're combined with other photosensitizing drugs. They can increase serum triglyceride (especially with alcohol consumption) and cholesterol levels, so they must be used cautiously in patients who are predisposed to hypertriglyceridemia. In diabetic patients, these drugs raise blood glucose concentrations.

Because retinoids are potent teratogens, women of child-bearing age must use contraceptive measures beginning at least 1 month before therapy and continuing at least 1 month after it ends.

Purpose and action
The exact mechanism of action for each drug is unknown. Isotretinoin reduces sebaceous gland size and activity. Etretinate acts much like vitamin A, promoting growth and regulating the proliferation and differentiation of epithelial tissues. Both drugs have antikeratinizing and anti-inflammatory actions.

Monitoring
Review the patient's medical history to identify high alcohol intake or a personal or family history of hypertriglyceridemia, obesity, or diabetes. Before therapy begins, obtain and review ordered laboratory tests, such as serum lipids, liver function tests, a complete blood count (CBC), and a pregnancy test. Ensure that the female patient of child-bearing age understands the importance of using contraceptive measures during and after therapy.

As ordered, monitor serum lipid levels at 1- to 2-week intervals until the patient's response to the retinoid is established (usually after 4 to 8 weeks), and review the results of liver function tests. With etretinate, liver function tests are usually performed every week or every other week for the first 2 months, and every 1 to 3 months thereafter. With isotretinoin, they're usually performed monthly. Other laboratory tests, such as a CBC or blood glucose test, may also be ordered, depending on initial test results, family history, or the patient's condition. Notify the doctor immediately of any abnormal test results.

Report any severe side effects, such as visual disturbances, rectal bleeding, severe headaches, nausea, or vomiting. If any of these occur, the doctor will probably discontinue therapy.

Home care instructions
• Tell the patient to stop taking the drug and to notify the doctor immediately if he experiences severe side effects. Advise him, though, that his skin condition will probably worsen before it improves.
• For the female patient of child-bearing age, emphasize the urgency of practicing birth control during therapy and for at least 1 month after it. Tell her to record the date of each menses and to notify the doctor and stop taking the drug immediately if she thinks she may be pregnant.
• Tell the patient not to donate blood during and for 30 days after retinoid therapy to prevent possible transfusion to a pregnant woman.
• To prevent elevated triglyceride levels, instruct the patient to refrain from consuming alcohol during therapy.
• Tell him to notify you or the doctor before taking any over-the-counter drugs. Warn against taking vitamin A or any vitamin supplements containing it.
• Caution the diabetic patient that retinoids may alter blood glucose levels. Emphasize the need for regular glucose testing and instruct him to call his doctor if he has difficulty controlling blood glucose.
• To minimize dry skin and mucous membranes, tell the patient to avoid any topical products containing alcohol, such as after-shave lotions, astringents, perfumed toiletries, and certain mouthwashes. Also tell him to avoid products containing benzoyl peroxide, salicylic acid, or resorcinol, which may cause excessive peeling and dryness.
• Recommend petrolatum for cracked and dry lips, a bland emollient for relief of skin dryness, and chewing gum to stimulate salivation. For dry eyes, suggest artificial tears. If the patient wears contact lenses, advise switching to glasses for the duration of therapy.
• Remind the patient to limit sun exposure, since retinoids can cause increased sensitivity to sunlight.

Silver Sulfadiazine

Possessing a broad spectrum of antimicrobial activity, this topical sulfa drug helps treat or prevent wound infection—most often in patients with second- or third-degree burns. It's also used to treat large denuded areas of skin caused by bullous disease. What's more, it serves as an artificial barrier for compromised skin.

Silver sulfadiazine is contraindicated in patients with impaired hepatic or renal function, since it's metabolized in the liver and excreted by the kidneys. In addition, the drug inactivates topical proteolytic enzymes and therefore shouldn't be used with them. Because the drug may cause kernicterus, it shouldn't be given to pregnant women, premature infants, or term infants within the 1st month of life. It's also contraindicated in patients with a known hypersensitivity to sulfa drugs or a known deficiency of glucose-6-phosphate dehydrogenase, in whom it may precipitate hemolysis.

A nurse normally applies silver sulfadiazine using sterile technique or reverse isolation. She applies a layer 2 to 3 mm thick to all debrided, cleansed, or burned areas once or twice a day or when the unguent is accidentally removed. A dressing isn't required.

Purpose and action
Silver sulfadiazine is bactericidal for gram-negative and gram-positive organisms. It's used to retard bacterial growth and hasten healing in superficial lesions.

Monitoring

Check for rashes or other skin reactions and for complaints of pruritus or burning. Be alert for and report systemic effects, especially when the drug is applied to large areas of compromised skin. These effects may include vomiting, diarrhea, headache, and fatigue.

Assess the patient for signs of blood dyscrasias, such as sore throat, fever, pallor, purpura, jaundice, or weakness. Also assess for early signs of Stevens-Johnson syndrome: high fever, severe headache, stomatitis, conjunctivitis, rhinitis, urethritis, or balanitis. If any signs of this syndrome occur, notify the doctor since drug withdrawal is necessary.

Evaluate the patient's renal function and be on guard for decreased urinary output, hematuria, flank pain, or generalized abdominal pain. Record intake and output and encourage fluids to promote drug excretion and prevent crystalluria.

Home care instructions

Silver sulfadiazine is usually applied to burn victims in the hospital. As a result, no treatment-related home care instructions are required.

SURGERY

Moh's Micrographic Surgery

One of the newest techniques for excising basal and squamous cell carcinomas, Moh's micrographic surgery involves serial excision and histologic analysis of cancerous or suspected cancerous tissue (see *Moh's Surgery: Excising Tumors a Step at a Time*). This surgery offers several advantages over wide resection. First, it minimizes the size of the scar, a vital consideration in facial surgery. In addition, it helps prevent recurrence: basal cell carcinomas spread in a fingerlike pattern, and simple superficial excision often fails to remove all malignant tissue. The procedure can usually be performed in a single day in a doctor's office; hospitalization is required only if the lesion is extremely large or dangerously located.

Basal cell carcinomas are particularly responsive to Moh's surgery. The procedure usually isn't necessary for a primary, well-localized tumor of recent origin. It is indicated, however, if the lesion has been present for a long time; is extremely large; is adjacent to important organs, such as the eyes; is in an area that's difficult to visualize, such as the ear; or is in an area where recurrence or extensive invasion is likely, such as the nasolabial folds adjacent to the alae. In addition, Moh's surgery is the preferred treatment for recurrent skin cancer.

The cure rates with Moh's surgery are impressive: about 96% for basal cell carcinoma and 94% for squamous cell carcinoma. In addition, the treatment has been used successfully for basal cell carcinomas of the morpheaform, sclerotic, infiltrating, and basosquamous types.

Moh's surgery has two common complications: bleeding and facial scarring. Bleeding is easily controlled with direct pressure; the devastating psychological effects of a large facial scar or defect are more difficult to treat and require considerable support from you and from the patient's family.

Purpose

To remove basal and squamous cell carcinomas.

Preparation

Keep in mind that the patient awaiting this procedure is likely to be extremely anxious about his cancer, the surgery's outcome, and his appearance after sur-

MOH'S SURGERY: EXCISING TUMORS A STEP AT A TIME

A lengthy but highly effective procedure, Moh's surgery involves a series of excisions and histologic analyses designed to detect and remove all cancerous tissue.

STEP 1
Moh's surgery begins with a simple excision of the visible tumor, along with a margin of skin.

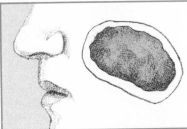

STEP 2
Once the tumor is excised, the doctor or nurse sketches a map of the defect, indicating its orientation and nearby anatomic landmarks.

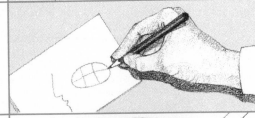

STEP 3
In the laboratory, the tissue is cut into sections for histologic analysis. Corresponding sections are drawn on the map.

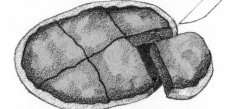

STEP 4
After reading the histologic results, the doctor marks on the map those sections containing cancerous tissue.

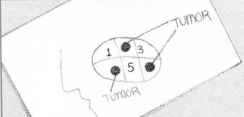

STEP 5
Then the doctor removes additional tissue from the margins where cancerous tissue was found.

Steps 3 through 5 are repeated until all tissue is microscopically identified as cancer-free.

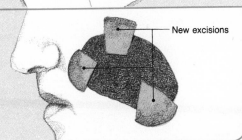

New excisions

gery. So be sure to provide emotional support and give him the opportunity to express his fears. Many family members may also require reassurance and appropriate information. If necessary, give them a chance to express their concerns and answer any questions they may have.

Review the patient's history, noting especially allergies and hypersensitivities (especially to epinephrine and xylocaine), cardiac disease, or ongoing anticoagulant therapy. Be sure the patient understands that the surgery typically takes many hours, most of which will be spent waiting for histologic results. Reassure him that a long wait doesn't mean his cancer is especially serious. Similarly, tell him that he shouldn't worry if the doctor performs numerous excisions: it simply means that he's making conservative excisions in an attempt to preserve as much normal tissue as possible.

Explain that the doctor will use electrocauterization to control bleeding and that a grounding plate will be affixed to the patient's leg or arm to complete the circuit between the cautery pencil and the generator. Reassure the patient that he won't feel anything from the ground. Warn him, however, to expect an unpleasant burning odor.

Once you've prepared the patient, assemble the equipment. Usually, you'll open the scalpel, blade, curette, and forceps and place them on the tray, leaving the other instruments in their sterile packets, to be opened as needed. Add sterile gauze, a drape, alcohol swabs, and the anesthetic (usually xylocaine with epinephrine) to the tray. In addition, have a container available to transport the specimen to the laboratory. And label an index card with the patient's name, date, stage of excision, lesion type, and location.

Procedure

After the doctor administers the anesthetic and it has taken effect, position the patient comfortably and place the grounding pad on his leg or arm. Then drape the surgical area and adjust the lights.

As the doctor excises the visible tumor with margins, apply direct pressure to the site to prevent bleeding. After the tissue has been excised, place it on a telfa pad, apply a dressing over the operative site, and escort the patient to the waiting room. Then you or the doctor will draw a map of the lesion, showing anatomic landmarks and the orientation of the wound. Next, take the specimen to the laboratory.

In the laboratory, the doctor or technician divides the specimen into sections, freezes them, and places them on slides for staining and microscopic analysis. Using these slides, the doctor marks the areas of malignancy on the map.

If malignant cells are found in the tissue margin, return the patient to the treatment room so that the doctor can excise additional tissue from the affected area. This process of excision and histologic analysis continues until all tissue margins are free of malignancy.

Once the tumor has been excised, the doctor will either repair the site or leave it open to heal. Sometimes plastic surgery is necessary. If surgical repair isn't going to be performed, cleanse the wound with hydrogen peroxide and apply an antibiotic ointment and a pressure dressing.

Monitoring and aftercare

During the procedure, be alert for any signs of distress or discomfort. Assess the patient's level of pain and provide analgesics, as ordered.

Periodically check the dressing for excessive bleeding. If it occurs, remove the dressing and apply pressure over the site for 20 minutes.

Home care instructions

• Tell the patient to leave the dressing in place for 24 hours. However, if he experiences frank bleeding, he should reinforce the bandage and apply direct pressure to the wound for 20 minutes, using clean gauze or a clean washcloth. If this measure doesn't control bleeding, he should call the doctor.

• Warn the patient not to remove the original dressing for 24 hours but to change the dressing once daily thereafter. If bleeding occurs, he should reinforce the dressing and apply pressure. However, if the bleeding doesn't stop, he should notify the doctor.

• Instruct the patient to be alert for signs of infection, such as redness, warmth, or extreme tenderness, and to notify the doctor if any of these signs occur.

• Advise the patient to refrain from alcohol consumption, use of aspirin or anticoagulants, or excessive exercise for 48 hours to prevent bleeding and promote healing.

• Recommend acetaminophen for discomfort.

• Instruct the patient to return for follow-up appointments for examinations or reconstructive surgery.

Laser Surgery for Skin Lesions

The highly focused and intense light of lasers can be used to treat many types of dermatologic lesions. Laser surgery offers several advantages: it's an outpatient procedure, usually performed in a doctor's office under local anesthesia; its effects can be controlled precisely, sparing normal tissue and promoting faster healing; and it helps prevent postsurgical infection since it actually sterilizes the operative site during the procedure.

Two types of lasers are used in dermatology: argon lasers and CO_2 lasers. The blue-green light of argon lasers is absorbed by the red pigment of hemoglobin. Therefore, blood vessels absorb much more energy from the argon laser than do surrounding tissues. As the light energy is transformed to heat

energy, it coagulates small blood vessels and ablates superficial vascular lesions, while leaving surrounding tissues relatively unaffected.

One important application of the argon laser is for port wine stains, which are otherwise untreatable. Although complete removal of the stain occurs in only a small number of patients, a satisfactory degree of lightening and flattening can be achieved in most. Telangiectasias, other hemangiomas, and venous lakes also respond to argon laser surgery.

The CO_2 laser emits an invisible beam in the far infrared wavelength; water absorbs this wavelength and converts it to heat energy. This laser helps treat warts and malignancies. And although it's not as selective in its effects as the argon laser, its narrow beam can be used to coagulate blood vessels. Thus, it too can be used to treat port wine stains, facial telangiectasias, and spider angiomas as well as to remove tattoos.

In yet another application, the CO_2 laser beam can be focused to a fine point and used in place of a scalpel. Besides its sterilizing effects, the laser seals tiny blood vessels as it cuts, providing a virtually bloodless operative field.

In general, laser surgery is safe, although bleeding and scarring can result. The most pronounced hazard to patients and medical personnel alike is eye damage or other injury caused by unintended reflection of the beam. For this reason, anyone in the surgical suite, including the patient, must wear special goggles to filter laser light. In addition, the surgeon must use special nonreflective instruments, access to the room must be strictly controlled during surgery, and all windows must be covered.

Purpose

• To treat port wine stains, telangiectasias, venous lakes, spider angiomas, warts, malignancies, pyogenic granulomas, acquired angiomas, angiomas

of disseminated blue-rubber nevus, lymphangiomas, or keloids
● To remove tattoos.

Preparation

Your major responsibility in laser surgery is patient support and teaching. Explain how the laser works and why the surgeon is using it. Show the patient the machine and outline the procedure to help allay his concerns.

Explain that the laser causes a wound similar to a burn and that this wound can be deep. Warn the patient to expect a pungent odor and smoke during the procedure and that the surface of the wound will appear charred afterward. Tell him that some of the eschar will be removed during the initial postoperative cleaning and that more will gradually dislodge at home.

Before the procedure begins, prepare the tray, including a local anesthetic. Although pain is minimized by the laser's selective effects, the surgeon will usually administer a local anesthetic. Also place dry and wet gauze on the tray. The dry gauze will be used during the procedure to control bleeding. Some of the wet gauze will be placed around the operative area to protect healthy tissue; the rest will be used to abrade and remove any eschar, which would otherwise inhibit laser wavelength absorption.

Some surgical instruments may be required: a curette, for example, is sometimes needed for wart removal and tissue forceps are often used for keloid excisions. Ensure that all instruments are nonreflective.

If the surgical suite has windows, ensure that shades or blinds don't allow light to enter. Cover all reflective surfaces, such as stainless steel fixtures. Also, remove any flammable materials since the lasers spark tissue.

When the surgeon's ready to begin, position the patient comfortably, drape him, and place protective gauze around the operative site. Make sure that everyone in the room—including the patient—is wearing safety goggles. Lock the door to keep unprotected persons from inadvertently entering the room.

Procedure

After the surgeon administers the local anesthetic and it takes effect, activate the laser's vacuum. The CO_2 laser has a vacuum hose attached to a separate machine, which is used to clear the surgical site. The vacuum has a filter that traps and collects much of the vaporized tissue. Change the filter whenever there's a decrease in suction, and follow your institution's guidelines for filter disposal.

The surgeon uses the laser beam much as he would a scalpel to cut away the lesion. After he has completed the procedure, apply direct pressure over any bleeding wound for 20 minutes.

Monitoring and aftercare

Initial wound care varies, depending on the procedure. However, if the wound continues to bleed, notify the doctor. If it doesn't, first clean the area with a cotton-tipped applicator dipped in hydrogen peroxide. Then cut a nonadhering dressing to size. Spread a thin layer of antibiotic ointment on one side of the dressing. Place the ointment side over the wound and secure the dressing with micropore tape.

Home care instructions

● Tell the patient to dress his wound daily, following the same procedure that you used. Tell him that he can take showers but that he mustn't immerse the wound site in water.
● Tell him that, if bleeding occurs, he should apply direct pressure on the site with clean gauze or a washcloth for 20 minutes. If pressure doesn't control the bleeding, he should call the doctor immediately.
● If the patient's foot was operated on, tell him to keep it elevated and to walk as little as possible, since pressure can inhibit healing.
● Warn the patient to protect the wound from exposure to the sun, to avoid changes in pigmentation.

• Explain that he should keep the wound clean and bandaged until the first postoperative visit, which is usually about 10 days after surgery.

Cryosurgery

A common dermatologic procedure, cryosurgery refers to the destruction of tissue by the application of extreme cold. Often performed in the doctor's office, it's used to treat actinic and seborrheic keratoses, leukoplakia, molluscum contagiosum, condyloma acuminatum, verrucae, and sometimes basal cell epitheliomas and squamous cell carcinomas. It can be performed quite simply, using nothing more than a cotton-tipped applicator dipped into liquid nitrogen and applied to the skin, or it may involve a complex cryosurgical unit (CSU).

Cryosurgery offers several advantages over conventional excision of dermatologic lesions: it is easy to perform, usually requires no anesthesia (since the cold itself has an anesthetic effect), and causes epidermal-dermal separation *above* the basement membranes—which, in turn, prevents scarring after reepithelialization. Complications of cryosurgery, when they occur, are usually minor. They include hypopigmentation (from destruction of melanocytes) and secondary infection. Rarely, the procedure may damage blood vessels, nerves, and tear ducts.

Cryosurgery's success depends on the type of lesion, the extent and depth of the freeze, and the duration between freezing and thawing. A slow thaw destroys lesions most effectively.

Liquid nitrogen and nitrous oxide (N_2O) are the most commonly used cryogens, but some CSUs employ carbon dioxide or Freon. At a temperature of $-196°$ C., liquid nitrogen is by far the most powerful cryogen. It's especially useful for treating malignancies, which

resist cold well because of their vascularity. N_2O is often favored for less extensive procedures, since the surgeon can more easily control its effects.

When freezing superficial lesions, the doctor can often determine the correct temperature and depth of freezing simply by palpating and observing the lesion. When treating skin cancers, however, he uses thermocouple needles and a tissue temperature monitor (pyrometer) to be sure that tissue at the deepest part of the lesion has been adequately frozen. In these cases, the nurse is often responsible for operating the needles and pyrometer.

Contraindications to cryosurgery include an underlying cryoglobulinemia, cryofibrinogenemia, cold intolerance, Raynaud's disease, cold urticaria, pyoderma gangrenosum, collagen and autoimmune disease, concurrent dialysis or immunosuppressive drug therapy, platelet deficiency, blood dyscrasias, multiple myeloma, and agammaglobulinemia.

Purpose
To destroy diseased tissue by the application of extreme cold.

Preparation
Most patients will be unfamiliar with cryosurgery, so briefly explain the procedure, its intended purpose, and the appearance of the site postoperatively. Outline the basic steps of the procedure to the patient. If the doctor is using a pressurized delivery system, show the patient the equipment and explain how it works. If thermocouple needles will be used, also show them to the patient and explain their purpose.

Ask the patient if he has any known allergies or hypersensitivities, especially to lidocaine, iodine, or cold. Tell him that the povidone-iodine solution used to cleanse the treatment area causes temporary staining.

Tell the patient that he'll initially feel cold, followed by burning, during the procedure. Caution him to remain as still as possible to prevent inadvertent

POSITIONING THERMOCOUPLE NEEDLES

During cryosurgery, you may be responsible for positioning thermocouple needles. These needles measure the temperature of the tissue at its tip and help the doctor gauge the depth of freezing—a vitally important factor when destroying cancerous lesions. The needle may be placed in any of several positions. At top, it's shown inserted at an angle so that its tip rests about 5 mm below the base of the tumor to give a direct reading of tissue temperature. When used in this fashion, the temperature reading may be affected by chilling of the shaft within the frozen tissue, but the error isn't likely to be significant. On the bottom, the probe is placed about 5 mm to one side of the frozen tissue at a depth of about 3 mm. In this position, it will register the same temperature as the probe at left, since both probe tips are about the same distance from the frozen tissue.

Precise temperature measurement can be difficult, since a variation of only 1 mm in the probe's position can translate into a difference of 10 to 15 C. degrees. For that reason, you'll usually place two or more probes in different areas to increase the accuracy of the reading.

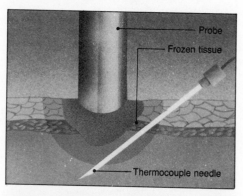

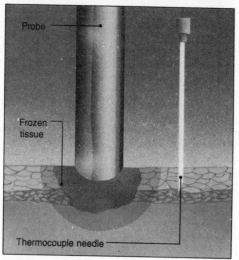

freezing of unaffected tissue.

After providing the patient with this overview, gather the necessary equipment. Make sure the cryogen is available (some institutions have a large container of liquid nitrogen, from which smaller insulated bottles are filled for surgery), as well as cotton-tipped applicators or the CSU. If you'll be using thermocouple needles and a pyrometer, obtain them as well, and make sure that they're sterile and in proper working order. You may also need tape to secure the needles to the base of the lesion, and you'll need a watch or clock with a second hand to time the thaw and freeze cycles accurately. Also obtain the local anesthetic, alcohol swabs, and gauze.

Some surgeons use gentian violet or a surgical marker to delineate the margins of the lesion. If necessary, obtain the appropriate marker.

Position the patient comfortably. If necessary, shield his eyes or ears to prevent damage.

Procedure

The surgeon may give a local anesthetic, depending on the type of procedure. After it takes effect, cleanse the operative site with povidone-iodine solution. If the surgeon is using thermocouple needles, assist him as he inserts and secures them into the base of the tumor (see *Positioning Thermocouple Needles*).

The surgeon uses the cotton-tipped applicator or the CSU to freeze the lesion. He may refreeze a tumor several times to ensure its destruction; for each cycle, monitor and record the number of seconds that elapse until the tissue reaches −20° C. and the number of seconds that it takes the tissue to thaw.

Monitoring and aftercare

After cryosurgery, cleanse the area gently with a cotton-tipped applicator soaked in hydrogen peroxide. Because cryosurgery doesn't cause bleeding, you needn't apply a bandage. In fact, occlusive dressings are contraindicated.

If necessary, apply an ice bag to relieve swelling and give analgesics to relieve pain, as ordered. Cryosurgery may cause considerable pain, especially if it was performed on or near the lips, eyes, eyelids, tongue, or plantar surfaces of the feet. Generalized headache may persist for more than an hour after freezing of a scalp tumor.

Home care instructions

● Tell the patient to expect pain, redness, and swelling and that a blister will form within 6 hours of treatment. Ordinarily, it will flatten within a few days and slough off in 2 to 3 weeks. Serous exudation may follow during the 1st week, accompanied by the development of a crust or eschar.
● Warn the patient that the blister may be large and may bleed. Warn him not to touch it, to promote healing and prevent infection. Tell him that, if the blister becomes uncomfortable or interferes with daily activities, he should call the doctor, who can decompress it with a sterile blade or pin.

● Emphasize the importance of calling the doctor immediately if he experiences extreme pain, a widening area of erythema, oozing (of other than serous material), or fever.
● Tell him to cleanse the area gently with soap and water, alcohol, or a cotton-tipped applicator soaked in hydrogen peroxide, as ordered.
● To prevent hypopigmentation, instruct him to cover the wound with a loose dressing when he's outdoors. After the wound heals, he should apply a sunblock over the area.
● If the patient had a cancerous lesion destroyed, urge him to have regular checkups since skin cancers may recur.

Skin Grafts

Skin grafts cover defects caused by burns, trauma, or surgery. They're indicated when primary closure isn't possible or cosmetically acceptable; when primary closure would interfere with functioning; when the defect is on a weight-bearing surface; or when a skin tumor is excised and the site needs to be monitored for recurrence. Grafting may be done using a general or local anesthetic. It may be performed in the operating room or under sterile conditions at bedside. Occasionally, it's performed on an outpatient basis for extremely small facial or neck defects.

Types of skin grafts include *split-thickness* grafts, which consist of the epidermis and a small portion of dermis; *full-thickness* grafts, which include all of the dermis as well as the epidermis; or *composite* grafts, which also include underlying tissues, such as muscle, cartilage, or bone. The thickness of the graft largely depends on the defect to be covered, with thicker grafts used for larger defects. If the blood supply is poor at the recipient site, a thinner graft is used because less time is required for revascularization. No matter which type of graft is used, the procedure's success depends on re-vascularization. The graft initially sur-vives by direct contact with the underlying tissue, receiving oxygen and nutrients through existing lymph, but it eventually will die unless new blood vessels develop. In split-thickness grafts, revascularization usually takes 3 to 5 days; in full-thickness grafts, it may take up to 2 weeks.

Grafts are contraindicated if the defect lacks a sufficient blood supply; for that reason, they can't be applied directly over bare tendon, bone, cartilage, nerves, large fat deposits, or tissue damaged by X-rays. Relative contraindications include arteriosclerosis, venous stasis, previous surgery, and cosmetic considerations; however, in these patients, skin grafts may be the only treatment available to close a large defect. Complications include graft failure because of inadequate blood supply, hematoma formation, poor contact between the graft and wound bed, or infection.

Purpose

To close a skin defect, thereby pre-venting infection, restoring function, and relieving pain.

Preparation

Because successful skin grafting be-gins with a good graft, take steps to preserve potential donor sites. Provide meticulous skin care: turn or reposition the patient every 2 hours, provide range-of-motion exercises and mas-sage, maintain good preoperative nu-trition, dry areas completely after bathing, and watch for reddened areas or other signs of irritation.

Also assess the recipient site. The graft's survival depends on close con-tact with the underlying tissue, and ideally the recipient site should be healthy granulation tissue, free of es-char, debris, or the products of infec-tion.

The patient undergoing skin grafting usually requires a great deal of emo-tional support both before and after the procedure. Make sure his expectations are realistic; many patients expect to look better immediately after the sur-gery. Warn the patient that he won't see the final results for at least a year and that immediately after surgery, normal contours may be distorted by tissue re-action, suture lines may be reddened, and the color of the newly transplanted skin may differ somewhat from that of surrounding skin. Also explain to members of the patient's family what to expect, and enlist their help in pro-viding psychological support for the patient.

Explain postsurgical routines to the patient. Tell him that you'll be inspect-ing the graft frequently after surgery, to ensure that it's adhering to the un-derlying tissue, and warn him that he'll be immobilized after the grafting pro-cedure, to keep the graft from becom-ing dislodged or strangled. Also tell him that the original dressing will re-main in place for a day or two and that it will be rather bulky and awkward.

Follow the doctor's orders or insti-tutional policy to prepare the donor and recipient sites for surgery. In many hos-pitals, the donor site is washed twice with soap and water, with the final shave and scrub done in the operating room; the recipient site may receive three or more dressing changes before grafting, with the last one including application of a topical antibiotic.

If the grafting is being done at bed-side, gather the required equipment, including a local anesthetic, a der-matome, a surgical tray, and dressing materials. Drape the donor site and, if ordered, administer the local anes-thetic, being careful not to raise wheals. On concave donor sites, the doctor may infiltrate saline solution or an anesthetic to elevate the skin.

Procedure

Grafts may be harvested using a free-hand knife technique or a dermatome, depending on the doctor's preference.

Prepare the skin while the anesthetic takes effect. The Padgett dermatome

REVIEWING BIOLOGICAL DRESSINGS

Biological dressings function much like skin grafts, preventing infection and fluid loss and easing the patient's discomfort. However, they're only temporary; eventually the body rejects them. And, if the underlying wound hasn't healed, these dressings must be replaced with a graft of the patient's own skin. Here's a comparison of the four types of biological dressings and their uses.

TYPE AND SOURCE	USE AND DURATION	NURSING CONSIDERATIONS
Homograft (allograft) Harvested from cadavers	Used to debride untidy wounds, to protect granulation tissue after escharotomy, to protect excisions, to serve as a test graft before skin grafting, and to temporarily cover burns when the patient doesn't have sufficient skin for immediate grafting. They're usually rejected in 7 to 10 days.	• Observe for exudate. • Watch for local and systemic signs of rejection.
Heterograft (xenograft) Harvested from animals (usually pigs)	Used for same purposes as a homograft. Also used to cover meshed autografts, to protect exposed tendons, and to cover burns that are free of eschar and only slightly contaminated. Heterografts are usually rejected in 7 to 10 days.	• Wound may be dressed or left open. • Watch for signs of rejection.
Amnion Made from amnion and chorionic membranes	Used to protect burns and to temporarily cover granulation tissue awaiting an autograft. Must be changed every 48 hours.	• Apply only to clean wounds. • May be left open to the air or covered with a dressing.
Biosynthetic Woven from man-made fibers	Used to cover donor graft sites; to protect clean, superficial burns and excised wounds awaiting autografts; and to cover meshed autografts. Must be reapplied every 3 or 4 days.	• Biosynthetic dressings are permeable to antimicrobials, so they don't have to be removed to treat the wound. Elastic and durable, they adhere to wound surfaces until they are removed or slough off by spontaneous reepithelialization.

uses an adhesive cement to bond the skin to a rotating drum; clean both the skin and the drum with acetone or ether to remove all traces of moisture and grease. Motor-driven dermatomes simply require that the donor site be lubricated with sterile mineral oil or a sheet of semipermeable film.

After the skin is prepared, the doctor harvests the graft while an assistant provides traction and positions the skin. The doctor places the harvested grafts in a basin of isotonic solution, then smooths them out, epidermal side down, on sterile wrapping paper.

To position the graft, the doctor places it—still attached to the wrapping paper—on the recipient site, using the edge of the paper as a handle. After positioning it and smoothing it out, he removes the paper and trims the graft to fit. Then he sutures or staples it in place and covers it with fine mesh gauze. Next, he or his assistant applies a pressure dressing and covers it with an outer dressing.

For split-thickness grafts, the doctor or assistant applies a dressing to the donor site, with a layer of fine mesh gauze in direct contact with the wound. Full-thickness grafts are closed with sutures or staples and dressed.

Monitoring and aftercare

Meticulous postsurgical care is vital for graft survival. Position the patient so that he's not lying on the graft and, if possible, keep the graft area elevated and immobilized. Modify your nursing routine to protect the graft; for example, never use a blood pressure cuff over a graft site. For burn patients, omit hydrotherapy while the graft heals. Administer analgesics as necessary, and help the patient use nonpharmacologic pain-reduction techniques.

The doctor will change the first dressing, usually 24 to 48 hours postoperatively, and may change the dressings for the next several days as well, to assess the graft. Afterward, you'll be responsible for dressing changes.

Use sterile technique when changing a dressing, and work gently to avoid dislodging the graft. Clean the graft site with warm saline solution and cotton-tipped applicators, leaving the fine mesh gauze intact. Aspirate any serous pockets with a sterile needle and syringe by clipping the bleb and dabbing it with gauze or by rolling the fluid to the edge of the wound with a cotton-tipped applicator. If you note any hematomas, exudate, or purulent drainage, carefully remove the fine mesh gauze, clean the graft, and remove the exudate. To prevent contamination of healthy tissue, never roll out infectious drainage. Afterward, saturate fresh fine mesh gauze with the prescribed topical agent and apply it to the graft. Cover and secure it with Kerlix. After the graft has healed, clean it with soap and water and apply prescribed moisturizing cream.

If ordered, apply scarlet red ointment to the donor site and cover it with fine mesh gauze. Then apply an elastic gauze bandage soaked in peroxide and normal saline solution. Change the bandage every 6 to 8 hours until the dressing or donor site stops oozing. Then remove it altogether and allow the fine mesh gauze to dry.

After the gauze has dried, remove it and wash the crusts off the wound with soap and water. However, if you see evidence of infection, soak the dressing off and dress the wound with a local anti-infective agent, such as silver sulfadiazine. If necessary, use a heat lamp to hasten drying of the area.

Apply the prescribed cream daily to the healed donor site to keep it pliable.

Home care instructions

● If grafting is done as an outpatient procedure, emphasize to the patient that the graft site must be immobilized to promote proper healing.
● Tell the patient not to disturb the dressings on the graft or donor site for any reason. If they need to be changed, instruct him to call the doctor.
● Tell him to apply cream to the healed graft several times a day to keep the skin pliable and aid scar maturation.
● Because sun exposure can affect pigmentation of the graft, tell the patient to limit his time in the sun and to use a sunblock on all grafted areas.
● Explain that after scar maturation is complete, the doctor may use other plastic surgery techniques to improve the graft's appearance.

DEBRIDEMENT, BATHS, AND LIGHT TREATMENTS

Debridement

Debridement is the mechanical, chemical, or surgical removal of necrotic tissue from a wound. Although this procedure can be extremely painful, it's necessary to promote healing and prevent infection of burns and skin ulcers.

Mechanical debridement includes wet-to-dry dressings, irrigation, hydrotherapy, and bedside debridement. Wet-to-dry dressings are appropriate for partially healed wounds with only slight amounts of necrotic tissue and minimal drainage; they're most commonly used to treat ulcers rather than burns. The nurse or doctor places a wet dressing in contact with the lesion and covers it with an outer layer of bandaging. As the dressing dries, it sticks to the wound. When the dried dressing is removed, the necrotic tissue comes off with it. Wet-to-dry dressings have a number of disadvantages. They cause considerable pain, must be changed frequently, and may lead to destruction of newly healed skin.

Irrigation of a wound with an antiseptic solution cleanses tissue and removes cell debris and excess drainage. It also helps a wound heal properly—from the inside outward to the skin surface—and prevents abscess formation. After a wound is irrigated, it's usually packed to absorb any additional drainage.

Hydrotherapy—often referred to as "tubbing" or "tanking"—involves immersion of the patient in a tank of warm water and intermittent agitation of the water. It's usually performed on burn patients and allows relatively atraumatic wound debridement, dressing changes, removal of previously applied topical agents, and general body cleaning. A nurse usually performs hydrotherapy with the assistance of a physical therapist.

Bedside debridement of a burn wound involves careful prying and cutting of loosened eschar (burned tissue) with forceps and scissors to separate it from viable tissue beneath. "Bedside" debridement isn't always done at the bedside. Depending on the size and severity of the burn, it may be done during hydrotherapy or afterward in the dressing room. One of the most painful types of debridement, it may be the only practical means of removing necrotic tissue from a severely burned patient.

Chemical debridement uses Debrisan hydrophilic wound-cleaning beads or topical debriders, which absorb exudate and particulate debris. These agents also absorb bacteria and thus reduce the risk of infection. They're often used for decubitus and stasis ulcers, traumatic infected surgical wounds, and sickle cell ulcers. Sometimes chemical and mechanical debridement are combined by saturating bandages with medications, such as aluminum acetate, potassium permanganate, or hydrogen peroxide.

Surgical debridement, done under general or regional anesthesia, affords the fastest and most complete debridement but is usually reserved for burn patients or those with extremely deep or large ulcers. Often performed with skin grafting, it carries the risk of sepsis, if the wound is grossly infected at the time of excision, as well as hemorrhage and the usual risks of surgery.

In any type of debridement, fluid and electrolyte imbalance and infection may occur.

Purpose

To remove necrotic tissue from a wound, thereby promoting healing, preparing an area for grafting, or preventing secondary infection.

Preparation

Explain to the patient that debridement will remove dead tissue from his burn or ulcer. Discuss the type of debridement he'll undergo and reassure him that analgesics will be provided, if needed. To help the patient cope with the pain of debridement, teach him relaxation techniques.

Now gather the equipment (see *How to Debride a Wound*, pages 578 and 579). If ordered, administer an analgesic 20 minutes before the procedure. Then position the patient comfortably, providing maximum access to the site.

Procedure

Perform the debridement as quickly and gently as possible. See *How to De-*

HOW TO DEBRIDE A WOUND

All debridement methods have the same goal: to remove necrotic tissue and promote healing of burns and ulcers. The particular method used depends on a number of factors, including the type and extent of injury and the patient's overall condition. Here's how these different methods of debridement are performed.

Wet-to-dry dressings

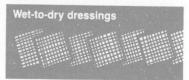

When changing a wet-to-dry dressing, you'll need a sterile bowl, sterile gauze, wetting solution, an outer dressing, and two pairs of sterile gloves. To begin, first loosen and lift the outer layer of the old dressing and discard it. Then clean the wound well. Next, open the sterile bowl's wrapper and use it as a sterile field. Open the sterile gauze and put it into the bowl; pour enough wetting solution into the bowl to dampen the gauze. Then open the outer dressing and drop it onto the sterile field.

Now put on sterile gloves and gently remove the dressing that has adhered to the wound. Discard the old dressing and gloves.

Put on a fresh pair of sterile gloves. Remove the gauze from the bowl and wring out excess moisture. (If the gauze is too wet, it won't dry completely before the next dressing change and thus won't effectively debride the wound. In addition, the excess moisture may macerate the wound tissue.) Place the moistened gauze over the wound and gently pack it in. Then apply the outer dressing and remove your gloves. Secure the dressing with tape or wrap it with kling.

Irrigation

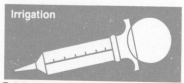

To irrigate a wound, you'll need to obtain the prescribed irrigating solution. If it isn't prepared in the pharmacy, dilute the irrigant with the proper amount of sterile water or sterile saline solution, as prescribed. Use aseptic technique when preparing the solution. You'll also need a sterile container, a rubber catheter and syringe, and an emesis basin or bed-saver pad to protect the bed linens.

Begin by removing the soiled dressing and establishing a sterile field. Then pour the prescribed amount of irrigating solution into the sterile container. Fill the syringe with irrigating solution and connect it to the rubber catheter.

Gently insert the catheter into the wound until you feel resistance. Then instill a slow, steady stream of solution into the wound until you've emptied the syringe. Make sure the solution flows from the clean to the dirty area of the wound to prevent cross-contamination. As you withdraw the syringe, pinch the catheter to avoid contaminating the equipment with aspirated drainage.

Repeat the irrigation until you've administered the prescribed amount of solution or until the solution returns clear. Be sure you've irrigated all areas of the wound and note the amount of solution that returns.

While cleansing the area around the wound, keep the patient in the same position to permit further drainage into the basin. Finally, pack the wound, if ordered, and apply a sterile dressing.

Bedside debridement

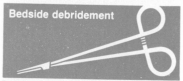

Besides wound-cleansing materials, you'll need forceps, scissors, and gauze sponges to perform bedside debridement. During the procedure, keep the patient warm and avoid exposing large areas of his body to prevent chilling and fluid loss.

To begin, remove the dressing, using sterile technique, and cleanse the wound. Debride an area no more than 4″ × 4″ (10 cm × 10 cm) at a time, and work as quickly as possible. Limit the procedure to a maximum of 20 minutes at a time.

Pick up the loosened edges of the eschar with forceps and examine it. Then, using scissors, cut the dead tissue away from the wound. Leave roughly a ¼″ margin of remaining eschar to avoid cutting into viable tissue. Bleeding should be minimal; if it occurs, apply gentle pressure with a 4″ × 4″ gauze sponge. However, if bleeding persists, notify the doctor and maintain pressure until he arrives; he may need to ligate bleeding vessels.

Hydrotherapy

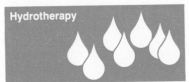

Before beginning hydrotherapy, clean and disinfect the tub, the room, and the equipment to prevent cross-contamination. Place the liner in the tub and fill the tub with water warmed to 98° to 104° F. (36.7° to 40° C.). Add the prescribed chemicals, which may include sodium chloride (to maintain isotonicity and prevent dialysis and irritation), potassium chloride (to prevent potassium loss), calcium hypochlorite detergent (to help prevent infection), and an antifoaming agent. Make sure the treatment room is warm enough to keep the patient from being chilled.

Finally, gather the same equipment and supplies that you'd use for bedside debridement, as well as towels. Keep in mind that hydrotherapy should be limited to 20 or 30 minutes, to prevent hypothermia and fluid and electrolyte imbalance.

Begin by taking and recording the patient's vital signs. If possible, weigh him to establish a baseline. If the patient's dressing is to be changed, remove and dispose of the outer dressing. Leave the inner dressing in place.

Next, help the patient into the tub. (If he isn't ambulatory, use a plinth and hydraulic lift system.) After the patient soaks for 3 to 5 minutes, remove the rest of the gauze dressings. If ordered, place the agitator into the water and turn it on.

Cleanse all unburned areas and provide general hygiene; then gently scrub the burned areas with gauze pads or sponges to remove topical agents, exudates, necrotic tissue, and other debris. Next, debride the wound as described in "Bedside debridement," above.

When the treatment has been completed, spray-rinse the patient's entire body to remove any remaining debris. Pat dry the unburned areas of his body, working quickly to prevent the patient from becoming chilled. Then transport the patient to the dressing area, and perform further debridement there if necessary. Apply sterile dressings.

Help the patient dress and escort him back to his room. Take his vital signs and weight (to detect fluid loss), and record the condition of the wound.

Chemical debridement

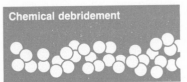

To perform chemical debridement, you'll need dextranomer, 4″ × 4″ gauze sponges, a plastic dressing, a rubber bulb and syringe, normal saline solution, and a sterile container.

Begin by gently irrigating the wound and the surrounding tissue with normal saline to remove any dextranomer remaining from the previous application. Blot the area, leaving it slightly moist. Then pour the dextranomer into the wound, forming a layer at least 3 mm thick. Cover the wound with gauze sponges and apply the transparent plastic dressing.

Between dressing changes, monitor the dextranomer's color through the plastic dressing. When it turns from white to gray or yellow—usually after 6 to 8 hours—it's time for a new application.

Also watch for and report the formation of viable nonoozing granulation tissue, which indicates the need to decrease the frequency of chemical debridement. Expect to see some inflammation from the dextranomer. If it's excessive or if signs of infection appear, notify the doctor immediately.

Surgical debridement

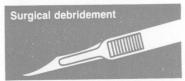

In surgical debridement, of course, you won't take as active a role as in other methods. In the operating room, the doctor may perform one of two procedures, depending on the depth and extent of the wound. In the first, tangential excision, he uses a dermatome or knife to remove sequential layers of dead tissue until he reaches viable tissue. In the second, fascial excision, he removes all injured tissue and underlying fat down to the fascia, using a scalpel, avulsion, or a laser.

In addition to the usual preoperative and postoperative monitoring, be especially alert for blood loss—which can quickly progress to hypovolemic shock—and signs of septicemia.

bride a Wound, pages 578 and 579, for details of mechanical, chemical, and surgical debridement.

Monitoring and aftercare

Assess the patient's pain level, both from his own reports and from such signs as restlessness, increased muscle tension, and rapid respirations. Provide additional analgesics, as ordered.

During dressing changes, note the amount of granulation tissue, necrotic debris, and drainage. Be alert for signs of wound infection. Report such signs immediately, since infection in compromised patients can quickly grow to life-threatening proportions.

Assess the patient's fluid and electrolyte status, especially if he has burns. Weigh him daily, maintain accurate intake and output records, and closely monitor laboratory test results. Watch for and report signs of electrolyte imbalance, such as poor skin turgor, cardiac disturbances, tremors, weakness or spasms, or confusion.

If the patient's limb was debrided, keep it elevated to promote venous return—especially for stasis ulcers.

Home care instructions

Because debridement is performed only in the hospital, it doesn't require any home care directions.

Therapeutic Baths
[Balneotherapy]

Therapeutic baths help treat psoriasis, atopic eczema, exfoliative dermatitis, bullous diseases, and pyodermas. Four types are commonly used: antibacterial, colloidal, emollient, and tar (see *Comparing Therapeutic Baths*). Besides promoting relaxation, they permit treatment of large areas. Because they can also cause dry skin, pruritus, scaling, and fissures, they should be limited to 20 or 30 minutes.

Purpose

• To cleanse the skin, loosen or remove crusts or scales, and relieve pruritus
• To deliver topical medications or hydrate the stratum corneum to allow penetration of topical medications.

Preparation

Explain the purpose of the bath to the patient and answer any questions he may have. Tell him that you'll respect his privacy but that, for safety reasons, he must leave the door unlocked. Point out the location of the call bell.

Make sure the tub and tub area are clean and that a soiled-dressing bin is available. Also make sure the room is warm enough; close the windows if necessary. Then gather the necessary supplies, including a good supply of clean towels, a washcloth (for psoriatic patients), a bath thermometer, a disposable bath mat, a clean gown and robe, slippers, and the medication to be added to the bath.

Place the bath mat in the tub and run the bath. Use a bath thermometer to ensure that the water temperature is about 97° F. (36° C.). Then carefully measure and add the medication to the water to achieve the prescribed dilution. Mix the water and medication well to prevent a sensitivity reaction. Hang an "occupied" sign on the door.

Procedure

Bring the patient to the treatment room and ask him to remove his clothes. Help him into the tub and position him comfortably, with as much of his body covered as possible. Place folded towels behind his head and, if he's short, place a bath stool or metal box in the tub so that he can brace his feet.

Caution the patient not to stand in the tub. Have him soak for 20 or 30 minutes. Then help him out of the tub. To prevent chills, instruct him to dry himself quickly by patting gently with a towel until his skin is damp dry. Apply ordered topical medications immediately, since they're absorbed better when the skin is damp. Assess his skin

COMPARING THERAPEUTIC BATHS

TYPE	AGENTS	PURPOSE
Antibacterial	Acetic acid Hexachlorophene Potassium permanganate Povidone-iodine	Used to treat infected eczema, dirty ulcerations, furunculosis, and pemphigus.
Colloidal	Aveeno colloidal oatmeal Aveeno colloidal oatmeal, oilated Starch and baking soda	Used to relieve pruritus and to soothe irritated skin. Indicated for any irritating or oozing condition, such as atopic eczema.
Emollient	Bath oils Mineral oil	Used to cleanse and hydrate the skin. Indicated for any dry skin condition.
Tar	Bath oils with tar Coal tar concentrate	Used to treat scaly dermatoses, sometimes in combination with ultraviolet light therapy. Loosens scales and relieves pruritus.

and note any improvement or reaction. If necessary, help him dress and escort him back to his room.

Monitoring and aftercare
Check the patient frequently while he's in the tub. If he's elderly or debilitated, stay with him throughout the bath.

Home care instructions
• Provide the patient with instructions and outline safety precautions. Explain that the therapeutic agents may make the tub slippery and that a bath mat is a necessity. Tell him that overly hot water can increase pruritus and scaling, and urge him to use a bath thermometer to measure water temperature.
• Explain to the patient that the average home bathtub holds 150 to 200 gallons of water, and that he should measure his medication accordingly. Tell him to mix the water well to prevent a reaction to the medication.
• If he has dry skin, mention that soap is drying. Explain that normal skin requires bathing only every other day, with soap applied only to the underarms, groin, and bottoms of feet.
• Remind the patient that friction during or after a bath can damage his skin. Unless he suffers from psoriasis, instruct him to wash himself with his bare hands instead of using a washcloth. Tell the patient with psoriasis to use a washcloth to loosen crusts, but only after he has soaked for 15 or 20 minutes. Instruct all patients to gently pat themselves dry with a clean towel, leaving the skin slightly damp.
• Tell the patient to report any increase in pruritus, oozing, erythema, or scaling to the doctor, and remind him to return for follow-up visits.

Ultraviolet Light Treatments

Ultraviolet light helps treat psoriasis, mycosis fungoides, atopic dermatitis, and uremic pruritus. It decreases epidermal cell proliferation, probably by inhibiting DNA synthesis. Two different ultraviolet light wavelengths, A and B, are used therapeutically. Ultraviolet light B (UVB) is the component of sunlight that causes sunburn. Ultraviolet light A (UVA) has no effect on normal skin, but the drug psoralen creates artificial sensitivity to it by binding with the DNA in epidermal basal cells. The combination of psoralen with UVA is known as PUVA therapy, or photo-chemotherapy.

UVB, which has been used for more than 50 years, usually provides long remissions from psoriasis. Treatments are typically given daily until the psoriasis clears and then one to three times a week for maintenance.

PUVA takes longer than UVB. Initially, it's given every other day until psoriatic lesions clear—typically after 4 to 8 weeks. Afterward, the patient may require maintenance therapy.

Ultraviolet light therapy can be done in the hospital, in a doctor's office, or at home. Typically, the light source is a bank of high-intensity fluorescent bulbs, set into a reflective cabinet. (At home, a small sunlamp may be used.)

Overexposure of the skin to ultraviolet light can result from prolonged treatment, inadequate distance between the patient and light source, use of photosensitizing drugs, or overly sensitive skin. Eye damage can be prevented by using gray or green polarized lenses during UVB therapy or UV-opaque sunglasses during PUVA therapy. The patient undergoing PUVA therapy should wear these glasses during daylight hours after treatment, since psoralen remains in eye tissue for a prolonged period.

Long-term effects of treatment are basically the same as for excessive sun exposure: atrophy and aging of the skin and an increased risk of skin cancer. These can be minimized by using emollients and a sunscreen.

Contraindications to PUVA and UVB therapy include photosensitivity diseases, use of photosensitivity-inducing drugs, a history of skin cancer, previous skin irradiation (since it can induce skin cancer), and cataracts or loss of a lens secondary to cataract surgery.

Purpose
To treat psoriasis and other skin disorders by decreasing epidermal cell proliferation.

Preparation
Explain to the patient that ultraviolet light treatments produce a mild sunburn that will help clear up skin lesions. With UVB, the erythema appears within 4 to 6 hours; with PUVA, it may not become evident for 48 to 72 hours. In either case, it should disappear within another 24 hours. Tell the patient that mild dryness and desquamation will follow within 1 to 2 days.

Review the patient's history for photosensitivity diseases, skin cancer, or previous radiation treatments. Ask about current use of photosensitizing drugs, such as anticonvulsants, certain antihypertensives, phenothiazines, salicylates, sulfonamides, tetracyclines, tretinoin, various cancer chemotherapeutic drugs, and others.

Perform a thorough skin examination. If the patient will be undergoing PUVA therapy, tell him to take psoralen with food 2 hours before treatment. Emphasize the importance of wearing UV-opaque sunglasses when he's outdoors for the remainder of the day because psoralen's effects persist for about 12 hours. Tell him to report any signs of overexposure, such as painful and excessive erythema and blistering. Also have him report the absence of erythema, which indicates the need to increase psoralen dosage.

Before therapy begins, the doctor will determine the proper dosage. For PUVA, the initial dosage is usually 0.5 joules/cm^2 (which requires 1 to 8 minutes of exposure), depending upon the patient's skin type and pigmentation. For UVB, the doctor calculates the patient's minimal erythema dose.

Procedure
To begin therapy, tell the patient to disrobe and to put on a hospital gown. Have him remove the gown or bare just the treatment area once he's in the phototherapy unit. Make sure he's wearing protective goggles and that vulnerable areas of his skin are protected by a sunblock, towels, or the gown.

If the patient's undergoing local UVB

treatment, make sure he's positioned at the correct distance from the sunlamp or hot quartz lamp. For facial exposure with a sunlamp, position his face 12″ (30 cm) from the lamp. For exposure of areas on his body, position him about 30″ (76 cm) away. Also position him 30″ away if you're using a quartz lamp. After delivering the prescribed UVB dose, help the patient out of the unit.

Monitoring and aftercare
During therapy, make sure the patient has his goggles on at all times. If you're observing him through unit windows, wear goggles, too. If the patient's standing, tell him to report any dizziness.

Look for marked erythema, blistering, peeling, or other signs of overexposure 4 to 6 hours after UVB and 24 to 48 hours after UVA. If overexposure occurs, notify the doctor; he'll usually withhold treatment for a few days and then reinstitute it at a lower level of exposure.

If the doctor has prescribed tar preparations along with UVB, watch for signs of sensitivity, such as erythema, pruritus, or eczematous reactions.

Home care instructions
• To combat dry skin, encourage the patient to use emollients and drink plenty of fluids. Warn him to avoid hot baths or showers and to curb his use of soap, all of which promote dry skin.
• If the patient is undergoing PUVA treatments, review his schedule for taking psoralen. Explain that any deviation from it could result in burns or ineffective treatment. Emphasize the importance of wearing UV-opaque sunglasses when outdoors, for at least 12 hours after taking psoralen. Similarly, emphasize the need for yearly eye examinations to detect possible cataract formation.
• Tell the patient to notify his doctor before taking any drug, including aspirin, to prevent heightened photosensitivity.
• If the patient is using a sunlamp at home, tell him to first allow the lamp to warm up for 5 minutes and then to limit exposure to the time prescribed by the doctor. Instruct him to protect his eyes with goggles and to use a dependable timer or have someone in the room during therapy. Above all, *tell him never to use the sunlamp when he's tired;* some patients have fallen asleep under the warmth of the lamp and suffered severe burns.
• Mention to the patient that he can help relieve a localized burn by applying cool water soaks for 20 minutes or until skin temperature is cool. For larger burns, tepid tap water baths may be indicated, but have the patient check with the doctor first. After the bath, he can apply an oil-in-water moisturizing lotion; he shouldn't use a petrolatum-based product since it can trap radiant heat. For a severe PUVA burn, the doctor may prescribe prednisone.
• Tell the patient to limit natural light exposure, to use a sunblocker when he's outdoors, and to notify his doctor immediately if he discovers any suspicious lesions.

Selected References

Arndt, K. *Manual of Dermatologic Therapeutics,* 3rd ed. Boston: Little, Brown & Co., 1984.
Colman, W., and Coleman, W. *Outpatient Surgery of the Skin.* New Hyde Park, N.Y.: Medical Examination Pub. Co., 1983.
Demis, J. et al., eds. *Clinical Dermatology,* 4 vols. Philadelphia: J.B. Lippincott Co., 1986.
Epstein E., and Epstein, E., Jr., eds. *Techniques in Skin Surgery.* Philadelphia: Lea & Febiger, 1979.
Fitzpatrick, T., and Freedberg, I. *Dermatology in General Medicine,* 3rd ed. New York: McGraw-Hill Book Co., 1987.

18

Treating Trauma

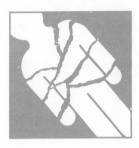

Treating Trauma

Introduction

Consider these grim statistics: trauma is the leading killer of Americans between the ages of 1 and 44. And the first hour after injury is the most critical. In fact, up to 75% of all fatalities occur within those crucial 60 minutes.

Despite statistics like these, your skills and expertise can help swing the odds of survival in the patient's favor.

Treatment stat

When caring for the trauma patient, you'll have to act swiftly and decisively. And you'll need to be conversant with a wide range of treatments. Suppose, for example, you're treating a patient with mutiple traumatic injuries. To promptly stabilize the patient and deter development or worsening of shock, you'll need to administer a vasopressor, such as norepinephrine. If he has a severed digit or limb, you'll need to control hemorrhage promptly and ensure that the severed segment is correctly prepared for possible replantation. Or if he has massive abdominal bleeding or a hemothorax, you may need to set up and operate an autotransfusion system so that you can reinfuse the patient's own blood.

For other trauma patients, you may be called upon to help correct thermal imbalances, such as hypothermia and hyperthermia. Treatments for these conditions span a wide range. In mild hypothermia, for example, you may be responsible for simply applying warm compresses and monitoring the patient's temperature. In severe hypothermia, you may need to infuse warmed I.V. fluids, warmed and humidified oxygen, and perhaps a warmed peritoneal dialysate. You may even be called upon to assist with extracorporeal blood warming.

In hyperthermia, your responsibilities are equally diverse. In mild cases, you may apply cold packs and monitor temperature. In severe cases, you may apply cooling blankets that come equipped with a rectal probe for continuous temperature monitoring.

Watch for warning signs

Besides performing or assisting with trauma treatments, you're also responsible for recognizing signs of complications. You'll need, of course, sharp assessment skills since complications of traumatic injury and its treatment often arise suddenly.

Consider, for example, cooling treatments for hyperthermia. If the patient experiences shaking chills, you'll need to discontinue the treatment and notify the doctor immediately. That's because chills increase the patient's metabolic rate, thereby elevating his body temperature to even more dangerous heights.

DRUG THERAPY

Vasopressors

By stimulating the sympathetic nervous system, vasopressors rapidly raise blood pressure and increase cardiac output, thereby improving perfusion of vital organs. In traumatic multisystemic injuries, they provide prompt stabilization and deter development or worsening of shock. As a result, they can sustain life until emergency treatments can correct the underlying problem. However, vasopressors should usually be given after hypovolemia has been corrected, to prevent peripheral vascular damage.

The five vasopressors used routinely include *dopamine, epinephrine, methoxamine, norepinephrine,* and *phenylephrine*. Except for epinephrine, their indications are similar: to correct acute hypotension caused by shock or anesthesia. Epinephrine, the drug of choice for treating anaphylactic shock, can also restore cardiac rhythm after cardiac arrest.

Because of their vasoconstrictive effects, vasopressors must be diluted and titrated precisely to prevent peripheral vascular damage and subsequent loss of digits. They should be given cautiously since extravasation into the surrounding tissue can cause necrosis. (See *Treating Extravasation*, page 588.) During injection or infusion, they require careful monitoring to detect blood pressure or pulse rate changes and other side effects.

Purpose and action
Vasopressors help stabilize patients with acute hypotension or shock. They stimulate or increase the effect of the hormones epinephrine and norepinephrine on alpha- and beta-adrenergic receptors within the sympathetic nervous system. However, because the vasopressors do not stimulate both classes of adrenergic receptors equally, their effects differ. Phenylephrine, for example, primarily stimulates alpha-adrenergic receptors, whereas dopamine stimulates both types of receptors as well as dopaminergic receptors.

Monitoring
Be sure to dilute the prescribed vasopressor in the correct solution (see *Comparing Vasopressors* for details). If possible, review the patient's medication regimen for possible interactions. For example, use of monoamine oxidase inhibitors in a patient receiving dopamine or phenylephrine may trigger hypertensive crisis. Similarly, use of tricyclic antidepressants with epinephrine, norepinephrine, or methoxamine may trigger hypertensive crisis. Concurrent use of phenytoin with dopamine may cause sudden hypotension and bradycardia.

During vasopressor administration, be alert for decreased urinary output, altered cardiac output or blood pressure, tachycardia, widened pulse pressure, and hypertension. If any of these effects occur, be sure to notify the doctor immediately. The drug may need to be discontinued or the dosage adjusted.

Check the patient's extremities frequently for changes in skin color and temperature and for the presence of distal pulses. Be especially alert if the patient has a history of occlusive vascular disease since he's at risk for distal necrosis and tissue sloughing.

When discontinuing I.V. administration of vasopressors, slow the infusion rate gradually and monitor the patient for sudden onset of hypotension. Continue to monitor vital signs for several hours after the drug is stopped.

Home care instructions
Because vasopressors are administered in emergencies, they don't require home care instructions.

COMPARING VASOPRESSORS

DRUG, ROUTE, AND INDICATIONS	CONTRA-INDICATIONS	ADMINISTRATION TIPS
Dopamine *I.V.:* to treat shock and correct hemodynamic imbalances	Ventricular fibrillation, uncorrected tachyarrhythmias, pheochromocytoma	• Mix just before use with normal saline solution (NSS), dextrose 5% in water (D_5W), or a combination of these. Discard after 24 hours or if discoloration occurs. Don't mix with alkaline solutions and don't give alkaline drugs through I.V. line containing dopamine. • Use a microdrip or infusion pump to control rate. Use large vein to reduce risk of extravasation. If it occurs, stop infusion and call doctor. • If diastolic pressure rises disproportionately, decrease infusion rate.
Epinephrine *I.V., into endotracheal tube, or intracardiac:* to restore cardiac rhythm in cardiac arrest. *S.C., I.M., or I.V.:* to treat bronchospasm, hypersensitivity, and anaphylaxis	Acute-angle glaucoma, shock (except for anaphylactic shock), coronary insufficiency, organic brain damage	• Mix just before use with NSS, D_5W, or a combination of these. Store in light-resistant container. Discard after 24 hours or if discoloration or precipitation occurs. • Avoid I.M. injection of oil solution into buttocks since gas gangrene may occur. • Massage site after injection to counteract possible local vasoconstriction. • If blood pressure rises too rapidly, give a fast-acting vasodilator.
Methoxamine *I.V. and I.M.:* to correct acute hypotension occurring during general anesthesia	Severe hypertension	• I.V. injection is usually given when systolic pressure falls below 60 mm Hg. It may be accompanied by I.M. injection for a prolonged effect. If systolic pressure exceeds 60 mm Hg, I.M. injection may be given. • Monitor blood pressure and cardiac rhythm. • Keep atropine available to correct bradycardia.
Norepinephrine *I.V.:* to restore blood pressure in acute hypotension	Mesenteric or peripheral vascular thrombosis, pregnancy, profound hypoxia, hypercarbia, hypotension caused by blood volume deficits, or during cyclopropane or halothane anesthesia	• Mix just before use with NSS and D_5W; don't mix solely with NSS. Discard solution after 24 hours. • Use a microdrip or infusion pump to control rate. Use large vein to minimize risk of extravasation. If it occurs, stop the infusion and call the doctor. Check for blanching along the course of the infused vein. • Keep atropine available to correct bradycardia, propranolol to correct arrhythmias. • During infusion, check blood pressure every 2 minutes until stable, then every 5 minutes.
Phenylephrine *I.V.:* to treat severe hypotension and shock	Acute-angle glaucoma, ventricular tachycardia, severe cardiovascular disease	• Mix with D_5W. • Monitor blood pressure frequently. Adjust infusion rate to maintain blood pressure slightly below patient's normal level, if known.

COMPLICATIONS

TREATING EXTRAVASATION

If you're administering norepinephrine or dopamine, be especially alert for signs of extravasation, such as pain, swelling, blanching, or discoloration, at the infusion site. If extravasation occurs, stop the infusion immediately. If possible, estimate the amount of extravasated solution and notify the doctor. Using a tuberculin syringe, he'll slowly and gently aspirate as much as possible of the infiltrated solution from the subcutaneous tissue. Then follow this plan of action.

Administer the antidote
To treat extravasation, most doctors order instillation of phentolamine. This drug combats the vasoconstrictive effects of norepinephrine or dopamine by dilating the peripheral vessels. It must be administered within 12 hours of extravasation to have this antidotal effect.
 If ordered, dilute 5 to 10 mg of phentolamine in 10 ml of normal saline solution. Then instill the solution into the area of extravasation.

Apply moist heat
Apply warm compresses to the area for 24 hours or as ordered. Besides promoting vasodilation, this measure will also reduce the patient's pain.

Provide ongoing monitoring
After treating extravasation, continue to monitor the patient for signs of tissue necrosis and sloughing, such as discoloration, pain or loss of sensation, swelling, or coldness at the site. Instruct him to report any of these signs.

Document the incident
Document the site of extravasation, the patient's signs and symptoms, and the estimated amount of infiltrated solution. Also specify the treatment given, the time you notified the doctor, and the doctor's name.

SURGERY

Repair of a Traumatic Amputation

In the past, traumatically severed digits or limbs usually spelled a life without the injured part for most patients. Today, however, microvascular surgery has dramatically reversed this unfavorable prognosis. Even when there is severe injury to the skin, muscle, bone, and blood vessels, doctors often attempt replantation if the nerves remain unscathed or minimally damaged. What's more, patients can regain a significant degree of function in the replanted limb or digit. To date, upper extremity replantations have proven more successful than lower extremity ones. This can be attributed partly to increased vascular flow.

Successful replantation, though, depends on several factors. First, the severed part must be kept moist, cool, and free from further contamination before surgery. Then, replantation must be performed and any complications, such as contractures, infection, or hemorrhage, must be avoided or promptly corrected. Once these obstacles have been overcome, the patient must undergo a lengthy and perhaps difficult rehabilitation program, attempting not only to recover use of the replanted part but also to learn to accept an altered body image and resume an independent life-style.

The repair of a traumatic amputation demands comprehensive preoperative and postoperative nursing care to prevent further injury to the affected part, to relieve the patient's pain and anxiety, and to reduce the risk of complications.

Purpose
To replant a fully or partially severed body part.

Preparation
A patient who has been given initial emergency treatment requires ongoing care and monitoring before microvascular surgery. Begin by giving an analgesic, as ordered.

If the patient's limb or digit has been completely severed, provide stump care. Make sure the wound is covered with a moist sterile pressure dressing. Elevate the stump, maintaining proper alignment, if possible. Place a light, loose ice bag on top of the stump to control bleeding. Apply pressure if bleeding continues, and keep a tourniquet available if severe bleeding occurs. Also, note the amount, nature, and location of drainage. Ensure that the severed part has been correctly prepared (see *Preserving an Amputated Part*).

If the patient has a large and incomplete amputation (the distal and proximal wounds remain connected by some potentially viable tissue and blood vessels), ensure that the affected area has been correctly prepared. Typically, the emergency room staff will have treated the amputation as an open fracture: the wound will have been cultured, irrigated, dressed with saline-soaked sterile gauze, and splinted to minimize discomfort and prevent motion and further injury. If all seems in order, elevate the affected part to promote venous return and minimize swelling. Help the patient assume as comfortable a position as possible, maintaining proper alignment.

Monitor the patient's vital signs, level of consciousness, and intake and output. Report any changes to the doctor.

Assess the patient for other injuries he may have sustained at the time of amputation. Draw a blood sample for typing and cross matching in case transfusion is required. Collect samples for routine laboratory tests, as ordered, and schedule an X-ray to help evaluate bone damage. Administer prophylactic antibiotics, as instructed. To prevent development of tetanus, verify that the patient has been immunized.

Because some patients will deny the

PRIORITIES

PRESERVING AN AMPUTATED PART

If you're called upon to preserve an amputated body part for replantation, you'll need to act quickly and correctly.

Protecting a partial amputation
Treat a partial amputation as you would an open fracture, using a rigid splint to immobilize the extremity. Here's how to proceed:
• Observe the damaged extremity for signs of fracture.
• Palpate the patient's pulse and check his sensory and motor function distal to the injury. Compare findings to those obtained on the uninjured side.
• Place moist sterile dressings over the site. Don't cover the wound with splinting materials.
• Immobilize at least one joint above and below the level of injury, taking care to pad all bony prominences.
• After splinting, again palpate the patient's distal pulse and test sensory and motor function distal to the injury.
• Keep the extremity cool by covering it with a plastic bag and then enclosing this in an ice-filled plastic bag. To prevent irreversible tissue damage, always protect the extremity from direct contact with ice. And never use dry ice.

Preserving a severed segment
Follow these directions to preserve a severed segment:
• Put on sterile gloves and flush the segment with normal saline or Ringer's solution. Avoid scrubbing or debriding it.
• Using sterile gauze, gently pat the segment dry. Then wrap it in saline-soaked sterile gauze and cover with a sterile towel.
• Place the wrapped part in a plastic bag and seal shut. Now place this bag inside an ice-filled plastic bag and seal.
• Label the plastic bag with the patient's name, identification of the amputated segment, and the date and time when cooling began.

severity of their injury, emphasize the need for surgery. Explain the replantation procedure and provide emotional support. Encourage the patient to express his feelings.

Procedure
In the operating room, the surgeon will examine the extent of damage and attempt to replant the severed part, if possible. He begins by approximating and stabilizing bone, usually by internal fixation. He identifies the veins and arteries, removes all clots, and assesses the patency of each vessel through angiography. Then he repairs the main nerve trunks and creates further meticulous anastomoses. Next, he repairs muscles and tendons, if possible, and covers all anastomosed sites with muscle to allow for optimal capillary and lymphatic regeneration.

After loosely suturing the skin, the surgeon may apply partial-thickness grafts. He may also perform a fasciotomy to prevent ischemia of major repaired vessels from muscle swelling. After completing these procedures, he applies a dressing over the site.

Monitoring and aftercare
Take the patient's vital signs and administer analgesics, as ordered. Regularly check his dressing for excessive bleeding or drainage. If hemorrhage occurs, apply direct pressure and notify the doctor immediately.

Frequently assess circulatory status and motor and sensory function in the most distal portion of the repaired part. Observe for swelling along fascial planes, a possible sign of compartment syndrome.

Because most traumatic amputations are contaminated, anticipate infection. The initial wound culture will reveal the pathogen. Based on the results, the doctor will adjust the antibiotic regimen, if necessary.

Continue I.V. fluids, as needed, to promote fluid replacement, tissue hydration, and electrolyte balance. Transfuse blood or administer a low-molecular–weight dextran, if required. Give oxygen, as ordered, to correct tissue hypoxia.

Home care instructions
• Instruct the patient and his family to watch for and report any unusual pain, bleeding, or signs of infection. Stress the importance of keeping the replantation site clean and dry to avoid skin breakdown, irritation, and infection.
• Explain any activity restrictions to the patient.
• Reinforce the need to follow the prescribed rehabilitation program to restore optimal function in the limb or digit. Help the patient and his family cope with the prospect of a lengthy rehabilitation. If necessary, refer them to a support group or suggest counseling.

AUTOLOGOUS TRANSFUSION

Autotransfusion

A procedure for collecting, filtering, and reinfusing the patient's own blood, autotransfusion is most commonly used for traumatic injury, such as hemothorax and massive abdominal bleeding. This procedure also allows treatment of primary injuries of the lungs, liver, chest wall, heart, pulmonary vessels, spleen, kidneys, inferior vena cava, and iliac, portal, and subclavian veins.

Although transfusion of homologous typed and cross-matched blood is used more commonly to restore hemodynamic equilibrium, autotransfusion possesses distinct advantages. For example, because of its autologous nature, autotransfusion eliminates the risk of disease transmission, transfusion reactions, and isoimmunizations. Moreover, it conserves blood bank supplies and provides a readily available source of compatible blood, saving time otherwise spent on typing and cross matching. This feature is especially important in treating trauma, where seconds count. Unlike bank blood, autologous blood has a normal temperature and pH, a high oxygen-carrying capacity due to high levels of 2,3-diphosphoglycerate, and normal clotting factors and levels of potassium and ammonia. Another special feature of autologous blood transfusion is its possible acceptability to patients whose religious beliefs prohibit transfusion of donor blood.

Despite these many advantages, autotransfusion has several potential complications, such as air embolism, which may result from faulty monitoring; coagulopathy; and enteric contamination. Occasionally, autotransfusion causes transient hemoglobinuria as a result of red blood cell trauma during collection.

Contraindications include fecal or urinary contamination of blood lost from hemorrhage; either of these makes the patient susceptible to bacterial growth and clotting, leading to sepsis, coagulopathies, and microemboli. Patients with coagulation defects, malignant neoplasms, or respiratory infection shouldn't undergo autotransfusion. Nor should patients with traumatic wounds over 4 hours old, since blood degradation occurs rapidly beyond that time.

Purpose
To correct hemodynamic imbalance through reinfusion of the patient's own blood.

Preparation
When you're preparing for autotransfusion, the patient may be unconscious. If he is, talk to him and touch him as you would any conscious patient.

Obtain baseline vital signs and ensure that basic life-support needs, including delivery of oxygen and administration of I.V. fluids, have been met. Collect the necessary equipment:

an I.V. pole or floor stand; a 50-ml bottle of the anticoagulant citrate-phosphate-dextrose (CPD); chest tubes for hemothorax or a drainage tubing set; a vacuum regulator (not needed if the autotransfusion system has an underwater seal unit); a canister; a sterile disposable blood liner with a 170-micron filter; and a microemboli filter with recipient set.

Now, set up the autotransfusion system. Remove the sterile liners from the package and stretch them to full length so that they expand in the canister when the vacuum is applied. Avoid contaminating the sterile spacer when capping the drainage port. While inserting the liner in the canister, snap the lid securely in place, placing the thumb tab directly over the canister to facilitate connection to suction. Connect the liner lid tubing with the sterile spacer to the canister tee. Attach the vacuum tubing to the opposite end of the canister tee. Temporarily occlude the tubing between the vacuum regulator and canister to set the vacuum pressure between 10 and 30 mm Hg; a higher setting increases hemolysis. Remove the protective cap from the patient port and attach the sterile proximal end of the drainage tubing with the anticoagulant connector to the patient port of the liner. Insert the volume-control set spike into the CPD bottle. Hang the bottle and prime the administration set. Remove the cap from the anticoagulant connector and attach the anticoagulant administration line. Run 100 ml of CPD into the liner to prevent clotting of blood.

Procedure
To collect blood, attach the proximal end of the drainage tubing to the chest drainage catheter. During drainage, add one part CPD to seven parts blood to avoid clotting.

To transfuse collected blood, clamp the patient's line to prevent pneumothorax when the vacuum is lost. Disconnect the patient and anticoagulant lines from the liner lid.

UNDERSTANDING
AUTOTRANSFUSION SYSTEMS

Several autotransfusion systems, such as the Sorensen and Bently systems, are commercially available. Typically, these systems contain a sterile canister that collects blood. The canister's liner contains two chambers separated by a 170-micron filter that traps aggregates of fibrin, red blood cells, platelets, and other potential thrombi.

Some systems also contain an underwater seal unit that allows collection of blood from the pleural cavity. This unit lets air escape from the pleural cavity and prevents its return, thereby maintaining negative pressure.

When the canister's liner contains 500 to 1,000 ml of blood, transfusion can take place. First, the liner is disconnected from the vacuum source and air is removed. Then the liner is inverted and a microemboli filter and transfusion tubing are attached.

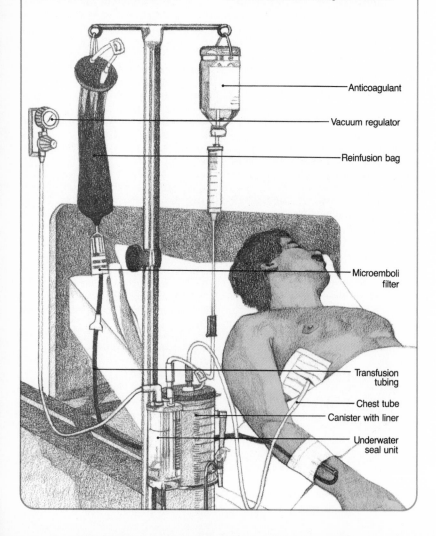

Anticoagulant

Vacuum regulator

Reinfusion bag

Microemboli filter

Transfusion tubing

Chest tube

Canister with liner

Underwater seal unit

Disconnect the liner lid tubing and sterile spacer from the canister tee; remove and discard the sterile spacer. Attach the liner lid tubing to the patient port, close the clamp, push up on the thumb tab to unsnap the liner lid, and remove the liner from the canister.

Invert the liner and raise the recessed stem at the bottom of the liner. Remove the cap and, using a twisting motion, insert the microemboli filter set into the liner port. Hold the filter and recipient set upright, open the clamp, and gently compress the bag to remove all air.

Close the clamp. Hang the liner, open the clamp, partly fill the drip chamber, and prime the tubing. Transfuse blood in the usual way.

Monitoring and aftercare

Monitor the volume of collected blood to prevent overflow. If you anticipate heavy bleeding, set up two canisters to eliminate changing the filter. Periodically shake the liner to mix the blood and anticoagulant thoroughly. Don't store blood in the liner; transfuse it within 4 hours of the start of collection.

Monitor the patient for signs of increased hemorrhaging. Continued hemorrhage may necessitate repeating the procedure or immediate surgery.

Assess the patient's airway, vital signs, urinary output, cardiac output, EKG, and level of consciousness, as well as the patency and infusion rates of all invasive lines. If such complications as hemolysis, thrombocytopenia, coagulopathies, sepsis, particulate and air emboli, and citrate toxicity occur, notify the doctor immediately.

Home care instructions

• If the insertion sites of chest and drainage tubes do not heal, instruct the patient on proper incision care and on keeping the incision clean and dry.

• Describe the signs of infection, such as fever, unusual soreness at the insertion site, and increased inflammation or redness. Tell the patient to report any such symptoms, or itching, to his doctor.

TREATMENTS WITH HEAT OR COLD

Rewarming Treatments

Used for hypothermia caused by exposure to cold, rewarming includes a range of treatments: from external application of a hot-water bottle to chest intubation and instillation of heated solution. The type of rewarming ordered depends on the degree of hypothermia and the patient's age and general health. In a healthy patient with mild hypothermia (core temperature of 90° to 94° F., or 32.2° to 34.4° C.), passive external rewarming, such as use of blankets, is indicated because it reduces heat loss by evaporation, convection, and radiation and allows spontaneous rewarming through generation of body heat. Passive rewarming also maintains peripheral vasoconstriction, reducing the risk of vascular collapse.

Active external rewarming, such as use of heating pads or a hypothermia blanket, may be ordered for moderate hypothermia or if passive rewarming fails to raise core temperature at least 1.8 F. degrees (1 C. degree) per hour. If a patient has severe hypothermia, active core rewarming techniques may be used to raise the patient's temperature rapidly. The doctor may order I.V. infusion of warmed fluids, administration of warmed oxygen, or an instillation of warmed dialysate into the peritoneum. In extremely severe hypothermia, he may insert a chest tube or perform a thoracotomy to instill heated normal saline solution or Ringer's lactate. Extracorporeal blood rewarming may also be initiated.

Complications during rewarming

may include ventricular fibrillation and vascular collapse, and core temperature can plummet after treatment is stopped. However, careful application of rewarming techniques and frequent monitoring help avoid such complications.

Purpose
To restore normal core temperature.

Preparation
If the patient has severe hypothermia, remove any wet clothing, check for frostbite, and prepare for active core rewarming, as ordered. Handle him gently to avoid ventricular fibrillation. In hypothermia, vasoconstriction shunts most of the patient's blood to the heart, lungs, and brain. As a result, the remaining blood in the extremities becomes cold, acidotic, and hyperkalemic. A sudden rush of this blood into the central circulation can cause ventricular fibrillation and even death. To avoid this, keep the patient as still as possible and don't allow him to exert himself.

If the patient isn't in immediate distress, explain that rewarming treatments will restore his body temperature to its normal level. Describe the specific treatment ordered by the doctor. Make sure the treatment room is warm and free of drafts. Have the patient put on a hospital gown without metal snaps to avoid heat injury. Cover him with blankets and wrap a towel around his head.

Now gather the necessary equipment. First, obtain a low-reading rectal thermometer or, better yet, a rectal probe that allows continuous temperature monitoring. Obtain towels for drying and adhesive tape or gauze for holding the equipment in place. Other necessary equipment may include a hot-water bottle with a utility thermometer to measure water temperature; an absorbent, protective cloth covering; an electric heating pad; an aquamatic K pad; a hypothermia blanket; and distilled water. Make sure dry bedding and warm blankets are in the patient's room.

If ordered, insert an I.V. line and warm dextrose 5% in water or dextrose 5% in normal saline solution. If ordered, insert an indwelling (Foley) catheter to monitor urinary output.

If you're using a hot-water bottle, check it for leaks by filling it with hot water. If no leaks appear, discard the water. Then fill the bag about halfway with water heated to 115° to 125° F. (46.1° to 51.7° C.) for adults or 105° to 115° F. (40.6° to 46.1° C.) for children and the elderly. Now squeeze the bag to expel any air, which may decrease flexibility and heat conduction.

If you're using an electrical heating device, check for frayed wires or damaged insulation. Also check an aquamatic K pad and hypothermia blankets for leaks, and clear the tubing of air, which could interfere with heat conduction. Because tap water leaves mineral deposits in the unit, use distilled water to fill these devices. Place the control unit on the bedside table, slightly above the patient so that gravity can assist water flow. Preheat the aquamatic K pad or hypothermia blanket so that the patient receives immediate benefit. Cover the device with an absorbent cloth to prevent possible tissue damage.

Just before rewarming, obtain baseline vital signs.

Procedure
If the patient has extremely severe hypothermia, the doctor may perform a thoracotomy or insert a chest tube and instill warmed normal saline solution or Ringer's lactate into the mediastinum. He may also initiate extracorporeal blood rewarming.

If the patient has severe hypothermia, infuse warmed I.V. fluids to decrease peripheral vasoconstriction and blood viscosity and to improve coronary perfusion, reducing the risk of arrhythmias. Give heated, humidified oxygen by mask, endotracheal tube, or intermittent positive-pressure breathing device. If ordered, assist with peritoneal dialysis, using dextrose 1.5% warmed to 110° F. (43.3° C.).

If the patient shows signs of frostbite (absence of skin blanching with application of pressure, pain, or possibly loss of sensation), handle the body part extremely carefully and quickly immerse it in warm water (100° to 108° F., or 37.8° to 42.2° C.) or wrap it with warmed, moist gauze. Avoid prolonged thawing, which increases cellular

damage in frostbite. Also avoid rubbing the area, to prevent further tissue damage.

If the patient has mild hypothermia, begin rewarming with the simplest measure: blankets. If the patient's core temperature doesn't rise at least 1.8 F. degrees (1 C. degree) after an hour, begin active external warming. Place a hot-water bottle or an electric heating pad on the blanket and over the patient's thorax. Or immerse the patient

_____COMPLICATIONS_____

GUARDING AGAINST HAZARDS OF REWARMING

Rewarming can contribute to severe and possibly life- or limb-threatening complications, especially if the patient's core temperature fell below 86° F. (30° C.) or if he experienced frostbite.

Monitor cardiac status
In severe hypothermia, closely monitor the patient's cardiac status. The reason? Atrial and ventricular fibrillation, premature ventricular contractions, and conduction blocks commonly occur when core temperature goes below 86° F. These arrhythmias are especially difficult to reverse until core temperature rises to 90° F. (32.2° C.), even with prompt defibrillation or administration of antiarrhythmics. For up to 24 hours after rewarming, the patient remains at risk for ventricular fibrillation. So be sure to have a defibrillator and sodium bicarbonate readily available.

Provide prophylaxis
To guard against pneumonia, the principal complication of hypothermia, administer antibiotics, as ordered.

Check intake and output
Monitor intake and output and give fluids, as ordered. Vasodilation and hyperemia may increase the patient's fluid needs during rewarming. At the same time, the patient remains susceptible to fluid overload. Observe for signs of pulmonary edema, such as crackles and distended neck veins.

Review laboratory data
Monitor blood studies, which characteristically reveal dehydration, electrolyte

imbalance, and acidosis. These should correct as the patient rewarms. If they don't, give potassium or sodium bicarbonate, as ordered.

Provide comfort and care for frostbite
Because frostbite causes considerable pain during thawing, administer analgesics, as ordered. Institute reverse isolation to prevent infection.

Monitor skin color in the affected area: a pink flush or skin that is warm and blanches when touched indicates a return of function; a mottled blue or purple skin indicates superficial frostbite; and gray suggests a deep frostbite.

Check pulses in the frostbitten part. If they're weak or absent after rewarming, the patient may have a thrombus. Observe for edema and persistent cyanosis or ischemia, which, along with worsening pain, may signal compartment syndrome. Notify the doctor immediately if any of these untoward signs occur.

Roughly 12 to 24 hours after exposure, inspect the frostbitten area frequently for skin blebs. Don't rupture the blebs, as they contain sterile fluid that helps to protect the underlying tissue.

Watch for other warning signs
Be alert for signs of thromboembolism, such as calf or chest pain, redness in the frostbitten area, or dyspnea. Observe for nasal or gum bleeding as well as for bleeding from an I.V. site. Such bleeding may result from increased viscosity and intravascular stasis. Notify the doctor if any of these complications occur.

in a warm-water bath. However, if the doctor has ordered a hypothermia blanket, apply lanolin over the area of the patient's skin that comes in contact with the blanket. Then place one blanket beneath the patient, with the top edge aligned with his neck. Use a sheet or bath blanket as insulation between the patient and the hypothermia blanket if no other cover is available. Insert the rectal probe and tape it in place to avoid dislodgment. If rectal insertion is contraindicated, insert the probe into the axilla and tape it in place. Plug the other end of the probe into the correct jack on the blanket's control panel. If necessary, place a sheet or a second hypothermia blanket over the patient to increase conduction by trapping heated air.

During rewarming, reposition the patient every 30 minutes, unless contraindicated, to prevent skin breakdown.

Monitoring and aftercare
Monitor vital signs and neurologic status every 5 minutes until core temperature reaches the desired level, then every 15 minutes until the temperature stabilizes or as ordered. Active core rewarming is typically discontinued when core temperature approaches 96° F. (35.6° C.) to avoid hyperthermia. After discontinuing rewarming, be alert for falling core temperature. If it occurs, notify the doctor; he may reinstitute rewarming.

Be alert for other possible complications of rewarming. (See *Guarding Against Hazards of Rewarming*, page 595.)

Generally, the patient's neurologic status improves as his core temperature rises. However, if you don't observe any improvement, assess for an underlying problem, such as head injury, sepsis, hypothyroidism, hypoglycemia, adrenal insufficiency, or uremia. Collect samples for thyroid function tests, serum cortisol levels, toxicology screening, and blood cultures, as ordered.

Home care instructions
• If appropriate, teach the patient how to prevent recurrence of hypothermia.
• If the patient had severe frostbite, recommend physical therapy.
• Evaluate the patient's home care needs. If you suspect the patient doesn't have adequate shelter or clothing, contact a social service agency. If the underlying cause is drug or alcohol abuse, recommend counseling.

Cooling Treatments

Used to aggressively correct hyperthermia, cooling treatments include both moist and dry forms. Moist cold, which provides deeper penetration, includes tepid or alcohol sponge baths, cold compresses for small areas, and cold packs for large areas. In severe hyperthermia, cold-water baths or, preferably, hyperthermia blankets (a type of dry cold) may be used. Other dry-cold methods include ice bags, aquamatic K pads, and chemical cold packs. Chilled saline enemas may control hyperthermia if other cooling treatments fail.

During cooling treatments, the patient's temperature and other vital signs must be monitored closely. Treatments typically cease when the patient's temperature falls to 102° F. (38.9° C.).

Cooling treatments should be used cautiously in patients with impaired circulation because of the risk of ischemia. They should be avoided altogether in infants, the elderly, and the arthritic.

Purpose
To lower body temperature, thereby preventing cellular death and organ damage.

Preparation
Begin by explaining the treatment and reassuring the patient that you'll make every effort to minimize any discomfort

associated with cold application. Gather the necessary equipment in the patient's room.

If you'll be using an ice bag, select the correct size and fill it with cold water to check for leaks. If you don't see any, empty the bag and fill it halfway with crushed ice, which allows you to mold the bag to conform to the patient's body. Squeeze the bag to expel residual air, fasten the cap, and wipe any moisture from the outside cover. Wrap the bag in a towel or blanket to prevent tissue trauma and to absorb condensation.

If you'll be using an aquamatic K pad, check for a frayed cord or damaged insulation. Fill the control unit two-thirds full with distilled water and check for leaks. Tilt the unit several times to clear air from the tubing. Then tighten the cap and check that the hoses between the control unit and pad are free of tangles. Place the unit on the bedside table, slightly above the patient so that gravity assists water flow. Set the temperature control to the lowest setting. Cover the pad with an absorbent, protective covering. Now turn the unit on and allow it to cool for about 2 minutes.

If you'll be using a chemical cold pack, follow the manufacturer's directions to activate the cold-producing chemicals. Select the correct size pack for the patient and securely wrap it in a cloth cover.

If you'll be using a cold compress or pack, first cool a container of tap water by placing it in a basin of ice or by adding ice to the water. Chill the water to 59° F. (15° C.) or as ordered and immerse the compress or pack.

If you'll be using a hyperthermia blanket, check for leaks in the control unit or blanket, broken plugs, and frayed wires. Prepare one or two blankets, as ordered, by wrapping disposable covers over them. The covers absorb perspiration and condensation, which, if left on the patient's skin, could possibly cause tissue damage. After connecting the blanket to the control unit, specify the manual or automatic setting, as needed, and the desired temperature. Next, turn the unit on and add distilled water to the unit reservoir. Allow the blanket(s) to cool and place the control unit at the foot of the patient's bed.

If you'll be giving a tepid sponge bath, place a bath thermometer in a basin of warm water. Add cool water until the temperature reaches 93° F. (34° C.). Obtain a supply of wash cloths. Also prepare a hot-water bottle and an ice bag.

If you'll be administering a chilled enema, place the solution container in a basin of ice water until it reaches the prescribed temperature.

Before proceeding with any cooling treatment, make sure the patient's room is warm and free of drafts. Obtain baseline vital signs and assess the patient's level of consciousness.

Procedure

To use an ice pack, an aquamatic K pad, or a chemical cold pack, place the covered device on the patient's groin or axilla and begin timing the application. Refill or replace the device, as necessary, to maintain the correct temperature. Change the protective cover when it becomes wet.

To use a cold compress or pack, place a waterproof pad under the treatment area. Remove the compress or pack from the water, wring it dry, and cover it with a waterproof cloth. Apply it to the patient and begin timing the procedure. Change the compress or pack as necessary, to maintain correct temperature.

If the patient has severe hyperthermia or if conservative measures have failed to lower temperature, you'll probably apply a hyperthermia blanket. Before doing so, apply lanolin over the area of the patient's skin that comes in contact with the blanket. Then place one blanket beneath the patient, with the top edge aligned with his neck. Use a sheet or bath blanket as insulation between the patient and the hyperthermia blanket if no other cover is available. Insert the rectal probe and tape it in place to avoid dislodgment. If rectal insertion is contraindicated, place the probe at the axilla and tape it in place. Plug the other end of the probe into the blanket's control panel. If necessary, place a sheet or a second hyperthermia blanket over the patient to increase cold transfer. Make sure the patient's head doesn't lie directly on the cold, rigid surface of the blanket. To minimize chills, wrap his hands and feet.

If you're giving a sponge bath, administer an antipyretic, as ordered, 15 to 20 minutes beforehand, or cover the patient's trunk with a wet towel for 15 minutes to facilitate more rapid cooling. If necessary, place a large fan near the patient to increase fluid evaporation from the skin, thus hastening cooling.

To give a tepid sponge bath, place a protective covering on the bed, have the patient undress, and cover him with a bath blanket. Place a covered hot-water bottle at his feet to help prevent chills. Also place a covered ice bag on his head to prevent headache and nasal congestion, which may occur as the rest of his body cools. To accelerate cooling, place moist washcloths over the major superficial vessels in the axilla, groin, and popliteal areas. Begin by bathing each extremity for about 5 minutes, then sponge the chest and abdomen for 5 minutes, and follow by bathing the back and buttocks for 5 to 10 minutes. Keep the patient covered, except for the area you're sponging. Maintain the desired water temperature by adding warm water to the basin. Also, change washcloths as they warm.

Monitoring and aftercare

During therapy, monitor the patient's rectal temperature continuously (if he has a rectal probe in place) or every 10 minutes. Keep in mind that overly rapid cooling may cause a decrease in the patient's level of consciousness, pupillary response, and cardiac output. If the patient develops shaking chills, discontinue the procedure and notify the doctor. Chills increase metabolism, thereby raising body temperature.

If you're using an ice bag, an aquamatic K pad, or a chemical cold pack, observe the treated area frequently for signs of tissue intolerance: blanching, mottling, graying, cyanosis, maceration, or blisters. Be alert for complaints of burning or numbness. Discontinue the treatment and notify the doctor if any of these complications develop.

If you're using a hyperthermia blanket, monitor the patient's vital signs and neurologic status every 5 minutes until the desired temperature is reached, and then every 15 minutes until his temperature stabilizes. Check the patient's intake and output hourly. Observe him regularly for color changes in skin, nail beds, and lips. If edema, induration, inflammation, pain, or sensory impairment occurs, discontinue the treatment and notify the doctor. Reposition the patient every 30 to 60 minutes, as tolerated, to prevent tissue breakdown. Keep the patient's skin and bed clothing free of moisture.

After removing the hyperthermia blanket, continue to monitor the patient's temperature until it stabilizes. Anticipate a decline of up to 5 F. degrees (2.8 C. degrees). If this occurs, continue to monitor vital signs, intake and output, and neurologic status every 30 minutes until the patient is stable for 2 hours and then as ordered. A hyperthermia blanket can cause sudden changes in vital signs, increased intracranial pressure, respiratory distress or arrest, oliguria, anuria, and shivering. If you observe any of these signs, notify the doctor and institute emergency measures, if needed.

If you're giving a sponge bath, check the patient's temperature, pulse, and respirations every 10 minutes. (Don't take axillary temperature because the cool compresses applied to the area will alter the readings. Take oral temperature cautiously since a chill may cause the patient to bite and break the thermometer.) If the patient's temperature doesn't drop within 30 minutes, notify the doctor. When the temperature decreases to 1 to 2 F. degrees (0.5 to 1 C. degree) above the desired temperature, discontinue bathing since the temperature will decline naturally at that point. Continue to monitor temperature until it's stable, and observe the patient for seizures. As with other cooling treatments, monitor for skin discoloration and changes in vital signs, especially a rapid, weak, or irregular pulse. If any of these changes occur, promptly stop the treatment, notify the doctor, and cover the patient.

Continue to monitor vital signs for several days after cessation of cooling treatments to detect recurrence of hyperthermia.

Home care instructions
• Advise the patient to avoid exposure to high temperatures since hypersensitivity to them may persist.
• Teach the patient the importance of maintaining adequate fluid intake and reducing activity in hot weather to avoid overheating.

ANTISHOCK DEVICE

Pneumatic Antishock Garment

By redirecting blood from the legs and abdomen to the brain, heart, and lungs, the pneumatic antishock garment (also called medical antishock trousers or a MAST suit) can successfully combat shock by increasing blood volume to vital organs by up to 30%. It's indicated when systolic pressure falls below 80 mm Hg or when it falls below 100 mm Hg and is accompanied by signs of shock. Developed during World War II, this garment can also control abdominal and lower extremity hemorrhage and help stabilize and splint pelvic and femoral fractures.

Today, most pneumatic antishock garments consist of three independent inflatable sections: the left leg, the right leg, and the abdominal section. Usually, a foot-operated air pump is used to inflate each section. (Earlier models of the garment had interconnecting sections that were inflated simultaneously.) Most garments also have independent pressure gauges to monitor each section, as well as pop-off valves to prevent overinflation. Another safeguard against overinflation is the Velcro closures, which crackle when pressure within the garment becomes dangerously high.

The inflated garment is typically kept in place for about 2 hours or until the patient's blood volume is restored, his condition stabilizes, or he's prepared for surgery. Complications include vomiting (from abdominal compression), skin breakdown after prolonged use, and potentially irreversible hypovolemic shock from overly rapid garment deflation.

Use of the garment is contraindicated in the patient with cardiogenic shock, congestive heart failure, pulmonary edema, chronic obstructive pulmonary disease, or tension pneumothorax. It should be used cautiously during pregnancy for treatment of postpartum hemorrhage or ruptured ectopic pregnancy.

Purpose
To restore blood pressure, promote hemostasis, or immobilize the pelvis and legs.

Preparation
After taking the patient's vital signs for a baseline, briefly explain the treatment to him, even if he's unconscious. Describe the compressing sensation that he'll experience as the garment's inflated. Reassure him that the garment won't impair his breathing and that

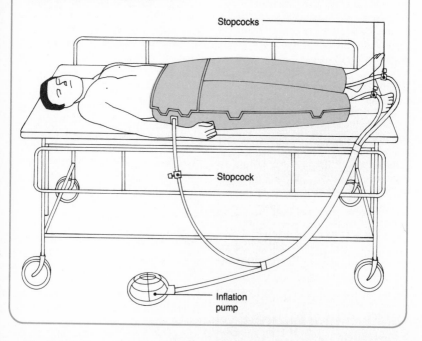

COMPLICATIONS

PREVENTING IRREVERSIBLE HYPOVOLEMIC SHOCK

Overly rapid deflation of the pneumatic antishock garment can trigger potentially irreversible hypovolemic shock by allowing blood to rush to the abdomen and legs. To prevent this complication, you'll need to *slowly* deflate each section—5 mm Hg at a time—when removing the garment. During this slow deflation, monitor the patient's blood pressure continuously.

Accidentally puncturing the garment or leaving its stopcocks open can also cause overly rapid deflation. To avoid punctures, carefully prepare the garment for use by unfolding it on a smooth surface. Also, pad any protruding foreign objects on the patient's body that might puncture the garment when it's inflated. After inflating the garment, inspect it carefully, verifying that all stopcocks are closed.

Stopcocks

Stopcock

Inflation pump

you'll monitor his condition minute by minute.

Mention that application of the garment increases pressure on the abdomen, which may cause him to vomit, urinate, or defecate. If ordered, insert a nasogastric tube and an indwelling (Foley) catheter to prevent or manage these effects.

Quickly assess the patient's injuries. Dress open wounds and fractures; stabilize and pad any protruding foreign objects that might puncture the gar-

ment when it's inflated. Be sure to leave spine boards in place.

Now, spread open the pneumatic antishock garment on a smooth surface or blanket. Take care not to puncture it. Open all stopcock valves and attach the foot pump.

Procedure
First, determine whether the patient can be turned from side to side, depending on his injuries. If he can't be turned, slide the garment under him.

If he can be turned, place the garment next to him and have another nurse help you logroll him onto it. You can also set up the garment on a gurney or stretcher, then transfer the patient onto it in a supine position. Make sure the upper edge of the garment fits just below the lowest rib to avoid pressure on the chest, which may impair lung expansion.

Wrap the garment snugly around the left leg, fastening the Velcro straps from ankle to thigh. Next, wrap the right leg, and, finally, the abdomen. Double-check the stopcocks to make sure they're all open, thus ensuring uniform inflation.

Inflate each leg of the garment, then the abdominal section, to about 20 to 30 mm Hg. Inflating the abdomen last prevents pooling of blood in the legs. Continue to inflate the garment slowly while monitoring the patient's blood pressure and pulse. Stop inflating when the patient's systolic pressure reaches the desired level, usually 100 to 110 mm Hg. Close all stopcocks to prevent air loss and accidental deflation. After the garment's properly inflated, initiate I.V. fluid replacement, as ordered.

Monitoring and aftercare
While the garment is still in place, monitor the patient's blood pressure, pulse, and respiratory rate every 5 minutes. Check his pedal pulse periodically, and notify the doctor if circulation to the patient's feet seems impaired.

Before removing the antishock garment, make sure that I.V. lines are patent and that emergency resuscitation equipment is readily available in case the patient's blood pressure drops. Deflate the garment one chamber at a time, beginning with the abdominal section. Slowly decrease the chamber pressure in 5–mm Hg increments over 30 to 60 minutes. Check the patient's blood pressure continuously during this slow deflation. If it drops, close the stopcock, reinflate the section, and increase I.V. fluids. If it remains stable, though, finish deflating the abdominal section. Then deflate each leg section of the garment individually, again in 5–mm Hg increments.

When the pneumatic antishock garment becomes loose enough, gently pull it off, as ordered. Or you can leave the garment in place for a few hours, in case reinflation becomes necessary.

Home care instruction
Mention to the patient that he may notice linear bruising where the inflated garment compressed clothing or skin folds.

Selected References

Benson, Maria L., and Benson, Don M. "Autotransfusion Is Here—Are You Ready?" *Nursing85* 15(3):46-49, March 1985.

Budassi, S., and Barber, J. *Mosby's Manual of Emergency Care: Practices & Procedures.* St. Louis: C.V. Mosby Co., 1984.

Donner, Howard. "Out in the Cold…Care of the Patient Who Is Injured in the Wilderness During the Winter," *Emergency Medicine* 17(21):20-24, 27-28, 30-31, December 1985.

Emergencies. Nurse's Reference Library. Springhouse, Pa.: Springhouse Corp., 1985.

Kunkel, D.B. "The Toxic Emergency—A Critical Look at Gut Decontamination," *Emergency Medicine* 17(3), 1985.

Nursing88 Drug Handbook. Springhouse, Pa.: Springhouse Corp., 1988.

Smith, David S. "Living Death: Don't Let Hypothermia Fool You into a Fatal Mistake…When Not to Assume that a Patient Is Dead," *RN* 46(1):48-51, January 1983.

19

Treating Pain

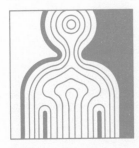

Treating Pain

Introduction

For centuries, pain has been contemplated by philosophers, theologians, and poets. But it wasn't until the 1960s, when Melzack and Wall proposed their gate control theory, that pain's physiologic and psychological components received close clinical study.

Acute versus chronic pain

Today, we understand that a treatment plan must take into account the differences between acute and chronic pain to be successful. Acute pain, usually caused by tissue damage from an injury or disease, may require cessation of activity to promote healing. If acute pain is untreated, reflex responses intended to promote healing may produce serious physiologic effects.

In acute pain, treatment aims to cure the disease or heal the causative injury. Palliative treatment may include drug therapy, surgery, applications of heat or cold, or psychological techniques for controlling pain.

Chronic pain may stem from prolonged pathology or dysfunction, as occurs in cancer or arthritis. Or it may be associated with psychopathology. It's strongly colored by the patient's emotions and his environment. In chronic pain, treatment aims to decrease or eliminate pain, to maintain or improve the patient's ability to conduct daily activities, and to reduce his need for nonessential medications. Typically, it requires a comprehensive approach. In mild chronic pain, treatment may simply combine ice massage and exercise. In severe chronic pain, though, a multidisciplinary program may be necessary to address the physiologic, psychological, and social components of the patient's condition.

Doing your part

As a nurse, you're responsible for assisting with or performing many pain-control measures. For example, in traditional pharmacologic and surgical treatments, you'll provide patient support and education, monitor therapeutic effects, and supply emotional support. In psychological pain-control techniques, such as relaxation, you'll teach the patient how to perform the technique and help him overcome any obstacles. In a comprehensive pain-management program, you'll complete a thorough pain assessment, provide patient education, address behavioral problems, and perform or monitor trials of pain-control techniques.

But whatever the treatment, keep in mind that there's no substitute for empathetic understanding of the patient's needs and condition. You can't feel his pain, of course, but you can let him know that you recognize his suffering—and that you care.

DRUG THERAPY

Nonnarcotic Analgesics

The nonnarcotic analgesics consist of nonsteroidal anti-inflammatory drugs (NSAIDs) and *acetaminophen*. The NSAIDs, in turn, include *aspirin, ibuprofen, indomethacin, naproxen, naproxen sodium, phenylbutazone,* and *sulindac*. Both NSAIDs and acetaminophen produce antipyretic and analgesic effects, and the NSAIDs also produce anti-inflammatory effects. Because all of these drugs differ in chemical structure, they vary in their onset of action, duration of effect, and method of metabolism and excretion.

Nonnarcotic analgesics treat mild to moderate pain. If combined with narcotic analgesics, they can also relieve moderate to severe pain while allowing a reduced dosage of narcotics. However, unlike the narcotic analgesics, these drugs don't cause physiologic dependence. They commonly treat postoperative and postpartum pain, headache, myalgias, arthralgias, dysmenorrhea, and cancer pain.

The chief side effects of NSAIDs include GI irritation, hepatoxicity, nephrotoxicity, and headache. GI irritation and bleeding occur more commonly with NSAIDs (except perhaps for ibuprofen and naproxen) than with acetaminophen.

Acetaminophen may be used in place of aspirin and other NSAIDs in peptic ulcer or bleeding disorders. But long-term, high-dose use of acetaminophen may lead to hepatic damage.

NSAIDs shouldn't be used in patients with aspirin sensitivity—especially in those with the triad of allergies, asthma, and aspirin-induced nasal polyps—because of the risk of bronchoconstriction or anaphylaxis. Some NSAIDs are also contraindicated in renal dysfunction, hypertension, GI inflammation, or ulcers. Since aspirin increases prothrombin and bleeding times, it's contraindicated in hemophilia and other bleeding disorders. It shouldn't be given with anticoagulants or other ulcerogenic drugs, such as corticosteroids, and should also be avoided in patients scheduled for surgery within 1 week. Acetaminophen is contraindicated in an allergy to the drug.

Purpose and action

NSAIDs apparently reduce pain by inhibiting prostaglandin synthesis at the tissue level. (See *How NSAIDs Reduce Pain*.) Acetaminophen reduces pain by interfering with prostaglandin synthesis in the CNS and by blocking pain impulse generation in the peripheral nervous system. This action probably results from inhibition of prostaglandin synthesis; or it may also result from the inhibition of the synthesis or action of other substances in the periphery.

Monitoring

Before giving a nonnarcotic analgesic, check the patient's history for a previous hypersensitivity reaction, which may indicate hypersensitivity to a related drug in this group.

If the patient's taking an NSAID, ask about any GI irritation. If it occurs, the doctor may reduce the dosage or discontinue the drug.

In long-term therapy, report any abnormalities in renal and liver function studies. Also monitor hematologic studies and evaluate complaints of nausea or gastric burning. Be alert for signs of iron deficiency anemia, such as pallor, unusual fatigue, or weakness.

Home care instructions

● If the patient's taking an NSAID, instruct him to immediately report rash, dyspnea, confusion, blurred vision, nausea, bloody vomitus, or black, tarry stools. These may indicate an overdose, hypersensitivity, or GI bleeding.

HOW N.S.A.I.D.s REDUCE PAIN

After an injury, cells release bradykinin precursors and histamine, and arachidonic acid is formed. Bradykinin stimulates nerve endings to produce a pain impulse. Histamine triggers inflammation and edema, also stimulating pain receptors.

As part of this normal reaction to cellular injury, the enzyme prostaglandin synthe-tase acts on arachidonic acid, leading to formation of prostaglandins. The prostaglandins, in turn, sensitize peripheral pain receptors to bradykinin and histamine.

NSAIDs inhibiit prostaglandin synthesis, thus reducing local tissue sensitivity to bradykinin and histamine. As a result, pain and inflammation are reduced.

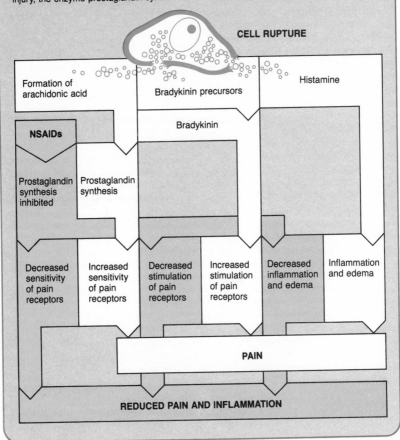

CELL RUPTURE

Formation of arachidonic acid

Bradykinin precursors

Histamine

NSAIDs

Bradykinin

Prostaglandin synthesis inhibited

Prostaglandin synthesis

Decreased sensitivity of pain receptors

Increased sensitivity of pain receptors

Decreased stimulation of pain receptors

Increased stimulation of pain receptors

Decreased inflammation and edema

Inflammation and edema

PAIN

REDUCED PAIN AND INFLAMMATION

• If the patient's taking acetaminophen, tell him to immediately notify the doctor for any signs of an overdose: nausea, vomiting, abdominal cramps, or diarrhea.

• To minimize the GI upset that may occur with NSAIDs, instruct the patient to take his medication with food or a full glass of water. Afterward, he should remain upright for 15 to 30 minutes to reduce esophageal irritation. If he experiences gastric burning or pain, tell him to notify the doctor.

• Explain that some NSAIDs may cause increased bleeding time. Urge the patient to avoid injury, which could cause bleeding.

• Reassure the patient that tinnitus—a

dose-related effect of aspirin—is reversible. However, if it persists, he should notify the doctor, who may reduce the dosage.

• Caution the patient that dizziness may occur with ibuprofen, naproxen, or sulindac. Explain that he should drive or use machinery cautiously until he knows his response to the medication.

• If the patient misses a dose, advise him to take it as soon as he remembers. However, if the next dose is less than 4 hours away, he should skip the missed dose and return to his regular schedule. He shouldn't double-dose.

• In long-term use of any nonnarcotic analgesic, emphasize the need for periodic blood tests to detect nephritis and hepatotoxicity.

Narcotic Analgesics

The narcotic analgesics include both opiates and opioids. Opiates refer to natural opium alkaloids and their derivatives; opioids refer to synthetic compounds with varied chemical structures. Morphine is the prototype for both types of narcotic analgesics.

Narcotic analgesics can be classified as agonists or agonist/antagonists. Agonists, such as *morphine, codeine, hydromorphone, levorphanol, meperidine, methadone,* and *propoxyphene,* produce analgesia by binding to CNS opiate receptors. Agonist/antagonists, such as *buprenorphine, butorphanol, nalbuphine,* and *pentazocine,* also produce analgesia by binding to CNS receptors. When another narcotic is present, these drugs act as antagonists, blocking narcotic effects and causing withdrawal symptoms.

Narcotic analgesics provide relief from moderate to severe pain. In fact, the narcotic agonists may be the drugs of choice for severe chronic cancer pain. The agonist/antagonist drugs, in contrast, have limited use in cancer. That's because many of them are available only in parenteral forms. And with increasing doses, they produce hallucinations and other psychotomimetic effects. In the narcotic-dependent patient, they may produce withdrawal symptoms.

Other indications for narcotic analgesics include pain in acute MI, pulmonary edema, cough, and GI and urinary tract disorders. They're also used as preanesthetics.

Narcotic analgesics can be given by various routes: oral, I.M., I.V., epidural, or intrathecal. For most patients, oral administration is preferred. I.M. administration, though usually effective, can result in erratic absorption, especially in debilitated patients. In severe pain, as in an anginal attack, I.V. administration may be chosen for its rapid onset and precise dosage control. However, sudden, profound respiratory depression and hypotension can occur with this route. Continuous I.V. infusion has been used successfully in some cancer patients. (See *Understanding Patient-Controlled Analgesia Systems.*)

Narcotic analgesics can cause severe side effects, such as respiratory depression. As a result, they're contraindicated in severe respiratory depression and should be used cautiously in chronic obstructive pulmonary disease. Because they're metabolized by the liver and excreted through the kidneys, they should also be used cautiously in hepatic or renal impairment. And since they increase intracranial pressure, they should be used cautiously, if at all, in head injury or in any condition that raises intracranial pressure. Also, they can induce miosis, which, in patients with head injury, can mask pupil dilation, an important indicator of increased intracranial pressure. Other side effects include drowsiness, dizziness, nausea, vomiting, sweating, flushing, constipation, and cough suppression.

Prolonged use of these drugs can lead to increased tolerance and physiologic

UNDERSTANDING PATIENT-CONTROLLED ANALGESIA SYSTEMS

Patient-controlled analgesia (PCA) systems provide an optimal narcotic dose while maintaining a constant serum concentration of the drug.

A PCA system consists of a syringe-type injection pump piggy-backed into an I.V. or subcutaneous infusion port. By depressing a button, the patient can receive a preset bolus dose of a narcotic. (The doctor programs the bolus dose and the "lock-out" time between boluses, thus preventing overdosage.) The device automatically records the number of times the patient depresses the button, thus helping the doctor to adjust drug dosage.

The PCA system may allow a reduction in drug dosage, perhaps because a patient typically feels he has more control over his pain. And he's reassured to know that an analgesic is quickly available.

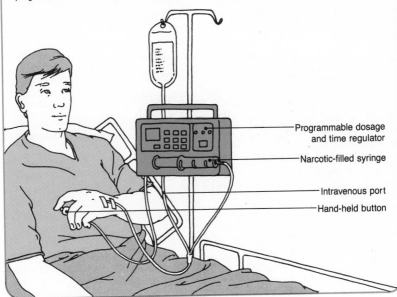

Programmable dosage and time regulator

Narcotic-filled syringe

Intravenous port

Hand-held button

and psychological dependence. Therefore, they shouldn't be used for chronic pain in nonmalignant disorders.

Purpose and action

Narcotic analgesics relieve acute and chronic pain by diminishing the patient's perception of pain and his emotional response to it. They do this by binding with CNS opiate receptor sites.

Monitoring

Before giving a narcotic analgesic, review the patient's medication regimen for use of other CNS depressants, such as barbiturates. Concurrent use of another CNS depressant enhances drowsiness, sedation, disorientation, and fear.

During administration, check the patient's vital signs and be alert for respiratory depression. If his respiratory rate declines to 10 breaths/minute or less, call his name and touch him, and instruct him to breathe deeply. If your attempts to rouse him fail or if you observe confusion or restlessness, notify the doctor and prepare to provide oxygen. If ordered, administer a narcotic antagonist, such as naloxone.

If the patient experiences persistent nausea and vomiting during therapy, notify the doctor, who may reduce the dosage or change the medication. As ordered, give the patient an antiemetic, such as hydroxyzine.

To help prevent constipation, administer a stool softener, and if necessary, a senna derivative laxative. Also provide a high-fiber diet, and encourage fluids, as ordered. Regular exercise may also promote motility.

Because narcotic analgesics can cause postural hypotension, take measures to avoid accidents. For example, keep the bed's side rails raised. If the patient is mobile, help him out of bed and assist him with ambulation.

Encourage the patient to practice coughing and deep-breathing exercises to promote ventilation and prevent pooling of secretions, which could lead to respiratory difficulty.

Evaluate the effectiveness of the drug. Is the patient experiencing relief? Does his dosage need to be increased because of persistent or worsening pain? Is he developing a tolerance to the drug? Remember that the patient should receive the smallest effective dose over the shortest period of time. However, narcotic analgesics shouldn't be withheld or given in ineffective doses for fear of iatrogenic dependence. Psychological dependence occurs in less than 1% of hospitalized patients.

Home care instructions
• Explain to the patient that the prescribed drug is most effective when taken before pain becomes intense.
• Advise him to consult his doctor if the drug becomes less effective in relieving pain. Stress that he shouldn't increase the dose or the frequency of administration.
• Tell him that if he misses a dose he should take it as soon as he remembers. However, if it's almost time for the next dose, he should skip the missed dose. Warn him never to double-dose.
• Instruct the patient's family to notify the doctor immediately if they detect

signs of an overdose: cold, clammy skin; confusion; severe drowsiness or restlessness; slow or irregular breathing; pinpoint pupils; or unconsciousness. Teach them how to maintain respirations until help arrives.
• Advise the patient to get up slowly from bed or a chair because the drug can cause postural hypotension.
• Tell him to eat a high-fiber diet, to drink plenty of fluids, and to take a stool softener, if prescribed.
• Caution against drinking alcohol since it enhances CNS depression.
• Tell him to contact the doctor before stopping the drug since a gradual dosage reduction may be necessary to avoid withdrawal symptoms.

Tricyclic Antidepressants

Primarily used to treat depression, tricyclic antidepressants (TCAs) also effectively relieve chronic arthritis pain, postherpetic neuralgia, diabetic neuropathy, headaches, facial pain, and back pain from neurologic and musculoskeletal disorders. Although all TCAs can help relieve chronic pain, the more serotonergic drugs, such as *amitriptyline* and *doxepin*, may prove more effective than the more noradrenergic ones, such as *desipramine* and *trimipramine*.

TCAs shouldn't be used during recovery from acute MI since they can produce arrhythmias, sinus tachycardia, and prolonged myocardial conduction time. They're also contraindicated in patients using monoamine oxidase (MAO) inhibitors because hyperpyretic or hypertensive crisis, severe seizures, coma, or death can occur. And TCAs shouldn't be used in acute angle-closure glaucoma; even therapeutic doses may precipitate an attack.

TCAs should be used cautiously in

the elderly, who may exhibit increased sensitivity to these drugs' anticholinergic, sedative, and hypotensive effects. Because TCAs are metabolized by the liver and excreted by the kidneys, they should be used cautiously in renal or hepatic dysfunction. What's more, because they lower the seizure threshold, they should be used cautiously in seizure disorders.

Purpose and action

Exactly how TCAs relieve pain isn't known, but one theory holds that they have a direct analgesic effect, or that they potentiate the analgesic effects of other drugs. They achieve this by increasing the availability of the neurotransmitters norepinephrine and serotonin, which act to inhibit pain impulse transmission. A second theory proposes that TCAs' action in chronic pain relates to their mood-elevating effects. Research studies have shown a correlation between decreased depression (depression is a common symptom in chronic pain) and pain relief.

Monitoring

Before giving TCAs, review the patient's medication regimen for possible interactions. Concurrent use of TCAs and MAO inhibitors, for example, can cause life-threatening effects.

During therapy, monitor for cardiac effects, including an irregular pulse rate, tachycardia, bradycardia, and blood pressure changes. Also be alert for hyperpyretic or hypertensive crisis. Report any of these symptoms to the doctor; he may discontinue the drug.

Notify the doctor immediately if the patient develops symptoms of an overdose. Such symptoms include severe drowsiness, confusion, dyspnea or labored respirations, fever, vomiting, and cardiac effects.

Assess for dry mouth and a metallic taste. Dry mouth may cause erosion of the gingiva and teeth, especially in middle-aged and elderly patients. During long-term therapy, monitor liver and renal function studies and notify

HYDROXYZINE: ADJUVANT PAIN RELIEF

When given with narcotic analgesics, hydroxyzine may enhance analgesic effects and reduce the anxiety component of pain.

If you're giving hydroxyzine parenterally, remember to administer it by deep I.M. injection into a large muscle mass, preferably the upper outer quadrant of the buttock or midlateral thigh. Avoid S.C. administration since this route causes tissue damage. Also avoid I.V. administration since this route causes hemolysis.

If the patient's taking oral hydroxyzine, warn him to notify the doctor immediately if he feels faint or extremely drowsy. These symptoms may indicate an overdose or an interaction with other drugs, such as tricyclic antidepressants. The doctor may need to adjust the dosage.

Instruct the patient to follow the prescribed administration schedule carefully. If he misses a dose, he should take it as soon as possible, but he shouldn't double-dose. Finally, warn the patient against drinking alcohol during hydroxyzine therapy because severe CNS depression may result.

the doctor of any abnormalities.

Home care instructions

● Instruct the patient to notify the doctor and stop the drug if he experiences confusion, severe drowsiness, fever, hallucinations, restlessness and agitation, seizures, breathing difficulty, an unusually fast, slow, or irregular heartbeat, unusual fatigue, weakness, or vomiting. If any of these occur, the patient may require hospitalization to monitor cardiac and respiratory function.

● Tell the patient to report eye pain, blurred vision, constipation, urinary retention, muscle stiffness, or twitching. Any of these symptoms may require a dosage adjustment or drug discontinuation.

● Explain that a once-a-day dose, taken at bedtime, will lessen these drugs' sedative effect. Tell the patient that morning sedation is temporary and may decrease if he takes the dose earlier in

the evening (rather than at bedtime).
• Tell him to get up slowly from a lying or sitting position. However, if weakness or dizziness persists or worsens, instruct him to notify the doctor.
• Advise the patient to guard against weight gain, since these drugs can cause an increased appetite and a craving for sweets. Tell him to weigh himself weekly. If he gains weight, suggest a weight-loss or maintenance diet.
• To relieve dry mouth, suggest the use of ice chips or dietetic candy, along with good oral hygiene.
• Advise the patient to use a strong sunblocking agent until he's certain of his response to sun exposure. Photosensitivity is possible.
• Instruct him to avoid using alcohol since increased CNS depression will occur.
• Explain that if he misses a dose, he should take it as soon as possible. However, if he remembers within 4 hours of the next dose, he should skip the missed dose and return to his regular schedule. He should never double-dose. If the patient misses more than one dose, he should notify the doctor.
• Instruct the patient not to stop the drug on his own. Explain that the doctor will reduce the dosage gradually to avoid worsening his condition and precipitating withdrawal symptoms, such as headache, nausea, vomiting, and vivid dreams.
• Stress the importance of keeping appointments for follow-up studies, such as an EKG, a complete blood count, a blood glucose test, glaucoma testing, blood pressure monitoring, and renal and liver function tests.

Anticonvulsants

The anticonvulsant drugs *carbamazepine* and *phenytoin* may help relieve acute neuropathic pain. Carbamazepine, in fact, is the drug of choice for pain in trigeminal and glossopharyngeal neuralgia. However, if this drug fails to provide relief, phenytoin may be given with it.

These anticonvulsants prove most effective against sharp, lancing pain, reducing the frequency and severity of painful attacks. But they're less effective against steady, persistent pain.

The chief side effects of carbamazepine and phenytoin include CNS and hematologic reactions and GI upset. Carbamazepine shouldn't be used in patients with atrioventricular (AV) block, blood dyscrasias, or bone marrow depression because it will exacerbate these conditions. And since this drug resembles tricyclic antidepressants chemically, it's contraindicated in patients with sensitivity to those drugs. Likewise, phenytoin should be avoided in patients with a hypersensitivity to other hydantoins. And since phenytoin may reduce serum thyroxine concentrations, it should be used cautiously in impaired thyroid function.

Both drugs should be used cautiously in cardiac disorders, diabetes mellitus, and glaucoma. And because they're metabolized in the liver and excreted by the kidneys, they should be used cautiously in renal or hepatic impairment. In addition, they should be used cautiously during pregnancy since they're associated with malignancies and congenital defects.

Purpose and action
Carbamazepine and phenytoin have an incompletely understood mechanism of action. They may, however, relieve pain by decreasing the synaptic transmission of pain impulses.

Monitoring
Before administering carbamazepine or phenytoin, check the patient's medication regimen for possible interactions. Concurrent administration of tricyclic antidepressants or anticoagulants, for instance, can reduce the effectiveness of anticonvulsants, thus requiring a dosage adjustment. Use of acetaminophen increases the risk of

hepatotoxicity, requiring close monitoring of liver function tests.

During therapy, monitor the patient for drowsiness, dizziness, ataxia, or GI upset. These side effects, though typically transient, may require a dosage reduction. To minimize these effects, the doctor may initiate therapy using a low dosage, increasing it gradually until a therapeutic response is obtained.

Be alert for and report any signs of CNS toxicity, including slurred speech, weakness, and behavioral changes. Check for fever and easy bruising, signs of rare but life-threatening hematologic reactions. If any of these signs occur, stop the drug immediately and notify the doctor.

Home care instructions

• Tell the patient to take a missed dose as soon as he remembers, unless the next scheduled dose is less than 4 hours away. Stress that he shouldn't double-dose. If he misses more than one dose, he should notify the doctor.

• Tell the patient to report sore throat, fever, mouth ulcers, or easy bruising. These symptoms could indicate hematologic toxicity, requiring discontinuation of therapy.

• To relieve dry mouth, suggest the use of ice chips or dietetic candy.

• Inform the patient of the need for periodic tests, such as a complete blood count, liver and renal function studies, and ophthalmologic tests. If he's taking phenytoin, he may also need thyroid function and serum calcium tests.

• If the patient's taking carbamazepine, he may experience photosensitivity. Caution him to use a sunblocker or wear protective clothing when outdoors.

• If the patient's taking phenytoin, explain the importance of regular dental checkups and meticulous oral hygiene to avoid gingivitis, a common side effect of this drug.

• Mention that every few months the doctor will attempt to reduce or discontinue therapy. Caution the patient not to discontinue it on his own.

Topical Anesthetics

The topical drugs *benzocaine, dibucaine, dyclonine, ethyl chloride, lidocaine, pramoxine,* and *tetracaine* anesthetize the skin and mucous membranes. These drugs provide relief from the pain caused by sunburn, minor burns, pruritus, and other dermatologic conditions. They can be applied to the mucous membranes of the rectum, vagina, urethra, and bladder before invasive procedures. In addition, they're used to suppress the gag reflex before endoscopy and to anesthetize the pharynx, larynx, and trachea before intubation.

Topical anesthetics can cause CNS and hypersensitivity reactions as well as local reactions, such as contact dermatitis. They shouldn't be applied to any infected area because of a decreased or absent anesthetic effect. They're contraindicated in severe, extensive skin disorders involving abraded or broken skin.

Purpose and action

Topical anesthetics produce a local loss of sensation by temporarily blocking conduction of pain impulses.

Monitoring

Before applying a topical anesthetic, ask the patient if he has a history of hypersensitivity to the drug. If he does, notify the doctor, who may substitute a different topical anesthetic.

After applying the anesthetic, observe the patient for CNS reactions, such as drowsiness, blurred vision, or seizures. Report any of these to the doctor.

Home care instructions

• Emphasize the importance of applying the topical anesthetic correctly to avoid toxic effects.

• Inform the patient using viscous lidocaine that it may make swallowing difficult. As a result, he should avoid eating or drinking for 1 hour after application to prevent aspiration.

• If the patient forgets to apply the anesthetic, instruct him to apply it as soon as possible. However, if it's almost time for the next application, he should skip the missed one and return to his regular schedule.

• Advise him to discontinue the agent and contact the doctor if his condition worsens, if it doesn't improve in several days, or if a rash, swelling, or an infection occurs.

Nerve Blocks

Used for moderate to severe pain, nerve blocks can serve as a treatment of choice, such as for reflex sympathetic

COMPARING NERVE BLOCKS

NERVE BLOCK	INDICATIONS
Subarachnoid Most commonly given in the lumbar region to interrupt sensory motor and autonomic components of nerves	• Diagnostic before surgery or a neurolytic block • Postamputation pain • Visceral pain • Cancer pain
Epidural Most commonly given in the lumbar region to interrupt sensory motor and autonomic components of nerves; onset is slower than with subarachnoid block	• Radicular pain • Postoperative pain • Causalgia • Reflex sympathetic dystrophy • Visceral pain
Paravertebral somatic nerve May be given in the cervical, thoracic, or lumbar region to interrupt sensory and pain pathways	• Prognostic before surgery or a neurolytic block • Neuralgia • Cancer pain • Causalgia • Vertebral fracture pain
Sympathetic ganglion nerve Most commonly given in the stellate ganglion, celiac plexus, or lumbar sympathetic nerves to eliminate vasomotor, sudomotor, and visceromotor hyperactivity and to inhibit activity of the neuroaxis responsible for some chronic pain states	• Causalgia • Postherpetic neuralgia • Visceral pain • Phantom pain • Acute herpes zoster
Peripheral nerve Most commonly given at the intercostal nerves, the lateral femoral cutaneous nerve, or the sciatic nerve to interrupt sensory and pain pathways	• Rib fracture or hip pain • Postherpetic neuralgia • Postoperative pain • Meralgia paresthetica
Local infiltration (trigger point injection) Given to interrupt sensory and pain pathways in a muscle in which palpation produces pain	• Costal chondritis • Myofascial pain • Pyriformis syndrome

dystrophy, or provide symptomatic relief, such as for the pain of certain cancers. They anesthetize specific nerves to block the conduction of pain impulses through the CNS. The most common agents used are local anesthetics, such as *bupivacaine, etidocaine, lidocaine, procaine,* and *tetracaine.* (If inflammation is present, a steroid may be added.) These nerve-blocking agents may be injected into the subarachnoid or epidural space, paravertebral so-

matic or sympathetic ganglion nerve, peripheral nerve, or nerve endings.

Bupivacaine and etidocaine provide the most prolonged analgesia. Bupivacaine, which produces neural blockage for 18 to 24 hours, affects sensory fibers more than motor ones. Etidocaine, which is less toxic than bupivacaine in equipotent solutions, affects motor fibers more than sensory ones.

In terminal illness, though, local anesthetics may fail to relieve severe pain. And if all other treatments have proven ineffective, neurolytic agents, such as alcohol or phenol, may be injected to damage nerve pathways, thereby blocking pain transmission. But these agents act unpredictably and may produce only transient relief at best.

Nerve blocks can cause complications, such as puncture of the dura, subarachnoid space, or a blood vessel during injection. Dural puncture can lead to headache, whereas subarachnoid puncture can cause severe cardiovascular complications and respiratory failure. Puncture of a blood vessel can cause hemorrhage.

Absorption of a sufficient amount of anesthetic into the bloodstream may produce systemic effects. Absorption increases in vascular areas, such as the upper respiratory passages, the urethra, and the large venous plexus of the caudal canal. Most reactions occur within 10 minutes of injection. Rarely, injection causes anaphylaxis.

Nerve blocks are contraindicated in local infection, bleeding disorders, concurrent anticoagulant therapy, and deafferentation syndromes.

Purpose and action
To provide analgesia by interrupting pain pathways.

Preparation
Reinforce the doctor's explanation of the procedure and answer the patient's questions. Also, ask if he has ever had an adverse reaction to any local anesthetic. Inform him that the duration of the procedure depends on the type

SPECIAL CONSIDERATIONS

- May block more segments than necessary.
- May preview effects of neurolytic injection.
- Complications include motor weakness, paralysis, meningitis, dysesthesias, neuropathies, arachnoiditis, and myelopathy.

- Appropriate concentration of local anesthetic can produce sensory and vasomotor block *without* involving skeletal muscles.
- Complications include hypotension and headache.

- Sensory and motor functions are affected similarly.
- Muscle weakness or paralysis and loss of proprioception and touch sensation may result in a practically useless limb.
- Cervical injection may cause vertebral artery puncture and phrenic and vagus nerve block. Thoracic injection may cause pneumothorax.
- Chemical neuropathy may occur in neurolytic block with alcohol.

- A successful block causes vasodilation and suppresses the galvanic skin reflex.
- Complications of *stellate ganglion block* include phrenic or laryngeal nerve paralysis and pneumothorax. Complications of *celiac plexus block* include hypotension. Complications of *lumbar sympathetic block* include hemorrhage, hypotension, sexual impotence, and block of lumbar somatic nerves.

- Appropriate concentration of local anesthetic affects sensory fibers but not motor conduction.
- Can cause pneumothorax and hemorrhage.

- Useful for localized pain.

MANAGING REACTIONS TO NERVE BLOCKS

During administration of a local anesthetic, systemic reactions can occur, resulting from improper administration technique, inadvertent injection of the anesthetic into a blood vessel, or an overdose.

Before a nerve block is performed, be sure to insert an I.V. line and gather resuscitation equipment. Also keep these drugs available: thiopental sodium, succinylcholine, diazepam, ephedrine, and phenylephrine. If you detect a reaction, use the guidelines listed below.

Treating a mild reaction
A mild reaction may produce dysarthria, light-headedness, tinnitus, headache, tachycardia, or tachypnea. If any of these occur, the doctor will stop the injection. Then you'll need to provide oxygen, monitor the patient's vital signs and, if ordered, administer appropriate drugs.

Treating a moderate reaction
In a moderate reaction, the signs and symptoms of a mild reaction progressively worsen. You may also detect confusion, muscle twitching, seizures, and hypertension. If any of these effects occur, the doctor will stop the injection. You'll need to take immediate action to prevent anoxia and CNS hyperactivity: ensure a patent airway, provide mechanical ventilation, and administer drugs, as ordered.

Treating a severe reaction
Be alert for loss of consciousness, hypotension, bradycardia, and respiratory depression. If untreated, the patient will succumb to cardiac arrest and respiratory failure, resulting in death.

If any of these effects occur, the doctor will stop the injection. You'll need to ensure a patent airway and provide mechanical ventilation. Then rapidly infuse I.V. fluids, give drugs as ordered, and elevate the patient's legs above the level of his heart.

of nerve block used and that he'll be awake and alert during the injection. If he's nervous, he may be given a sedative to help him relax. Instruct him not to move during the injection to confine the local anesthetic and avoid injury. Tell him to report any pain to the doctor. Lastly, make sure he has signed a consent form.

Establish a baseline for pain. Using a scale of 0 (for no pain) to 10 (for the worst pain imaginable), ask the patient to estimate the severity of pain. Also record any evidence of hypalgesia or other sensory changes, motor dysfunction, or reflex abnormalities.

Ensure that monitoring and resuscitation equipment are close by and that epinephrine, bronchodilators, and antihistamines are readily available. Prepare the nerve block tray with a variety of needle sizes. Also prepare the injection site, and if ordered, insert an I.V. line. Then position the patient (usually lying down) to reduce the risk of syncope.

If the patient will be receiving a neurolytic block, position him as ordered. If he'll be receiving an alcohol injection, warn him that painful paresthesias may occur during injection. If he'll be receiving phenol, tell him to expect a warm, tingling sensation in the involved dermatomes.

Procedure

After the patient has been prepared, the doctor inserts the needle into the appropriate area, and may use fluoroscopy to verify proper placement. Before injection, he carefully attempts aspiration to prevent inadvertent intravascular or intrathecal injection.

Once proper needle placement has been verified, the doctor injects a test dose. If no adverse reactions occur, he injects the remainder of the anesthetic, usually in small increments. After the doctor completes the injection, he removes the needle and applies pressure over the site. The patient meanwhile remains recumbent for the specified time and then returns to his room.

Monitoring and aftercare

After a nerve block, closely observe the needle insertion site for bleeding or hematoma formation every 30 minutes for 4 hours. Immediately notify the doctor if either occurs. Also monitor the patient's vital signs; report hypotension, dyspnea, or a change in pulse rate.

After an *epidural* nerve block, have the patient maintain the lateral position for 30 minutes so that the ensuing hypalgesia is confined mostly to the dependent side. After an *intrathecal* block, reevaluate motor function and bowel and bladder function for 24 to 48 hours. After *stellate ganglion* and *intercostal* nerve blocks, auscultate the lungs to rule out pneumothorax.

If the patient has had a *cervical plexus* block, caution him to lift his head and body slowly when rising since extensive vasodilation commonly causes severe orthostatic hypotension. If the patient experiences severe orthostatic hypotension after a *neurolytic* block, apply an abdominal binder and administer an oral vasopressor, as ordered.

Evaluate the effects of the nerve block by comparing current pain levels to baseline ones. Also review the patient's medication requirements. If appropriate, the narcotics dosage should be reduced gradually to avoid withdrawal symptoms. Be aware, too, that patients with cancer may have pain in areas that haven't been blocked and may still need analgesics.

Home care instructions

● If the patient is discharged with an anesthetized extremity, advise him to change position every 30 minutes to prevent skin breakdown. Tell him to move cautiously to avoid falls.

● Instruct the patient to immediately report any bleeding, fainting, difficulty breathing, or decreased motor function.

● If a neurolytic block causes sexual impotence or bladder or bowel dysfunction, refer the patient to the appropriate specialist.

SURGERY

Cordotomy

By destroying sensory pathways that carry pain impulses to the brain, cordotomy relieves severe, intractable cancer pain in the thorax, abdomen, and lower extremities. However, this surgical procedure doesn't guarantee pain relief, and its complications can be severe. What's more, a significant percentage of cordotomies lose their effectiveness in 1 to 5 years since new pain pathways may develop after the original pathway has been interrupted. As a result, this surgery is usually reserved for patients whose pain is unresponsive to more conservative treatments and for those with a life expectancy of under 2 years.

A cordotomy may be achieved by one of two approaches: an open surgical procedure under general anesthesia or a percutaneous procedure under local anesthesia. An open cordotomy involves transection of the spinothalamic tract on the side opposite the pain. It provides pain relief below the level of transection. Percutaneous cordotomy, a closed technique, uses radio frequency coagulation to create a lesion on the anterolateral spinothalamic tract, thereby providing pain relief below the lesion. The percutaneous approach is preferred: its results compare favorably with the open approach and it's easier to perform, safer, and more precise. An open approach may be indicated in a patient unable to tolerate testing procedures while awake or one with anatomic changes in the cervical spine, such as severe arthritis.

Cordotomy can cause severe complications, such as neurologic dysfunction, respiratory distress, bladder dysfunction, and sexual impotence. It can also cause permanent loss of some sensations in the zone of analgesia.

Purpose
To relieve severe, intractable pain by preventing transmission of pain impulses to the brain.

Preparation
Provide a clear explanation of the surgery—its benefits and risks—to the patient and his family. Explain that after surgery the patient won't feel pain, temperature, or other sensations within the zone of analgesia. Inform the male patient that impotence commonly occurs after the surgery.

If the patient's undergoing a percutaneous cordotomy, explain that he'll be awake during the procedure. (If he's having an open surgical approach, he'll be under anesthesia.) Inform him that muscle tests will be performed throughout the procedure and that he should immediately alert the surgeon to any sensations of pain, pressure, or weakness. Explain that after surgery he'll lie flat in bed for 12 to 24 hours. Teach him the log-rolling maneuver and coughing and deep-breathing techniques to help prevent respiratory complications. And make sure the patient or a responsible family member has signed a consent form.

To serve as a baseline, take the patient's vital signs, evaluate the motion, strength, and sensation of each extremity, and obtain arterial blood gas measurements.

Help position the patient. In percutaneous cordotomy, proper positioning and the patient's cooperation are crucial since electrode placement must be precise. Then prepare the incision site.

Procedure
If the patient's having an *open cordotomy*, he's given a general anesthetic and placed in a sitting or prone position, depending on the level of the procedure. The surgeon performs a laminectomy to expose the spinal cord, then makes a small incision through the spinothalamic tract in the anterolateral quadrant of the cord. He closes the dural flap with fine sutures, then closes the laminectomy wound, and applies a pressure dressing. After the procedure, the patient is taken to the recovery room.

If the patient's having a *percutaneous cordotomy*, he'll lie supine with his head immobilized by a head holder and a pad placed beneath his shoulders to extend his neck. After administering a local anesthetic, the surgeon inserts a cannula into the patient's neck below and behind the mastoid process. He then injects radiopaque material and inserts an electrode through the cannula, guided by fluoroscopy, into the spinal cord.

To verify electrode placement, the surgeon stimulates the electrode, observing the patient's motor responses. Then he uses radio frequency currents to make a lesion at the desired spinal cord level. (Warn the patient when the current is being passed because the local anesthetic may not be completely effective.) After forming the lesion, the surgeon withdraws the electrode, sutures the incision, and applies a pressure dressing. Then the patient is returned to his room to recover from the local anesthetic.

Monitoring and aftercare
Throughout the procedure, you'll assist in testing motor function to reduce the risk of motor deficit. You'll also test muscle groups, observing for weakness. Severe weakness could indicate improper electrode placement or simply that the muscle is too weak to withstand the procedure. If you detect weakness, alert the doctor immediately. He'll discontinue the procedure.

After the cordotomy, keep the patient lying flat for the specified time. If he has had cervical incisions, keep his neck in a neutral position; don't use pillows to elevate his head. If the patient has had a thoracic cordotomy, you may turn him to the prone position.

DEALING WITH COMPLICATIONS OF CORDOTOMY

After cordotomy, complications may be numerous and severe. They include respiratory distress, hemorrhage, bladder dysfunction, and loss of temperature, pain, and fine tactile sensations in the affected area. Use these guidelines to help you deal with cordotomy's possible complications.

Respiratory distress
Have the patient cough and deep-breathe every 2 hours. Observe for labored breathing, weakened voice, confusion, and drowsiness.

Monitor the patient's respiratory pattern while he's asleep. He may breathe well while awake but may experience progressive hypercarbia and hypoxia while he's asleep. If periods of apnea or decreased respirations occur, wake the patient and have him breathe deeply. Provide oxygen during his sleep, if ordered.

Monitor the patient's arterial blood gases and be prepared to give mechanical ventilation. Notify the doctor of any respiratory distress.

Hemorrhage
Inspect the patient's dressing every 15 minutes for the first hour postoperatively, then every 30 minutes for the next 4 hours. Don't remove the dressing unless so ordered. Notify the doctor if drainage increases.

Monitor the patient's vital signs, especially blood pressure. If he remains hypotensive for more than 2 hours, notify the doctor. If he's severely hypotensive or symptomatic, contact the doctor right away.

Monitor for decreased neurologic function every few hours for 48 hours postoperatively. Assess motor and sensory function and report paresthesias and any decrease in movement, strength, or sensation. A deficit could indicate hemorrhage, requiring emergency surgery.

Bladder dysfunction
Check for urinary retention and notify the doctor if the patient hasn't voided in 8 hours. As ordered, instruct the patient to sit or stand to void, or institute intermittent catheterization.

If the patient has permanent urinary retention or requires an indwelling (Foley) catheter for a prolonged period, begin a bladder training program.

Loss of sensation
Reassure the patient that this is normal after a cordotomy. Turn him at least every 2 hours and feel his skin regularly for temperature changes. Overly cool skin can indicate compromised circulation, increasing the risk of skin breakdown.

Teach the patient to inspect his skin for breakdown and to wear loose clothing to avoid impairing circulation. To avoid burns, tell him to check bath water temperature with a thermometer.

Assess the patient for complications. (See *Dealing with Complications of Cordotomy.*)

Home care instructions
• Explain to the patient that he may feel numbness or tingling in the area of analgesia.
• Remind him that the loss of sensation in areas affected by the cordotomy requires taking special precautions. Teach him to inspect his skin, using a hand mirror to view hard-to-see areas, since skin integrity may be compromised in areas of insensitivity. Also instruct him to protect himself against temperature changes and weather extremes, and have him test bath or shower water with a thermometer. Advise him to avoid wearing constrictive clothing, which may impair circulation in the area of analgesia.
• Inform the patient that temporary paresis is common and that weakness may persist on the affected side. Warn him to guard against falls caused by weakness.
• Explain that some degree of impotence occurs in most postcordotomy patients. Provide emotional support and refer the patient to a specialist in sexual dysfunction.

• Reinforce the family's understanding that the analgesic effects of a cordotomy may diminish with time and that pain may return. Explain that repeating a cordotomy at another level is usually no more successful than the first procedure.

NERVE STIMULATION

Transcutaneous Electrical Nerve Stimulation

A useful approach for relieving both acute and chronic pain, transcutaneous electrical nerve stimulation (TENS) uses a mild electrical current to stimulate nerve fibers to block the transmission of pain impulses to the brain. The TENS unit consists of a portable, battery-powered generator that sends a mild current through electrodes placed on the skin at points determined to be related to the pain.

TENS is used to treat chronic back pain and pain after knee, hip, or lower back surgery. However, TENS may relieve any postoperative pain since it promotes healing by increasing blood flow near the electrodes. Other indications include dental pain, labor pain, pain from peripheral neuropathy or nerve injury, postherpetic neuralgia, reflex sympathetic dystrophy, musculoskeletal trauma, arthritis, and phantom limb pain.

The few adverse effects of TENS therapy relate to skin irritation and pruritus caused by the electrodes, the conductive gel, or the adhesive used to secure the electrodes. Electrical burns, caused by improper electrode placement, can also occur. Although TENS therapy presents few risks, the electrodes should never be placed over the carotid sinus nerves or over laryngeal or pharyngeal muscles. Likewise, the electrodes shouldn't be placed on the eyes; and they should never be located on the pregnant uterus, since this treatment's safety during pregnancy hasn't been determined.

This technique is contraindicated in patients with pacemakers, and the current may also interfere with EKG or cardiac monitoring. What's more, TENS shouldn't be used for pain of unknown etiology since it may mask a new pathology.

Purpose
To reduce pain by sending electrical impulses through the peripheral nerves to block transmission of pain impulses to the brain.

Preparation
After the doctor orders the TENS trial, show the patient the TENS unit. Inform him that he will have electrodes attached to his skin and will feel a tingling sensation when the controls are turned on. Explain that the controls will be adjusted to specified settings or to those most comfortable and effective. Advise him to use the unit for at least a week before deciding if it helps reduce his pain.

Assess the patient's level of pain to use as a baseline. Then assemble the TENS unit, lead wires, and electrodes, making sure that alcohol wipes, electrode gel, and tape are available. Determine the locations for electrode placement. This is crucial and can mean the difference between pain relief or increased pain. (See *Positioning TENS Electrodes.*)

Procedure
The physical therapist or specially trained nurse performs treatments with TENS. Treatments may be given three or four times daily for 30 to 45 minutes, for periods of 6 to 8 hours, or intermittently at the patient's discretion.

POSITIONING T.E.N.S. ELECTRODES

Typically, electrode placement varies even though patients may have similar complaints. The illustrations show three combinations of electrode placement (indicated by black squares) and areas of nerve stimulation (shown in color) for low back and leg pain.

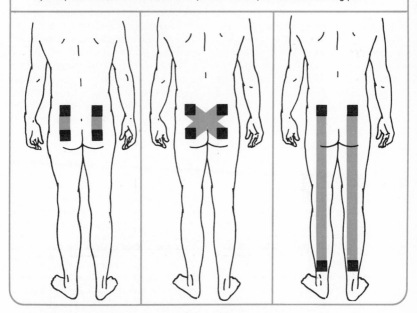

When you're ready to begin, make sure that the skin beneath the electrode sites is intact. Clean it with an alcohol wipe and dry well. Shave the area, if necessary.

Next, apply a small amount of electrode gel to the bottom of each electrode to improve conductivity. (Omit this step if the electrodes are pregelled.) Place the electrodes on the skin and secure with tape (some are self-adhering), leaving at least 2″ of space between the electrodes to prevent burns. Be sure the controls on the control box are turned to the "off" position. Attach the lead wires to the electrodes, and plug them into the control box. Set the pulse width and rate as recommended. Turn on the unit and adjust the intensity until the desired effect is achieved. Now secure the unit to the patient.

After the prescribed duration of treatment, turn the unit off and remove the electrodes. Wash and dry the patient's skin.

Monitoring and aftercare

Assess the patient for signs of excessive or inadequate stimulation. Muscle twitching may indicate overstimulation, whereas an inability to feel any tingling sensation may mean that the current is too low. If the patient complains of pain or intolerable paresthesias, check the settings, connections, and electrode placements. Adjust the settings, if necessary. If you must relocate the electrodes during treatment, first turn off the TENS unit. After treatment, be sure to clean the unit and replace the battery pack.

Evaluate the patient's response to each TENS trial and compare the results. Also use your baseline assessment to evaluate the effectiveness of the procedure.

Home care instructions

• If the patient will be using the TENS unit at home, have him demonstrate the procedure, including electrode placement, the setting of the unit's controls, electrode removal, and proper care of the equipment.

• Explain that he should strictly adhere to the prescribed settings and electrode placements. Warn against using high voltage, which may increase pain, and against using the unit for pain of unknown etiology. Also tell the patient to notify the doctor if pain worsens or develops at another site.

• If skin irritation occurs, instruct the patient to keep the area clean and apply soothing lotion. However, if his skin breaks down, he should notify the doctor. Explain that irritation may be decreased by leaving the electrodes in place during the day between treatments. Inform him that nonallergenic electrodes, such as those made with karaya gum, are available if skin irritation worsens.

• Make sure the patient understands that he should remove the unit before coming in contact with water to avoid possible electrocution.

Acupuncture

This ancient Chinese practice, first introduced in the United States in the 1800s, continues to be viewed skeptically by many Western pain experts. They point to the absence of controlled scientific studies and to acupuncture's philosophical origins. According to Chinese thinkers, acupuncture corrects a disharmony between yin and yang, the complementary life forces that flow through channels, or meridians, in the body. This disharmony, say the Chinese, creates illness and pain.

Some Western researchers, though, view acupuncture favorably, but for a different reason than the Chinese. Using the gate control theory of pain, they suggest that the needles used in acupuncture stimulate large sensory nerve fibers that carry pain-inhibiting impulses, thereby blocking impulses from the smaller pain-conducting fibers at the spinal level. Researchers also suggest that acupuncture's analgesic effects result from triggering the release of opioid-like compounds, such as enkephalins and endorphins.

Despite the ongoing controversy over acupuncture's merits, this technique may be used for pain with an inflammatory component, such as tenosynovitis or bursitis, and muscle spasm. It's also used to relieve diverse types of pain that fail to respond to more conventional treatments. Such pain includes postherpetic neuralgia, diabetic neuropathy, causalgia, reflex sympathetic dystrophy, osteoarthritis, rheumatoid arthritis, headache, low back and cervical pain syndromes, and temporomandibular joint syndrome.

Typically, acupuncture causes few complications if performed correctly. Possible complications include hyperemia or hematoma at a needle insertion site, light-headedness, syncope, puncture of a vital organ and, rarely, infection.

Acupuncture should be avoided in patients with profound immunodeficiency or bleeding disorders or certain psychiatric disorders, such as paranoia, which may preclude the use of any elective invasive procedure. In pregnancy, acupuncture may be contraindicated because of the risk of precipitating contractions. Electrical acupuncture should be used with caution in patients with pacemakers.

Purpose

To relieve pain caused by inflammation, neuralgia, back strain, and many other conditions.

Preparation

Reinforce the therapist's explanation of the procedure and its risks. Explain that the therapist will insert thin needles into the skin and that the patient may feel sensations of pin pricks, warmth, dizziness, and stinging or a dull, aching throb. Mention that as treatment progresses, he'll probably be able to tolerate more stimulation. Tell him to report increasing discomfort. Mention that the first treatment may provide only temporary relief or none at all but that the duration of pain relief should lengthen with successive treatments.

Assess the patient's level of pain to serve as a baseline. Position him as ordered (usually lying down). Assemble the necessary equipment and ensure that all needles are sterile. Then cleanse the skin at the needle insertion sites.

Procedure
The therapist places 6 to 18 needles under the skin at the appropriate points. Needles may be inserted directly into a painful area as well as in areas remote from the pain. Once the needles are in place, the therapist stimulates them, either electrically or manually. Then he removes them.

Monitoring and aftercare
After acupuncture, observe the needle insertion sites for hematoma formation. If a hematoma occurs, apply pressure and reassure the patient. Have him sit up or stand slowly to avoid syncope or light-headedness.

If needles were inserted in the patient's thorax, carefully assess for signs of pneumothorax, such as dyspnea or tachypnea.

Compare the patient's level of pain to pretreatment levels.

Home care instructions
• Teach the patient to identify signs of local infection, such as redness, swelling, and discharge. Explain that infection is unlikely, but that if it occurs, he should notify the therapist immediately.
• Instruct the patient who has had needles placed in the thorax to immediately report any shortness of breath or

INQUIRY

QUESTIONS PATIENTS ASK ABOUT ACUPUNCTURE

Does acupuncture work?
Yes, for some patients. In fact, some achieve permanent and complete relief from pain. Others, though, experience only temporary relief or, worse yet, no relief at all. If you don't feel an improvement after a reasonable number of sessions, you should probably stop the treatment.

Can acupuncture cure the cause of my pain?
That depends on the cause. Some therapists think acupuncture may stimulate the body's anti-inflammatory response and help resolve conditions like tendonitis and bursitis. However, acupuncture isn't a cure-all. Most therapists believe it relieves pain but doesn't eliminate the cause.

How do I find an acupuncturist?
Because acupuncture was first introduced in the United States without scientific backing, therapists who aren't doctors dominate the practice. And the established medical community doesn't always accept their methods. If you're serious about undergoing acupuncture treatments, look for a doctor trained in acupuncture or for an acupuncturist who practices with a doctor. You might also ask your doctor for the name of a reliable practitioner.

painful breathing.
• Have the patient note the duration and effectiveness of pain relief, and instruct him to report his observations at the next appointment. For full effect, 8 to 16 treatments may be required. However, if analgesia hasn't occurred after a reasonable number of sessions, the therapist may terminate treatment.

TREATMENTS WITH HEAT OR COLD

Heat Treatments

An age-old remedy, heat relieves pain by promoting sedation and muscle relaxation. By causing vasodilation, heat helps restore nutrition to the cells and facilitates the elimination of waste products, such as bradykinin, histamine, and prostaglandins, from muscle. It also raises the pain threshold of sensory nerve endings and thus may break the pain-spasm-pain cycle. What's more, heat increases the extensibility of connective tissue, thereby reducing pain during activity. Commonly used for superficial muscular pain, heat may also be used to relieve pain caused by arthritis or muscle trauma.

Heat treatments include superficial and deep heat. Superficial heat comes in many forms, such as *hot-water bottles*, *heating pads*, *aquamatic K pads*, *heat lamps*, and *hot packs*. Deep-heat treatments, which require specially trained personnel and equipment, include ultrasound and diathermy. *Ultrasound*, the most common deep-heat treatment, directs focused sound waves through soft tissue to deep structures, such as bone, where they're absorbed and converted into heat. *Diathermy* uses high-frequency current to generate heat in some part of the body.

Because heat causes vasodilation, it is contraindicated in bleeding disorders and should be avoided in traumatic injury. In addition, deep-heat therapy shouldn't be used in patients with metal implants because of the risk of local tissue damage.

Heat treatments should be used cautiously in patients with sensory impairment, heat intolerance, or impaired renal, cardiac, or respiratory function. Patients with impaired arterial or venous circulation have a decreased ability to dissipate heat effectively, thereby reducing their tolerance.

Purpose
To relieve pain by relaxing muscles and promoting sedation.

Preparation
Explain the specific heat treatment to the patient. Tell him that a treatment session usually lasts 20 to 30 minutes for dry or deep heat and 15 to 20 minutes for moist heat. (The maximum treatment time is 45 minutes.) Also tell him how often treatments will be performed. (They may range from two or three times daily to two or three times weekly.) Find out if the patient has any metallic implants.

Assess the patient's pain level, his need for analgesics, and his activity level. Tell him to report any pain during treatment and, if necessary, to remove the heating device himself.

For a superficial heat treatment, assemble and check the necessary equipment. (See "Rewarming Treatments" in Chapter 18 for directions on preparing hot-water bottles, heating pads, and aquamatic K pads.) For a hot pack, heat sterile saline solution in hot water to a temperature of 131° F. (55° C.); then pour the heated solution into a sterile basin. Using sterile technique, soak a compress in the basin.

For a heat lamp, check for a frayed cord and make sure the bulb is of the correct wattage. Expose only the treatment area since vasodilation will chill the patient.

Procedure
If you're using a hot-water bottle, an aquamatic K pad, or an electric heating pad, position the patient comfortably, apply the device, and begin timing the procedure. Secure the device with gauze. Remember to pay special attention to the patient's skin condition, checking it every 5 minutes and removing the device if you notice exces-

sive redness, blistering, or maceration. End the treatment after 20 to 30 minutes, dry the patient's skin, and redress the site if necessary.

If you're using a hot pack, place a linen-saver pad beneath the treatment area and position the patient. Spread petrolatum (sterile, if necessary) over the affected area but don't apply it to broken areas. Now remove the compress from the basin and wring out excess solution (using sterile gloves or forceps for a sterile procedure). Apply the compress and, after a few seconds, check the area for excessive redness or maceration. (Use sterile forceps or gloves, if needed.) Then mold the compress firmly to the skin, and apply and secure a waterproof cover. Check the patient's skin every 5 minutes for signs of tissue intolerance, removing the device if you observe redness or maceration. Remove the compress after 15 to 20 minutes and discard it. Finally, dry the patient's skin and redress the area, if needed (using sterile technique, if necessary).

If you're using a heat lamp, position the patient and place the lamp beside him. Measure and adjust the neck of the lamp so that the light bulb is the correct distance from his skin. In most cases, allow 14" (35.6 cm) for a 25-watt bulb, 18" (45.7 cm) for a 40-watt bulb, and 24" to 30" (61 to 76.2 cm) for a 60-watt or higher bulb. Time the application and check the lamp position and the patient's skin every 5 minutes. Turn off the lamp after 20 to 30 minutes and redress the area, if necessary.

If the patient's having a deep-heat treatment, he'll go to the physical therapy department, where a therapist will direct ultrasound waves at the painful area for 20 to 30 minutes.

Monitoring and aftercare

Regardless of the method used, you'll need to monitor the patient for burns. In the debilitated patient, be alert for cardiovascular or respiratory effects. Take vital signs periodically until the patient's response to treatment is clear.

If the patient is elderly, neurologically impaired, disoriented, confused, or insensitive to heat, stay with him throughout the treatment. Check the treatment site frequently to avoid complications, such as edema, maceration, and blisters.

Remember to never continue a heat treatment for longer than 45 minutes. By this time, maximum vasodilation has occurred. Continued use causes vasoconstriction, reversing the effects of therapy. Similarly, to avoid vasoconstriction, allow at least 1 hour between treatments.

Home care instructions

● If the patient will be performing heat treatments at home, provide clear instructions and have him demonstrate the correct technique.

● Teach the patient safety measures, such as checking equipment carefully before use. Caution him against lying or sleeping on or near the heating device, to prevent burns. Also instruct him to secure the device with gauze—never with safety pins; heated metal can cause burns or electric shock. Warn him against exposing electrical heating devices to water because of the risk of electric shock.

● Instruct the patient to follow the doctor's orders precisely for the duration and frequency of treatment.

● Tell him to check his skin every 5 minutes during treatment. (Sensory-impaired patients should be especially cautious.) He should report any unusual redness or blistering to the doctor. Also have him report any increase in pain or skin breakdown.

Cold Treatments

Long used to treat acute pain from sprains, strains, and spasms, cold treatments have recently been used to relieve chronic pain. They're useful in most pain-producing disorders, except those involving vasoconstriction.

These treatments work because cold reduces nerve conduction velocity, producing analgesia by decreasing the number of pain impulses reaching the brain. It may also stimulate the large nerve fibers at the spinal cord or brainstem level, inhibiting the influence of the smaller fibers that carry pain impulses. What's more, cold produces peripheral vasoconstriction followed by vasodilation to maintain tissue viability at low temperatures. At the same time, cold decreases the release of pain-producing substances.

Cold can be delivered in many ways. In an *ice massage*, a block of ice is massaged directly over the painful area. In the *ice bag* technique, plastic, cloth, or rubber bags are filled with ice cubes or crushed ice and applied directly to the area. Other types of cold therapy include *cold immersion*, *cold compresses*, *chemical cold packs*, and an *aquamatic K pad*.

Cold treatments are contraindicated in peripheral vascular disease, a history of frostbite in the affected area, or any form of cold allergy, such as hives. They should be used cautiously, if at all, in collagen diseases and Raynaud's disease.

Purpose
To produce local analgesia.

Preparation
Describe the cold treatment to the patient. Explain that sessions usually last 10 to 30 minutes. Tell him that he may experience four stages of sensory changes: cold, burning, tingling, and numbness. Explain that these sensations don't indicate tissue damage, nor do they predict therapeutic effects. Explain that the first few treatments may not be noticeably effective, but that significant analgesia (lasting from 15 minutes to several hours) can be achieved with repeated treatments.

Assess the patient's pain level. Cau-

tion him to immediately report any new or unusual discomfort during treatment. Instruct him to remove the cold device himself, if necessary.

Now assemble the equipment. For an ice massage, prepare ice in a plastic tub (for example, a margarine tub) or in a paper cup with a popsicle stick for a handle. For cold immersion, pour cold tap water (or sterile saline solution) into a basin and add pieces of ice. The water temperature should be about 59° F. (15° C.). (To prepare an icebag, cold compress, chemical cold pack, or aquamatic K pad, see "Cooling Treatments" in Chapter 18.)

Procedure
To use ice massage, place a linen-saver pad beneath the treatment area. Wrap the ice in a cloth or hold the stick and rub in a circular or back-and-forth motion over the painful area. Avoid bony prominences and use light to moderate pressure. If the patient is anxious, apply the ice at 30-second intervals, gradually increasing the interval until he can tolerate continuous massage. End the treatment when he reports numbness or after 10 minutes. Then dry the treatment area.

To perform cold immersion, place a linen-saver pad beneath the basin. Immerse the painful area in the basin and time the treatment. Keep the area immersed for the specified time (usually 20 minutes), then remove and dry the area. (For directions on using an ice bag, a cold compress, a chemical cold pack, or an aquamatic K pad, see "Cooling Treatments" in Chapter 18.)

Monitoring and aftercare
During therapy, observe the patient for signs of frostbite or hypersensitivity, such as blanching, mottling, urticaria, flushing, or syncope. Observe the site every 5 minutes for signs of tissue intolerance, including blanching, mottling, or graying. If the patient shivers or complains of new, unusual, or intolerable pain, discontinue the treatment and notify the doctor.

If the patient is elderly, neurologically impaired, or insensitive to cold, stay with him during the treatment and check the site often to avoid complications, such as mottling and blisters.

Never allow a cold treatment to continue for more than 30 minutes or an ice massage more than 10 minutes since reflexive vasodilation will occur and probably increase the pain. The incidence of side effects may also increase.

Home care instructions
• Tell the patient not to exceed the recommended duration of treatment because frostbite and burns may result.
• Instruct him to report any change in symptoms or pain location, and any mottling, grayness, or blanching.
• If the patient's recovering from an injury, inform him that cold-induced numbness can be deceiving—an absence of pain doesn't necessarily indicate recovery. Caution him to move the injured area carefully and to avoid strenuous activity until healing is complete.
• Inform the patient that ice massage may be used in conjunction with a home exercise program recommended by a physical therapist.

BEHAVIORAL AND RELAXATION TECHNIQUES

Cognitive Pain-Control Techniques

Behavior modification and relaxation techniques, including biofeedback, distraction, guided imagery, hypnosis, and meditation, help the patient reduce the suffering associated with pain. (See *Comparing Methods for Managing Pain*, page 626.) These "mind-over-pain" techniques allow the patient to participate in his treatment and to achieve a degree of control over pain. They're virtually risk-free and have few contraindications. However, if the patient has a significant psychiatric problem, relaxation techniques should be taught by a psychotherapist.

Purpose
To reduce pain by promoting relaxation or a behavioral change.

Preparation
Begin by performing a thorough assessment, evaluating environmental factors, family relationships, and any psychosocial considerations that may intensify pain or anxiety. And since the success of these techniques depends largely on the patient's motivation and commitment, you'll need to convince him that they do, indeed, work. Keep in mind that the patient with a sensorium clouded by disease or medication may be incapable of following instructions.

If the patient's using *meditation*, suggest that he repeat a word or a phrase or stare at an object until he's relaxed. While relaxed, he may feel warmth, heaviness, lightness, or tingling.

If he's using *distraction*, tell him that this technique can involve almost any activity—reading a book, listening to music, or simply talking. Mention that the more absorbed he becomes in the activity, the less pain he's likely to feel.

If he's using *guided imagery*, inform him that the more vivid the image, the better the results. Encourage him to choose vivid images associated with peaceful and calming memories and feelings from his own experience.

For *hypnosis*, tell him that the type of technique varies with the therapist.

If the patient's using *biofeedback*, inform him that he'll be connected to a monitor that will measure changes in his blood pressure, pulse, and skin temperature. These readings will help determine his level of relaxation.

When using *behavior modification*, explain to the patient that you and he

COMPARING METHODS FOR MANAGING PAIN

TECHNIQUE	ADVANTAGES	DISADVANTAGES
Behavioral Pain Control		
Behavior modification Reinforces behavior to increase activity level, reduce concentration on pain, and enhance a healthy life-style	• Improved self-esteem. • Increased activity and productivity. • Decreased preoccupation with pain, suffering, and disability.	• Requires trained personnel and the cooperation of everyone involved, especially the family. Personnel unfamiliar with treatment plan may inadvertently undo its good effects. • May be best suited for pain clinics. • Requires exploration of environmental and social problems that cause or worsen pain. Otherwise, relief may be short-term.
Relaxation Techniques		
Biofeedback Gives immediate feedback on biological processes affected by relaxation, such as temperature and muscle tension	• Enhances control over muscle tension. • Some people benefit most from immediate feedback.	• Patient may become dependent on biofeedback machine to achieve relaxation. • Patient may "fight" the machine, becoming more tense.
Distraction Removes attention from pain, focusing instead on some other activity, such as knitting or reading. Most effective when multiple senses are involved.	• Easily taught.	• Difficult if pain is unrelenting, unpredictable, and severe.
Guided imagery Encourages the imagining of a peaceful, pleasant scene, thereby providing a substitute for pain sensations.	• Patient can relive or experience peaceful, comfortable memories/feelings to the exclusion of pain and suffering.	• Requires a vivid imagination and excellent concentration.
Hypnosis Concentrates the patient's attention on something other than pain. Since the mind can truly concentrate on only one thing at a time, pain is no longer the center of attention.	• May change the patient's perception of pain, create a sense of control, and provide long-lasting relief. • Posthypnotic suggestion can maintain pain relief.	• If hypnosis triggers a traumatic memory, it may increase the patient's anxiety and pain. • Patient becomes dependent on the therapist.
Meditation Focuses concentration on the art of breathing and on a single number, object, or phrase to produce relaxation.	• Does not require a vivid imagination. • Focuses attention away from pain. • May be especially useful while waiting for an analgesic to work.	• Immediate results unlikely.

will identify and modify patterns of behavior that contribute to or reinforce pain.

Procedure

Because these techniques require concentration, begin when pain is absent or mild, if possible. However, if pain is persistent, begin with short, simple exercises and build on the patient's abilities. First, have him remove or loosen restrictive clothing, dim the lights, and keep noise to a minimum.

For muscle *relaxation*, instruct the patient to alternately tighten and relax the muscles of a specific muscle group, concentrating on tension and relaxation. Repeat for all groups. (If tensing a muscle group is painful, move on to the next group or repeat another group.)

For *distraction*, instruct the patient to listen to music, using a headset, and to focus on an object or on the imagery evoked by the music, keeping time to the beat and increasing the volume when pain worsens. Or he can sing, read a book, or try rhythmic breathing.

For *guided imagery*, have the patient concentrate on a soothing image while you describe the sensations, such as the smell of grass or the warmth of the sun.

For *hypnosis*, the therapist may employ various techniques, such as symptom suppression to block awareness of pain or symptom substitution, which allows a positive interpretation of pain.

For *biofeedback*, the patient uses the relaxation technique he finds most helpful. While connected to a biofeedback machine, the patient recognizes and controls the relaxation process, taking his cues from the device's audible tones, flashing lights, or digital readouts.

For *behavior modification*, identify behaviors that reinforce pain, suffering, and disability, such as being overly dependent on others or using a cane when it's not medically indicated. Also help the patient define his goals, such as decreasing his dependence on others, and use appropriate reinforcements to achieve the desired behavior patterns.

Monitoring and aftercare

Remember to be consistent. And be sure that all staff members understand and reinforce the chosen approach.

If the patient becomes upset at his inability to concentrate and relax, have him stop and try again later. End each session on a positive note—for example, by pointing out improvements.

Home care instructions

● Advise the patient with overwhelming psychosocial problems to seek help in psychotherapy. Any gains in pain management may be quickly lost unless he deals with these factors.

● Suggest that the patient continue to use pain-control techniques after his pain has resolved, since they may help relieve everyday stress.

Selected References

Aronoff, G.M., ed. *Evaluation and Treatment of Chronic Pain.* Baltimore: Urban & Schwarzenberg, 1985.

Foley, K.M. "The Treatment of Cancer Pain," *New England Journal of Medicine* 313(2):84-95, July 11, 1985.

Moulin, D.E., and Coyle, N. "Spinal Opioid Analgesics and Local Anesthetics in the Management of Chronic Cancer Pain," *Journal of Pain and Symptom Management* 1(2):79-86, Spring 1986.

Principles of Analgesic Use in the Treatment of Acute Pain and Chronic Cancer Pain: A Concise Guide to Medical Practice. Washington, D.C.: American Pain Society, 1987.

Warfield, C.A. "Patient-Controlled Analgesia," *Hospital Practice* 20(7):32L-P, July 15, 1985.

20

Treating Mental and Emotional Problems

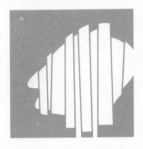

Treating Mental and Emotional Problems

Introduction

Keeping current with treatments for mental and emotional problems can sometimes seem like an unending challenge. After all, the diagnostic classification of mental disorders has undergone drastic changes within the past decade. Certain treatments, such as electroconvulsive therapy, have come in and out of vogue, and new antidepressant drugs have appeared on the therapeutic horizon. What's more, psychotherapeutic approaches, such as milieu therapy, have changed the climate at some of our psychiatric institutions. Despite changes like these, many major treatment considerations remain the same.

The patient
Obviously, patients vary in their personalities, symptoms, and motivation. All of these factors affect their ability to comply with prescribed therapy. And these personal variations can also cause patients to respond to treatment in drastically different ways even though they may be afflicted with the same disorder. The moral: What helps one patient may not necessarily help another patient.

The therapist
Just as patients differ, so do therapists. Whether the therapist's a psychiatrist, psychoanalyst, psychologist, social worker, or psychiatric clinical nurse specialist, each brings preconceptions about what type of therapy works best. And each carries a distinctive style into therapy. One therapist may assume the position of a neutral observer while another may be overtly directive.

Combination therapy
Successful therapy commonly relies on using two or more forms of treatment. For example, a behavioral therapist might combine drug therapy and desensitization to treat a phobia. Another therapist might use electroconvulsive therapy followed by antidepressant drugs to treat major depression.

An expanded nursing role
Nurses today are playing an ever-larger role in all types of psychiatric treatments. Besides fulfilling the traditional task of administering drugs and monitoring their effects, nurses can act as primary therapists in milieu therapy. Or they may direct certain types of behavior therapies. In detoxification programs, they may offer guidance and support while monitoring for compliance with abstention from the abused substance.

In short, as treatments for mental and emotional problems evolve, nurses' roles become increasingly varied and important.

DRUG THERAPY

Benzodiazepine Anxiolytics

Benzodiazepines, a group of structurally related synthetic drugs, gained popularity in the early 1960s, replacing barbiturates as the treatment of choice for anxiety. Today most clinicians still prefer benzodiazepines to barbiturates. The reasons? First, benzodiazepines act more predictably than barbiturates and produce fewer side effects with therapeutic doses. They also have less potential for dependence and abuse and for interaction with other drugs. In overdoses, they produce less toxicity.

Benzodiazepines are used preoperatively to relieve anxiety and provide sedation, light anesthesia, and anterograde amnesia. They're also used to manage agitation associated with acute alcohol withdrawal, to treat anxiety disorders, and to provide short-term relief of anxiety. However, benzodiazepines aren't usually recommended for anxiety associated with the stress of everyday life.

Nine drugs make up the family of benzodiazepine anxiolytics: *alprazolam, chlordiazepoxide hydrochloride, clorazepate dipotassium, diazepam, halazepam, lorazepam, midazolam hydrochloride, oxazepam,* and *prazepam.* Choice of a specific drug for treatment depends on the doctor's clinical experience, the patient's response, the desired route of administration, and the drug's price. It also depends on the drug's pharmacokinetic profile, especially the absorption rates of the parent compound and the biotransformation and elimination rates of active metabolites. For example, in a patient with depressed renal or hepatic function, any of three benzodiazepines—alprazolam, lorazepam, or oxazepam—might be prescribed since each has a relatively short duration of action and no active metabolites.

Chief side effects of benzodiazepine anxiolytics include subtle cognitive impairment, anterograde amnesia, ataxia, and diminished fine motor coordination and reaction time. And, although benzodiazepines have been proven safe and effective for both short- and long-term treatment, they can cause psychological and physiologic dependence. When taken with alcohol or other CNS depressants, they can lead to increased CNS depression and possibly death.

Because dependence occurs most commonly in patients with a history of alcohol and drug abuse, the benzodiazepines should be avoided in these patients, if possible. They should be used cautiously in patients with suicidal tendencies and in those whose history indicates that they may increase dosage on their own initiative. Benzodiazepines are contraindicated in patients with a hypersensitivity to at least one of the drugs. Usually, they're also contraindicated in patients with acute closed-angle glaucoma but may be given to patients receiving treatment for chronic open-angle glaucoma. Intravenous administration should be avoided for patients in shock or coma or with depressed respiration.

Purpose and action
Benzodiazepines relieve anxiety by depressing the CNS. However, the precise sites and mechanisms of their action are still somewhat unclear. Apparently, the benzodiazepines amplify or facilitate the inhibitory presynaptic and postsynaptic action of gamma-aminobutyric acid—a major neurotransmitter—by interacting with specific neuronal membrane receptors in the ascending reticular activating system. This interaction increases inhi-

bition and blocks both cortical and limbic arousal when anxiety stimulates the brain.

Monitoring

When they're given intravenously, benzodiazepines may produce apnea, hypotension, bradycardia, or cardiac arrest, especially in elderly or severely ill patients and in those patients who have limited pulmonary reserve or unstable cardiovascular status. As a result, always keep resuscitation equipment nearby when using this administration route. After I.V. injection, watch for redness, swelling, or pain at the injection site.

Keep in mind that benzodiazepines may make the patient feel drowsy, dizzy, light-headed, clumsy, unsteady, or less alert than normal—especially if he is elderly or debilitated or has hepatic disease or low serum albumin levels. (Young children and infants are also usually more sensitive to the CNS effects of benzodiazepines.) Even if the patient takes the drug at bedtime, he may feel drowsy or less alert on arising. Typically, these effects occur during the first few days of therapy and then subside. If therapy begins in the hospital, take measures to protect the patient from falls, such as raising side rails and instructing him to request assistance when ambulating.

Monitor liver and kidney function tests and blood counts regularly during long-term therapy, especially if the patient has hepatic or renal disease. Check his drug history to see if he's taking cimetidine, which may interact with certain benzodiazepines. Specifically, cimetidine delays plasma clearance of alprazolam, chlordiazepoxide, clorazepate, diazepam, prazepam, and probably halazepam by interfering with their oxidative metabolism. To compensate for this, the doctor may need to reduce the benzodiazepine dose. Cimetidine doesn't interact with lorazepam or oxazepam because these drugs are metabolized by conjugation with glucuronic acid.

Home care instructions

● If the patient thinks that the drug isn't working effectively, warn him not to increase the dose on his own. Doing so enhances his risk of drug dependence.

● Describe side effects that the patient should watch for and report immediately. These include confusion or depression, blurred vision, ataxia, and unusual fatigue or weakness. Tell him to make sure that he knows how he reacts to this drug before he drives, operates machinery, or does any other task that requires him to be alert and coordinated.

● If the patient experiences GI upset, advise him to take the drug with or immediately after meals.

● Warn the patient that this drug will accentuate the effects of alcohol and other CNS depressants. Stress that he shouldn't consume alcohol while on benzodiazepine therapy. Explain that consuming alcohol or taking other CNS depressants may lead to unconsciousness and possibly death.

● Inform him that cigarette smoking may interfere with benzodiazepine therapy. Although the mechanism is unclear, smoking apparently speeds the drug's metabolism, thereby decreasing its effectiveness.

● If the patient is taking the drug regularly and misses a dose, tell him to take it right away if he remembers within an hour or so of the missed dose. However, if he doesn't remember until later, have him skip the missed dose and return to his regular dosing schedule. He shouldn't double-dose.

● If the patient is taking the extended-release form of diazepam, tell him to swallow the capsules whole. He shouldn't crush, break, or chew them before swallowing.

● If the patient will be taking this drug regularly for a prolonged period, explain that the doctor will check his progress at least every 4 months to assess the need for continued therapy. Warn him not to stop taking the drug abruptly without his doctor's approval.

• Tell the patient that after he stops taking this drug, his body may need time to adjust—especially if he took the drug in high doses or for a prolonged period. This adjustment may take just a few days or up to 3 weeks. Have him notify his doctor if he experiences withdrawal symptoms: unusual irritability or nervousness, incoordination, or weakness.

Antipsychotics
[Major tranquilizers, neuroleptics]

Antipsychotics treat a wide variety of disorders, including schizophrenia, organic psychoses, and the manic phase of bipolar disorders. They're also used for acute psychotic symptoms, such as paranoia, hostility, combativeness, hallucinations, and persistent delusions. The most commonly used classes of antipsychotics include the *phenothiazines*, such as chlorpromazine and fluphenazine, and the *butyrophenones*, such as haloperidol. Less commonly used classes include the *thioxanthenes*, such as chlorprothixene and thiothixene, the *dihydroindolones*, such as molindone, and the *dibenzoxazepines*, such as loxapine.

Patients receiving antipsychotic drugs require careful monitoring for compliance and adverse reactions. Major reactions vary, depending on the drug class, but may include excessive sedation, extrapyramidal symptoms, orthostatic hypotension, and anticholinergic effects.

Purpose and action
Antipsychotics relieve psychotic symptoms and provide sedation by decreasing levels of the neurotransmitters norepinephrine and dopamine, which have been associated with psychosis and mania. (See *How Chlorpromazine Relieves Schizophrenic Symptoms.*)

Monitoring
Carefully observe the patient for adverse reactions. *Extrapyramidal symptoms*, such as ataxia and tremors, occur most commonly with piperazine phenothiazines, haloperidol, thiothixene, molindone, or loxapine. *Sedation* occurs most commonly with chlorpromazine, triflupromazine, or piperidine phenothiazines. *Orthostatic hypotension* occurs with chlorpromazine and thioridazine, and *anticholinergic effects*, such as dry mouth, occur with promazine, triflupromazine, or thioridazine.

If the patient experiences extrapyramidal symptoms, reassure him that they're typically reversible. If ordered, administer an antiparkinsonian drug, such as diphenhydramine or benztropine mesylate. These symptoms usually subside within 3 months. If they persist, the doctor may discontinue the antipsychotic drug or reduce its dosage. However, if the patient experiences an acute dystonic reaction, administer diphenhydramine or benztropine I.M. or I.V., as ordered, and maintain airway clearance and adequate hydration. If the patient's receiving long-term drug therapy, watch for tardive dyskinesia, a potentially irreversible syndrome characterized by rhythmic, involuntary movements of the tongue, face, mouth, jaw, and extremities. If you detect this syndrome, notify the doctor immediately.

If the patient experiences excessive sedation, take appropriate precautions, such as raising the side rails of his bed and assisting him with ambulation. Also, monitor the patient's blood pressure to detect orthostatic hypotension. If it occurs, advise him to rise slowly from a sitting or lying position to avoid dizziness or light-headedness.

If the patient experiences a dry mouth while taking an antipsychotic drug, provide hard candy or sugarless gum. If he becomes constipated, increase his fluid intake and provide a stool softener. If he gains weight, help

HOW CHLORPROMAZINE RELIEVES SCHIZOPHRENIC SYMPTOMS

Schizophrenia purportedly results from excessive CNS levels of the neurotransmitter dopamine. As shown here, chlorproma-zine blocks neuron binding sites, thereby reducing dopamine absorption and relieving schizophrenic symptoms.

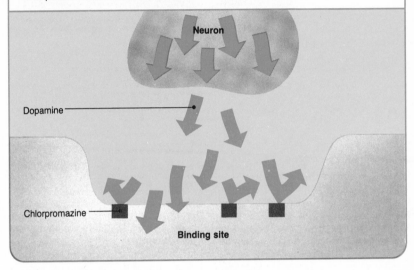

him select low-calorie foods and maintain adequate nutrition.

Be alert for an acute reaction, such as neuroleptic malignant syndrome, a rare but possibly fatal syndrome that can arise after an initial dose or after prolonged treatment. Suspect neuroleptic malignant syndrome if the patient experiences respiratory distress, fever, hypertension or hypotension, incontinence, and rigidity and weakness. Other signs include pallor, fatigue, and tachycardia or an irregular pulse. Provide supportive and symptomatic treatment.

Because antipsychotic drugs can cause leukopenia and agranulocytosis, be sure to monitor the patient's complete blood count and differential throughout therapy. Because these drugs can also produce hepatic impairment, check the results of liver function studies and observe for jaundice. Also check for tachycardia or EKG changes, which can indicate the need for dosage adjustment.

Review the patient's current medication regimen for possible interactions. Barbiturates, for example, may reduce the therapeutic effect of phenothiazines. Lithium, commonly used with haloperidol during early treatment of acute manic episodes, may cause irreversible neurotoxicity with continued use.

Home care instructions

• Instruct the patient to make up a missed dose if he remembers within 2 hours of the scheduled administration time. If more than 2 hours elapse, advise him to skip the dose altogether and to take the next dose as ordered. Warn against doubling the next dose.

• Inform the patient to report a sore throat, fever, or weakness immediately. These symptoms may indicate blood dyscrasias.

• Tell him to use caution when driving or performing tasks that require alertness until he can predict his response to the medication.

• Warn against excessive exposure to the sun to reduce the risk of phototoxicity.

• If dry mouth occurs, advise the patient to use throat lozenges for symptomatic relief.

• If the patient's receiving an antipsychotic, such as chlorpromazine, that can cause orthostatic hypotension, suggest that he rise slowly from a lying or sitting position. If he's taking antacids and a phenothiazine, instruct him to separate doses of these drugs by at least 2 hours. If he's taking a liquid phenothiazine, warn against skin contact with the drug since contact dermatitis may occur.

• Tell the patient to avoid alcohol because it can cause increased sedation.

• Have the patient check with his doctor before discontinuing the drug. Patients are usually weaned gradually; abrupt withdrawal may cause nausea, vomiting, trembling, and dizziness.

Monoamine Oxidase Inhibitors

Three monoamine oxidase (MAO) inhibitors—*isocarboxazid*, *phenelzine*, and *tranylcypromine*—are used to treat depression when tricyclic antidepressants and electroconvulsive therapy are ineffective or contraindicated. Both isocarboxazid and phenelzine have a delayed therapeutic effect, with the patient showing improvement roughly 4 weeks after the start of therapy. Tranylcypromine usually produces therapeutic effects within a few days; however, tranylcypromine has a higher incidence of CNS stimulation than other MAO inhibitors.

MAO inhibitors are used sparingly because of their serious side effects, including orthostatic hypotension, severe headache, and hypertensive crisis.

They're contraindicated in children because of potential growth retardation and in geriatric patients because of increased risk of cerebrovascular accidents. They're also contraindicated in patients with cardiovascular disease or impaired renal or hepatic function.

When caring for the patient receiving an MAO inhibitor, your key responsibility will be the prevention or monitoring of side effects.

Purpose and action

To reduce CNS levels of catecholamines (dopamine, norepinephrine, and epinephrine), thereby relieving depression.

Monitoring

Ensure that the patient's diet doesn't include caffeine or tyramine-containing foods and that his medication regimen doesn't include drugs that interact with MAO inhibitors. (See *Hazards of Using MAO Inhibitors with Other Agents.*) Warn visitors not to give the patient coffee, chocolate, alcohol, over-the-counter drugs, or other restricted products. Ingestion of any of these can cause hypertensive crisis. If this crisis does occur, discontinue the MAO inhibitor immediately and slowly give 5 mg of phentolamine I.V. Reduce fever by external cooling.

Regularly monitor the patient's blood pressure and liver function tests since MAO inhibitors can cause hypotension, hypertension, and hepatitis. Observe for unusual sweating; fever; cold, clammy skin; enlarged pupils; increased sensitivity to light; and an unusually rapid or slow heartbeat. Tell the patient to report severe dizziness or chest pain, light-headedness, nausea, vomiting, or a stiff or sore neck. Also tell him to report persistent constipation, urinary difficulty, dizziness or light-headedness, drowsiness, or dry mouth.

If the patient becomes constipated, increase his fluid intake and provide a stool softener, if ordered. Give throat lozenges to help relieve dry mouth. To alleviate orthostatic hypotension, instruct the patient to rise slowly and sit on the bed or a chair before standing.

Home care instructions
• Instruct the patient not to change the dosage or stop the drug. Remind him that therapeutic effects may take several weeks.

• Tell him to take a missed dose if he remembers within 2 hours of the scheduled administration time; otherwise, he should skip the missed dose. Recommend not taking the drug close to bedtime because of possible insomnia.

• Teach the patient and his family what foods to avoid, and remind them that

INTERACTIONS

HAZARDS OF USING M.A.O. INHIBITORS WITH OTHER AGENTS

AGENT	EFFECT	NURSING ACTIONS
Alcohol	Increased sedation, decreased metabolism	• Instruct patient to avoid alcohol.
Analgesics	Severe hypotension or hypertension, excitation, sweating, rigidity, coma, convulsions, or death	• Allow 14 days after discontinuing monoamine oxidase (MAO) inhibitor before giving analgesics. • Administer one quarter of usual narcotic dose, if necessary.
Anesthetics	*General:* potentiated hypertensive and hypotensive effect and increased CNS depression. *Local:* severe hypertension. *Spinal:* potentiated hypotensive effect	• Stop MAO inhibitor 14 days before surgery. • If emergency surgery is required, reduce narcotic or other premedication dose to one quarter of usual amount. • Adjust anesthetic dose according to the doctor's instructions.
Anticoagulants	Increased anticoagulant effect	• Monitor clotting time.
Anticonvulsants	Changes in pattern of epileptiform seizures	• Monitor vital signs. • Observe for symptoms of CNS depression and changes in epileptiform seizures.
Antidepressants (tricyclic)	Severe seizures, hyperpyretic crisis, hypertensive crisis, or death	• Avoid concurrent administration. Allow 2 to 4 weeks after discontinuing MAO inhibitor before giving these antidepressants.
Antidiabetic agents (oral or insulin)	Enhanced hypoglycemic effect	• Monitor blood and urine glucose levels. • Watch for hypoglycemic symptoms. • Reduce dosage of the hypoglycemic agent, if ordered.
Antihistamines	Increased sedation, decreased metabolism	• Instruct patient to avoid use of over-the-counter (OTC) drugs.

(continued)

INTERACTIONS

HAZARDS OF USING M.A.O. INHIBITORS WITH OTHER AGENTS *(continued)*

AGENT	EFFECT	NURSING ACTIONS
Antihypertensives with CNS depressant effects (clonidine, guanabenz, methyldopa, metyrosine, and pargyline)	Increased CNS depression, possible decreased antihypertensive effect, hypertension	• Monitor for hypertension.
Antiparkinsonian agents	Potentiated atropine-like action, sudden hypertensive crisis	• Allow 2 to 4 weeks after discontinuing MAO inhibitor before giving these agents.
Anxiolytics	Increased sedation, decreased metabolism	• Watch for and report symptoms of CNS depression.
Caffeine-containing preparations	Cardiac arrhythmias and severe hypertension	• Instruct patient to avoid coffee, tea, chocolate, cola, or OTC "stay-awake" products.
Cerebral stimulants	CNS excitation, hypertension, fever, cardiac arrhythmias	• Allow 2 to 4 weeks after discontinuing MAO inhibitor before giving these drugs.
Diuretics	Worsened hypotension	• Monitor blood pressure. • Teach ways to reduce hypotension.
Other MAO inhibitors	Worsened side effects and hypertensive crisis	• Do not give two MAO inhibitors. • Allow 2 weeks before switching to another MAO inhibitor.
Tyramine-containing foods and beverages	Sudden, severe hypertensive crisis	• Advise patient to avoid tyramine-containing products during therapy and for up to 14 days after its cessation. These products include nonprocessed, aged cheese; red wines; beer; soy sauce; monosodium glutamate; pods of Chinese broad beans; chocolate; licorice; pickles; herring; chicken livers; snails; raisins; and yogurt. • In a hypertensive crisis, administer phentolamine.

dining out is no exception. Emphasize that the patient's restricted diet must be maintained for at least 2 weeks after cessation of therapy to allow for regeneration of monoamine oxidase. Describe the signs of hypertensive crisis, and tell the patient to go to a hospital emergency room immediately if any signs occur.

• Emphasize the need to avoid nonprescription drugs to prevent a possible dangerous interaction with the MAO inhibitor.
• Warn the patient not to get up suddenly from a kneeling, sitting, or lying position.
• Advise him to delay elective surgery or dental work until 2 weeks after dis-

continuing therapy. Suggest that he carry a medical identification card in case he needs emergency treatment.
• Refer the patient to an outpatient treatment center for continued support.

Tricyclic Antidepressants

Tricyclic antidepressants (TCAs) are currently the drugs of choice for treating major depression and dysthymic disorder. The reason: their comparatively low incidence of side effects. The seven TCAs most widely used include *imipramine, desipramine, amitriptyline, doxepin, nortriptyline, protriptyline,* and *amoxapine.* (Also see *Trazodone: Alternative to Tricyclics.*)

Tricyclic antidepressants should be administered cautiously to suicidal patients since an overdose can occur with as little as 10 times the regular daily dose. They should also be given cautiously to patients with acute closed-angle glaucoma, benign prostatic hypertrophy, cardiovascular disorders, or urinary retention.

Purpose and action
To relieve depression by reducing CNS levels of dopamine and epinephrine while raising levels of norepinephrine or serotonin or both.

Monitoring
Expect patient improvement in 10 to 14 days after the start of therapy; the full effect usually takes 30 days. However, keep in mind that side effects, such as dry mouth, drowsiness, and dizziness, can begin immediately. Monitor the depressed patient with a psychotic disorder for worsened hallucinations or delusions. If symptoms worsen, reduce the TCA dosage, as ordered. Also observe the patient for mood swings or suicidal tendencies.

Check the patient's alertness and

TRAZODONE: ALTERNATIVE TO TRICYCLICS

The first of a new class of antidepressant drugs, trazodone provides an alternative treatment for major depression. Compared to tricyclics, it has fewer cardiovascular effects, producing only slight changes in blood pressure. Its side effects, drowsiness and dizziness, usually subside after the first few weeks of treatment. Like the tricyclics, its therapeutic effects are noticeable after 10 to 14 days and fully present after 30 days.

If your patient will be receiving trazodone, advise him to take the drug after meals or a light snack to increase absorption and reduce dizziness. Warn against using alcohol or other depressants since severe CNS depression can occur. If the patient's male, urge him to discontinue the drug and notify the doctor if he experiences priapism.

---

psychomotor coordination before he drives or engages in any activity requiring fine-motor coordination. If the patient's elderly, be alert for increased sensitivity to the sedative and hypotensive effects of TCAs. If the TCA causes constipation, increase the patient's fluid intake and administer a stool softener, as ordered.

Check the patient's vital signs, watching for orthostatic hypotension, tachycardia, and hypertension. Instruct the patient to rise slowly from a lying or sitting position and to sit momentarily before rising. Monitor the patient's EKG for any changes during therapy.

Review the patient's medication regimen for possible interactions. Concurrent use of barbiturates, for example, can diminish the TCA's antidepressant effect. Monoamine oxidase inhibitors may cause severe excitation, seizures, and hyperpyrexia, especially in high doses. Steroids, oral contraceptives, and methylphenidate all potentiate the effects of TCAs. Observe the patient receiving these drugs and adjust dosages, as ordered.

Home care instructions

• Inform the patient that side effects usually subside within 2 to 3 weeks of the start of therapy. Encourage him to continue taking the drug as long as side effects don't worsen. Warn against stopping it abruptly. Suggest hard candy or sugarless gum to relieve dry mouth. If drowsiness remains a problem, the doctor may advise taking the entire daily dose at bedtime.

• Tell the patient to take a missed dose if he remembers within 2 hours of the scheduled administration time; otherwise, he should skip the missed dose.

• Warn the patient to avoid alcohol since CNS depression can occur.

• Advise him to consult his doctor before taking any over-the-counter drug.

• Weight gain often presents a problem because TCAs increase appetite while decreasing metabolism. As a result, advise the patient to weigh himself weekly; if he gains too rapidly, suggest reducing his caloric intake.

Antimanics

The drugs *lithium carbonate* and *lithium citrate* act as mood stabilizers, reducing the severity or frequency of manic episodes. Because these drugs have a narrow therapeutic margin of safety, regular determinations of blood levels are necessary to prevent toxicity. If such determinations can't be made, lithium is contraindicated. It's also contraindicated in renal or cardiac dysfunction and during pregnancy because of possible teratogenic effects. This treatment should be used cautiously in patients with a history of fluid retention and in those who use diuretics or follow low-salt diets.

Purpose and action

To prevent or control mania by reducing norepinephrine levels. (See *How Drug Therapy Combats Mania and Depression.*)

Monitoring

Check lithium levels 8 to 12 hours after the first dose and then every 2 to 3 days until the doctor reduces the dosage (usually when the patient's manic symptoms abate). Thereafter, check levels weekly the first month and then monthly. Draw blood samples before the morning dose to avoid spuriously high readings. Watch for symptoms of toxicity, including drowsiness, slurred speech, twitching, increased tremors, vomiting, and staggering. If any of these occur, discontinue lithium, as ordered.

If your patient's receiving haloperidol during initial lithium therapy, carefully observe for extrapyramidal symptoms. Also review his medication regimen for other possible interactions. Diuretics, for example, increase renal reabsorption of lithium and can lead to toxicity. Carbamazepine, probenecid, indomethacin, methyldopa, and piroxicam potentiate lithium's effect. In contrast, aminophylline, sodium bicarbonate, and sodium chloride promote lithium excretion.

Monitor the patient's EKG, electrolyte levels, and thyroid, renal, and hematologic studies during therapy. That's because lithium can cause reversible EKG changes, arrhythmias, hypotension, and leukocytosis. Prolonged use can cause renal toxicity and suppress thyroid hormone levels, requiring replacement therapy. Watch for an enlarged thyroid gland or unusual fatigue or weakness.

If your patient's diabetic, check glucose levels regularly. Lithium may cause transient hyperglycemia, requiring increased dosage of a hypoglycemic drug. Instruct the patient to report nausea, polyuria, increased thirst, mild weakness, and hand tremors. If these side effects don't diminish after a few days, consult the doctor about lowering the lithium dosage.

Home care instructions

• Tell the patient that lithium produces its full effect 1 to 3 weeks after the start of therapy.

HOW DRUG THERAPY COMBATS MANIA AND DEPRESSION

Mania and depression stem from abnormal levels of the neurotransmitter norepinephrine. Excessive levels cause mania while insufficient levels lead to depression.

The illustration here shows how antidepressant and antimanic drugs achieve their therapeutic effects. The antidepressant isocarboxazid, for example, inhibits mono-amine oxidase, an enzyme that breaks down norepinephrine, thus raising norepinephrine levels. The tricyclic antidepressant imipramine blocks the reabsorption of norepinephrine, achieving the same effect. In contrast, the antimanic drug lithium promotes reabsorption of norepinephrine, thereby lowering levels.

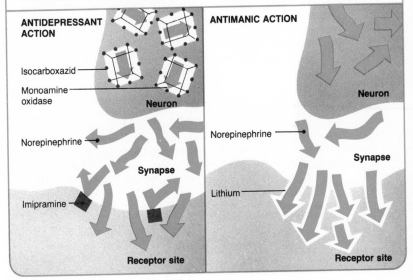

ANTIDEPRESSANT ACTION

Isocarboxazid
Monoamine oxidase
Neuron
Norepinephrine
Synapse
Imipramine
Receptor site

ANTIMANIC ACTION

Neuron
Norepinephrine
Synapse
Lithium
Receptor site

• Instruct him to return for regular lithium level tests. Warn him and his family that lithium toxicity can occur easily. If toxic effects do occur, the patient should skip one dose and call his doctor. He shouldn't stop the drug abruptly.

• Unless the doctor prescribes the sustained-release form, tell the patient to take lithium at regular intervals. If he misses a dose, he may take the missed dose within 2 hours of the prescribed time. After that, he should not make up the dose nor double the next one.

• If the patient experiences persistent hand tremors during therapy, the doctor may have him take the majority of the daily dose at bedtime. Also, instruct the patient to reduce caffeine intake.

• Advise the patient not to take any over-the-counter drugs without first checking with his doctor.

• Instruct him to drink 2,500 to 3,000 ml of fluid daily and to avoid excessive salt intake, which enhances lithium excretion and reduces the drug's effectiveness.

• If the patient experiences GI upset, suggest that he take lithium with a glass of water after meals or a snack.

• Tell him to contact his doctor if vomiting, diarrhea, or excessive perspiration occurs. Advise against strenuous exercise, particularly in hot weather. Also warn against taking sodium-containing antacids. Excessive loss of body fluids can require lithium dosage adjustment.

• Inform the patient that lithium causes weight gain. Advise him to weigh himself daily. If he gains weight, teach him how to reduce his caloric intake while maintaining sound nutritional habits.

Cerebral Stimulants

Cerebral stimulants—such as *amphetamine sulfate, methylphenidate hydrochloride, dextroamphetamine sulfate, and pemoline*—are the drugs of choice for treating attention-deficit disorder with hyperactivity (ADDH). They may be used alone or along with psychological treatments and educational or social modifications.

Beginning 2 to 3 weeks after therapy starts, cerebral stimulants achieve their paradoxical calming effect in a child with hyperkinesia. This calming effect increases the child's attention span, curbs his impulsiveness, and assists socialization. Relieving the distressing symptoms of ADDH also increases the child's amenability to adjunctive psychotherapy and educational modifications.

Before the start of treatment, the child should undergo a complete physical examination and have a psychological history taken. During treatment, he'll need close supervision because of the potential for drug dependence.

All cerebral stimulants are contraindicated in children under age 3 and in those with severe cardiac disease. Two cerebral stimulants, methylphenidate and pemoline, are also contraindicated in children under age 6 because of the increased risk of Gilles de la Tourette's syndrome.

Purpose and action
To treat ADDH by promoting nerve impulse transmission through the release of epinephrine stored in nerve terminals in the brain.

Monitoring
Observe the child for signs of excessive stimulation, such as a rapid pulse, hypertension, and nervousness. A reduced dosage may relieve such symptoms.

Because methylphenidate and pemoline may precipitate Gilles de la Tourette's syndrome and amphetamine may intensify symptoms of this disorder, be sure to observe the child for tic, echolalia, coprolalia, and motor incoordination, especially at the start of therapy.

If the child's diabetic, regularly check his glucose level because cerebral stimulants may alter his insulin requirements. Also review his medication regimen for possible interactions. Concurrent use of monoamine oxidase inhibitors, for example, could cause life-threatening hypertensive crisis. Antacids, acetazolamide, and sodium bicarbonate increase the effects of cerebral stimulants; phenothiazines and haloperidol decrease them.

If the child's receiving long-term therapy, be sure to check his height and weight regularly to detect growth retardation.

Home care instructions
● Inform the patient's parents to give their child his medication at least 6 hours before bedtime to prevent insomnia and after meals to reduce appetite suppression.
● If the child misses a dose, explain that it may be taken only within 2 hours of the scheduled administration time and that the next dose should be taken as ordered.
●Warn the parents to restrict the child from any activities that require alertness or good motor coordination until his CNS response to the drug has been determined.
● Instruct them to avoid giving him chocolate, colas, or other caffeinated products. These enhance the effects of most cerebral stimulants.
● Warn the parents against suddenly discontinuing the medication after long-term use. Acute rebound depression will occur unless the dose is lowered gradually.

• Remind the parents that cerebral stimulants are addictive and should be kept in a secure location.

COUNSELING

Psychotherapy

Simply stated, psychotherapy refers to the psychological treatment of mental and emotional disorders. This term may be applied to a range of approaches—from Freudian psychoanalysis of the patient with an obsessive-compulsive disorder to family therapy for the anorexia nervosa patient and her parents. It may probe the unconscious and explore the significance of dreams or may address family dynamics and problematic social relationships. (See *Understanding Types of Psychotherapy*, pages 642 and 643.) Regardless of the approach, psychotherapy aims to change a patient's attitudes, feelings, or behavior. To promote this change, the therapist may use reinforcement, persuasion, suggestion, reassurance, and support.

The therapist's role may vary from observer to participant. However, the success of therapy doesn't usually hinge on the therapist assuming any specific role. Instead, it depends largely on the compatibility between patient and therapist, the treatment goals selected, and the patient's commitment. The therapy itself may last only one session or may span several years.

Purpose
To effect positive changes in a patient's attitudes, emotions, or behavior.

Preparation
Review the patient's psychiatric history, treatment history, and current psychiatric status to help assess his needs. Explain the therapeutic techniques to him and help him establish a treatment goal.

Maintain the confidentiality of information the patient shares with you unless, of course, he plans to harm himself or someone else. Typically, you'll share with the therapist only that information which the patient wants shared.

Procedure
Depending on his beliefs and training, the therapist selects an approach to meet the patient's needs. For instance, the therapist may choose *reinforcement*, which strengthens the appropriate behavior by fear of punishment or the anticipation of a reward. Or if a strong rapport exists between therapist and patient, the therapist may use *suggestion* (or *persuasion*) to implant an idea or a belief in the patient's mind as a means of effecting change. The therapist may also direct discussion of the patient's ideas and feelings to achieve *abreaction*, the emotional relief obtained by mentally reliving or bringing into consciousness a long-repressed, painful experience. Therapists will commonly combine these and other techniques to achieve treatment goals.

Monitoring
During psychotherapy, observe the patient for signs of increased distress, depression, anxiety, and restlessness. If the patient feels uncomfortable with therapy, he may display loss of appetite, irritability, or insomnia. Reassure the patient that talking about his feelings will help relieve distress. And be sure to reinforce any gains that the patient has made.

Home care instructions
• Refer the patient to a self-help group, if appropriate.
• Instruct the patient to contact his therapist if distressing symptoms recur.

UNDERSTANDING TYPES OF PSYCHOTHERAPY

INDIVIDUAL THERAPY

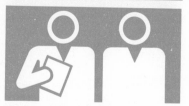

Seeks to change patient's behavior throughout a number of individual counseling sessions. Involves mutually agreed-upon goals, with the therapist mediating the patient's disturbed patterns of behavior to promote personality growth and development.

Duration and uses
Short or long term. Useful if patient develops personal distress or dissatisfaction in his relationships with co-workers, family, or friends.

Nursing actions
• Listen well and provide emotional support.
• Assist patient in handling distress.

CRISIS THERAPY

Helps patient develop adequate coping skills to resolve an immediate, pressing problem. Allows the patient to return to the level of functioning that existed before the crisis. Usually involves just the patient and therapist, but may include family members.

Duration and uses
Usually lasts from 1 session to 6 months. Useful when the patient must handle a current situation but seems incapable of doing so. The crisis can be a developmental one, such as a marriage or death of a family member, or a situational one, such as a natural disaster or illness.

Nursing actions
• Listen well and offer support.
• Provide opportunities for catharsis.
• Communicate hope.
• Set limits on demonstrative behavior.

Behavior Therapy

Used by psychologists, specially trained nurses, and others, this form of therapy assumes that problem behaviors are learned and, through special training, can be unlearned and replaced by acceptable ones. Unlike psychotherapy, it doesn't attempt to uncover the reasons for problem behaviors. In fact, it tends to deemphasize the patient's thoughts and feelings about them.

The behavioral approach relies on a cluster of therapies, rather than on just

one, to change a behavioral pattern. Commonly used therapies include desensitization, assertiveness training, flooding, token economy, positive conditioning, and social skills training. Suitable for adults or children, behavior therapies can be used for an individual or for groups of patients with a similar problem.

Behavior therapies may employ different techniques, such as positive or negative reinforcement, shaping, modeling, punishment, or extinction. *Positive reinforcement* increases the likelihood of a desirable behavior being repeated by promptly praising or rewarding the patient when he performs it. In contrast, *negative reinforcement*

GROUP THERAPY

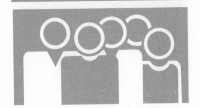

Guided by a psychotherapist, this permits a group of people (ideally 4 to 10) experiencing similar emotional problems to discuss their concerns with group members as a means of effecting personality changes.

Duration and uses
Duration varies from a few weeks in acute episodes requiring hospitalization to several years. Useful in treating addictions.

Nursing actions
• Support the group effort.
• Observe and document any changes in patients' behavior.
• Reinforce positive changes.

FAMILY THERAPY

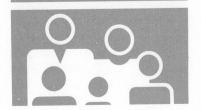

Seeks to alter relationships within the family to change problematic behavior of one or more members.

Duration and uses
Short or long term. Useful in treating adjustment disorders of childhood or adolescence, marital discord, and abuse situations.

Nursing actions
• Listen well and provide emotional support.
• Reinforce positive changes.
• Try to remain nonjudgmental.

---

involves the removal of a negative stimulus only after the patient provides a desirable response. *Punishment*, of course, discourages problem behavior by inflicting a penalty, such as temporary removal of a privilege. Although difficult to sustain, *extinction* is a technique that simply ignores undesirable behavior—provided, of course, that the behavior isn't dangerous or illegal. Another technique, *shaping,* initially rewards any behavior that resembles the desirable one. Then, step by step, the behavior required to gain a reward becomes progressively closer to the desired behavior. *Modeling* provides a reward when the patient imitates the desired behavior.

Purpose
• To remove problem behaviors or replace them with more appropriate ones
• To strengthen acceptable behaviors.

Preparation
Before therapy begins, determine that the patient is amenable to behavior therapy. Consider his age, intellectual function, and mental status. Review with the therapist what behavior requires alteration and why.

Counsel the patient about what behaviors need changing, the goals of therapy, and the techniques used to accomplish them. Make it clear exactly what's expected of him and what he can expect from the health care staff.

UNDERSTANDING TYPES OF BEHAVIOR THERAPY

Behavior therapy is a broad term that includes desensitization, flooding, token economy, assertiveness training, positive conditioning, and social skills training.

DESENSITIZATION

The treatment of choice for phobias, desensitization slowly exposes the patient to something he fears. It's most successful when used with other psychological treatments since phobias reflect unresolved conflicts. In practice, desensitization teaches the patient to use deep breathing or another relaxation technique when confronted with a staged series of anxiety-producing situations. If your patient's undergoing desensitization, provide reassurance and review relaxation techniques. Monitor his response to each anxious situation and emphasize that he needn't proceed to the next one until he feels ready.

FLOODING

Also called implosion therapy, flooding can provide rapid relief of phobias, such as travel phobias. Like desensitization, it involves direct exposure to an anxious situation. Unlike desensitization, it doesn't employ relaxation techniques. Instead, it assumes that anxiety and panic can't persist and that confrontation helps the patient overcome fear.

If your patient's undergoing this therapy, monitor him for signs of excitation, such as elevated blood pressure and heart rate. If fainting or another extreme reaction occurs, remove the patient from the anxiety-producing situation. Assess for signs of psychological trauma.

TOKEN ECONOMY

In this treatment, the therapist rewards acceptable behavior by giving out tokens, which can be used as currency for some privilege or object. He can also withhold or rescind tokens as punishment or to avert undesirable behavior. If you're part of this therapy, monitor the patient for appropriate behavior. Provide or withhold rewards consistently and promptly.

ASSERTIVENESS TRAINING

Using the techniques of positive reinforcement, shaping, and modeling, assertiveness training aims to reduce anxiety. It teaches the patient ways to express feelings, ideas, and wishes without feeling guilty or demeaning others. You can help the patient by modeling appropriate behaviors and by suggesting situations in which he can be more assertive.

POSITIVE CONDITIONING

Building on the principle of desensitization, this therapy attempts to gradually instill a positive or neutral attitude toward a phobia. Used effectively for patients with sexual problems, positive conditioning first introduces a pleasurable stimulus, such as music. Then the patient is encouraged to heighten the pleasurable stimulus by associating other pleasurable experiences with it. Next, the therapist introduces the phobic stimulus along with the pleasurable one. Gradually, the patient develops a positive response to the phobia.

If your patient is undergoing positive conditioning, reinforce relaxation techniques and provide encouragement.

SOCIAL SKILLS TRAINING

Using shaping and modeling techniques, this therapy helps patients develop or regain skills for forming relationships. Used mainly for institutionalized, acutely ill, and mentally retarded patients, its success hinges on consistent reinforcement.

Procedure

Depending on his beliefs and training, the therapist selects one or more behavioral therapies for the patient or group. See *Understanding Types of Behavior Therapy* for information on how each of these therapies is typically carried out.

Monitoring and aftercare

Your most important task will be monitoring the patient throughout therapy, reinforcing acceptable behaviors, and discouraging unacceptable ones. If unacceptable behaviors persist, inform the therapist. He may need to try another technique.

Home care instructions

● If appropriate, teach the patient's family the basic techniques used to correct problem behaviors. Encourage them to institute this therapy if these behaviors persist.

● Recommend an outpatient therapist to help reinforce desirable behaviors and to respond to patient or family problems or questions. Remember that family members, friends, co-workers, and community members often tolerate problem behavior or seem reluctant to interfere.

Milieu Therapy

Whether employed in the hospital or in a community setting, milieu therapy refers to the use of the patient's environment as a tool for overcoming mental and emotional disorders. Specifically, the patient's surroundings become a therapeutic community, with the patient himself involved in planning, implementing, and evaluating his treatment as well as in sharing with staff and other patients the responsibility for establishing group rules and policies. The staff, in turn, assume a different role. They usually wear street clothes instead of uniforms, keep units unlocked, and run activities in a community room, which is the center for meetings, recreation, and meals. They also provide individual, group, and occupational therapy.

Nurses play a key part in milieu therapy. They work closely with psychiatrists and social workers, planning programs, assisting with therapy, and sharing observations and suggestions for modifying treatment plans.

What type of patient qualifies for milieu therapy? First, he must be able to participate in group activities. And he must show a willingness to accept responsibility for his daily activities. His goal will be to function in a socially and emotionally appropriate way so that he may progress to a transitional or halfway house. Then, if he progresses in this less structured environment, he may return to the outside community ready to apply the positive behaviors and skills he has learned.

Purpose

To promote behavioral change and personal growth in a controlled therapeutic community so that the patient can function effectively in the outside community after discharge.

Preparation

Explain the purpose of milieu therapy to the patient, stating what you expect of him and how he can participate in the therapeutic community. Orient him to the community's routines, such as the schedule for various activities. Introduce him to other patients and staff.

Procedure

The patient follows a schedule that's typical of life outside the therapeutic community. He also attends individual and group therapy sessions, goes to group meetings, and learns to interact appropriately with staff and other patients.

Monitoring and aftercare

Regularly evaluate the patient's symptoms and therapeutic needs. Oversee his activities, encouraging him to keep a schedule typical of life outside the hospital. Also encourage him to interact with others so he doesn't become withdrawn or feel secluded. Point out the importance of respecting others and his environment.

Home care instructions

If the patient eventually returns to the outside community, encourage him to keep follow-up appointments with his therapist.

WITHDRAWAL FROM ABUSED SUBSTANCES

Detoxification

Detoxification refers to withdrawal from prolonged dependence on alcohol or drugs. Designed to help the patient maintain abstinence, detoxification programs offer a relatively safe alternative to self-withdrawal, which is difficult and often dangerous. Performed in outpatient centers or in special units, detoxification programs provide symptomatic treatment as well as counseling or psychotherapy on an individual, group, or family basis.

Alcohol withdrawal, requiring total abstinence, usually proves more severe and potentially deadly than drug withdrawal. Its symptoms vary from morning hangover in mild alcoholism to delirium tremens—a condition of severe distress marked by menacing hallucinations, gross uncontrollable tremors, extreme restlessness, vomiting, profuse diaphoresis, and elevated pulse rate and blood pressure.

Drug withdrawal may be achieved by gradually lowering the dosage of the abused drug or by substituting a drug with similar action; for example, methadone may be substituted for heroin.

If these options aren't available, treatment is supportive and symptomatic.

Treating patients undergoing detoxification requires compassion and commitment. Because substance abusers have a low self-esteem and commonly try to manipulate people, you'll need to recognize their attempts at manipulation and to control your natural feelings of anger and frustration.

Purpose

To help the patient achieve abstinence from alcohol or drugs while providing supportive and symptomatic care.

Preparation

If the patient is in acute distress, inform him that he'll receive immediate treatment. If he isn't in acute distress, perform a psychosocial evaluation to examine his family and social life. The patient will probably rationalize his abuse or minimize its extent. If possible, substantiate what he tells you with family members or friends. Also determine the patient's motivation for successful detoxification and form an opinion about his support systems. Deeply motivated patients with strong support systems are most apt to overcome their substance abuse.

Next, take a medical history to find out if the patient has a history of any psychiatric disorder, drug or alcohol abuse, seizures, or delirium. The doctor will probably order a neurologic workup as well as a urinalysis, a complete blood count, liver function tests, serum electrolyte and glucose levels, and a chest X-ray. Obtain urine and blood samples for alcohol and drug screening to provide information on the most recent ingestion. Together, the medical and psychosocial evaluations help determine the type of treatment and whether the treatment will be provided on an inpatient or outpatient basis.

Procedure

If the patient is in acute distress, provide a quiet, softly lit environment to avoid overstimulation and agitation, which can cause tremors. Remove any potentially harmful objects from the room. (See *Treating Drug Intoxication*.)

If the patient's undergoing alcohol withdrawal and experiences delirium tremens, give antianxiety agents, anticonvulsants, and antidiarrheals or antiemetics, as ordered. Monitor his mental status, vital signs, and lung sounds every 30 minutes. Orient him to reality since he may be having hallucinations. If he's combative or disoriented, restrain him. Take seizure and suicide precautions. If ordered, give I.V. glucose for hypoglycemia and thiamine and other B-complex vitamins for nutritional deficiencies.

If the patient is undergoing opioid withdrawal, detoxify him with methadone, as ordered. To ease withdrawal from opioids, depressants, and other drugs, provide nutritional support, suggest mild exercise, and teach relaxation techniques. If appropriate, temporarily administer sedatives or tranquilizers to help the patient cope with anxiety, depression, and/or insomnia.

After withdrawal from alcohol or drugs, rehabilitation is needed to prevent recurrence of abuse. For the alcoholic, rehabilitation may include aversion therapy, using a daily oral dose of disulfiram, and supportive counseling or individual, group, or family psychotherapy. For the drug abuser, it may include psychotherapy.

Monitoring and aftercare

Encourage the patient's participation in rehabilitation programs and self-help groups. But be alert for any continued substance abuse after admission to the detoxification program. Carefully administer any prescribed medications to prevent hoarding by the patient, and closely monitor visitors, who might bring the patient drugs or alcohol from the outside. If you suspect any abuse, obtain a blood and urine sample for screening and report any positive findings to the doctor.

Because resistance can be lowered in drug or alcohol abuse, observe the patient for signs of infection. Also watch for signs of vitamin deficiency and malnutrition. With the dietitian's

---

TREATING DRUG INTOXICATION

Sometimes drug abusers enter detoxification programs requiring emergency treatment, typically for an overdose of narcotics, barbiturates, cocaine, or amphetamines.

OPIOID OVERDOSE

Your immediate goal is to prevent shock and maintain respirations. Intubate the patient and give oxygen, I.V. fluids, and plasma expanders. Also give naloxone to reverse CNS depression.

BARBITURATE OVERDOSE

Like treatment of opioid overdose, treatment of barbiturate overdose aims to prevent shock and maintain respirations. It may also include gastric lavage or induction of vomiting if the patient ingested the drug within 4 hours. Or it may include administration of activated charcoal followed by a cathartic to eliminate the toxic drug. Extreme intoxication requires dialysis.

COCAINE INTOXICATION

Because cocaine's cardiotoxic, monitor the patient's heart rate and rhythm. If ventricular defibrillation or asystole occurs, institute cardiopulmonary resuscitation and defibrillation.

Provide supportive care. For example, give an antipyretic to reduce fever, an anticonvulsant to prevent seizures, and propranolol to treat tachycardia.

AMPHETAMINE OVERDOSE

If the drug was taken orally, induce vomiting or perform gastric lavage. Or give activated charcoal and a sodium or magnesium sulfate cathartic. Also give mannitol to induce diuresis, pentobarbital to prevent or control seizures, haloperidol or chlorpromazine to treat agitation, and phentolamine to lower blood pressure. To acidify the patient's urine, give ammonium chloride or ascorbic acid I.V.

help, ensure that the patient maintains an adequate diet. Offer bland foods if he experiences GI distress.

If the patient exhibits impaired mobility, assist him with ambulation, as necessary, and encourage bed rest until he regains stability.

Home care instructions

• Patients who return to a social setting where substance abuse is common are likely to have a relapse. As a result, encourage professional and family support after the patient leaves the detoxification program.

• Emphasize to the patient that he needs to join an appropriate self-help group, such as Alcoholics Anonymous or Narcotics Anonymous, for support and encouragement. Recommend that the patient's spouse or mature children accompany the patient to group meetings. Also, refer the patient's family to a support group, if necessary.

• Stress to the patient that he ultimately must accept responsibility for avoiding abused substances.

ELECTROSHOCK

Electroconvulsive Therapy

Electroconvulsive therapy (ECT), also referred to as electroshock therapy, was first introduced in 1937 as the primary treatment for all types of emotional disorders. Early misuse of this treatment (because of ignorance or the unavailability of proper anesthesia) resulted in severe memory loss, fractures, and death.

Today, ECT is recognized as a legitimate treatment for major depression when tricyclic antidepressants are con-

traindicated or faster onset is warranted. It's also used for acute mania and, to a lesser degree, for acute schizophrenia when psychotropic drugs are ineffective. The number of treatments varies with the disorder's severity and the patient's response; however, treatments are usually given two or three times a week, with an interval of 48 hours between sessions.

In ECT, an electrical stimulus travels through electrodes placed on the patient's temples, causing a generalized tonic-clonic seizure. The electrodes are placed unilaterally since some authorities believe bilateral placement causes greater memory loss and confusion. The resulting seizure reduces hypothalamic stress and stimulates biogenic amine metabolism.

Although ECT can cause arrhythmias and even death, untreated depression can carry a higher mortality because of suicide. However, ECT is contraindicated in recent myocardial infarction with cardiac decompensation, CNS tumors, organic brain syndrome, and aortic aneurysm. This treatment should be used cautiously during pregnancy and old age and in patients with glaucoma or cardiac disease.

Purpose

To alleviate major depression or other severe mental disorders by inducing a generalized tonic-clonic seizure.

Preparation

Explain the treatment to the patient and his family, including its risks, its expected effects, and the use of anesthesia. Correct any misconceptions they may have and allow them to voice their fears and hopes. Next, have the patient sign a consent form and prepare him for a complete physical examination and electroencephalography.

Stop any psychotropic drugs the day before ECT to prevent any interactions. Restrict foods and fluids after midnight to prevent aspiration while under anesthesia. Just before ECT, ask the patient to void to prevent incontinence during the induced seizure. If he wears dentures, ask him to remove them to prevent airway obstruction. Ensure that emergency resuscitation equipment is available.

Procedure
Administer atropine or another anticholinergic agent, as ordered, to prevent bradycardia or asystole. Next, give a short-acting barbiturate, such as methohexital, to anesthetize the patient. To induce muscle relaxation and prevent fractures, the doctor will probably ask you to administer succinylcholine.

Now place a rubber block between the patient's teeth because his jaw muscles will contract during the induced seizure. Provide oxygen through a face mask. If ordered, apply a blood pressure cuff to an extremity to prevent the muscle relaxant from reaching it. This will allow you to accurately assess the extremity for tonic-clonic movement once the stimulus is given.

After you apply the electrodes to the patient's temple, the doctor will apply the electrical stimulus, causing a seizure lasting about 30 seconds and unconsciousness lasting several minutes.

Monitoring and aftercare
After the patient awakens, remove the electrodes and help to orient him. Calling him by name, let him know that the treatment is complete. Reassure him, as necessary.

Until the patient becomes oriented, keep the bed's side rails raised. Check the patient's vital signs until they return to normal. Also monitor cardiac rhythm.

Ask the patient if he's experiencing headache or nausea. If he reports discomfort, administer analgesics or antinausea drugs, as ordered.

Home care instructions
● If the patient receives ECT as an outpatient, make sure a family member or companion provides transportation home. Inform the patient that he mustn't drive or operate machinery until confusion and drowsiness completely subside. In addition, he may resume his daily activities only when he feels physically able.
● Remind the patient's family or companion that temporary anterograde and retrograde amnesia and mild confusion can occur after ECT. These symptoms usually diminish or disappear within 8 weeks.
● Encourage the patient's family to support the patient once he's home. Allay their fears and encourage them to make sure the patient follows the doctor's orders and keeps follow-up appointments.

Selected References

Appleton, W.S. "Fourth Psychoactive Drug Usage Guide," *Journal of Clinical Psychiatry* 43:12-27, January 1982.
Diagnostic and Statistical Manual of Mental Disorders, 3rd ed. Washington, D.C.: American Psychiatric Association, 1981.
Drug Information for the Health Care Provider, vol. 1, 7th ed. Rockville, Md.: United States Pharmacopeial Convention, 1985.
Holloway, H.C., et al."Recognition and Treatment of Acute Alcohol Withdrawal Syndromes," *Psychiatric Clinics of North America* 7(4):729-42, December, 1984.
Nursing88 Drug Handbook. Springhouse, Pa.: Springhouse Corp., 1988.
Rawls, W.N., "New Drug Evaluations: Trazodone," *Drug Intelligence and Clinical Pharmacy* 16:7-12, January 1982.
Wilmer, H.A., "Defining and Understanding the Therapeutic Community," *Hospital Community Psychiatry* 32(2):95-99, February 1981.

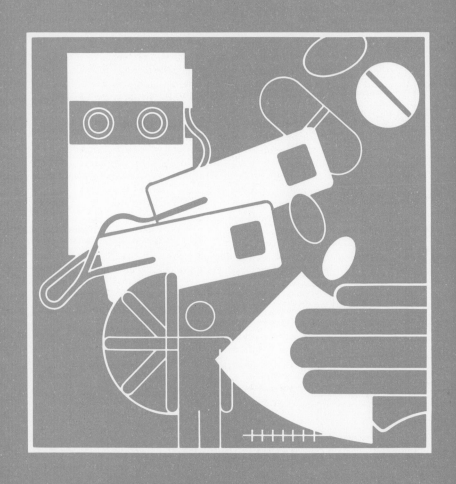

Appendices and Index

Selected Treatments

This appendix supplements the main text of *Treatments*, which provides comprehensive information on more than 300 surgeries, diets, drug regimens, and other therapies. In contrast, this appendix summarizes key considerations for treatments that require limited, but significant nursing action.

A

Activated charcoal. An adsorbent used as an antidote for oral poisoning by certain drugs, chemicals, and toxins, including phenol and acetaminophen. The drug should be given within 30 minutes of an overdose or poison ingestion. The powder form is most effective, but the patient may resist taking it. To make it palatable, mix it in water to form a thick syrup, then add soda or juice. If ipecac syrup is ordered, give activated charcoal after emesis to prevent binding to ipecac.

Allopurinol. A xanthine oxidase inhibitor used to correct hyperuricemia. Indications include gout, hyperuricemia secondary to malignancies or blood dyscrasias, and elevated uric acid levels during chemotherapy. Obtain baseline complete blood count and hepatic and renal function test results before therapy. Monitor these and serum uric acid levels during therapy. Maintain urine output of at least 2 liters a day, with a neutral or alkaline pH. Watch for anemia, agranulocytosis, cataracts, retinopathy, hepatitis, or altered liver function. Give the drug with or after meals to manage GI effects. Discontinue the drug if a rash develops.

Antiembolism stockings. Elastic stockings applied to the legs to improve venous return. The stockings are most often used to prevent deep vein thrombosis in immobilized patients. Measure the patient's legs to ensure proper fit. Instruct him to apply stockings with short pulls, and to smooth them between pulls to prevent folds and rolls, which act as tourniquets.

Antimalarials. Agents used to prevent or treat malaria, such as chloroquine and hydroxychloroquine. For malarial prophylaxis, these drugs are given before, during, and after travel to areas where the disease is endemic.

Arterial ligation. A surgical procedure used to control epistaxis when nasal packs have failed to do so. A common ligation site is the internal maxillary artery. Preoperatively, assess the patient's respiratory status and ensure a patent airway. Postoperatively, watch for bleeding and replace fluids, as ordered. Using a flashlight, check the posterior pharynx to detect blood or slippage of the nasal packing placed after ligation.

Arthrodesis. Fusion of a joint by bone graft, osteotomy, or use of internal fixation devices. It's most commonly performed on the ankle, knee, hip, or spine to relieve pain that accompanies motion. It may also be done to restore stability to a joint when supporting ligaments can't be repaired, or to correct a deformity by realigning a joint at the level of fusion. An external fixation device or a cast may be applied after the procedure. Postoperatively, watch for infection, swelling, and signs of a fat embolism. With internal fixation, be alert for signs of nonunion, avascular necrosis, and failure of fixation devices. With external fixation, watch for loose pins or infection at pin sites. If a cast is in place, check circulation and skin integrity.

Artificial urinary sphincter. A surgically implanted device used to control incontinence—usually after other treatments have failed. It consists of a urethral cuff, a balloon reservoir in the lower abdomen, and a pump in the scrotum or labia. The patient remains continent while the cuff is inflated, and initiates voiding by squeezing the pump to move fluid from the cuff to the balloon. Preoperatively, evaluate the patient's ability to understand pump mechanics, his manual dexterity, and his motivation to use the device. Explain that he'll remain incontinent until the surgeon activates the sphincter at a follow-up visit, usually in about 6 weeks.

Arytenoidectomy. Surgical excision of the arytenoid cartilage. Indications include vocal cord paralysis or rheumatoid arthritis of the cricoarytenoid joints that results in midline fixation of the arytenoid cartilage. Perform a thorough preoperative respiratory assessment. Monitor respiratory status after surgery, comparing findings to baseline.

B

Bladder fulguration. Electrocoagulation of blood vessels or lesions within the bladder. Indications for this procedure include bleeding after surgery and carcinoma in situ (lesions 2″ [5 cm] or less). Bleeding sites or lesions are visualized by cystoscopy and coagulated using an electrode that conducts a high-frequency electrical current to the target tissue. Afterward, provide catheter care and monitor urine for color, amount, and presence of clots.

C

Calcitonin. A synthetic hormone used to treat hypercalcemia, postmenopausal osteoporosis, and Paget's disease of bone. It inhibits bone resorption and increases calcium excretion. Keep epinephrine handy during administration if skin testing hasn't been done. After injection, observe the patient for signs of hypocalcemic tetany or hypercalcemic relapse. Monitor serum calcium levels.

Chloramphenicol. A broad-spectrum antibiotic used only to treat severe infections that are resistant to other antibiotics, such as ampicillin-resistant typhoid fever. Because of the risk of fatal blood dyscrasias, monitor the patient's complete blood count daily. Instruct him to report nausea, vomiting, diarrhea, fever, confusion, sore throat, or mouth sores.

Clindamycin. An antibiotic used for septicemia and severe infections caused by staphylococci, streptococci, pneumococci, and susceptible anaerobic bacteria. Its common side effects include rash, nausea, diarrhea, and abdominal pain. Don't give antiperistaltic drugs for diarrhea since they'll worsen it. Tell the patient to take the oral form with a full glass of water to prevent dysphagia. Monitor vital signs, since fever and hypotension can occur. Also monitor renal, hepatic, and hematopoietic function during long-term therapy. Warn the patient to report abdominal cramps, excessive diarrhea, or bloody stools.

Cochlear implant. Cochlear placement of an electrode connected to an external coil. This treatment for bilateral sensorineural hearing loss is still considered experimental. Sounds are received by the coil and conducted into the bony labyrinth by the electrode. After implantation, the patient can't hear normally but can detect such sounds as the ringing of a telephone and can perceive the cadence and volume of speech. To prevent unrealistic expectations about hearing acuity, reinforce the patient's understanding of the potential outcome.

Colonic lavage. Irrigation of the colon with an enema containing about 1 liter of tap water. It's performed in patients with liver dysfunction and portal-systemic encephalopathy to help rid the bowel of protein. It's also used to treat severe constipation.

Continent vesicostomy. A form of urinary diversion most commonly used in infants who have neurogenic bladder associated with hydronephrosis and hydroureter. The surgeon closes the urethra and, using a portion of the bladder wall, forms a suprapubic stoma and creates a nipple valve. Accumulated urine in the bladder presses on the nipple valve, preventing urine leakage. Urine is drained through the nipple valve, using a catheter. After healing, bladder emptying requires intermittent suprapubic catheterization.

After surgery, change the dressing and provide catheter and stoma care. Teach the patient or his parents how to irrigate the tubes, change the dressing, and use drainage bags.

Continuous slow ultrafiltration (CSU). A method of continuous hemofiltration used to correct fluid overload in a patient who doesn't require dialysis. Indications include congestive heart failure and pulmonary edema. CSU avoids hypovolemia and removes little or no solute. Hemodialysis access and gravity flow are used. Care measures are similar to those for patients receiving hemodialysis.

Credé's maneuver. Continuous manual application of downward pressure over the suprapubic area to expel urine. Teach the patient how to perform this maneuver.

Cromolyn sodium. A mast cell inhibitor used to treat allergic rhinitis, asthma (maintenance therapy only), and allergic conjunctivitis. As a powder (inhaled) and a solution (nebulized), it's used to prevent bronchospasm related to exercise, cold air, and environmental factors. As an ophthalmic solution, the drug's full therapeutic effect may not be evident for several days. Instruct the patient to avoid wearing soft contact lenses while using the ophthalmic solution.

D

Decortication of the lung. Surgical removal of the visceral pleura performed when the lung fails to reexpand spontaneously after drainage of an empyema—indicating that adhesions are anchoring the lung to the visceral pleura. Preoperatively, give oxygen and perform chest physiotherapy every 2 hours. Turn the patient frequently and monitor arterial blood gas levels. Postoperatively, continue to follow the preoperative regimen and maintain chest tube drainage.

Dental soft diet. A nutritionally adequate diet consisting of soft foods. It's given to patients who can't chew foods well because of missing teeth or poorly fitted dentures. Foods include milk; eggs; cheese; soup; soft fruits, such as bananas; cooked or pureed vegetables; cubed, minced, or ground meat or fish; and soft bread. Ensure that selections are varied to make the diet appetizing.

Dermabrasion. Abrasive planing of the epidermis and dermis. It's done to smooth scarring and to remove hyperplastic tissue or tattoos. It's also used to treat keratoses, adenoma sebaceum of tuberous sclerosis, milia, and rhinophyma. Small areas are sprayed with a freezing agent, such as ethyl chloride, and immediately abraded. Antibiotic ointment is then applied and covered with Telfa dressings, which the patient usually removes after 24 hours. After dermabrasion, teach the patient how to perform wound care, remove dressings, and recognize signs of infection. Inform him that his skin will feel tight as it heals. Tell him to avoid exposure to sun, wind, and temperature extremes.

E

Ear irrigation. Gentle instillation of normal saline solution, alcohol, or oil into the external audi-

654

tory canal, using a bulb, rubber bulb, or Pomeroy syringe. Used to soften and remove impacted cerumen or to dislodge a foreign body, the treatment must be done carefully to avoid tympanic membrane rupture, vertigo, or skin maceration. It's contraindicated if the patient has a cold, fever, ear infection, ruptured tympanic membrane, or a foreign object embedded, such as a dry bean, that will swell during irrigation.

With the patient seated and his head tilted slightly forward and toward the affected side, direct a stream of solution against the posterior ear canal wall. Keep the syringe tip pointed upward and toward the posterior wall, so the solution flows forward to carry debris from the ear.

Electrodesiccation. Destruction of tissue by electric current. It's used with manual curettage for treating benign and malignant growths on skin and mucous membranes, such as verrucae, nevi, basal cell epitheliomas, and squamous cell carcinomas in situ. A lesion is infiltrated with a local anesthetic, curetted until pinpoint capillary bleeding occurs, and then desiccated. Afterward, clean the wound with hydrogen peroxide and apply an antibiotic ointment and a dressing. Provide instructions for wound care and recognition of infection.

Epididymectomy. Surgical removal of the epididymis performed when conservative treatments have failed to control inflammation. Through an incision made in the anterior scrotum, the testis is brought out and the epididymis is separated from it and removed. A pressure dressing is applied, and a scrotal drain may be placed. Postoperatively, place a folded towel under the scrotum to keep it elevated, as ordered. Provide analgesics, as ordered, and change the dressing as needed.

Escharotomy. Lengthwise incision through an eschar. It's usually performed without anesthesia for circumferential third-degree burns of the extremities, trunk, or neck to allow skin to expand as edema forms. Packing, cautery, or suturing may control bleeding. Before and after treatment, monitor blood flow in affected extremities with Doppler ultrasound. Afterward, check for bleeding. Watch for respiratory distress if escharotomy was performed on the trunk or neck.

Esophageal bougienage. Introduction of a thin, flexible cylindrical cannula (a bougie) into the esophagus to dilate a stricture. In the early stages of stricture development, the patient swallows graded tapered bougies until stricture is adequately opened. In advanced stages, bougienage preserves esophageal patency by daily introduction of a larger bougie until the esophageal lumen is stable. After treatment, observe for signs of bleeding and esophageal obstruction. Keep suctioning apparatus nearby.

Ethambutol. A bacteriostatic drug used in adjunctive treatment of pulmonary tuberculosis. It's effective against the active tubercle bacillus because it interferes with cell metabolism. Before therapy, test the patient's visual acuity since ethambutol may cause optic neuritis. Tell him to report vision changes promptly. Reassure him, though, that vision gradually returns after stopping therapy. Give the drug with food to minimize GI upset. Monitor serum uric acid levels.

External nasolacrimal massage. Maneuver employed with a Honan cuff before cataract and other eye surgeries to lower intraocular pressure. Or massage may be done manually to treat congenital nasolacrimal duct obstruction. This method requires application of firm pressure over the inner aspect of the upper orbital area, moving downward to the inner canthus. You'll perform massage or teach the patient or a family member to do it. Stress good hand washing to prevent infection. During massage, observe the eye for excessive tearing, exudation, or crusting.

Extracranial-intracranial bypass surgery. Anastomosis of the superficial temporal artery (or possibly the occipital, meningeal, or subclavian artery) to a branch of the middle cerebral artery. Used to treat bilateral occlusive carotid artery disease, it's especially helpful in internal carotid occlusion and middle cerebral artery stenosis. After surgery, blood flows from the external carotid system to the circle of Willis via the donor arteries, bypassing the internal carotid system or the stenotic portion of the middle cerebral artery.

Eyelid resection. Partial or complete removal of the upper or lower eyelid. It's done for treatment of malignant tumors or for cosmetic reasons. Preoperatively, explain reconstructive surgery, if appropriate. Postoperatively, help the patient adjust to having vision in one eye (due to the eye patch). Administer methyl cellulose drops and ointment, if ordered, to prevent eye irritation and inflammation. Long-term use of an eye patch, shield, or glasses may be necessary.

Eyelid scrubs. Removal of mucus, crust, scaling, and exudate by applying a warm soak to the eyelid. The soak may use warm water, diluted baby shampoo, 0.1% selenium sulfide solution, or normal saline solution. Use aseptic technique (sterile, if ordered). Have the patient lie supine to keep the soak in place. Tell him to avoid rubbing his eyes to prevent spreading infection.

Eye patching. Application of a pad and shield to the eye. It's done to protect the eye from dust, wind, and light; to promote comfort; and to eliminate diplopia. Before patching, cleanse the eye and apply any ordered medication. Have the patient close both eyes while you place the pad, taking care to avoid contaminating it. Secure the pad with an attached strap or with three pieces of tape. Change the pad daily or more often if there's drainage from the eye. Place a plastic or metal shield over the pad, if needed, to prevent external pressure or eye injury.

F

Fasciotomy. Longitudinal incision into the fibrous membrane (fascia) that separates, covers, and supports muscles. It may be done after burn injuries to detect viable muscle or to treat compartment syndrome. In compartment syndrome, immediate treatment is needed to prevent permanent nerve damage and muscle necrosis. The procedure relieves pressure on the compromised nerve and helps restore blood supply to the muscle. The wound may be left open temporarily to allow for further swelling. Provide meticulous wound care and perform a careful circulatory assessment after the procedure.

Fertility drugs for men. *Clomiphene*, a synthetic steroid, spurs spermatogenesis by increasing levels of luteinizing hormone and follicle-stimulating hormone. *Human chorionic gonadatropin (HCG)* can be used alone or along with clomiphene and menotropins to promote spermatogenesis in men with hypogonadatropic hypogonadism by stimulating testicular androgen production.

Fistulectomy and fistulotomy. Excision and incision of an anal fistula, respectively. Fistulotomy is preferred for deep fistulas. Both procedures leave a wide saucer-shaped wound. Postoperatively, focus on pain control: apply warm compresses or dressings soaked in witch hazel, and have the patient take a sitz bath four times a day. To prevent constipation, monitor his diet and administer stool softeners and laxatives, as ordered. Provide a protected pillow or thick foam-rubber cushion for the patient to sit on.

Flucytosine. An antifungal drug used for severe systemic infections caused by susceptible strains of *Candida* or *Cryptococcus*. Before treatment, obtain hepatic, renal, and hematopoietic studies. During treatment, monitor test results. Warn the patient that nausea, vomiting, and diarrhea may occur. Give capsules over a 15-minute period to reduce nausea and vomiting.

Fructose- and sucrose-free diet. A diet that eliminates all sources of fructose, sucrose, and sorbitol. It's used for hereditary fructose intolerance and fructose 1,6-diphosphate deficiency. The diet eliminates all fruits, vegetables, and their juices, along with all products that contain sugar, corn syrup, or invert sugar.

G

Galactose-free diet. A diet that eliminates all milk and dairy products, organ meats (such as liver), and monosodium glutamate. It's used for patients who lack an enzyme that converts galactose to glucose in the liver. In infants, soy- or meat-based formula substitutes for breast or bottled milk. Children may eat foods, such as baked goods, that contain small amounts of milk. Pregnant women, though, must follow the diet rigidly to prevent fetal damage.

Garren gastric bubble. An experimental device used to treat morbid obesity. The bubble, a durable balloon about 3″ (7.6 cm) in diameter, is inserted into the stomach through flexible nasogastric tubing and then inflated. Properly positioned, it reduces stomach capacity, thus limiting food intake and promoting weight loss. Although this treatment is safer than gastroplasty or gastric bypass, its complications include ulceration and perforation of the stomach and intestinal obstruction. Postoperatively, encourage the patient to eat small meals.

Gastric bypass. Placement of a row of sutures to close off the fundus from the body of the stomach, with creation of an anastomosis between the fundus and a jejunal loop to allow food to pass through the GI tract. This experimental treatment for morbid obesity reduces stomach capacity by about 85%. Postoperatively, encourage the patient to eat small meals.

Gastroesophageal reflux repair. Surgical correction of gastroesophageal reflux by wrapping the upper end of the stomach around the esophagus. This high-pressure barrier effectively prevents backflow of stomach contents into the esophagus. Preoperatively, assess the frequency, severity, and quality of the patient's pain, as well as measures that relieve it. Postoperatively, monitor his tolerance of the initial clear liquid diet and his progression to regular food. Check for difficulty swallowing, which may result from edema at the surgical site but will subside in a few days. Administer analgesics, as ordered.

Gastroplasty. Placement of a row of staples to close off the fundus from the body of the stomach. A small opening left between the fundus and body allows passage of food through the GI tract. This experimental treatment for morbid obesity reduces stomach capacity, thereby limiting intake, and slows food passage. Encourage the patient to eat small, well-balanced meals.

Griseofulvin. An antifungal drug used systemically to treat major tinea infections of the skin and nails. Instruct the patient to take the drug with meals. Advise him that it's most easily absorbed and causes the least GI upset when it's taken after a high-fat meal. Warn him to avoid exposure to strong sunlight because photosensitivity can occur. In addition, tell him to report hives, rash, or pruritus. Caution against using alcohol during therapy.

H

Hemin. An enzyme inhibitor, isolated from red blood cells, that limits porphyrin synthesis. It's used to induce prolonged remission in porphyria. Reconstitute the solution immediately before use; it has a short life span, and chemical decomposition occurs rapidly. Side effects include phlebitis, coagulopathy, leukocytosis, and fever. Monitor the patient's urine output closely since renal failure may occur with high doses. Assess his neurologic status frequently to determine the effectiveness of therapy.

Hemoperfusion. Passage of blood through an adsorptive system, such as a column containing activated charcoal, to remove drugs. Common indications are liver failure and drug overdose. The selection of adsorbent material depends on the drug to be removed.

Hemorrhoid reduction. Placement of a rubber band at the base of a hemorrhoid, resulting in necrosis and sloughing of tissue distal to the band in about 7 days. It's indicated when internal hemorrhoids bleed persistently or prolapse. Postoperatively, promote comfort with analgesics, warm compresses, and sitz baths. Give stool softeners and encourage fluids and dietary fiber to prevent straining during defecation.

Hepatitis B immune globulin (H-BIG). An immunoglobulin solution derived from persons who have antibodies to hepatitis B surface antigen. It's used with hepatitis B vaccine to prevent or modify symptoms after exposure to hepatitis B— for example, after needle stick by a contaminated syringe or after contaminated blood splashes the eye or mucous membranes. H-BIG is given I.M. within 7 days of exposure. Watch for signs of anaphylaxis.

High-carbohydrate diet. A diet that increases carbohydrate intake from a usual level of 100 to 200 g per day to 300 to 400 g per day. It includes increased intake of such foods as pasta, rice, bread, cereals, and sweet potatoes. The diet serves as part of a high-calorie regimen for patients who need to gain weight, and it's beneficial for patients with a variety of diseases. For example, increased carbohydrate intake can provide additional energy in cystic fibrosis.

High-phosphorus diet. A diet that increases phosphorus intake to treat hypophosphatemia caused by intestinal malabsorption, prolonged or excessive use of phosphate-binding antacids, I.V. hyperalimentation, severe burns, or alcoholism. High-phosphorus foods include eggs, meat, fish, milk, and carbonated beverages. Vitamin D supplements should be given concurrently to increase phosphorus absorption. Monitor the patient's serum calcium levels during therapy and watch for muscle twitching and tetany.

High-potassium diet. A diet that increases potassium intake through ingestion of meat, milk, vegetables, whole grains, and fruits (especially bananas, oranges, and prunes). It's used for patients who have burns and injuries, diabetic ketoacidosis, or adrenal tumors. It's also given to patients who have inadequate dietary potassium intake or are undergoing long-term therapy with a diuretic that doesn't spare potassium.

Monitor the patient's heart rate during therapy, since hypokalemia can cause tachycardia, and hyperkalemia can cause heart failure. If the pa-

tient has severe potassium deficiency, encourage small, frequent feedings of potassium-rich foods, since his appetite may be poor. If ordered, administer potassium supplements and provide potassium-containing salt substitutes.

Hyperbaric oxygenation. Administration of 100% oxygen in a pressurized chamber. Used for years to manage decompression in divers and aviators, this treatment is today used for crush injuries (to promote healing where ischemia is present), burn injuries (to decrease fluid loss), radiation necrosis, gas gangrene (to inhibit growth of anaerobic organisms such as clostridia), smoke inhalation, and carbon monoxide poisoning. To prevent fire in the hyperbaric chamber, ensure that all clothing and linens are cotton and that electrostatic equipment isn't being used. Orient the patient to the chamber's confined space to avoid claustrophobia. During treatment, watch for signs of oxygen toxicity, which can be prevented by breathing room air.

I

Interleukin-2 (IL-2). A glycoprotein produced by antigen-stimulated human lymphocytes. IL-2 mediates many immune responses. For example, it acts as a growth factor that stimulates the development of cytotoxic T cells, sometimes called natural killer cells. Biosynthetic IL-2, an experimental agent, is given primarily to patients with advanced cancer to determine if it boosts killer cell development enough to destroy the malignancy. Routes of administration include I.V. bolus, continuous infusion, injection, and peritoneal instillation. Possible side effects and toxic reactions include confusion, pulmonary edema, oliguria, anemia, and high fever.

Intrauterine intraperitoneal transfusion. Transfusion of blood into the fetal peritoneal cavity to treat hemolytic disease of the newborn. Transfusion begins at 24 to 30 weeks' gestational age to prolong fetal survival and continued intrauterine development. It may be required every 2 weeks until delivery. With treatment, about 50% of affected fetuses survive and develop normally.

With ultrasound guidance, the doctor inserts a needle transabdominally into the amniotic sac and injects contrast medium. After the fetus swallows the contrast medium, its GI tract is visualized by X-rays. The doctor then injects packed RBCs directly into its peritoneal cavity. The RBCs enter the fetal circulation through the lymphatic vessels and great veins.

Ipecac syrup. An emetic used to induce vomiting after ingestion of poison. Ipecac should always be administered in the syrup concentration. (Fluid extract of ipecac is 14 times more concentrated, and inadvertent use may cause death.) Its use is strongly contraindicated in patients who have a depressed level of consciousness or gag reflex (risk of aspiration) or have ingested caustic substances (further risk of esophageal or mediastinal injury) or petroleum distillates or volatile oils (risk of aspiration followed by bronchospasm, pulmonary edema, or pneumonia). After you administer ipecac syrup, give water, milk, or soda; vomiting should occur within 20 minutes. If not, repeat the dose. If two doses don't induce vomiting, gastric lavage may be necessary. Don't give a third dose because ipecac may cause cardiac arrhythmias if absorbed by the GI tract. If ordered, administer activated charcoal after the patient vomits.

Islet cell transplant. A technique in which cells from the islets of Langerhans are implanted into the peritoneum or transfused into the liver through the portal vein. It's used experimentally to treat diabetes mellitus and to prevent diabetes in patients who have had a pancreatectomy. Complications include portal hypertension and disseminated intravascular coagulation. Preoperatively, teach the patient about the procedure and its possible complications. Stress its experimental nature. Postoperatively, watch for signs of infection, since immunosuppressants may be given. Prevent respiratory infection by frequent turning and coughing and deep-breathing exercises. Monitor vital signs. Also, monitor blood glucose levels and perform urine testing or bedside glucose monitoring, as ordered.

Isometric exercises. Contraction and relaxation of muscles without movement of the associated body segment. It's the preferred method to maintain muscle strength and tone when immobility is necessary—for example, following hip or knee surgery or when the patient has a long leg cast. As ordered, teach the patient to perform these exercises with the unaffected extremity. They're performed 5 times per hour initially and increased to 20 times per hour as tolerated.

J

Jejunoileal bypass. A surgical procedure that connects the proximal segment of the jejunum to the distal ileum. Used to treat morbid obesity, it's performed infrequently because of its severe complications, such as fluid volume deficit, electrolyte imbalances, chronic diarrhea, and liver failure. Postoperatively, monitor serum electrolyte levels closely, since hypovolemia can develop quickly. Replace fluids and electrolytes as ordered. Monitor intake and output, including feces, to evaluate fluid and electrolyte balance.

K

Kegel exercises. Contraction and relaxation of the perineal muscles—a conservative treatment for stress incontinence. Instruct the patient to stop and start the urinary stream several times when she voids and to do the exercises at least 4 times a day, with 10 to 12 repetitions each time. Tell her to sit in a chair with her knees apart and feet flat on the floor to facilitate exercising the correct muscles.

Keratolytic agents. Topical keratin-dissolving agents, including salicylic acid, resorcinol, sulfur, benzoyl peroxide, tretinoin, coal tar, and ammoniated mercury. They're used to treat psoriasis, seborrheic dermatitis, acne, verrucae, corns, and calluses. Generally, systemic effects are rare because of limited percutaneous absorption. Prolonged use of salicylic acid, however, may lead to toxicity; signs and symptoms include tinnitus, nausea, and vomiting.

Explain correct application, avoiding mucous membranes because these agents are irritants. Inform the patient that erythema, scaling, and dryness commonly occur. Tell him to report severe tenderness. Watch for local side effects, especially contact dermatitis.

Ketoconazole. A broad-spectrum antifungal agent used to treat systemic fungal infections, such as candidiasis, histoplasmosis, chromomycosis, oral thrush, and coccidioidomycosis. Because ketoconazole may produce severe hepatotoxicity, it shouldn't be used for less serious infections. Be alert for jaundice, unusual fatigue, dark urine, or pale stools. Monitor hepatic enzyme levels and report any signs of hepatic dysfunction. Warn the patient that nausea commonly occurs early in treatment; tell him to take the drug with meals.

L

Labyrinthectomy. Removal of the bony labyrinth and the footplate of the stapes. It's indicated in Ménière's disease for patients with severe vertigo and little or no hearing. The procedure destroys cochlear and vestibular function.

Preoperatively, inform the patient that he may have some vertigo after treatment but that it should subside within 2 months. During recovery, tell him to ask for assistance when walking to avoid injury. Inform him that antinausea drugs will be available, as ordered. Postoperatively, be alert for episodes of vertigo and nausea and vomiting. Implement safety measures, especially during periods of vertigo. Administer antibiotics, as ordered, to prevent inner ear infection.

Lactulose-induced catharsis. Evacuation of the bowels after administration of lactulose, a semisynthetic disaccharide. It's used to treat portal systemic encephalopathy and sometimes to relieve constipation. Lactulose decreases serum ammonia levels by 25% to 50%. It acidifies colonic contents, attracting ammonia from the blood and converting it to the ammonium ion. Metabolites of lactulose then act as a laxative, and the ammonium is excreted. As ordered, relieve rectal pain from frequent bowel movements with witch-hazel-soaked pads, warm sitz baths, or local anesthetics in cream or suppository form.

Laser neurosurgery. Use of a carbon dioxide laser to dissect, coagulate, or vaporize CNS tissue. Beam intensity and exposure time determine results. Vaporizing intensity is used with solid brain tumors. Coagulating and dissecting intensities are used to correct arterial malformations or remove vascular tumors. Postoperatively, monitor neurologic status and vital signs frequently. Position the patient's head at a 30-degree angle to promote venous drainage and decrease cerebral perfusion. Immediately report signs of increased intracranial pressure.

Leukapheresis. Separation and removal of abnormal or excessive white blood cells. It's a supportive treatment in chronic diseases, such as lymphatic leukemia and multiple sclerosis. Side effects include hemorrhage, seizures, hypotension, and electrolyte imbalance.

Lipolysis. Cosmetic surgical technique for suctioning small amounts of fat through skin incisions. It's used to change body contours. A cannula attached to a suction pump is inserted through a small incision, and fat is sucked out when the pump is turned on. The patient wears a snug elastic bandage or garment for 6 to 8 weeks, until underlying tissue heals. Fat doesn't reappear; however, the treatment is most successful in patients under age 40, whose skin is elastic enough to reshape over the affected area.

Preoperatively, inform the patient that muscle aches, bruising, swelling, and a burning sensation may be present for 2 months after treatment. Postoperatively, watch for hypovolemia from excessive blood or fluid loss. Monitor temperature and check the incisional area for redness and excessive warmth. Report any complaints of numbness, tingling, or pain to the doctor.

Liquid diet. A diet of foods that are liquid at room temperature. Clear or full liquid diets are given after surgery or in acute GI disturbances since they minimize fecal matter. However, because these diets may not be nutritionally complete, they're used for short durations and may be supplemented with vitamins and minerals.

A *clear* liquid diet consists of tea, fruit juices, broth, carbonated beverages, gelatins, and fruit ices. It supplies water and prevents thirst and dehydration. The patient normally takes small, frequent sips of fluid throughout the day.

A *full* liquid diet contains liquids and foods that are liquid at room temperature. It also includes pureed meats and vegetables. Used as a bridge from a clear to a regular diet, the liquid diet may be given to patients who are too sick to chew.

Litholapaxy. Crushing and removing a calculus from the urinary bladder. After cystoscopic inspection, the doctor inserts appropriate instruments to crush and remove the calculus. Afterward, an indwelling catheter may be inserted. Hematuria commonly occurs but should clear in 48 hours. Perforation of the bladder and urethral stricture formation are possible complications. Give prophylactic antibiotics, as ordered, and provide catheter care, if appropriate.

Lovastatin. A fungal metabolite, representing a new class of cholesterol-lowering agents. Lovastatin enhances the removal of circulating low-density lipoproteins (LDLs) and reduces LDL production. The drug effectively treats familial hypercholesteremia when used with ileal bypass, other cholesterol-lowering agents, or liver transplantation.

Low-phosphorus diet. A diet that decreases phosphorus intake to correct hyperphosphatemia. Indications include renal failure, overuse of phosphate-containing cathartics and enemas, hypoparathyroidism, and excessive phosphate treatment. Ingestion of milk and other dairy products, meat, fish, and carbonated beverages is limited. The diet also includes vitamin D and calcium supplements and aluminum hydroxide taken with meals to bind phosphorus and prevent absorption from the GI tract.

During therapy, be alert for severe constipation, from aluminum hydroxide. Encourage a high-fiber diet. Give stool softeners and laxatives, if needed. In renal failure, observe for muscle excitability and tetany, and monitor serum calcium and phosphorus levels. Encourage fluids, if tolerated, to limit mineral precipitation.

M

Massage. Passive or active manipulation of specific muscle groups or extremities. It's used for pain relief, stress reduction, and prevention of complications related to disuse of an extremity or muscle group.

Mastoidectomy. Removal of diseased mastoid cells (cortical, or simple, mastoidectomy) or the mastoid bone (radical or modified radical mastoidectomy). Common indications include acute and chronic infections of the mastoid bone or cholesteatoma. The surgeon may use a postauricular approach (most common) or an endaural approach. Advances in antibiotic therapy have reduced the number of mastoidectomies performed in recent years.

In a *simple* mastoidectomy, the surgeon makes a postauricular incision, opens the mastoid antrum, and removes diseased bone cells with a drill. Before surgery, tell the patient that surgery won't change his hearing. Postoperatively, check for bleeding, dizziness, nausea, and vomiting. Be alert for signs of infection.

In a *radical* mastoidectomy, all diseased bone is removed along with any cholesteatoma that's present. In addition, diseased ossicles (except for the stapes) and the tympanic membrane are removed. Then the bony wall between the mastoid and middle ear is removed. Before surgery, inform the patient that he may have dizziness or vertigo afterward and that medication will be available to alleviate these symptoms. Encourage him to call for assistance when walking to prevent injury. After surgery, observe facial movements; they'll be limited on the involved side if surgery affected the facial nerve. Monitor for bleeding, dizziness, and vertigo.

In a *modified radical* mastoidectomy, part of the tympanic membrane and malleus are retained to allow for later reconstructive surgery.

Monoclonal antibodies. Tumor-specific antibodies used experimentally in cancer treatment. They're produced by hybridomas—cultured cells consisting of antibody-producing cells (usually from mice) and cancer antigens. Monoclonal antibodies are often used alone, but some researchers are trying to attach chemotherapeutic agents to them to increase cytotoxic specificity. Complications include toxic reactions to impurities and circulating tumor-associated antigens, as well as the production of antimouse antibodies. Rapid administration may lead to toxic reactions characterized by wheezing, hypotension, and rashes. Have resuscitation equipment available in case of anaphylactic reaction. Keep records of the effects of treatment.

N

Nasal polypectomy. Removal of polyps from the nose with a snare or blunt forceps. A part of the lining covering the ethmoid sinuses may also need to be removed. After polyp removal, an anterior nasal pack impregnated with antibiotics or petrolatum is inserted. The packing is removed about 48 hours after surgery. Postoperatively, monitor vital signs and ensure a patent airway. Check for dislodging of the nasal pack by examining the back of the patient's throat with a flashlight. Offer sedatives or analgesics, as ordered. Warn the patient that blowing his nose may dislodge clots and cause bleeding.

Niclosamide. An anthelmintic used to treat infection by beef, dwarf, or fish tapeworm. Tell the patient to take the drug with food to prevent GI upset. Instruct him to chew the tablets thoroughly before swallowing. In addition, warn him not to drive or operate machinery if he feels dizzy, drowsy, or light-headed.

Nicotine resin complex (Nicorette). Nicotine chewing gum used as a substitute source of nicotine during the behavioral modification phase of a smoking cessation program. Tell the patient to chew slowly and pause whenever he feels a tingling in the mouth to promote slow, even nicotine release. Light-headedness, nausea, vomiting, and GI upset may occur with overly rapid nicotine absorption. Tell him not to chew more than 30 pieces each day. His desire to smoke should decrease in 1 to 2 months.

O

Oophorectomy. Removal of one (unilateral) or both (bilateral) ovaries. Unilateral oophorectomy is usually performed to remove a malignancy. Bilateral oophorectomy is usually performed with hysterectomy and bilateral salpingectomy to treat severe endometriosis, fibromyoma, or pelvic inflammatory disease. It results in onset of menopause.

Osteoplasty. Plastic or reconstructive surgery to rebuild bone. It may be used with osteotomy. Plastic reconstruction may require the use of cement to bind bone grafts in the rebuilding process. If a limb is involved, it's usually placed in a cast for 2 to 3 weeks. Weightbearing is generally permitted in 7 to 10 days, unless bone damage is extensive and a second procedure is planned.

Osteotomy. Division of bone, performed to permit realignment. Originally, it was used to correct the bowleg deformity of rickets. Now, it's commonly used to provide pain relief in osteoarthritis or spinal correction in spondylitis. Surgical techniques vary, depending on the bone and tissue involved at the selected site. A deformity can be corrected and pain relief provided by removing a wedge of bone or by cutting the bone and realigning it. Internal fixation (such as pins, screws, or nails and a plate) is used to maintain the newly corrected position. Prepare the patient for inactivity while the bone reknits after surgery. He may have a cast for 2 to 3 weeks.

Ovarian wedge resection. Removal of one third to one half of an ovary. It's done primarily to correct infertility due to polycystic ovaries. Removing a section of the ovary preserves its function.

Oxamniquine. An anthelmintic drug used to treat all stages of *Schistosoma mansoni* infection. Effective against immature and mature worms, the drug should be administered with food to prevent nausea and vomiting. Other side effects include dizziness, drowsiness, headache, and skin rashes. Warn the patient not to drive or operate hazardous machinery if he feels dizzy or drowsy. Tell him that reddish orange discoloration of the urine is normal and harmless.

P-Q

Pancreas transplant. Transplantation of a pancreas from a cadaver donor. Candidates for this experimental treatment include insulin-dependent diabetics with progressive secondary complications but normal renal function, or diabetics who have end-stage renal disease and have already received a renal transplant. Transplantation aims to achieve better control of carbohydrate metabolism, glucose homeostasis, and secondary lesions associated with diabetes mellitus. Cyclosporine is used postoperatively to reduce the risk of rejection.

Preoperatively, teach the patient about the surgery and postoperative care. Afterward, encourage coughing and deep breathing and watch for signs of rejection. Assess vital signs and check blood or urine glucose levels, as ordered.

Pancreatin. A preparation (extracted from animal pancreas) containing amylase, lipase, and trypsin, the most abundant pancreatic enzymes. It's indicated for conditions in which these enzymes are diminished or absent, such as chronic pancreatitis and mucoviscidosis. Pancreatin is administered in enteric-coated capsules to prevent its destruction by pepsin. Give with food.

Paracentesis. Aspiration of ascitic fluid from the peritoneal cavity. A treatment for severe respiratory distress, it's also used prophylactically before peritoneal dialysis or abdominal surgery. Before paracentesis, obtain vital signs and have the patient void. During the procedure, help him maintain proper position and assess his response to fluid removal. Monitor his blood pressure frequently. After the procedure, help the patient into a comfortable position. Be alert for respiratory compromise, pallor, hypotension, and tachycardia. Check the dressing frequently for drainage.

Parotidectomy. Removal of parotid gland lobes, which lie superficial to the facial nerve. The surgeon makes an incision below the angle of the jaw, resects the lobes, inserts a drain, closes the wound, and applies a pressure dressing. Complications include facial asymmetry caused by nerve damage. Postoperatively, check for facial asymmetry by asking the patient to smile, show his teeth, and purse his lips. Make sure he maintains good oral hygiene to prevent infection. If chewing causes pain, administer an analgesic before meals, as ordered, and provide a soft diet. Monitor intake and output.

Pelvic exenteration. Removal of a woman's rectum, distal sigmoid colon, urinary bladder, distal ureters, internal iliac arteries and veins, reproductive organs, pelvic lymph nodes and peritoneum, levator muscles, and perineum. Uncommonly performed, it may be indicated in extensive metastatic disease. Nursing care is complex: it includes measures associated with abdominal hysterectomy, abdominoperineal resection with colostomy, and ileobladder resection with cutaneous ureterostomy. Provide emotional support for the patient and her partner, and evaluate their need for psychological counseling.

Penectomy. Excision of the penis. This is treatment for penile carcinoma, a relatively uncommon cancer. The extent of tissue removal depends on the site of the tumor and its potential for lymphatic spread. Partial amputation may be performed if the tumor is distal to the bulbous urethra; resection is done about 1″ (2.5 cm) proximal to the tumor. With partial penectomy, a urethral catheter is left in place for up to 10 days. With total penectomy, a perineal urethrostomy is peformed. Because penile carcinoma can be psychologically devastating to the patient, provide ongoing support and recommend counseling. Postoperatively, provide emotional support as well as physical care. Follow all catheter care basics and provide aseptic wound care. To prevent deep venous thrombosis and leg edema, apply antiembolism stockings. Encourage the patient to walk and to elevate his legs at rest.

Peripheral neurectomy. Excision of part of a peripheral nerve to relieve pain when malignancy affects that particular nerve. It's used infrequently because of possible side effects, including persistence of pain, numbness, and dysesthesia. The procedure results in loss of motor and sensory function. Preoperatively, perform a neurologic assessment and record the frequency, onset, duration, and type of pain. Administer analgesics, as ordered, to keep the patient comfortable and reduce preoperative stress. Postoperatively, perform frequent neurologic assessments. Record the patient's response to treatment, and be alert for pain. Provide instructions on safety precautions and care related to neural function loss.

Phenazopyridine. An anesthetic that relieves the burning and cramping sensation of urinary tract infections, such as cystitis and urethritis, and pain caused by trauma, surgery, or the use of instruments. It's often given with sulfonamides. Side effects include nausea, urine discoloration, and yellow skin and sclera.

Phlebotomy. Controlled removal of blood from the patient. It's used mainly to reduce blood volume, red cell mass, and iron stores in hemosiderosis. It may be used to treat diseases that increase red cell mass, such as polycythemia vera. A venipuncture is performed, and the required amount of blood is withdrawn. Watch for signs of a reaction to the change in circulating blood volume.

Phototherapy. Therapeutic use of ultraviolet or visible wavelengths of light. Use of blue visible light in infantile hyperbilirubinemia causes photoisomerization of bilirubin, which is then readily excreted in bile and urine. Ultraviolet light is also used to treat proliferative skin diseases.

Phrenic pacing. Electrical stimulation of the phrenic nerve by electrodes implanted in the thoracic diaphragm. Indications include chronic dysfunction of the respiratory control center and muscle paralysis. It may be used with noninvasive ventilatory support measures, such as a rocking bed. Obtain baseline information regarding air volume exchanges when the patient occupies various positions (for example, supine and side lying) during phrenic pacing. Instruct the patient to report signs of hypoventilation, such as morning headaches, increased fatigue, and worsened dyspnea. Observe his mental status, respiratory rate and rhythm, quality of breath sounds, skin color, and circulatory status.

Plateletpheresis. Extraction of excessive or abnormal platelets to treat thrombocytosis. A cell separator processes the patient's blood, removes unwanted platelets, and returns other blood components to the circulation. This treatment supplements other measures. As with other apheresis techniques, such complications as hemorrhage, seizure, hypotension, cardiac irregularities, and electrolyte imbalance can occur.

Podophyllum resin. A caustic agent that inhibits cell division and other processes, eventually causing cell death. It's used to treat molluscum contagiosum, warts, and benign epithelial growths. Inform the patient that application of podophyllum usually results in minor discomfort and skin irritation. Protect uninvolved skin. If the resin is accidentally applied to normal tissue, remove it with acetone, alcohol, or tape remover, and wash the area with soap and water.

Polypectomy. Excision of a polyp. In patients with colorectal polyps, preoperative care may include bowel preparation to clear the intestinal tract. Afterward, assess for abnormal rectal bleeding. Administer stool softeners, and encourage increased dietary fiber.

After excision of esophageal polyps, evaluate respirations and swallowing frequently. Keep suctioning equipment at the patient's bedside.

Probenecid. A uricosuric agent used to treat chronic gout. It increases excretion of uric acid by inhibiting reabsorption of urates in the renal tubules. This drug also inhibits excretion of penicillins and cephalosporins and may be used to increase their serum levels for therapeutic purposes. As ordered, restrict foods containing purine, such as anchovies and sardines, liver, sweetbreads, peas, and lentils. Give the drug with milk, food, or antacids to reduce GI distress. To help prevent urate calculi, make sure the patient drinks 2 to 3 liters of fluid per day, and alkalinize the urine with sodium bicarbonate or potassium citrate, as prescribed. Watch for side effects, such as headache, dizziness, urinary frequency, and signs of hypersensitivity.

Proctectomy. Excision of the rectum, usually by an abdominoperineal resection and requiring a colostomy. Preoperatively, prepare the bowel. Afterward, give analgesics, as ordered. Assess the dressing for drainage. Maintain nasogastric suction and decompression of the stomach. Provide colostomy care.

Pyelolithotomy. Formerly, the most common procedure for removing renal calculi. The advent of endoscopic urologic procedures and extracorporeal shock-wave lithotripsy has greatly reduced its use. Following a flank incision, the ureter is commonly tied off to prevent calculi particles from entering the ureter, and the renal pelvis is incised. The surgeon then removes the calculi and irrigates the renal pelvis with a saline solution to remove all fragments. Postoperatively, monitor drainage: expect serosanguinous fluid and some urine from the incisional drain and bloody urine from the indwelling catheter. Auscultate for bowel sounds and be alert for paralytic ileus. If this occurs, a nasogastric tube may need to be inserted. Keep the incision site clean and dry, and make sure the incisional dressing is changed at least once in every shift.

Pyrimethamine. An antimalarial typically used with sulfadoxine to treat chloroquine-resistant falciparum malaria. It's also used in weekly doses as a malaria prophylactic and suppressive agent. Combined with a sulfonamide such as sulfadiazine, it's used to treat toxoplasmosis. If the patient's taking a high dose, give the drug with meals or snacks to reduce GI upset. Also monitor his complete blood count to detect anemia.

R

Rabies immune globulin. Gamma globulin obtained from the plasma of persons who have antibodies to rabies. It's used to prevent rabies or lessen its severity after a serious exposure, such as a deep animal bite (especially around the head). Usually administered with rabies vaccine, it isn't useful when signs of rabies are present. Monitor for signs of anaphylaxis.

Rectal tube insertion. A single-lumen catheter temporarily used to remove flatus from the lower large intestine. Long-term use may impair anal sphincter tone. Remove the tube after bowel movements and clean it daily to ensure patency. Use warm compresses, local anesthetics, and sitz baths, as ordered, to relieve anal discomfort.

Reverse Trendelenburg's position. Placement of the patient in a supine or semiprone position with his head elevated about 30 degrees and his legs slightly lowered. It's used to decrease intracranial venous pressure in head injury. Other indications include copious airway secretions, gastric reflux, and increased comfort in advanced pregnancy or extreme obesity. Observe the patient's extremities for signs of decreased circulation. If his legs are cold, mottled, or discolored or his pedal pulse is weak, reposition him to facilitate blood flow. Observe for skin breakdown on the hips or buttocks.

Rhizotomy. Chemical or surgical interruption of the sensory pathways of a spinal nerve. It's performed to relieve intractable pain, but results are unpredictable. If possible, a nerve block should be done to demonstrate the effects before this drastic treatment. Preoperatively, do a complete neurologic assessment. Inform the patient that treatment numbs the area innervated by the affected nerve but doesn't always relieve pain. Before a sacral rhizotomy, inform him that incontinence and loss of sexual function may occur. Postoperatively, monitor neurologic status to detect complications early. Provide analgesics, as ordered. Explain precautions for skin care in the numbed area and the need to avoid temperature extremes and prolonged pressure.

Ribavirin. A systemic antiviral drug used to treat respiratory syncytial virus and influenza B viral infections. It's given by aerosol to hospitalized high-risk infants and young children with severe lower respiratory tract infections. (The oral form is given to children who require ventilatory assistance.) The patient may feel dizzy, weak, or lightheaded. Be alert for blurred vision; itching, redness, or swelling around the eyes; and increased photosensitivity.

Rotating tourniquets. Use of pressure cuffs on the extremities according to a system of rotation in which each cuff is released for 15 minutes every hour while the other three remain inflated. No longer in common use, this treatment aims to reduce venous return in congestive heart failure so that right ventricular output, left ventricular work load, and pulmonary congestion decrease. To perform this treatment, take a blood pressure reading and apply the pressure cuffs as high as possible on the extremities. Inflate three of them to 10 to 20 mm Hg below the patient's systolic blood pressure. Deflate one cuff every 15 minutes and inflate another. During the procedure and after tourniquet removal, assess blood pressure, skin color and temperature, and peripheral pulses. Upon discontinuation, release one cuff at a time to prevent fluid overload.

S

Salpingectomy. Removal of one (unilateral) or both (bilateral) fallopian tubes. Unilateral salpingectomy is most commonly done for ectopic pregnancy, to remove a fallopian tube that has ruptured or may soon rupture. Bilateral salpingectomy, usually performed with hysterectomy and bilateral oophorectomy, helps treat severe endometriosis, fibromyoma, and pelvic inflammatory disease. Nursing care is the same as for hysterectomy. However, it may also include administration of antibiotics to treat pelvic inflammatory disease or peritonitis caused by tubal rupture.

Sclerotherapy. Injection of a sclerosing agent into bleeding esophageal varices through a fiber-optic endoscope. The injected agent causes a collapse of the varix, with eventual thrombosis and sclerosis. This procedure has been used therapeutically and prophylactically—to treat bleeding and nonbleeding esophageal varices. Complications include aspiration pneumonia, upper GI bleeding, and esophageal rupture. After the procedure, observe the patient closely for signs of bleeding. Place aspiration apparatus and emergency lavage equipment at the patient's bedside.

Sinus washes. Irrigation of the nares and sinuses, usually with a saline solution, to treat chronic sinusitis related to reactive airway disease. Sinus washing is usually performed twice a day to clear the nasal airway and sinuses of secretions and debris. It may be followed by a steroidal nasal spray to decrease inflammation. Before instilling the sinus wash, clean the external nares to prevent propulsion of the debris into the sinuses. Warn the patient that he may taste the solution as it washes into the oropharynx.

Sitz bath. A perineal bath, using a basin filled with tepid or hot water. It's used to promote healing of a perineal wound, to decrease edema, or to relieve perineal pain. Most institutions have sitz bath basins that fit into toilet seats. For heat application, water temperature should be 110° to 115° F (43° to 46° C.). Water temperature for other sitz baths should be 94° to 98° F. (34° to 37° C.).

Monitor the patient for weakness or dizziness during treatment. Cover him with a blanket or towel to prevent vasoconstriction and maintain privacy. If he's left unattended, place the bathroom call light close by. Because of possible vasodilation, help the patient back to bed after the procedure.

Sleep therapy. Use of an extended period of drug-induced sleep—usually 18 to 24 hours—to interrupt a pattern of headaches refractory to medication. The choice of a specific hypnotic drug depends on the doctor's preference and the patient's status. Flurazepam, secobarbital, chloral hydrate, and glutethimide are equally effective in inducing and maintaining sleep. When pain is also present, an analgesic may also be given.

Before treatment, reinforce the doctor's explanation of the procedure. Obtain a sleep history to help identify specific routines or aids that help the patient fall asleep, such as use of two pillows, a favorite quilt or pillow, or specific hygienic practices, such as brushing and flossing his teeth. The procedure can be made more natural by incorporating these. During therapy, monitor the patient's vital signs and EKG.

Soft diet. A diet of soft-cooked, easily digestible foods. Acting as a bridge between liquid and normal diets, a soft diet can benefit patients recovering from surgery or those who have acute infection, fever, or GI disturbances. Nutritionally adequate, the diet contains foods that are low in residue and mildly spiced and seasoned. These include milk and milk products, mild soft cheese, eggs, refined breads and cereals, all beverages, and such cooked meats as lean pork, turkey, and chicken. The diet excludes fried foods, nuts, seeds, and dry coarse cereals. Although the patient may tire of this bland diet, encourage him to eat enough each day to meet his caloric needs.

Sorbitol-induced catharsis. Use of sorbitol to induce rapid bowel evacuation. When concentrated in the GI tract, sorbitol will draw water and electrolytes into the lumen, resulting in catharsis. It's used for this purpose in hepatic encephalopathy.

Explain the procedure to the patient. After the procedure, treat anorectal discomfort with warm soaks, sitz baths, and local anesthetics, as ordered.

Sulfasalazine. A combination of sulfapyridine and salicylic acid, used in treating ulcerative colitis and regional enteritis. Inflammation caused by ulcerative colitis tends to improve significantly. The drug should be administered in evenly divided doses over each 24-hour period. Common side effects include anorexia, headache, nausea, and GI distress. Evaluate the patient's response and be alert for side effects.

Sympathectomy. Surgical or chemical interruption of a portion of the autonomic pathways. Possible side effects include neuralgia, tenderness, hyperalgesia, hyperpathia, paradoxical gangrene, and disturbance of sexual function. Aggressive physical therapy restores mobility and strength to the affected area, improves skin appearance, and resolves edema.

Preoperatively, perform a complete neurologic assessment and obtain a pain history. Explain the procedure to the patient. Advise him that medication will be available for postoperative pain.

Postoperatively, assess the patient's neurologic status. Check pulses, skin color, and capillary refill time to detect paradoxical gangrene. Report changes in neurologic or vascular status to the doctor immediately. Be alert for neuralgia, which may appear 7 to 10 days after surgery; it can be treated with carbamazepine or diphenylhydantoin. Make the patient comfortable by limiting physical activity, repositioning, and initiating relaxation techniques, such as guided imagery. Begin passive or active range-of-motion exercises as soon as the patient can tolerate them.

T

Teflon injection. Injection of Teflon into a paralyzed vocal cord to improve the voice. This causes the vocal cord to swell and move toward the midline. This technique has also been used for individuals who experience aspiration as a result of vocal cord paralysis. Speech therapy may be needed postoperatively.

Tendon treatments. *Tenotomy,* the partial or total severing of a tendon, may be performed to correct contractures. *Tendon lengthening* may be performed to correct such deformities as severe clawfoot. *Tendon transfer* may be used, for example, after rupture of the extensor pollicis longus tendon in the hand. *Tendon grafting* may be performed to replace damaged tendons. *Tenodesis,* in which a tendon is fixed to a joint to act as a tether, is another procedure. After tendon surgery, the patient's joint may be immobilized in a splint or cast.

Tetanus antitoxin. Serum obtained from the blood of horses who have developed antibodies to tetanus. In a patient with an uncertain immunization history, it's used to prevent tetanus from wounds contaminated with *Clostridium tetani.* Because many persons are allergic to horse serum, tetanus antitoxin should be used only when tetanus immune globulin is unavailable. An intradermal sensitivity test should be done before administration. Monitor for anaphylaxis.

Tetanus immune globulin. A human immune serum used for passive tetanus prophylaxis in patients who aren't immunized or have an uncertain immunization history. Given I.M. at the same time as tetanus antitoxin, it produces effective levels of circulating antibodies for 3 weeks or more than the toxoid. Monitor for anaphylaxis.

Therapeutic touch. An alternative therapy used to enhance other pain control treatments or to increase patient tolerance of painful stimuli. It involves the use of touch to provide comfort and nonverbal support to the patient. Therapeutic touch may decrease feelings of isolation, hopelessness, and fear, all of which may intensify the patient's perception of pain. Use therapeutic touch with or immediately after other measures to control pain. Also incorporate it into daily nursing care, say, in early morning or at night, when feelings of fear and isolation may be intense. Involve family members in the treatment.

Thiabendazole. An anthelmintic most effective against threadworms and pinworms, but also used against hookworms, roundworms, and whipworms. Because the drug has a broad spectrum of activity, it's especially useful in mixed infestations. In treating trichinosis, it decreases fever, muscle pain, and eosinophilia but apparently doesn't eliminate larvae from muscle tissues. Side effects may include GI upset, dizziness, drowsiness, or foul-smelling urine.

Thymectomy. Removal of the thymus gland. It's commonly used in uncomplicated myasthenia gravis that doesn't respond to drug therapy. It's also indicated for patients with a thymoma. Preoperatively, advise the patient that even if remission occurs, it takes weeks or even months before improvement occurs. Postoperatively, perform chest physiotherapy and suction every 2 hours. Examine the incision site every 4 hours. In myasthenia gravis, resume anticholinesterase drugs, as ordered, and monitor response.

Tick removal. Application of a greasy or thick substance, such as petroleum jelly or nail polish, over the tick may cause it to drop off. It can also be removed with tweezers by grasping it close to the skin and pulling carefully. Don't squeeze it. After removal, wash the site with soap and water and apply antiseptic or antibiotic ointment.

Transcutaneous emobilization. Used to control intractable bleeding in diverticular disease. The vessel involved is identified by angiography and injected with hemostatic agents, such as oxidized cellulose. After injection, monitor the catheter insertion site in the groin for bleeding, and check the distal pulse.

Transfer factor. A dialyzable extract of human lymphocytes that's capable of transferring cell-mediated immunity. In this experimental procedure, lymphocytes are removed from a donor who tests strongly positive for a certain type of cell-mediated immunity. They're then processed and injected into the patient, achieving striking results in some viral, fungal, and other infections. The procedure is also used for AIDS and some cancers. Maintain aseptic technique when giving transfer factor to reduce the risk of infection in the patient, who is given immunosuppressants. Assess his vital signs and response to therapy.

Truss. A pad made from a firm, solid material that's held in place over a hernia with a belt. It's used to prevent a hernia from protruding when the patient is standing. An improperly applied truss may cause skin irritation and breakdown and strangulation of the hernia.

Teach the patient to perform a daily assessment of the hernia, including manual reduction and inspection of the skin covered by the truss. Advise him to remove the truss at bedtime and to reduce the hernia manually before applying the truss.

U

Ureteral reimplantation. Surgical removal of the ureter from the bladder and its subsequent replantation, usually superior to the original site. Most commonly performed in children, it treats ureterovesical reflux, distal ureteral stricture, and injuries to the lower ureter. Postoperatively, watch for signs of catheter obstruction. Give antispasmodics, as ordered, to relieve bladder spasms. Before discharge, explain the signs of urinary tract infection to the patient. Tell him to expect fatigue as well as incisional discomfort.

Ureteral stent. A small tube used to divert urine temporarily from the renal pelvis to the bladder or an external collection bag. It can be used to bypass an obstruction and to maintain patency of the urinary tract until stenosis or edema subside. The stent is placed internally or externally with the aid of a cystoscope. An internal stent is held in place by a coil or J-like bend at either end. An external stent is a straight tube that extends from the renal pelvis through the ureter and bladder and exits at the urinary meatus. It's usually taped to an indwelling catheter.

With both stents, a crystalline buildup may occur. The stent, like any foreign body, may contribute to infection or become dislodged. Watch for signs of obstruction and urinary tract infection, including flank pain, chills, and fever.

Ureterolithotomy. Removal of a calculus from the ureter, using an abdominal or flank incision. Endoscopic procedures and extracorporeal shock-wave lithotripsy have significantly curtailed use of this major invasive procedure. When a flank incision is used, be alert for severe flank pain if the patient doesn't have an internal stent; this indicates possible ureteral obstruction. Report it immediately. Expect urine leakage through the incisional drain for up to 1 week. With an abdominal incision, postoperative care is much the same as that after any major surgery.

Before discharge, explain care measures for the incision, activity restrictions, warning signs of urinary tract infection, and the need for adequate hydration. Tell the patient to notify the doctor if urine continues to drain from the incision site for more than a week.

Urinary meatotomy. A surgical procedure performed in the course of treating urinary stenosis to allow normal flow of urine from the bladder through the urinary meatus. Use of a urethrotome is an alternative to urinary meatotomy. The urethrotome is inserted into the urinary meatus and the inelastic area is cut. Postoperative complications include bleeding and recurrence of stenosis. Apply xylocaine ointment for pain.

Uvulopalatopharyngoplasty. Excision of soft tissue in the upper airway to treat obstructive sleep apnea and heavy snoring. It's most effective in correcting an obstruction at the level of the velum or oropharynx. Preoperatively, monitor respiratory status and ensure a patent airway. Postoperatively, observe for bleeding and nasal regurgitation, monitor respiratory status, and ensure a patent airway.

V-Y

Vancomycin. An antibacterial drug used to treat gram-positive infections. Effective against severe staphylococcal infections, it's used in patients who are allergic to penicillin or the cephalosporins and have endocarditis, osteomyelitis, pneumonia, or septicemia. It's usually given by slow I.V. infusion, using a dilute solution. Monitor for "red neck syndrome," a maculopapular rash on the face, neck, and trunk. Evaluate renal and auditory function since the drug's nephrotoxic and ototoxic.

Vidarabine. An antiviral agent available as an ophthalmic ointment and an I.V. preparation. It's used topically for herpes simplex keratitis and parenterally for herpes simplex encephalitis. It's also used for herpes zoster infections in immunodeficient patients. With topical use, notify the doctor if tearing, photophobia, or eye irritation or pain develops. With parenteral use, expect such effects as nausea, diarrhea, dizziness, and confusion. Assist the patient with ambulation, if necessary. Monitor his complete blood count for decreases in hemoglobin, hematocrit, white blood cells, and platelets.

Z

Zinc gelatin boot. A compression dressing for venous ulcers, consisting of alternate layers of bandage and a paste of gelatin, zinc oxide, and glycerin. It stimulates and maintains healthy tissue in the skin surrounding varicose ulcers. Healing may take 3 months.

When this boot is ordered, evaluate the ulcer, palpate the dorsalis pedis pulse, and check capillary refill, skin temperature, and color before boot application. Explain to the patient that full ambulation is permitted. Cleanse the ulcer and dry the leg thoroughly.

To apply the boot, pad the instep and ankle with cotton and wrap the bandage in overlapping turns in a figure-eight pattern. Mold the case during application until it's even and smooth, with a cut beneath the knee to avoid constriction. The dressing, which hardens as it's applied, should be changed once a week. The day after application, check the toes for edema, cyanosis, and decreased sensation.

Disorders and Their Treatments

This alphabetically organized appendix summarizes treatments for about 600 disorders. Organized by *disorder,* it complements the main text, which is organized by *treatment.*

You can use this appendix to find out how disorders are treated. Then, if you want to read further about a specific treatment, consult the index for its location in the main text.

A

Abdominal aortic aneurysm. Resulting from weakness in the elastic fibers of the aortic wall, an abdominal aneurysm requires drug therapy or surgery, depending on its size and the extent of concurrent cardiovascular disease. Antihypertensives, such as captopril and hydralazine, reduce blood pressure, thereby decreasing aortic wall tension and the risk of aneurysmal rupture. Usually, however, the aneurysm requires resection and replacement of the damaged aortic section with a Dacron graft.

Abortion. In a spontaneous abortion (which occurs without known cause before the fetus can survive outside the womb), the patient may require hospitalization to control severe hemorrhage. If the abortion is incomplete, she may require a dilatation and curettage.

Abruptio placentae. Treatment aims to deliver a viable infant (possibly by cesarean delivery), to control hemorrhage and restore lost blood volume with Ringer's lactate or a blood transfusion, and to assess and correct coagulopathy.

Acceleration-deceleration cervical injury. Typically the result of a rear-end automobile collision, this traumatic injury responds to bed rest, application of a soft cervical collar, administration of nonsteroidal anti-inflammatory drugs, and heat therapy.

Achilles tendon contracture. Prolonged immobility (even 2 to 3 weeks) may result in deformity responsive only to z-tenotomy, which allows further stretching by cutting the tendon.

Acne vulgaris. Topical or systemic treatment depends on the severity and location of lesions and the patient's response. Topical applications of benzoyl peroxide, topical antibiotics, tretinoin, sulfur, resorcinol, or salicylic acid produce a mild erythema and peeling, helping lesions dry and heal. However, systemic antibiotics, such as tetracycline and erythromycin, may be necessary. Less commonly used drugs include sulfones, hormones, corticosteroids (for a brief period), and retinoids (reserved for severe acne, because of their numerous side effects).

Acquired immune deficiency syndrome (AIDS). At present, no curative treatment exists for this syndrome, which is caused by the human immunodeficiency virus. However, investigational drugs, such as azidothymidine (AZT), prolong survival in some patients. Treatment typically aims to remedy associated opportunistic infections. *Pneumocystis carinii* pneumonia requires treatment with co-trimoxazole. Oral candidiasis responds to nystatin or clotrimazole or, if severe, to oral ketoconazole or I.V. amphotericin B. Treatment for herpes simplex virus calls for I.V. acyclovir.

Actinomycosis. Treatment for lesions occurring most commonly on the jaw, thorax, and abdomen consists of I.V. and oral penicillin therapy. If treatment is ineffective or the patient has a hypersensitivity to penicillin, such drugs as tetracycline, erythromycin, or cephalosporin may be given.

Actinic keratosis. Usually seen in elderly patients but also occurring more commonly in younger patients, this precancerous lesion requires treatment with topical fluorouracil, cryosurgery, excisional surgery, or dermabrasion.

Acute blood loss anemia. Treatment aims to restore blood volume with saline solution, Ringer's lactate, or a colloid solution. Loss of more than 40% of blood requires a transfusion of red cells and fresh-frozen plasma.

Acute bronchitis. Management consists of hydration, humidification of inspired air, cough suppressants (to help the patient rest), and symptomatic treatment of throat pain.

Acute intermittent porphyria. A high-carbohydrate diet may minimize attacks of neurologic dysfunction, and phenothiazines and meperidine may control the severe abdominal pain that characterizes this disorder of heme metabolism. Prophylactic injections of hemin may avert cyclic attacks.

Acute leukemia. Acute leukemia has two major categories: acute lymphoblastic leukemia (ALL) and acute nonlymphoblastic leukemia (ANLL). For ALL, initial treatment includes prednisone and vincristine. Prophylactic intrathecal methotrexate and cranial radiation prevent central nervous system leukemia. Subsequent systemic therapy is necessary to produce long-term remission. Currently, the most successful treatment regimen for ANLL uses daunorubicin or doxorubicin along with cytosine arabinoside or thioguanine or mercaptopurine. Single agents used to treat ANLL include cytosine arabinoside, hydroxyurea, daunorubicin, and cyclophosphamide. Alternative treatments involve massive leukopheresis and extracorporeal irradiation.

Local irradiation may be used as an adjunct when leukemic cells form tumors in the central nervous system or in other body areas. Administration of platelets and transfusion of packed red blood cells prevent hemorrhagic complications and correct anemia. Bone marrow transplantation and immunotherapy are being used increasingly, but with limited success.

Acute respiratory failure in COPD. Acute deterioration in chronic bronchitis or emphysema associated with respiratory infection or severe atmospheric pollution requires oxygen therapy or mechanical ventilation, endotracheal suctioning, chest physiotherapy, antibiotics, bronchodilators, and perhaps a short-term course of corticosteroids.

Acute transverse myelitis. Although no specific treatment exists for this disorder, corticosteroids may arrest myelitis related to multiple sclerosis. Antibiotics may be necessary for infection and narcotic analgesics for pain control of severe paresthesias. Supportive treatment in quadriplegic patients includes chest physiotherapy, and mechanical ventilation. Other important supportive measures include enteral feedings, parenteral nutrition, and I.V. therapy to maintain adequate nutrition, promote healing, and prevent skin breakdown. Laxatives, stool softeners, and intermittent catheterization may also be necessary.

Acute tubular necrosis. Recognition of contributing factors and prevention of nephrotoxic injury represent the best treatment. Otherwise, treatment is symptomatic. Intravenous hyperalimentation may correct severe catabolic states that accompany this disorder. Diuresis and large volumes of fluids can help flush debris from the kidneys. Dialysis may be necessary during the acute phase.

Adenoid hyperplasia. When chronic infection causes enlarged adenoids, resulting in nasal obstruction, treatment calls for adenoidectomy.

Adenovirus infections. For viral diseases of the respiratory tract, treatment is strictly symptomatic, including rest and increased fluids. Antibiotics treat bacterial complications.

Adrenal crisis. Initially, treatment for this abrupt decrease or total lack of adrenocorticoid hormones includes the administration of I.V. hydrocortisone to begin hormonal replacement. It also involves rapid administration of I.V. fluids to help prevent cardiovascular collapse, along with other antishock measures, such as oxygen and vasopressors. Later, hydrocortisone is given via intermittent I.V. infusion. As the patient's condition improves, oral corticosteroids are used in place of I.V. ones.

Adrenal hypofunction (Addison's disease). This condition requires hormonal replacement with hydrocortisone. If the patient has difficulty retaining sodium, drug therapy includes desoxycorticosterone or fludrocortisone. Supplemental therapy may consist of extra dietary salt or large divided doses of sodium chloride and frequent small feedings of high-carbohydrate, high-protein meals.

Adrenogenital syndrome. For congenital cortisol deficiency, treatment calls for glucocorticoids to suppress ACTH. With 21-hydroxylase deficiency, about 50% of children also need mineralocorticoid replacement. Female children with ambiguous genitalia may require plastic surgery.

In adult females, the syndrome usually relates to excessive androgen production from polycystic ovaries (Stein-Leventhal syndrome). Therapy involves genetic counseling, correction of ovarian problems, and suppression of ACTH with cortisol or prednisone.

Adult respiratory distress syndrome (ARDS). The severe ventilation-perfusion imbalance and decreased lung compliance that characterize ARDS require correction of the underlying cause and severe arterial hypoxemia. Mechanical ventilation with adequate FIO_2 and PEEP is usually necessary to support gas exchange. High-dose corticosteroids may decrease or reverse damage from pulmonary capillary leakage.

Affective disorders. Treatment for a dysfunctional mood disturbance may include lithium, tricyclic antidepressants or monoamine oxidase inhibitors, or antipsychotic agents such as haloperidol. Psychotherapy is also necessary.

Alcoholism. In acute withdrawl, treatment involves I.V. glucose, increased fluids, thiamine, reality orientation, antianxiety agents, anticonvulsants, antiemetics, and antidiarrheals, as needed. Long-term measures include deterrent therapy and supportive counseling.

Allergic purpura. In this nonthrombocytopenic purpura with allergic symptoms, treatment is symptomatic, including corticosteroids to relieve inflammation associated with joint and abdominal pain, dialysis to treat renal failure, and possibly immunosuppressive therapy.

Allergic rhinitis. Primary treatment for allergic rhinitis—the body's response to airborne allergens—calls for identification and avoidance of the allergen. It also includes antihistamines and ephedrine or pseudoephedrine (often used with antihistamines to counteract drowsiness and relieve nasal congestion). Short-term topical or systemic corticosteroid therapy may relieve symptoms of the inflammatory response. Long-term treatment may include desensitization with extracts of the allergen.

Alport's syndrome. Currently, no treatment exists to cure this hereditary kidney disease, which causes nephritis and hearing loss. Dialysis or renal transplantation is usually necessary to treat chronic renal failure. Hearing aids may be used to improve audition.

Alzheimer's disease. No treatment exists for this degenerative neurologic disease. Oral physostigmine, choline, and lecithin produce only transient improvement in memory. Chlorpromazine and haloperidol may control agitation and hallucinations. Support and counseling help family members.

Amebiasis. This protozoal intestinal infection can also produce hepatic abscess and infection of the lungs, pleural cavity, pericardium, and peritoneum. Treatment consists of oral metronidazole for intestinal and extraintestinal sites and diiodohydroxyquin to eliminate intraluminal encysted organisms. Needle aspiration may reduce abscess size. Supportive measures include fluid and electrolyte replacements.

Amenorrhea. The absence of menstruation may result from congenital, structural, or endocrine abnormalities. Treatment relates to the cause, such as decreasing stress or exercise, or taking oral contraceptives to resolve ovarian cysts and restore menstruation.

Amputation. Emergency treatment aims to minimize blood loss and prevent hypovolemic shock. Steps to stem bleeding include application of direct pressure and sometimes cold compresses. Measures to replace fluids include administration of normal saline, crystalloid, and colloid solutions and blood transfusions as needed. Surgery may include microsurgical replantation, reconstruction (if possible), or wound closure to form a stump.

Amyotrophic lateral sclerosis. In this progressive degenerative disorder, supportive therapy may include gastrostomy tube feedings, mechanical ventilation, and drugs, such as atropine, to dry secretions.

Amyloidosis. In this chronic condition, abnormal deposits of amyloid occur in various body tissues. In its secondary form, the condition exists with a degenerative disease, such as tuberculosis or osteomyelitis. Treatment centers on the cause; otherwise, it's mainly supportive. For example, corticosteroids and immunosuppressants reduce inflammation.

Anal fissure. Conservative measures include laxatives, bowel retraining, corticosteroid-containing suppositories, and possibly anal dilation. Surgical removal of the fissure and hemorrhoidectomy may be necessary.

Anaphylaxis. This acute allergic reaction requires immediate treatment with epinephrine to reverse the effects of massive histamine release. In an especially severe reaction, oxygen therapy and endotracheal intubation may be necessary to combat progressive hypoxia, and aminophylline to relieve bronchospasm. Persistent respiratory distress requires I.V. corticosteroids. Antihistamines relieve urticaria.

Angioedema. Treatment aims to eliminate contact with trigger factors or, if this is impossible, to desensitize the patient to them and to relieve symptoms with oral corticosteroids. In acute laryngeal angioedema, epinephrine should be given subcutaneously along with supplemental oxygen. Tracheostomy may be necessary.

Ankylosing spondylitis. Characterized by inflammation of the cartilaginous joints between the vertebral bodies and of the spinal gliding joints, this disorder usually progresses upward from the lumbar vertebrae. Therapy aims to help the patient maintain an erect posture. It includes periodic rest on a flat surface, avoidance of muscle strain and fatigue, physical therapy with emphasis on postural and breathing exercises, analgesics, and nonsteroidal anti-inflammatory drugs. If conservative measures fail, wedge osteotomy removes part of the vertebrae.

Anorectal abscess and fistula. This localized infection in the pararectal spaces typically leads to fistula development. Sitz baths and analgesics relieve discomfort. Surgery involves incision and drainage of the abscess and excision of a fistula. Antibiotics treat infection.

Anorectal strictures. Resulting from intraluminal inflammation caused by ulcerative colitis, Crohn's disease, or radiation therapy, most strictures resolve once the local inflammation subsides. Treatment consists of anti-inflammatory drugs, such as sulfasalazine and adrenal corticosteroids. Permanent strictures, which result from scarring, may require surgical dilation or dissection.

Anxiety disorders. Treatment may include psychotherapy, behavior therapy, milieu therapy, or drug therapy with anxiolytics, such as chlordiazepoxide.

Aplastic or hypoplastic anemias. Resulting from congenital or acquired bone marrow failure, aplastic anemia requires bone marrow transplant, if severe. Prednisone may treat moderate cases (because of an immunosuppressive effect on the toxin that destroys the bone marrow cells), and androgen therapy is used for a mild form. To minimize infection and hemorrhage, therapy may also consist of isolation, blood transfusions, and avoidance of invasive procedures.

Appendicitis. In acute appendicitis, prompt appendectomy is necessary. A perforated appendix requires surgical drainage and removal followed by antibiotic therapy.

Arnold-Chiari syndrome. Treatment for this congenital deformity may include surgical placement of a shunt, upper cervical laminectomy, and enlargement of the foramen magnum to provide symptomatic relief and possibly arrest progression of the anomaly. It also involves surgical release of adhesions to relieve tethering of the spinal cord and prevent cranial nerve involvement.

Arousal dysfunction. Stemming from a variety of causes, inhibited sexual desire requires professional counseling. Such treatment generally includes sex education, anxiety reduction, enhancement of communication skills, and sensate focus exercises.

Arterial occlusive disease. The sudden interruption of arterial blood flow, resulting from embolism, thrombosis, or injury, necessitates immediate embolectomy, thrombectomy, or bypass grafting if it threatens a limb. In arterial occlusion caused by an embolism, long-term warfarin therapy may be necessary.

Ascariasis. This helminthic infection of the small intestine responds to mebendazole.

Aspergillosis. If invasive, this disorder requires I.V. amphotericin B, sometimes combined with rifampin or flucytosine. Allergic aspergillosis requires desensitization and corticosteroids. In the pulmonary form, local excision of the lesion is necessary if hemoptysis occurs.

Asthma. Management of chronic asthma includes avoidance of causative factors and drug therapy to promote immediate relief during attacks and long-term bronchial relaxation. In acute attacks, treatment consists of inhaled $beta_2$-selective agonists followed by a continuous I.V. infusion of aminophylline. If the patient doesn't respond, I.V. steroids may be added. Long-term therapy includes theophylline compounds and $beta_2$-adrenergic inhalers or oral preparations.

Atelectasis. Bronchiole blockage may cause alveolar collapse leading to hypoxemia. Treatment includes coughing and deep-breathing exercises, incentive spirometry, and intermittent positive-pressure breathing treatments or, if necessary, a continuous positive airway pressure using a mask.

Atherosclerosis. Treatment aims to control hyperlipidemia and hypertension and to identify and remove risk factors through patient education. Currently, no specific treatment exists to cure this disorder or reverse its effects.

Atopic dermatitis. Characterized by intense itching and cutaneous changes, this disorder requires the identification, elimination, and avoidance of any allergens or irritants. High doses of antihistamines, cool compresses, and medicated tub baths may relieve pruritus. Topical corticosteroids treat inflammation.

Ataxia-telangiectasia. No treatment exists for the progressively severe ataxia and frequent sino-pulmonary and other infections in this disorder. Bone marrow transplantation has been tried. Therapy aims to prevent respiratory infection.

Atrial fibrillation. When decompensation occurs, cardioversion can convert atrial fibrillation to sinus rhythm. Quinidine and procainamide can also convert the arrhythmia but may facilitate atrioventricular nodal conduction and increase the ventricular rate.

In *paroxysmal atrial fibrillation*, treatment focuses on controlling the ventricular rate while waiting for the paroxysm to reverse spontaneously. Cardiac glycosides, beta-adrenergic blockers, and verapamil generally increase atrioventricular nodal refractoriness and slow the ventricular rate. As soon as a sinus rhythm is obtained, cardiac glycosides or beta-adrenergic blockers can maintain the ventricular rate.

Atrial flutter. Cardioversion may correct this arrhythmia. Type I antiarrhythmic drugs may also correct it, but these drugs may raise the ventricular rate. Cardiac glycosides, quinidine, or procainamide may control the ventricular rate and prevent recurrent atrial flutter.

Atrial septal defect. Surgical correction of this congenital anomaly is recommended for children aged 3 to 6 with uncomplicated disease who exhibit shunting, but it's not advised for patients with small defects and trivial left-to-right shunts or severe pulmonary vascular disease. Conservative measures include antiarrythmic drugs and treatment of respiratory infection and heart failure. Prophylactic antibiotics are necessary before dental procedures.

Attention deficit disorder. Treatment may include psychotherapy, special education, and drug therapy with cerebral stimulants, such as dextroamphetamine and methylphenidate.

B

Bell's palsy. Treatment of this facial palsy includes massage and electrotherapy to stimulate muscle activity and warm, moist compresses to relieve pain. A facial sling may prevent muscle stretching.

Benign prostatic hyperplasia. Characterized by urinary retention and chronic cystitis, this disorder may be initially treated with catheterization and antibiotics. The treatment of choice, however, is transurethral resection of the prostate (TURP). Perineal, suprapubic, or retropubic prostatectomy may be necessary if TURP can't be performed.

Berlock dermatitis. No treatment exists for this secondary reaction to photosensitization by furocoumarins present in many perfumes. To prevent this reaction, the patient must avoid prolonged exposure to the irritant.

Biliary cirrhosis. *Primary cirrhosis*, which results from chronic inflammation, requires systemic corticosteroids, androgens, and antihistamines to relieve pruritus; a reduction in long-chain dietary triglycerides to combat steatorrhea; a sodium-free diet and diuretics to combat ascites and edema; and fat-soluble vitamins to correct deficiencies. In *secondary cirrhosis*, surgery removes any mechanical obstruction that impairs biliary flow.

Bladder cancer. Treatment includes interstitial installation of chemotherapy, cystectomy, and radiation. Urothelial tumors of renal pelvis and ureters may need nephroureterocystectomy.

Blepharitis. Inflammation of the eyelid margins requires local antibiotics, such as sulfacetamide, gentamicin, or bacitracin. Corticosteroids decrease inflammation, and a 0.1% selenium sulfide solution or diluted baby shampoo can be used to clean the eyelids.

Blood transfusion reaction. An *immune reaction*, caused by hemolysis, may be intravascular or extravascular. Intravascular hemolysis requires immediate treatment with an osmotic diuretic, low-dose dopamine to support renal perfusion; volume expanders, such as 5% albumin, to correct shock; vasopressors to maintain blood pressure; placement in Trendelenburg's position; and platelet concentrates and fresh-frozen plasma to treat disseminated intravascular coagulation. Extravascular hemolysis requires avoiding additional tranfusions. Other immune reactions, such as febrile and allergic ones, require antipyretics or antihistamines.

A *nonimmune reaction* may stem from circulatory overload, massive tranfusion, infection, metabolic shock, embolism, or thrombophlebitis. Circulatory overload requires treatment with diuretics, such as mannitol. Some complications of massive transfusions may be avoided by giving platelet concentrates or fresh-frozen plasma with packed red blood cells. Calcium supplements may also be necessary.

Bone cancer. Treatment for *multiple myeloma*, the most common bone cancer, consists of radiation therapy and intermittent courses of vincristine, cyclophosphamide, and prednisone. In *osteogenic sarcomas*, amputation and radiation are the treatments of choice. Chemotherapy may also include doxorubicin, dactinomycin, high-dose methotrexate, or vincristine to re-duce the growth rate of tumor cells. In *chondrosarcomas*, radical excision is necessary. *Metastatic tumors* usually require palliative treatment, and local radiation and levodopa treat bone pain.

Botulism. Resulting from ingestion of food contaminated by a toxin produced by *Clostridium botulinum*, botulism requires administration of trivalent A, B, or E antitoxin (if the type is unknown) or U type specific antitoxin (if the type is known). Keep emergency airway equipment available in case the patient has respiratory difficulty. *Infant botulism* requires only symptomatic treatment since the botulinum antitoxin may cause anaphylaxis.

Brain abscess. Typically associated with ear or sinus infections, metastatic disease, osteomyelitis, endocarditis, or abscessed teeth, brain abscess calls for antibiotic therapy with penicillin G and chloramphenicol. Treatment also includes mannitol followed by dexamethasone to reduce intracranial pressure and anticonvulsants to prevent seizures. Surgical aspiration or drainage of the abscess may be needed if the lesion doesn't improve with antimicrobial therapy or if intracranial pressure increases despite treatment.

Breast cancer. Modified radical or total mastectomy removes primary tumors; modified radical mastectomy removes breast tissue with axillary dissection performed en bloc; total mastectomy removes the entire breast without any nodal resection; segmental mastectomy, tylectomy, and quadrantectomy are usually reserved for tumors less than 2 cm without apparent nodal involvement.

Nonsurgical measures include radiation therapy and adjunctive chemotherapy (commonly cyclophosphamide, methotrexate, and fluorouracil). If breast cancer has metastasized, single agents, such as fluorouracil, methotrexate, doxorubicin, or cyclophosphamide, may be used, but combination chemotherapy remains the treatment of choice. Hormonal therapy aims to decrease levels of estrogen and its precursors. Other treatments include administration of tamoxifen or diethylstilbestrol, adrenalectomy, or hypophysectomy.

Breast engorgement. To encourage the let-down reflex, breast massage and oxytocin nasal spray may be used. Nursing mothers may use hot packs or a hot shower to promote milk flow; bottlefeeding mothers should avoid heat. Comfort measures include ice packs applied between nursing periods, a good supportive bra with cotton straps, and analgesics, such as aspirin, acetaminophen, or codeine.

Bronchopulmonary fistula. This disorder most commonly results from high peak inspiratory pressures during mechanical ventilation, causing leakage of inspired air into the pleural space. Treatment requires chest tubes with an underwater seal and suction to remove air from the pleural space. Decreasing peak inspiratory pressures also promotes healing.

Bronchiectasis. Commonly caused by bacterial infection, bronchiectasis requires antibiotics. Complications may be minimized by chest physiotherapy and elimination of bronchial irritants, such as cigarette smoke. Surgical resection is necessary only for unresponsive localized lesions or extreme debilitation.

Brucellosis. Treatment of choice for this gram-negative infection includes oral tetracycline, I.M. streptomycin, and a high-calorie, high-protein diet.

Buerger's disease. Because tobacco chewing or smoking causes this disease, the only successful treatment is total abstinence from tobacco.

Burns. Treatment for minor burns may include oral fluids, analgesics, regular cleansing, topical drugs, and sterile dressings. Severe burns require immediate fluid replacement and prevention of infection with biological dressings and topical anti-infectives. Stabilization of the patient is the first priority, with subsequent skin grafting.

Bursitis. Local application of heat, immobilization, salicylates, nonsteroidal anti-inflammatory drugs, and intraarticular injections of corticosteroids relieve pain and inflammation. Occasionally, bursa aspiration may be used to reduce pain.

C

Candidiasis. Treatment includes topical nystatin for mucocutaneous infections, clotrimazole and miconazole for vaginal and other mucous membrane infections, and I.V. amphotericin B for invasive candidiasis. In severe infection, flucytosine may also be given.

Carbunculosis. In this disorder, painful, deep abscesses drain onto the skin surface, usually around several hair follicles. Treatment calls for a systemic antibiotic, such as oxacillin, or incision and drainage of lesions followed by application of a topical antibiotic.

Cardiac contusion. Commonly resulting from trauma, a nonpenetrating injury to the myocardial tissue may rupture valvular structures, atria, or ventricles, and cause pericardial effusion. Treatment depends on the area and extent of involvement. Valve rupture, for instance, requires surgical correction.

Cardiac tamponade. In this life-threatening condition, pericardiocentesis removes accumulated blood, thereby lowering intrapericardial pressure.

Cardiogenic shock. Resulting from any condition that significantly impairs left ventricular function and lowers cardiac output, cardiogenic shock requires constant monitoring of arterial pressure, pulmonary capillary wedge pressure, and cardiac output. It also requires oxygen therapy to minimize hypoxemia. Drug therapy may include cautious use of narcotics and vasopressors to relieve pain and maintain coronary perfusion. An intraaortic balloon pump may need to be inserted to promote effective pumping and decrease cardiac workload. Fluid replacement may be necessary to correct hypovolemia.

Carpal tunnel syndrome. Initial measures include shaking the hands, immersing them in warm water, or splinting the hand and forearm nightly to relieve pain. Local corticosteroid injection may also help. When conservative measures fail, surgical decompression of the nerve becomes necessary.

Cataracts. *Acquired* cataracts require surgical extraction of the entire lens including the capsule (intracapsular) or extraction of the anterior capsule, nucleus, and cortex with retention of the posterior capsule (extracapsular). After surgery, the patient may need contact lenses or an intraocular lens implant to correct optical changes that occur with surgery. *Congenital* cataracts require immediate surgical removal of the anterior lens and lens cortex. Extended-wear contact lenses are usually required after surgery.

Celiac disease. To correct this disease, all gluten and wheat must be eliminated for several months. Adjunctive therapy includes vitamin supplements.

Cellulitis. Treatment for mild, early cellulitis caused by *Streptococcus* consists of penicillin G. Treatment for staphylococcal infections includes a penicillinase-resistant penicillin, such as oral oxacillin. For severe infections, treatment calls for a penicillinase-resistant penicillin, such as nafcillin I.V. Supportive care includes immobilization of the affected area and warm soaks to localize the infection.

Central sleep apnea. With cessation of respiratory effort and lack of air flow, treatment involves drug therapy with medroxyprogesterone and protriptyline, a nonsedating tricyclic antidepressant. Tracheostomy and nightly mechanical ventilation may be necessary if patients don't respond to medication. Weight loss is important for obese patients.

Cerebral aneurysm. Usually, surgical repair by ligation, clipping, or reinforcement with synthetic material or donor muscle should take place before the risk of rebleed and vasospasm occurs (about 7 days after the initial bleed). However, if surgery isn't possible, the patient should remain on bed rest, avoid stimulants and sources of stress, receive nonnarcotic analgesics, and maintain fluid balance. Treatment may also include calcium-channel blockers to prevent vasospasm, a fibrinolytic inhibitor to prevent hemorrhage from the aneurysm, and an anticonvulsant to prevent seizures.

Cerebral contusion. Usually resulting from a traumatic blow to the head, a cerebral contusion causes temporary cerebral dysfunction and petechial hemorrhage. Conservative treatment includes strict fluid control, nonnarcotic analgesics, and proper oxygenation. If the patient's intracranial pressure rises, hyperventilation and osmotic diuretics, dexamethasone, and anticonvulsants become necessary.

Cerebral palsy. This nonprogressive disease has no cure. Symptomatic treatments include stereotactic thalomotomy, implantation of cerebellar stimulators, peripheral nerve block, and orthopedic surgery to correct contractures. Supportive measures include braces for the extremities, frequent range-of-motion exercises and position changes, and good nutrition.

Cerebrovascular accident (CVA). Caused by an interruption of the oxygen supply to the brain, a CVA requires treatment to restore and maintain cerebral perfusion and prevent complications. The three most common types are thrombotic, embolic, and hemorrhagic. An evolving CVA may be arrested by continuous heparin infusion. Thromboendarterectomy, bypass graft, or long-term warfarin or antiplatelet therapy may be necessary.

Treatment for embolic CVA includes long-term anticoagulant therapy, correction of the underlying cause, and sometimes embolectomy. Hemorrhagic CVA and complications of thrombotic and embolic CVA require dexamethasone and mannitol, fluid restrictions, and careful positioning to minimize cerebral edema and control blood pressure.

Physical therapy and rehabilitation should begin immediately with passive range-of-motion exercises for paralyzed limbs, mobilization to prevent respiratory and skin complications, and speech therapy for aphasia or swallowing defects.

Cervical cancer. Successful treatment hinges on accurate clinical staging. Primary measures include surgical removal of tumors and local radiation therapy.

Chalazion. If asymptomatic, this cyst of the eyelid usually resolves spontaneously. Treatment for swelling and inflammation includes hot compresses and a topical antibiotic or sufonamide. If persistent or large, chalazia may require excision.

Chancroid. The treatment of choice for this sexually transmitted bacterial infection is a long-acting sulfonamide, such as sulfamethoxazole, and oral trimethoprim.

Chediak-Higashi syndrome. Currently, no specific therapy exists for this rare autosomal recessive childhood disorder. An accelerated phase of the disease, with lymphohistiocytic infiltration of multiple tissues, may be treated with corticosteroids and vincristine to retard organ infiltration by the lymphohistiocytes.

Chlamydial infections. These sexually transmitted genital infections require tetracycline or erythromycin.

Cholangitis. Bacterial infection of the bile duct responds to antibiotics. However, if pus and inflammatory debris obstruct the bile duct, immediate surgical correction and drainage are necessary.

Cholecystitis. In acute cholecystitis, cholecystectomy is mandatory. Before surgery, management includes the use of pain medications, such as meperidine or pentazocine; antibiotic therapy with ampicillin, cephalosporins, chloramphenicol, or aminoglycosides; and elimination of oral intake.

Choledocholithiasis. Treatment depends on the severity of symptoms but most often involves surgical removal of the gallstones.

Cholelithiasis. Cholecystectomy is necessary if the patient is symptomatic or suffering from complications of gallstone disease. Alternatively, chenodiol or ursodeoxycholic acid may be given to dissolve the gallstones.

Cholera. In this acute enteric disease, the sudden onset of profuse watery stools, vomiting, rapid dehydration, and circulatory collapse requires rapid fluid replacement to correct dehydration and electrolyte imbalance—oral if the patient is conscious, or I.V. if the patient is unable to take oral solutions. To treat the infection, tetracycline is the antibiotic of choice. In pregnancy, ampicillin is used in its place.

Choriocarcinoma. This highly malignant trophoblastic neoplasm responds to methotrexate and actinomycin D, which may be used alone or with radiation therapy.

Chronic granulocytic leukemia (CGL). Treatment consists of oral busulfan, cyclophosphamide, and phenylalanine mustard. Splenic irradiation has also been employed. Hydroxyurea may prevent evolution to the blastic phase. Although the blastic phase is refractory to most treatments, vincristine and prednisone may help achieve remission.

Chronic granulomatous disease. Antibiotics treat this inherited neutrophil defect. Prophylactic antibiotics may be successful but their use increases the risk of superinfections and the emergence of resistant organisms.

Chronic lymphocytic leukemia (CLL). Treatment is reserved for advanced disease with symptomatic lymphadenopathy, splenomegaly, or hematopoietic dysfunction. It may include lymph node or splenic irradiation and administration of chlorambucil or cyclophosphamide. Corticosteroids treat the autoimmune complications of CLL.

Chronic mucocutaneous candidiasis. These chronic, superficial candidal infections resist treatment, requiring correction, if possible, of immunologic defects or any predisposing factors. Topical antifungals include nystatin suspension, gentian violet, or amphotericin B rinses for oral lesions; imidazole creams or tablets for vulvovaginitis; and topical amphotericin B, imidazole, or nystatin powder for intertriginous areas.

Chronic obstructive pulmonary disease (COPD). In their early stages, these obstructive disorders (chronic bronchitis and emphysema) require elimination of contributing factors, such as smoking, air pollution, and infection, to decrease disease progression. Other measures include yearly vaccination against influenza and a pneumoccocal polysaccharide vaccination as indicated.

In patients with hypersecretion, chest physiotherapy is necessary. Drug therapy includes bronchodilators, such as theophylline and isoproterenol, and antibiotics to treat underlying infection. Pulmonary rehabilitation to improve self-care skills and exercise tolerance is essential.

Cirrhosis. Characterized by necrosis and fibrotic regeneration of hepatic cells, this disorder requires dietary therapy compatible with the patient's ability to metabolize protein, vitamin therapy to replace vitamins A, B complex, D, and K, and the administration of bile salts to facilitate absorption of these vitamins. Treatment also includes adequate rest, moderate exercise, removal of any toxins from the environment, and protection from infection. Alcohol is strictly prohibited.

Cleft lip and palate. A common congenital deformity, cleft lip and palate require surgical correction, but the timing varies depending on the type and severity of the deformity. Reconstruction may occur in stages.

Club foot. Early treatment is most successful. Ideally, serial corrective casts should be started in the first 2 to 3 days of life to maintain the foot in a more normal position. If casting is unsuccessful, surgical release of soft tissue on the posterior and medial aspects of the foot and ankle may be necessary.

Coarctation of the aorta. If uncomplicated, coarctation can be corrected surgically between ages 3 and 6. Such correction may involve resection and end-to-end anastomosis or subclavian flap angioplasty. A tubular graft or patch may be used for a lengthy constriction.

Coccidioidomycosis. Usually mild, this systemic fungal disease requires only bed rest and symptomatic treatment. Severe infection, though, requires I.V. amphotericin B.

Colorado tick fever. Tick removal and acetaminophen constitute treatment.

Colorectal cancer. The most effective treatment is surgical removal of the tumor, adjacent tissues, and any lymph nodes that may contain cancer cells. Preoperative radiation therapy may shrink the tumor and prevent metastases; fluorouracil may be used to treat liver metastases.

Common cold. Treatment, of course, is symptomatic, including rest, fluids, and analgesics. Decongestants and throat lozenges may also be used, but antibiotics are reserved for bacterial complications, such as pneumonia, sinusitis, and otitis.

Common variable immune deficiency. Treatment for this acquired agammaglobulinemia may include metronidazole, corticosteroids, and immunoglobulin replacement. Spruelike syndrome, a frequent complication, may require a gluten-free or lactose-free diet.

Compartment syndrome. Early treatment includes elevation of the extremity, application of cold packs, and administration of analgesics. Fasciotomy performed within 30 minutes of the onset of elevated pressure allows swelling without compression.

Complement deficiencies. Therapy for complement deficiencies aims to correct associated disorders since the deficiencies themselves have no known cure.

Congenital anomalies of the bladder, ureter, and urethra. *Partial or complete duplication of one or both ureters*, the most common ureteral anomaly, may need no treatment. In *ectopic ureteral orifice*, treatment includes ureteral replantation and nephroureterectomy. *Extrophy of the bladder* requires total bladder reconstruction. Often present with bladder extrophy, *epispadias* (with the urethral opening proximal to the glans on the dorsum of the penis) requires surgical repair during bladder reconstruction or later. Persistent *urachus*, another anomaly associated with the bladder, requires excision. Treatment for *posterior urethral valves*, an obstructive condition, involves valve destruction. *Hypospadias* (a disorder of the urethral meatus), *chordee* (dorsal curvature of the penis), and an *incompetent urinary sphincter* all require surgical repair. Eventually, a urinary diversion may be necessary if attempts to correct incontinence are unsuccessful.

Congenital hip dysplasia. Treatment depends on the severity and duration of the dislocation. For infants younger than 3 months, it may consist of reduction and manipulation of the dislocation followed by holding the legs in abduction with double diapers or a splint-brace or harness to maintain reduction. For infants older than 3 months, closed reduction or bilateral skin traction may be needed to reduce the dislocation, followed by the use of a hip spica cast, splint, or brace to maintain the reduction. If conservative treatment fails, surgery involves open reduction and insertion of the femoral head into the acetabulum.

Congestive cardiomyopathy. Characterized by impaired systolic function, cardiomegaly, and congestive heart failure, congestive cardiomyopathy requires treatment with anticoagulants to decrease the risk of systemic embolization associated with this disorder. Limited activity, sodium restriction, diuretics, digitalis, and vasodilators may provide symptomatic relief in heart failure.

Antiarrhythmic agents, a permanent pacemaker, or a heart transplant may be necessary.

Congestive heart failure. Control of congestive heart failure involves reducing cardiac work load, enhancing cardiac contractility, and decreasing sodium and fluid retention. To reduce cardiac work load, treatment calls for reduced activity, rest, and administration of vasodilators. Digitalis strengthens myocardial contractility, leading to increased cardiac output, and dietary therapy and diuretics reduce excess fluid and sodium retention.

Conjunctivitis. For bacterial conjunctivitis, treatment may include topical agents, such as sulfacetamide, sulfisoxazole, erythromycin, or gentamicin, or systemic penicillin G or erythromycin. For conjunctivitis caused by irritation, treatment includes removal of irritants, such as contact lenses, medications, or dust.

Contact dermatitis. Allergic contact dermatitis represents a T-lymphocyte reaction, resulting in an eczematous reaction: erythema, edema, vesiculation, stinging, and pruritus. Effective treatment calls for identification and avoidance of the irritant or allergen and use of calamine lotion or medicated baths to help alleviate pruritus and promote the drying of lesions. Treatment also includes systemic antihistamines if pruritus is severe, topical or systemic corticosteroids, and application of Burow's solution for any secondary infection.

Copper deficiency anemia. Usually a secondary condition, this rare disorder requires I.V. replacement with copper sulfate, a well-balanced, high-copper diet, and supportive measures.

Corneal abrasion. Treatment involves eye irrigation with saline solution, local antibiotics, and avoidance of contact lens use. Artificial tears may relieve symptoms and reduce redness.

Corneal ulcer. Treatment may involve local antibiotics and atropine. Hot compresses decrease swelling, pain, and inflammation, and cortisone reduces inflammation. Antivirals are used for herpes simplex infection. If the ulcer impairs vision, a corneal transplant may be necessary.

Corns and calluses of the foot. Relief requires surgical paring of the lesion followed by intermittent debridement, using a 40% salicylic acid plaster. Intralesional steroids may reduce inflammation.

Coronary artery disease. Besides modification of risk factors, treatment includes symptomatic control with nitrates, beta-adrenergic blockers, and calcium channel blockers. If drug therapy proves ineffective, coronary artery bypass grafting or percutaneous transluminal coronary angioplasty may be necessary to prevent myocardial infarction.

Coronary artery spasm. Recognized as a causative factor in both angina pectoris and MI, coronary artery spasm may respond to calcium channel blockers, such as verapamil.

Cor pulmonale. Oxygen therapy is the primary treatment for the right ventricular hypertrophy associated with pulmonary hypertension. This relieves vasoconstriction that results from hypoxia. Symptomatic treatment includes diuretics and adequate ventilation to reverse the acidosis of CO_2 retention. Digoxin may treat arrhythmias, such as atrial fibrillation.

Corrosive esophagitis and stricture. Ingestion of a caustic substance, such as a strong alkali, may cause inflammation and infection of the esophagus followed by the development of strictures. Treatment for strictures involves passing a bougie into the esophagus to dilate it. If this is unsuccessful, surgical resection or bypass of the stricture may be necessary. If esophageal damage is extensive, gastrostomy may be necessary.

Crohn's disease. In this chronic intestinal inflammation, treatment involves sulfasalazine and corticosteroids to decrease inflammation. A low-residue diet with medium-chain triglycerides combats nutritional problems. Surgical resection is used for complications, such as bowel narrowing or obstruction.

Croup. This inflammation of the larynx and trachea requires treatment with cool mist, systemic hydration, and cough suppressants. Oxygen therapy and racemic epinephrine may also be necessary.

Cryptococcosis. This systemic fungal infection requires I.V. miconazole if it invades the meninges. I.V. amphotericin B and oral flucytosine represent an alternative treatment.

Cushing's disease. Treatment includes irradiation of the pituitary; partial destruction of the pituitary through cryotherapy, yttrium implant, or proton beams; or removal of pituitary microadenomas. If these measures fail, bilateral adrenalectomy is necessary, followed by lifelong hormonal replacement therapy.

Cutaneous larva migrans. Mild infection by the larvae of nematode parasites or hookworms responds to topical thiabendazole (2%) in dimethyl sulfoxide. More severe infestations require oral thiabendazole.

Cystic fibrosis. This severe hereditary lung disease requires daily chest physiotherapy and adequate hydration to prevent secondary respiratory complications that may lead to hypoxemia, pulmonary hypertension, and cor pulmonale. Antibiotics treat pulmonary infections, and bronchodilators relieve bronchospasm.

Cystinuria. An abnormally high urine concentration of cystine may cause mild cystinuria associated with calcium oxalate stones. This form of cystinuria requires increased fluids to maintain a 24-hour urine output of 3,000 ml and an alkaline ash diet (high in vegetables and fruits and low in protein) to produce an alkaline urine. A more severe form of cystinuria, associated with cystine stones, causes excretion of 5 to 10 times the normal amount of cystine in the urine. Initial treatment resembles that for the milder form of the disease but may also include cystine-binding drugs.

Cytomegalovirus infection. This viral disease can occur in the perinatal period, causing brain damage or death. No specific treatment exists, apart from symptomatic measures for fever, pain, and seizures.

D
Dacryocystitis. Acute inflammation of the lacrimal sac responds to local hot compresses and systemic antibiotics, such as erythromycin. Formation of an abscess requires incision and drainage.

Chronic dacryocystitis in infants calls for daily massage of the lacrimal sac and instillation of sulfacetamide. In children older than 6 months or in adults, probing of the lacrimal duct and passages may correct the obstruction. When probing is unsuccessful, dacryocystorhinostomy creates a connection between the lacrimal sac and the nose.

Decompression sickness. Also called "the bends," this painful condition results from an overly rapid change from high atmospheric pressures to low ones. It requires supportive measures, recompression, and administration of oxygen in a hyperbaric chamber.

Decubitus ulcer. Common treatments include pressure relief devices; topical applications, such as monosaccharides or heavy metal ions, antibiotic ointments, emollients, or hydrophilic absorption beads; biosynthetic dressings, such as Op-Site, Duoderm, or Vigilon; and nutritional support. Large areas of necrotic tissue, or eschar, require debridement. Hyperbaric oxygenation is currently undergoing clinical trials. Prevention and early detection remain the preferred defense.

Dermatitis. Treatment for chronic dermatitis includes elimination of known allergens and decreased exposure to irritants. It also involves topical corticosteroids, antihistamines, and emollients. If blisters form, Burow's solution provides mild antibacterial action. Secondary infection requires systemic antibiotics.

Dermatomyositis. Supportive treatment includes high doses of a corticosteroid, such as methylprednisolone, and sometimes salicylates.

Dermatophytosis. Typically affecting the feet, groin, body, and scalp, minor ringworm lesions usually respond to exposure to the air and to topical antifungal agents, such as miconazole and clotrimazole. Systemic treatment with an antifungal-antibiotic agent, such as griseofulvin, may also be necessary.

Diabetes insipidus. Typically, this disorder requires S.C. or I.M. administration of vasopressin. Mild forms may respond to lypressin nasal spray. Chronic forms may need desmopressin acetate nasal spray.

Diabetes mellitus. For the *Type I* (insulin-dependent) patient, dietary therapy and insulin help regulate blood glucose levels. Rapid, intermediate, or long-acting insulins may be combined and given three or four times daily by S.C. injection, or continuous subcutaneous infusion may be used. For the *Type II* (non-insulin-dependent) patient, controlled caloric intake and weight loss may help control blood glucose levels. If dietary therapy alone doesn't work, an oral hypoglycemic drug may be added to encourage the body's own insulin production and increase glucose metabolism. In periods of illness or severe stress, the Type II diabetic may also need insulin.

DiGeorge's syndrome. Treatment includes a fetal thymus transplant, calcium administration with vitamin D or parathyroid hormone to control hypocalcemia, and surgical correction of congenital heart disease.

Diphtheria. Standard treatment includes diphtheria antitoxin (preceded by tests for hypersensitivity) and isolation if the patient is hospitalized. For adults, additional measures include I.M. penicillin G procaine or oral erythromycin, bed rest, maintenance of fluid and electrolyte balance, and monitoring for cardiac or neurologic complications.

Discoid lupus erythematosus (DLE). Some patients with this cutaneous form of systemic lupus erythematosus respond to antimalarials. Other measures include sunscreens to prevent rashes and topical, intralesional, and systemic glucocorticoids to treat them.

Dislocations and subluxations. Treatment varies with the severity of injury. A closed reduction may restore joint integrity. It's usually followed by joint immobilization with a sling or an elastic wrap. Analgesics may also be necessary.

Disseminated intravascular coagulation. Treatment aims to correct the underlying cause. It also includes administration of cryoprecipitate and fresh-frozen plasma to replace clotting factors and platelet transfusions to correct thrombocytopenia. Heparin therapy is controversial since it may increase the bleeding tendency.

Diverticular disease. In symptomatic diverticular disease without diverticulitis, treatment consists of a high-residue diet, bulk laxatives such as psyllium extract, mild sedatives, and anticholinergics to reduce sigmoid irritability. Diverticulitis requires a clear liquid diet, stool softeners, broad-spectrum antibiotics, and bed rest when perforation isn't a threat. Severe attacks require antibiotics and a temporary colostomy, followed later by an anastomosis.

Drug dependence. Acute drug intoxication requires symptomatic treatment, including fluid replacement, nutritional supplements, sedatives, anticholinergics, antidiarrheals, antianxiety agents, and use of detoxification agents specific to the abused drug. For example, methadone may be substituted for an abused opioid.
    To ease withdrawal, such measures as psychotherapy, exercise, relaxation, and nutritional support may be necessary. For opioid abusers, naltrexone and a support group, such as Narcotics Anonymous, may help users abstain.

Dysfunctional uterine bleeding. Small doses of estrogen given around the time of ovulation may prevent spotting. D & C or hormonal therapy treats endometrial hyperplasia; a progestational drug, such as medroxyprogesterone, used during the last part of the menstrual cycle, may regulate endometrial breakdown and control bleeding. Acute bleeding may require an oral contraceptive.

Dysmenorrhea. In the absence of pelvic pathology, treatment for primary dysmenorrhea (from an unknown cause) consists of mild analgesics—such as aspirin, nonsteroidal anti-inflammatory drugs, or oral contraceptives—which suppress ovulation. Secondary dysmenorrhea requires treatment for the underlying pathology.

Dyspareunia. If painful intercourse stems from a physical cause, treatment may include use of a water-soluble lubricant to relieve vaginal dryness and discontinuation of foams, creams, or jellies that cause irritation. Sex therapy is recommended for psychological causes.

E

Ear canal benign tumor. If growths interfere with hearing, they usually require surgical removal.

Eating disorders. In disorders such as anorexia nervosa and bulimia, dehydration and malnutrition require treatment. The patient's self-image may improve with behavior therapy and individual or family psychotherapy.

Ectopic pregnancy. Treatment aims to prevent shock and establish homeostasis. Usually, a laparotomy and salpingectomy are necessary to control hemorrhage and remove the involved fallopian tube and occasionally the ovary. (To preserve fertility, the tube may be left in place.) Antibiotics help treat septic infection.

Electric shock. Your first priority: separating the victim from the current source. If the electricity can't be turned off, pull the victim free from the wire with a nonconductive device (a dry, nonmetallic belt; a rope; or a loop of dry cloth or rubber). Don't touch him until after breaking contact with the electric current.
    Emergency measures include cardiopulmonary resuscitation, defibrillation, and I.V. administration of lactated Ringer's solution to maintain urine output of 50 to 100 ml/hr and mannitol to prevent renal shutdown. Burns and fractures require treatment as necessary.

Empyema. In pleural empyema, treatment consists of high doses of parenteral antibiotics and drainage of the pleural space.

Encephalitis. The antiviral agent vidarabine effectively treats herpes simplex encephalitis. Treatment of other forms is entirely supportive, including anticonvulsants to prevent seizures, dexamethasone to decrease cerebral edema, and I.V. fluids to maintain fluid and electrolyte balance.

Encephalocele. Protrusion of the brain through a congenital defect in the skull requires surgical removal.

Endocarditis. Treating this microbial infection of the heart's inner lining requires early antibiotic therapy. Otherwise, repair or replacement of the affected valve may be necessary.

Endometriosis. Treatment varies with the severity of symptoms and the patient's feelings about childbearing. An asymptomatic patient who doesn't wish to become pregnant requires only periodic observation. A patient with mild pain and the capacity to become pregnant may require analgesics. However, if she has severe pain and can postpone pregnancy, treatment may call for hormones such as danazol. High-dose oral contraceptives may also be prescribed to shrink endometrial tissue. Severe disease requires excision of endometrial implants or, if childbearing isn't a consideration, hysterectomy with bilateral salpingo-oophorectomy.

Enterobacterial infections. *E. enterobacter* usually responds to carbenicillin, piperacillin, ticarcillin, cefoxitin, moxalactam, tobramycin, amikacin, and methenamine. However, parenteral gentamicin is usually the drug of choice.

Enterobiasis. Pinworm disease requires treatment with oral pyrantel or mebendazole, examination of family members for signs of infestation, daily changes and careful washing of bed linen and underwear, and daily vacuuming of living areas for several days after treatment's start.

Epicondylitis (tennis elbow). Symptomatic treatment consists of complete rest of the affected joint, analgesics for pain, corticosteroid injections for acute exacerbations and, after activity, the use of ice packs.

Epidermolysis bullosa. Treatment aims to reduce or prevent even slight trauma, which produces blisters. This involves careful selection of clothing, especially shoes, to avoid shearing or trauma. When blisters develop, saline soaks along with topical antibiotics or corticosteroids may aid healing and prevent infection. Systemic corticosteroids can sometimes be used to reduce blistering.

Epididymitis. Treatment consists of antibiotics or, at times, epididymectomy.

Epidural hematoma. Emergency surgery is needed to drain large hematomas, usually through a burr hole. This may be followed by blood transfusions. Small epidural hematomas, which cause slight or no neurologic symptoms, may respond to dexamethasone, anticonvulsants, and rest.

Epiglottitis. Treatment of this fulminating condition may include insertion of an artificial airway, antibiotics, and antipyretics.

Epistaxis. A nosebleed requires firm pressure for 5 to 10 minutes or ice packs to arrest the bleeding. If these measures fail to stop bleeding, cauterization of the bleeding point with a silver nitrate stick or electrode may be necessary. Nasal packing may be needed.

Erectile dysfunction. If no physical cause exists, treatment may include sensate focus exercises or other forms of sex therapy, penile prostheses, or drug-induced erections.

Erythroblastosis fetalis. If this hemolytic disease is severe, intrauterine transfusion may be used to replace hemolyzed fetal red cells, and plasmapheresis may decrease circulating levels of maternal antibodies. After delivery, exchange transfusions are performed if the infant has isoimmune hemolytic anemia.

Esophageal atresia. Progressive dilation, temporary gastrostomy feedings, and surgical resection are common forms of treatment for narrowing of the esophagus.

Esophageal cancer. Surgery is the treatment of choice for resectable tumors. Other measures include chemotherapy, radiation therapy, and dilation procedures, such as insertion of prosthetic tubes.

Esophageal diverticula. Initial treatment for outpouchings of the esophageal wall includes a bland, soft diet; supportive positioning; and drug therapy with antacids, cholinergics, and cimetidine (to prevent gastric ulcer formation). Perforation, hemorrhage, or complete obstruction necessitates surgical removal of the diverticula. Associated motor abnormalities require a distal myotomy. Intramural diverticulosis may be treated with rubber dilators.

Exfoliative dermatitis. This inflammatory disorder requires protective isolation, hygienic measures (to prevent secondary bacterial infection), and colloidal baths, followed by application of topical corticosteroids and occlusive emollients. In severe cases, whole-body wet wraps induce vasoconstriction, thereby reducing heat loss. Other measures include increased fluids and protein, antihistamines, and systemic corticosteroids.

Exophthalmos. This abnormal protrusion of both eyes calls for dark glasses or shields to prevent irritation, methylcellulose eye drops to reduce redness, and orbital decompression to improve appearance. Antithyroid drugs, such as propylthiouracil, or surgery can correct the underlying disorder.

Eye cancer. In the early stages of *basal cell carcinoma*, excision can provide a cure. (Radiation may shrink the tumor but may also cause chronic keratitis.) Excisional biopsy is the preferred treatment for *squamous cell carcinoma* in the conjunctiva and adjacent tissue of the eye or orbit. However, when biopsy is impossible, radiation therapy should be used. Although resection may be performed, cortisone or radiation therapy is the usual treatment for lacrimal gland tumors, including *lymphoma, cystic adenoma, adenocarcinoma,* or *mixed cell tumors.* Local radiation may be used to shrink *choroid tumors,* which are mostly metastases. Iridectomy or enucleation is the preferred treatment for *melanoma* of the iris.

F

Fallopian tube cancer. Surgical resection is the treatment of choice.

Fanconi's syndrome. Symptomatic treatment includes vitamin D supplements, replenishment of lost fluids, electrolytes, and bicarbonate. If the syndrome causes end-stage renal failure, dialysis or kidney transplant becomes necessary.

Fat embolism. Corticosteroids, heparin, and ethanol therapy are effective in treating fat embolism. Treatment is supportive, but mortality is high.

Femoral and popliteal aneurysm. Treatment in the symptomatic patient consists of surgical repair.

Fibrocystic breast disease. Treatment may include the use of danazol, analgesics, vitamin E supplements, and padded bras. Caffeine restriction is also important. Surgical removal of the nodules may also be performed, but this doesn't prevent further nodule development.

First-degree atrioventricular block. No treatment's required for this arrhythmia unless progressive heart block ensues.

Flail chest. Caused by rib fractures, flail chest requires intubation and mechanical ventilation for severe pain or respiratory failure. Other measures include bronchodilators and, in nonventilator patients, incentive spirometry, coughing exercises, and intermittent positive-pressure breathing treatments to prevent atelectasis.

Folic acid deficiency anemia. Recommended treatment consists of oral or parenteral folic acid supplements and increased dietary folate (dark, leafy vegetables, fresh fruit, liver, and whole wheat bread). Treatment also includes correction of the underlying cause, such as a malabsorption disorder.

Folliculitis. Treatment involves thorough cleansing with soap and water; application of hot, wet compresses; and topical antibiotics such as bacitracin. Repeated infections may warrant systemic antibiotics.

Fractures. Closed reduction and manipulation can sometimes restore fracture fragments to their normal anatomic position. Extensive or complex fractures, however, require open reduction and perhaps fixation of bone fragments with metallic pins, wires, screws, or plates. Analgesics may be required for pain, especially in severe fractures accompanied by muscle spasms. Cast application follows open or closed reduction.

Frostbite. Treatment includes rewarming the affected part in tepid water (100 to 105° F., or 37.8 to 40.6° C.) followed by application of a bulky sterile dressing. If the toes are affected, cotton gauze should be placed between them. Fasciotomy may be necessary to decrease pressure from edema. Supportive measures consist of tepid beverages and analgesics. Antibiotic and tetanus prophylaxis may be necessary for any open skin wound. Gangrene may require amputation of the affected part.

Furunculosis. When the bacteria are susceptible, cutaneous abscesses or boils respond to penicillin or erythromycin.

G

Galactorrhea. Excessive flow or secretion of milk associated with Chiari-Frommel syndrome may respond to clomiphene. If galactorrhea stems from a pituitary microadenoma, it requires treatment with bromocriptine or transsphenoidal hypophysectomy.

Galactosemia. In this inherited metabolic disorder, treatment restricts galactose by eliminating milk, dairy products, organ meats, and monosodium glutamate from the diet.

Gallbladder cancer. When cancer is limited to the gallbladder, resection is the treatment of choice.

Gallstone ileus. Emergency laparotomy with enterolithotomy removes the gallstone that obstructs the small intestine.

Gas gangrene. For this soft-tissue infection, treatment involves high-dose I.V. penicillin, surgical excision, and debridement to remove necrotic tissue and foreign material. Hyperbaric oxygenation prevents multiplication of the anaerobic clostridia.

Gastric cancer. Surgical removal represents the only cure for gastric cancer, but chemotherapy with fluorouracil, doxorubicin, and mitomycin may shrink the tumor. Subtotal gastrectomy is used to remove a tumor of the distal or middle stomach, whereas distal esophagectomy and proximal gastrectomy are used to remove tumors of the proximal stomach. Palliative measures include iron and vitamin B_{12} replacement, analgesics, antiemetics, and dilation of obstructions with either surgery or stents.

Gastric lymphoma requires surgical excision and radiation. Radiation may also be used as treatment without surgery.

Gastritis. During acute attacks, conservative treatment calls for dietary modifications, rest, drug therapy (antacids, cimetidine, or anticholinergics), and parenteral nutrition. Complications, such as hemorrhage or peritonitis, may require surgery.

Gastroenteritis. Management of an acute attack involves fluid and electrolyte replacement, tube feedings as tolerated, sedation, and rest. Treatment also includes antibiotics if the etiology is bacterial. Severe complications, such as hemorrhage or obstruction, necessitate surgery. In chronic gastroenteritis, counseling may prove helpful in teaching the patient to manage stress.

Gastroesophageal reflux. Treatment includes antacids and histamine-receptor antagonists (cimetidine) to neutralize the regurgitated material. Dietary measures include elimination of fatty foods, coffee, chocolate, alcohol, and orange juice. In some patients, metoclopramide or bethanechol may raise sphincter pressure, hasten gastric emptying, and improve esophageal clearance. Patients should avoid eating 3 to 4 hours before bedtime, sleep in semi-Fowler's position, eliminate factors that may increase abdominal pressure, and lose weight, if appropriate. If these measures fail, surgery may be necessary.

Gastrointestinal hemorrhage. Intravenous or intraarterial infusion of vasoconstrictors, such as vasopressin, may stop persistent hemorrhage. Surgery may be necessary for resection of ulcerated tissue or correction of varices. Supportive measures include I.V. fluid replacement and blood transfusion.

Gaucher's disease. Supportive measures in this inherited disorder include vitamin and iron supplements, blood transfusion, and experimental enzyme replacement.

Genital herpes. Caused by herpes simplex type 2, this sexually transmitted infection requires bed rest and local application of heat to help alleviate pain. Administration of acyclovir reduces viral shedding, helps diminish pain, and accelerates healing.

Genital warts. Topical application of 20% podophyllum resin or benzoin eliminates small warts. Larger warts require removal or destruction by cryosurgery or electrocautery.

Giardiasis. The recommended treatment for this protozoan infection is metronidazole or quinacrine.

Gingivitis. Treatment consists of good oral hygiene and removal of irritations, such as ill-fitting dentures.

Glaucoma. In *open-angle glaucoma*, pilocarpine facilitates aqueous outflow, and epinephrine decreases the secretion of aqueous humor and also improves outflow. Acetazolamide also reduces the secretion of aqueous humor. If drug therapy fails to correct the condition, laser surgery, photocoagulation of the ciliary processes, trabeculectomy, or cauterization may be used to form a fistula between the anterior chamber and the subconjunctival space.

Angle-closure glaucoma initially requires treatment with acetazolamide to decrease intraocular pressure. After ocular congestion subsides, a peripheral iridectomy may remove aqueous humor from the posterior chamber.

In *congenital glaucoma*, goniotomy restores the patency of the trabecular meshwork and aqueous humor outflow.

Glomerulonephritis. Symptomatic measures include bed rest, immunosuppressants, and corticosteroids. Other measures may include correction of hypertension and fluid and electrolyte imbalance, dialysis, or kidney transplant.

Glossitis. Acetaminophen, an anesthetic mouthwash, and correction of the underlying cause (such as ill-fitting dentures) constitute treatment.

Glucose-6-phosphate dehydrogenase (G6PD) deficiency. In this X-linked trait, the patient must avoid certain drugs to prevent a hemolytic reaction. Severe hemolysis requires transfusion of red blood cells. .

Glycogen storage diseases. In *Type I*, the most common form, treatment consists of a low-fat diet and maintenance of glucose homeostasis through frequent feedings and continuous nocturnal nasogastric drip with a dextrose solution. No effective treatment exists for *Type II*, but *Type III* responds to frequent feedings and a high-protein diet. Treatment for *Type IV* includes a high-protein, high-calorie diet; bed rest; diuretics; sodium restriction; and paracentesis. *Types V, VI, VII,* and *VIII* don't require specific treatment.

Goiter. If caused by an iodine deficiency, goiter usually resolves with administration of iodone. If thyrotoxicosis occurs, treatment involves antithyroid agents, rest, and sometimes propranolol. When the patient becomes euthyroid, iodine administration may be resumed in small doses. Other drug therapy for goiter may include thyroid hormone administration (which can lead to thyrotoxicosis without strict medical follow-up) or ^{131}I in large doses. The patient will need to have surgery if the goiter presses on the trachea or esophagus or if it compromises the airway.

Gonococcal conjunctivitis. Caused by infection from the mother's cervix, this neonatal condition requires immediate saline irrigations of the eye and penicillin G. (Penicillin-resistant organisms respond to cefoxitin.) Prophylaxis involves ocular instillation of erythromycin ointment at birth.

Gonorrhea. This sexually transmitted infection responds to penicillin G procaine (or ampicillin or amoxicillin) and oral probenecid. For penicillinase-producing *Neisseria gonorrhoeae*, which is resistant to penicillin, and for penicillin-allergic patients, spectinomycin or cefoxitin is given along with oral probenecid.

Goodpasture's syndrome. Treatment may include plasmapheresis to remove antibodies, hemodialysis, immunosuppressants, and nephrectomy. Following nephrectomy, a kidney transplant may be tried after the anti-basement membrane antibodies disappear. Survival is rare even with early treatment.

Gout. Colchicine is the drug of choice for preventing and relieving acute attacks. Indomethacin and other nonsteroidal anti-inflammatory drugs are also effective. During remission, treatment consists of avoiding foods that precipitate attacks and maintenance doses of colchicine and uricosuric drugs or allopurinol to reduce serum uric acid levels.

Granulocytopenia. Treatment is aimed at the underlying cause, which may have been radiation or various drugs. It may include antibiotics to treat secondary infection. In addition, granulocyte transfusion may be necessary.

Granuloma inguinale. This chronic, progressive infection usually responds to tetracycline, gentamicin, or chloramphenicol.

Guillain-Barré syndrome. Thought to be an immunologic disease triggered by a viral infection, this syndrome requires plasmapheresis for rapidly progressive cases. If performed early, plasmapheresis may reduce the syndrome's severity. Other measures may include analgesics, corticosteroids, and mechanical ventilation. In long-term therapy, enteral or parenteral feedings, I.V. therapy, and vitamin supplements may be necessary to promote healing and myelin regeneration and to prevent secondary infection. Bulk laxatives, stool softeners, and intermittent catheterization may also be necessary.

H

Hallux valgus. Treatment depends on the degree of foot deformity. Sometimes a wider shoe or one contoured to the foot may help. Bunions may require surgical correction if they cause excessive pain. Occasionally, active range-of-motion exercises may decrease foot strain associated with guarding.

Hammer toe. Conservative treatment for this flexion deformity of the proximal interphalangeal joint (PIP) includes exercises such as passive stretching of the PIP joint, splinting of the affected toe, and wearing of shoes that conform to the shape of the foot and pad the joints. Failure of these treatments or increased pain may signal the need for surgery.

Headaches. Classic *cluster headaches* respond to methysergide, ergotamine, and prednisone. Chronic cases may respond to lithium; oxygen therapy is sometimes successful.

Mild *migraine headaches* require treatment with aspirin or small doses of codeine. Ergotamine in conjunction with promethazine or caffeine may effectively treat severe headache if given early. However, once pain becomes severe, meperidine or codeine may be necessary. Rest is often required after pain subsides. Propranolol, amitriptyline, methysergide, and belladonna alkaloids may prevent migraine attacks. Other measures may include meditation, acupuncture, relaxation, and biofeedback.

Treatment of *tension headache* focuses on relaxation of the muscles involved and stress management techniques. Heat, massage, sedatives, tranquilizers, and analgesics are effective supportive measures.

Hearing loss. *Sensorineural hearing loss* is irreversible. Hearing aids may help some patients. Occasionally, cochlear implants and cochlear stimulation may be performed.

In *conductive hearing loss,* antibiotics treat infection and stapedectomy corrects hearing loss caused by otosclerosis. Mastoidectomy may correct disease in the mastoid process, whereas myringoplasty closes a tympanic membrane perforation. Removal of cerumen, if present, with hydrogen peroxide or sodium bicarbonate irrigations can improve hearing.

Heat cramps. Administration of balanced electrolyte beverages correct fluid and electrolyte balance. Supportive measures include loosening restrictive clothing, resting in a cool area, and massaging muscles.

Heat exhaustion. Initial measures include moving the patient to a cool environment and giving a balanced fluid and electrolyte beverage. Subsequent measures include placing the patient in a shock position, loosening his clothing, massaging muscles, infusing normal saline or lactated Ringer's solution I.V. for severe cramps, and oxygen therapy, if needed.

Heatstroke. This requires I.V. fluids and oxygen therapy. Moist or dry cooling devices, such as ice packs and hypothermia blankets, lower body temperature. Diazepam or chlorpromazine controls shivering, whereas corticosteroids or mannitol treats edema.

Hemophilia. When hemorrhage occurs, treatment consists of replacement therapy with fresh-frozen plasma, cryoprecipitate, and Factor VIII and IX. Desmopressin acetate may increase plasma levels of Factor VIII in mild to moderate hemophilia. Development of an antibody against normal clotting factors requires an increased dose of Factor VIII, use of Factor IX, or plasmapheresis to reduce antibody levels.

Hemophilus influenzae. This infection usually responds to ampicillin or chloramphenicol. Vaccination should be performed between ages 18 months and 2 years.

Hemorrhoids. Stool softeners, sitz baths, and anesthetic creams or suppositories constitute initial measures. Hemorrhoidectomy may be needed for chronic, painful, or prolapsed hemorrhoids.

Hemothorax. Usually caused by chest trauma or an invasive procedure, this emergency requires chest tube insertion to drain accumulating blood. If bleeding is copious, transfusion helps prevent shock. Other measures consist of chest physiotherapy, oxygen therapy for atelectasis and hypoxemia from lung tissue compression by the hemothorax, and analgesics for easing deep breathing.

Hepatic encephalopathy. Treatment includes a protein-restricted diet, lactulose, neomycin or kanamycin enemas, hemodialysis, and exchange transfusion.

Hepatitis. Occurring in both viral and nonviral forms, hepatitis has no specific treatment. Supportive care consists of fluid replacement, activity restrictions, a high-calorie diet, avoidance of drugs metabolized by the liver, and administration of cholestyramine to relieve pruritus.

Hepatorenal syndrome. No effective treatment exists for this syndrome. Supportive measures include avoidance of nephrotoxic drugs, meticulous fluid replacement, and sodium restriction.

Hereditary angioedema. Characterized by recurrent attacks of colic and laryngeal edema, this disorder requires prophylaxis with synthetic androgens such as danazol. Antihistamines and sympathomimetics relieve symptoms.

Hereditary hemorrhagic telangiectasis. No definitive therapy exists. When necessary, patients receive iron supplements, transfusions, and treatment of bleeding episodes.

Hereditary spherocytosis. Splenectomy corrects this autosomal dominant anemia.

Herniated disk. Conservative treatment consists of bed rest, traction, and dry heat. Drug therapy includes muscle relaxants, such as diazepam and baclofen; narcotic analgesics; and dexamethasone to decrease swelling. If the symptoms don't resolve, laminectomy and, at times, spinal fusion can be used to stabilize the patient's vertebral column.

Herpangina. Supportive therapy—fluids, bed rest, and antipyretics—usually proves adequate for this acute viral disorder.

Herpes simplex. In this recurrent viral infection, therapy includes idoxuridine drops or ointment for eye infection, analgesics, and anesthetic mouthwashes for oral mucosal vesicles. Topical acyclovir treats mucocutaneous infection in immunocompromised patients. I.V. acyclovir helps treat severe infection.

Herpes zoster. Also known as shingles, this acute infection results from a reactivation of the varicella virus that causes chickenpox. To modify or prevent the disease, immunodeficient patients and nonimmune neonates require varicella-zoster immune globulin within 96 hours after exposure. Supportive treatment includes analgesics and corticosteroids. In the immunocompromised patient, vidarabine or acyclovir may be beneficial.

Hiatal hernia. A sliding hernia requires treatment with antacids and maintenance of an upright position after meals. A rolling hernia needs surgical repair.

Hirschsprung's disease. This congenital disease requires nasoenteric decompression or surgery to relieve intestinal obstruction.

Histoplasmosis. Amphotericin B is reserved for severe histoplasmosis because of its toxic effects. Ketoconazole may also be effective.

Hodgkin's disease. MOPP, the standard chemotherapeutic treatment, combines nitrogen mustard, vincristine, prednisone, and procarbazine. When this fails, ABVD (doxorubicin, bleomycin, vinblastine, and dacarbazine) can be used. Radiation therapy may also be used.

Hookworm disease. Mebendazole or pyrantel treats this disease. Iron supplements and an iron-rich diet correct associated anemia.

Huntington's disease. No cure is known. Symptomatic treatment includes tranquilizers, phenothiazines, and haloperidol.

Hyaline membrane disease. Characterized by respiratory failure after premature birth, this disease requires oxygen therapy for mild to moderate hypoxemia. In severe hypoxemia, continuous positive airway pressure is needed.

Hydatidiform mole. This placental anomaly necessitates dilation, curettage, and evacuation of the uterus or a hysterectomy. HCG levels require monitoring for one year.

Hydrocephalus. Ventricular shunting transports cerebrospinal fluid to the abdomen or elsewhere for absorption. Dexamethasone may be used to reduce cerebral edema.

Hydronephrosis. If surgical elimination of the causative obstruction isn't possible, treatment may include placement of a stent into the kidney from the bladder or insertion of a nephrostomy tube.

Hyperaldosteronism. If adenoma or carcinoma is the cause, treatment consists of unilateral adrenalectomy. With bilateral hyperplasia, treatment focuses on the use of the aldosterone-antagonizing diuretic spironolactone. Triamterene may also be used.

Hyperbilirubinemia. In infants, phototherapy is the recommended treatment. This disorder isn't considered harmful in other age groups.

Hypercalcemia. Treatment aims to correct the imbalance and prevent alterations in neuromuscular excitability. This disorder responds to hydration with normal saline solution and increased oral fluids.

Hyperchloremia. In this disorder, treatment involves administration of Ringer's lactate solution or I.V. sodium bicarbonate. It also includes resolution of the underlying condition.

Hyperemesis gravidarum. Treatment includes hospitalization in a pleasant, well-ventilated room and administration of parenteral fluids, electrolytes, sedatives, and vitamins. Depending on the disorder's cause, some women may require psychotherapy.

Hyperkalemia. Correction of the underlying condition may reverse this condition, but severe hyperkalemia requires infusion of 10% calcium gluconate to reduce myocardial irritability. In an emergency, sodium bicarbonate I.V. can cause potassium to shift back into the cells. Insulin and 10% to 50% glucose I.V. also promote the potassium shift. In addition, sodium polystyrene sulfonate with 70% sorbitol produces intestinal exchange of sodium and potassium ions. If necessary, hemodialysis or peritoneal dialysis can help remove excess potassium.

Hyperlipoproteinemia. In these lipid disorders, treatment aims to correct the cause. However, if no underlying disorder exists, a low-cholesterol diet helps treat types II, III, and IV. If dietary therapy alone isn't effective, lipid-lowering drugs, such as cholestyramine or clofibrate, are also given. In type I, weight reduction is necessary; the patient should also avoid alcohol, which may increase plasma triglycerides.

Hypermagnesemia. Therapy calls for increased fluids and, in an emergency, an injection of calcium gluconate, a magnesium antagonist. If excess magnesium can't be eliminated, dialysis may necessary.

Hyperparathyroidism. Surgical resection of benign single lesions is usually curative. Total parathyroidectomy is necessary if all glands are affected. A new technique—reimplantation of parathyroid tissue into the forearm muscles—may prevent postoperative hypocalcemia.

Hyperphosphatemia. Patients with excess phosphate should drink copious fluids and avoid phosphate-rich foods and soft drinks. Severe cases may require dialysis.

Hyperpituitarism. Gland removal or radiation therapy corrects this condition.

Hypersplenism. Treatment aims to correct the cause. Splenectomy is performed if severe granulocytopenia or thrombocytopenia exists.

Hypertension. *Essential hypertension* can't be cured, but it can be controlled by drug therapy with dietary and life-style changes. In mild hypertension, treatment may include a low-calorie, -sodium and -fat diet; regular exercise; relaxation; and cessation of smoking. If these measures fail to reduce blood pressure after 6 months, and if one or more unmodifiable risk factors are present, the patient should begin the stepped-care approach to drug therapy, starting with a thiazide diuretic, increasing to the maximum dose, as required. Beta-adrenergics, such as atenolol, may also be used, especially in the younger patient. If the diuretic alone isn't sufficient, a sympathetic inhibitor is added (for example, clonidine, methyldopa, metoprolol, nadolol, prazosin, propranolol, or rauwolfia). If a third drug is needed, a vasodilator such as hydralazine may be added. When these three fail to control blood pressure, and reasons other than drug failure have been ruled out, guanethidine, minoxidil, or captopril may be added in increasing doses or substituted for one of the previous drugs.

Treatment of *secondary hypertension*, the less common type, focuses on correcting the underlying cause. This may involve surgery, for example, to correct renal artery stenosis or to excise the pheochromocytoma.

Hypertensive crisis. Therapy involves two groups of drugs. Rapid-acting I.V. drugs with short-term effects make up the first group. These drugs include nitroprusside, diazoxide, and trimethaphan. Once blood pressure is controlled, an oral agent from the second group, such as hydralazine or clonidine, allows long-term blood pressure control.

Hyperthyroidism. Treatment aims to stop the excess secretion of thyroid hormone with propylthiouracil, methimazole, or iodine. Ablation of the gland is possible through radiation or surgery. Related ophthalmopathy requires prednisone, methylcellulose, diuretics, and eye glasses or plastic shields. Topical glucocorticoids relieve the discomfort of dermopathy.

Hypervitaminosis A. This condition quickly resolves by withholding vitamin supplements and excluding carotene-containing foods from the diet.

Hypervitaminosis D. Withdrawal of vitamin D results in gradual improvement. Glucocorticoids regulate hypercalcemia and prevent renal damage in severe hypervitaminosis.

Hypocalcemia. Treatment includes dietary therapy, oral supplements, or, if severe, I.V. infusion of calcium gluconate or calcium chloride.

Hypochloremia. Treatment involves oral replacement of chloride or administration of chloride-containing drugs and normal saline solution.

Hypoglycemia. A symptom of defective carbohydrate metabolism, fasting hypoglycemia requires correction of the underlying cause (tumors, liver damage, or cancer). The reactive type responds to a moderate-protein, moderate-carbohydrate diet and frequent, small meals. Concentrated sweets, alcohol, and caffeine should be avoided.

Hypogonadism. Treatment may consist of bromocriptine or removal of a prolactin-secreting pituitary tumor. True adult hypogonadism requires hormone replacement with testosterone, methyltestosterone, or fluoxymesterone.

Hypokalemia. Treatment consists of potassium chloride supplements.

Hypomagnesemia. Treatment includes magnesium supplements. Severe conditions require infusion of magnesium sulfate.

Hypoparathyroidism. Emergency treatment for acute hypoparathyroid tetany calls for administration of I.V. calcium and fluids and maintenance of an adequate airway. Follow-up treatment consists of calcium supplements, calciferol or dihydrotachysterol, and a high-calcium, low-phosphate diet.

Hypophosphatemia. Deficient patients should maintain a high-protein diet and take oral phosphate supplements. Severe cases require I.V. potassium phosphate.

Hypothermia. Active external and core rewarming help avoid potentially fatal ventricular fibrillation. Resuscitation attempts may continue for many hours.

Hypothyroidism. Treatment aims to restore a normal thyroid metabolic state with exogenous thyroid hormone replacement. This consists of gradually increasing doses of levothyroxine, liothyronine, liotrix, or thyroid USP. A sudden increase in thyroid hormone may lead to cardiac arrest. In acute hypothyroidism, especially

myxedema coma, I.V. levothyroxine with hydrocortisone is necessary.

Hypovolemic shock. Prompt blood and fluid replacement is necessary to restore intravascular volume and raise blood pressure. Emergency measures include infusion of saline solution, then plasma proteins, other plasma expanders, or lactated Ringer's solution to produce volume expansion until blood transfusion can be safely performed. In traumatic injury, autotransfusion can substitute for transfusion of bank blood. A pneumatic antishock garment may counteract bleeding and hypovolemia.

Additional measures include oxygen therapy, control of hemorrhage, maintenance of a patent airway, CPR, and placement of the patient in Trendelenburg's position.

I

Idiopathic hypertrophic subaortic stenosis. If calcium-channel blockers fail to reduce diastolic pressure, myotomy or myectomy may be necessary.

Idiopathic thrombocytopenic purpura (ITP). In *acute ITP*, corticosteroids promote capillary integrity but don't shorten the disorder's course. Platelet transfusions treat active bleeding but don't alter the platelet count. (I.V. immunoglobulin G has also been successful.) Splenectomy may be needed if the patient doesn't recover in 6 months. In *chronic ITP*, treatment includes corticosteroids and splenectomy. If surgery isn't successful, vincristine, cyclophosphamide, or azathioprine may be used.

Immunoglobulin A (IgA) deficiency. This disorder requires symptomatic treatment with antihistamines and alpha-adrenergics for respiratory infections, and dietary changes and diphenoxylate with atropine for chronic diarrhea. If transfusion is necessary, blood from an IgA-deficient patient should be used.

Impetigo. The recommended treatment for this contagious skin infection is penicillin or erythromycin.

Inactive colon. Therapy aims to correct the underlying cause.

Inclusion conjunctivitis. In newborns, treatment calls for topical tetracycline and systemic erythromycin. In adults, it consists of topical and oral tetracycline.

Infectious mononucleosis. This acute viral infection requires rest and analgesics for sore throat and fever. Corticosteroids are reserved for impending airway obstruction, thrombocytopenia, and hemolytic anemia.

Infectious myringitis. This disorder requires analgesics. Systemic and topical antibiotics prevent or treat secondary infection.

Infertility. Clomiphene or menotropins may induce ovulation in anovulatory women. And treatment of endometriosis, microsurgical repair of obstructed fallopian tubes, or drug therapy or surgery to stabilize thyroid function may correct the cause of infertility.

Treatment for male infertility may involve surgery to remove an obstruction to spermatic flow, chorionic gonadotropin to correct hormonal deficiency, or use of a mechanical sheath during intercourse to protect the sperm cells if antibodies from the patient's partner kill sperm cells.

Influenza. Amantadine provides prophylaxis against type A (but not type B) and may reduce its symptoms if given early. Supportive treatment includes rest, fluids, and *nonsalicylate* analgesics and antipyretics.

Inguinal hernia. Nonsurgical intervention includes manual reduction, use of an abdominal binder or truss, and weight loss. If these measures fail, or if the hernia is large and can become strangulated, herniorrhaphy is needed.

Intestinal lymphangiectasis. Marked by enteric loss of protein, edema, lymphocytopenia, malabsorption, and abnormal lymphatic channels in the small intestine, this disorder requires a low-fat diet or substitution of medium-chain for long-chain triglycerides.

Intestinal obstruction. Treatment includes nasoenteric decompression of the small intestine, I.V. therapy, nonnarcotic analgesics, antibiotics, and rest. If obstruction results from adhesions or hernia, surgery becomes necessary. In chronic obstruction, I.V. hyperalimentation, ileostomy, or temporary colostomy may be needed.

Intussusception. Surgical correction is necessary for this acquired intestinal obstruction.

Iodine deficiency. Treatment involves use of iodized salt or ingestion of shellfish and foods grown in iodine-rich soil.

Iron deficiency anemia. Oral iron preparations, combined with vitamin C to improve absorption, or parenteral iron help correct this anemia.

Irritable bowel syndrome. Symptomatic measures include natural bulk laxatives and increased fluids for constipation, diphenoxylate or paregoric for diarrhea. Other measures include phenobarbital, tranquilizers, or anticholinergics, and use of relaxation techniques, guided imagery, and exercise to relieve stress.

J

Juvenile rheumatoid arthritis. If aspirin and nonsteroidal anti-inflammatory drugs prove ineffective, gold salts, hydroxychloroquine, and

penicillamine may be tried. Physical therapy and exercise promote joint mobility. Good posture, gait training, and joint protection are beneficial. Splints may ease pain, prevent contractures, and maintain correct joint alignment.

K

Keratitis. If bacterial infection causes this corneal inflammation, treatment consists of cephalexin, gentamicin, or penicillin G. Fungal infection responds to miconazole and ketoconazole, whereas viral infection requires idoxuridine ointment or acyclovir. Keratitis caused by vitamin A deficiency requires a high-protein, high-carotene diet. If it stems from defects in tear flow, paralysis, or trauma, temporary tarsorrhaphy may be necessary.

Keratoconus. Contact lenses improve visual disturbances and provide a smooth anterior corneal surface. If these prove unsuccessful, corneal transplant may be necessary.

Kidney cancer. For *renal cell carcinoma* without obvious metastasis, treatment is a radical nephrectomy. For *nephroblastoma*, nephrectomy typically precedes multidrug chemotherapy.

Klinefelter's syndrome. Treatment for hypogonadism focuses on testosterone administration. No treatment exists for accompanying infertility.

Kyphosis. Conservative treatment includes exercises, bed rest on a firm mattress, and a brace to straighten the spinal cord until growth is complete. If these measures fail, corrective surgery includes a posterior spinal fusion, iliac bone grafting, and immobilization.

L

Labyrinthitis. Meclizine controls vertigo and high-dose antibiotics treat bacterial infections. Radical mastoidectomy or labyrinthectomy may be needed to remove the source of infection.

Laryngeal cancer. Small malignant lesions may respond to radiation therapy, but laryngectomy is usually required. Radiation may be used before surgery to shrink the tumor.

Benign laryngeal lesions—papillomas, cysts, neurofibromas, adenomas, or polyps—may be removed by thyrotomy, laryngoscopy, cryosurgery, or a lateral cervical approach.

Laryngitis. Treatment may include ampicillin to combat severe infections and prednisone to reduce inflammation and swelling. In an emergency, a tracheostomy or intubation can be used to maintain airway patency. In addition, removal of irritants, resting the voice, and humidification may help.

Legg-Calvé-Perthes disease. Treatment for this aseptic necrosis affecting the head of the femur includes removing the extremity from weightbearing and immobilizing it for 12 to 18 months.

Legionnaires' disease. Erythromycin and, if necessary, rifampin are the drugs of choice for this acute bacterial disease. Supportive measures include antipyretics, fluid replacement, and oxygen therapy, if necessary.

Leishmaniasis (cutaneous). Treatment includes parenteral antimonials, such as antimony sodium gluconate, or amphotericin B.

Leprosy. This progressive disease responds to rifampin, dapsone, and clofazimine.

Leptospirosis. Oral tetracycline or parenteral pencillin G helps treat this infection. Acetaminophen helps manage symptoms.

Lichen planus. Therapy aims to relieve pruritus with topical fluorinated steroids, occlusive dressings, intralesional corticosteroid injections, oatmeal baths, and antihistamines. Systemic corticosteroids may shorten the duration of the disease when given in the early acute stages. Retinoids shrink lesions but have potentially dangerous side effects. Rest and relaxation are important.

Listeriosis. Penicillin or ampicillin, possibly combined with gentamicin, treats most forms of listeriosis.

Liver abscess. Treatment consists of surgical drainage and antibiotics.

Liver cancer. Resection or a partial hepatectomy may be necessary for solitary hepatic lesions. Doxorubicin may provide temporary improvement. Transplantation is also an option, but liver cancer may recur afterward.

Lung abscess. Commonly caused by aspiration of an anaerobic organism, lung abscesses respond to antibiotics. Other treatments may include chest tube drainage of an associated empyema and chest physiotherapy.

Lung cancer. Treatment for Stage I and II non-small-cell lung cancers is pulmonary resection. Resection is also used for occult cancer, once it's localized. For Stage III cancer or for patients who refuse surgery, the recommended therapy is high-dose radiation. Combined therapy with radiation and surgery is still experimental. Treatment for disseminated nonsmall-cell cancer involves radiation and analgesics.

Initial treatment for small-cell cancer consists of various chemotherapeutic combinations, including CMC (cyclophosphamide, methotrexate, and CCNU) alternating with VAP (vincristine, doxorubicin, and procarbazine); CAV (cyclophosphamide, doxorubicin, and vincristine); CCMV (cyclophosphamide, CCNU,

methotrexate, and vincristine); or CAVP-16 (cyclophosphamide, doxorubicin, and VP-16). High-dose radiation may be used with chemotherapy or by itself.

Lung contusion. In severe cases, intubation and mechanical ventilation with FIo_2 and PEEP may be necessary.

Lyme disease. This tick-borne disease responds to tetracycline (in adults) or penicillin (in children). Early therapy may prevent or lessen complications.

Lymphocytopenia. Treatment aims to correct the underlying disorder.

Lymphogranuloma venereum. This sexually acquired infection responds to tetracycline or sulfonamides. Fluctuant buboes require aspiration.

M

Malaria. This infectious disease usually responds to chloroquine. Chloroquine-resistant malaria can be treated with quinine given along with pyrimethamine and a sulfonamide.

Mallory-Weiss syndrome. Emergency surgery may be necessary if ulcers at the gastroesophageal junction lead to rupture of the mucosa or submucosal wall.

Marfan's syndrome. This disorder of the connective tissue requires supportive measures, such as estrogen therapy in females and androgen therapy in males. Propranolol decreases myocardial contraction and subsequent stress on the aorta; however, surgery may be necessary if aortic or valvular disease develops. Because of the risk of endocarditis, a prophylactic antibiotic should be given before dental or invasive procedures.

Mastitis. Treatment includes intensive antibiotic therapy, analgesics, local heat, and a supportive bra with cotton straps. The mother may continue to lactate by using a breast pump or manual expression.

Mastoiditis. This acute inflammation of the mastoid area requires antibiotics, antihistamines, decongestants, bed rest, and fluid replacement. Recurrent or persistent infection or signs of intracranial complications indicate the need for simple mastoidectomy.

Meckel's diverticulum. This abnormality requires surgical excision of the diverticulum.

Medullary sponge kidney. Increased fluids should may be given to prevent infection and calculi formation.

Megaloblastic anemia. Treatment includes monthly administration of parenteral vitamin B_{12}

and daily doses of oral folic acid.

Ménière's disease. Recurrent attacks of vertigo accompanied by tinnitus and hearing loss require bed rest, a low-salt diet, and dimenhydrinate or meclizine. Atropine may be given in an acute attack. Long-term therapy may include vasodilators, diuretics, and, at times, sedatives. If these measures fail, ultrasound or cryotherapy applied to the horizontal semicircular canal, placement of a subarachnoid shunt, or labyrinthectomy may be attempted.

Meningitis. Antibiotics, the core therapy, are accompanied by bed rest, anticonvulsants, fluid management, and isolation.

Meningocele. Surgery corrects this meningeal protrusion.

Meningomyelocele. Removal of this spinal defect is cosmetic and doesn't improve neurologic function significantly. However, early repair prevents further neurologic compromise.

Mesenteric vascular occlusion. Bypass procedures or endarterectomy remove the occlusion, but resection may be needed to repair damaged bowel tissue. Anticoagulants may be used, too.

Metabolic acidosis. Treatment requires correction of the underlying cause. Reduced cerebrospinal fluid and blood pH require infusion of I.V. sodium bicarbonate or I.V. lactate, citrate, or acetate. In chronic metabolic acidosis, bicarbonate or citrate may be given orally.

Metabolic alkalosis. Therapy aims to correct the underlying cause. Administration of potassium chloride corrects hypokalemia, whereas normal saline solution promotes excretion of excess bicarbonate. In severe alkalosis, ammonium chloride may normalize the pH. Dialysis may also be necessary.

Motion sickness. Prochlorperazine and cyclizine treat vertigo and nausea in this disorder.

Mouth cancer. Tumor removal is necessary.

Multiple endocrine neoplasia (MEN). This disorder requires eradication of tumors in several endocrine glands and therapy to control residual symptoms. MEN I (Wermer's syndrome) calls for surgical removal of the affected gland, radiation treatment for pituitary tumors, and partial gastrectomy and administration of histamine-receptor antagonists to treat islet-cell lesions. MEN II (Sipple's syndrome) requires resection of pheochromocytomas and thyroid tumors. Unresectable malignant pheochromocytoma requires sympathetic blockers. MEN III requires tumor removal.

Multiple myeloma. Intermittent courses of vincristine, cyclophosphamide, and prednisone reduce the number of malignant cells. Radiation treats bone pain caused by fractures and reduces spinal compression by the tumor. Other measures include hemodialysis and antibiotics.

Multiple sclerosis. Although no cure exists for multiple sclerosis, ACTH and prednisone can decrease symptoms. Immunosuppressive drugs, such as azathioprine, may help arrest the disease. Plasmapheresis may prove helpful if other treatment fails. Supportive measures include intermittent catheterization, bethanechol, prophylactic antibiotics (co-trimoxazole) and acidifying drugs (vitamin C) to help prevent urinary tract infections, and baclofen or dantrolene to treat spasticity.

Mumps. Symptomatic treatment includes analgesics, antipyretics, and fluids.

Muscular dystrophy. No cure exists for this progressive muscle disease. Treatment is limited to general supportive care, including the use of light, functional braces.

Muscle-tendon rupture. Ice bags reduce swelling, immobilization prevents further damage, and surgery may be necessary to reattach the muscle and tendon. Immobilization may last 6 to 9 months in severe cases.

Myasthenia gravis. In this disorder, anticholinesterase drugs, pyridostigmine, and neostigmine increase the amount of acetylcholine available at the neuromuscular junction. Atropine counteracts muscarinic effects. Because acetylcholine receptor antibodies may originate in the thymus gland, thymectomy may be performed. In severe myasthenia gravis, treatment may involve corticosteroids and immunosuppressants. Plasmapheresis may remove antibodies directed against acetylcholine.

Mycosis fungoides. Treatment involves topical application of mechlorethamine and photochemotherapy with psoralens and ultraviolet light. Systemic chemotherapy may cause regression of tumor cells.

Myelitis. Anti-inflammatory agents may prove helpful in this acute spinal inflammation. Nutritional supplements and I.V. therapy may be necessary to maintain body weight and promote healing. Other supportive treatment includes chest physiotherapy, bulk laxatives, stool softeners, adequate hydration, frequent turning, and range-of-motion exercises.

Myocardial infarction. Sudden blockage of a coronary artery, causing myocardial necrosis, calls for narcotic analgesics for pain and sedation and oxygen therapy for dyspnea. Treatment may also include lidocaine to correct arrhythmias, atropine to correct heart block, and nitroglycerin, calcium channel blockers, or isosorbide dinitrate to reduce cardiac workload. If MI occurred within 6 hours, thrombolytic drugs may be infused. Other possible measures include insertion of an intraaortic balloon pump to help correct cardiogenic shock, dobutamine to reduce cardiac contractility, percutaneous transluminal coronary angioplasty, and beta-adrenergic blockers to prevent reinfarction.

Myocarditis. Besides antibiotic therapy for the underlying cause, myocarditis requires administration of antiarrhythmic drugs and a cardiac glycoside to prevent heart failure. Life-threatening complications require corticosteroids. Bed rest, oxygen therapy, sodium restriction, and diuretics may also be necessary.

Myxedema coma. Treatment aims to support vital functions while restoring euthyroidism. Such treatment involves maintenance of a patent airway, intubation, and mechanical ventilation. It also includes thyroid replacement with levothyroxine, I.V. fluids, corticosteroids, and glucose. The hypothermic patient requires gentle, passive rewarming.

N

Narcolepsy. Treatment includes analeptics, such as dextroamphetamine, and tricyclic antidepressants. Short naps during the day can promote normal function.

Nasal deformities. Surgery may be necessary to preserve a patent airway.

Nasal papillomas. These cauliflower-like epithelial tumors require surgery.

Nasal polyps. These grape-like herniations require surgery.

Near-drowning. Begin emergency treatment and life support measures immediately, adding other treatments as needed. If the victim's abdomen is distended, insert a nasogastric tube. Give sodium bicarbonate to thwart acidosis, corticosteroids to reduce cerebral edema, antibiotics to prevent infection, and bronchodilators to relieve bronchial spasms. Since the person may have increased lung fluid even after being pulled from the water, observe him in the hospital.

Nelson's syndrome. Metyrapone, mitotane, or cyproheptadine may be given to reduce ACTH secretion. Pituitary irradiation may help. Eventually, surgical excision will probably be needed.

Nephrotic syndrome. The goal of treatment is to prevent or correct complications of the underlying disease. It commonly includes corticosteroids, antibiotics, and diuretics. Additional measures include a high-protein diet to replace the copious protein lost in the urine and elevation of the feet to aid circulation. Dialysis or kidney transplant may be necessary in end-stage disease.

Neurofibromatosis (von Recklinghausen's disease). Soft and bony growths require excision and sometimes cosmetic surgery.

Neurogenic arthropathy. Patients with this axial and peripheral joint disease need nonnarcotic analgesics, and crutches, splints, or braces to reduce joint pressure.

Neurogenic bladder. Treatment includes antibiotics to prevent infection and catheterization to avoid urinary retention. If possible, patients should use intermittent self-catheterization and fluid restriction; others require an indwelling (Foley) catheter. Baclofen may be given to quiet a spastic bladder.

Nezelof's syndrome. Aggressive antibiotic therapy is needed to battle opportunistic infections associated with this childhood immunodeficiency. Monthly injections of gamma globulin, thymic factor, or transfer factor can prolong health. Bone marrow transplants are occasionally successful.

Nocardiosis. Common in patients with immunodeficiency, this chronic bacterial infection begins in the lungs and later forms abscesses in the brain, liver, and elsewhere. Patients require complete bed rest and 12 to 18 months of treatment with co-trimoxazole, high doses of other sulfonamides, ampicillin, or erythromycin. Abscesses require surgical drainage.

Nodal rhythm. An asymptomatic patient needs no treatment. A symptomatic, hypotensive patient may need a pacemaker. If the patient has bradycardia, atropine should be given.

Nodal tachycardia. Treatment may include stimulating the vagus nerve, giving such drugs as propranolol, quinidine, or digitalis (unless you suspect digitalis toxicity), and performing elective cardioversion.

Non-Hodgkin's lymphomas. Treatment includes localized radiation for early lymphoid malignancies and chemotherapy for later stages, especially II and IV. Drug therapy may include mechlorethamine (nitrogen mustard), vincristine, prednisone, and procarbazine. In patients with diffuse histology, C-MOPP (cyclophosphamide, vincristine, prednisone, and procarbazine) or BACOP (cyclophosphamide, vincristine, prednisone, bleomycin, and doxorubicin) regimens may be used. When drug treatment fails, whole body irradiation may be necessary.

Nonspecific nongonococcal genitourinary infections (NGU). The patient and all sexual partners should take oral tetracycline (except pregnant women), erythromycin, or streptomycin followed by a sulfonamide. Women should use sulfa vaginal cream. If cervicitis develops, cryosurgery may be necessary.

Nummular dermatitis. Treatment includes topical corticosteroids (sometimes combined with ultraviolet therapy and tar compounds), antihistamines to reduce itching, and systemic antibiotics. Additional measures include reduced exposure to skin irritants and caution against overdrying. Because systemic corticosteroids may have severe side effects, they're used only after other measures have failed.

O

Obesity. Initial treatment should target underlying conditions, such as tumor of the hypothalamus. Second-line treatment includes a low-calorie diet, exercise, and behavior modification. Treatment for morbid obesity may involve psychotherapy, hypnosis, drugs, gastric stapling, jejunoileal bypass, or the gastric bubble.

Obstructive sleep apnea. To clear the airway, patients should sleep with head and neck flexed and lose weight, if needed. If these measures are ineffective, other treatments include medroxyprogesterone, continuous positive airway pressure, tracheostomy, uvulopalatopharyngoplasty, or tonsillectomy and adenoidectomy.

Orbital cellulitis. Treatment includes immediate I.V. antibiotics in severe cases, oral chloramphenicol and nafcillin in mild to moderate cases, and sometimes surgical drainage of an abscess or infected sinus.

Orchitis. Testicular inflammation requires antimicrobials and, when mumps is involved, diethylstilbestrol to relieve pain, swelling, and fever. Suggest that the patient elevate the scrotum using a towel, stay in bed, wear an athletic supporter, and take analgesics.

Organic brain dysfunction. Depending on the cause and symptoms, treatment may include an antipsychotic drug like haloperidol, plus therapy for the patient and family.

Orgasmic dysfunction. Counseling is the primary treatment for this usually psychogenic problem. Sensate focus exercises and sex education may be helpful as well.

Osgood-Schlatter disease. Initial treatment for this disorder includes immobilizing the affected knee for 6 to 8 weeks with an elastic support, cast, or splint. If this measure fails, further treatment includes removing or fixing the epiphysis or drilling holes through it to encourage new vessel growth.

Ornithosis. Tetracycline is the drug of choice; second choices include penicillin G procaine and chloramphenicol.

Osteoarthritis. Anti-inflammatory drugs and analgesics can reduce pain and joint inflammation, whereas hot packs and hot paraffin dips can relieve any wrist or hand pain. Stress and tension-producing activities should be avoided. Synovectomy and joint replacement may be necessary in advanced cases.

Osteogenesis imperfecta. Heroic efforts are needed to prevent repeated fractures. Padded bedside rails and extra pillows provide protection during sleep. Kneepads, helmets, and other protective gear should be worn during strenuous activities.

Osteomyelitis. Treatment for this bone infection includes I.V. antibiotics and surgical drainage.

Osteoporosis. Calcium supplements and regular exercise can help halt degenerative bone changes. Estrogen supplements may decrease the rate of bone resorption.

Otitis externa. Treatment includes hot, damp compresses or a heating pad on the affected ear, acetaminophen for mild pain (codeine for severe pain), and antibiotic ear drops with or without hydrocortisone to clean the ear canal.

Otitis media. Ampicillin and amoxicillin are the drugs of choice; cefaclor and co-trimoxazole are good substitutes for patients allergic to penicillin. Bed rest and acetaminophen are sufficient for mild cases; codeine and antibiotic/corticosteroid drops are necessary for more severe cases. Decongestants may be helpful. Myringotomy may be needed to relieve extreme pain or a bulging tympanic membrane.

Otosclerosis. Stapedectomy or fenestration can improve hearing.

Ovarian cancer. Treatment includes surgical removal of the tumor and ovaries plus multidrug chemotherapy. Radiation may also be used; immunotherapy is experimental.

Ovarian cysts. Depending on the type of cyst involved and the patient's history and drug tolerance, treatment may aim to facilitate ovulation with clomiphene or progesterone or suppress ovulation with oral contraceptives. Continued symptoms or a ruptured cyst will necessitate surgical excision or wedge resection.

P

Paget's disease (osteitis deformans). For mild cases of this rare bone disease, treatment includes analgesics plus a diet high in protein, vitamin C, and calcium. For progressive cases, treatment includes the hormones calcitonin and etidronate to reduce bone resorption plus the cytotoxic antibiotic plicamycin.

Pancreatic cancer. Treatment includes bypass

surgery to unblock the biliary tract and sometimes chemotherapy and high-dose radiation to prolong life.

Pancreatitis. Treatment for the acute stage includes I.V. fluids, nothing by mouth, perhaps nasogastric suction, narcotic analgesics, atropine, and calcium if the patient is deficient. After stabilization, treatment shifts to a low-fat diet and avoidance of alcohol. Unresolved pseudocysts or abscesses require surgery.

Parainfluenza. This self-limiting infection may require acetaminophen and bed rest.

Paralytic ileus. Urge the patient to move about and give no food or fluids until peristalsis returns. If paralytic ileus occurs postoperatively, the patient may need cholinergic drugs. If it lasts more than 48 hours, he may need nasoenteric suctioning.

Parkinson's disease. The most effective treatment is levodopa; combining it with carbidopa can increase its effect at lower doses. Treatment may include other dopaminergic agents, such as amantadine and bromocriptine. If drug therapy fails, stereotactic surgery can be used as a last resort to still tremors.

Parotitis. Treatment includes parotid gland massage, antibiotics, and frequent use of mouthwash and throat lozenges. Surgical drainage is needed for an abscess.

Paroxysmal atrial tachycardia. Have the patient hold his breath, lean forward, or press on the carotid sinuses. If the arrhythmia continues, give a cardiac glycoside and a sedative, as ordered.

Patent ductus arteriosus. Preterm infants with symptoms of congestive heart failure will need indomethacin to inhibit prostaglandin production or surgery to ligate the ductus. Full-term infants usually survive without treatment but, barring complications, will need corrective surgery after reaching age 2.

Pediculosis. Patients should apply a lotion or shampoo of lindane as directed and remove dead lice and nits with a fine-toothed comb. They must wash all clothes and bedding in hot water.

Pelvic inflammatory disease. Two I.M. injections of penicillin G procaine combined with oral probenecid can generally resolve this bacterial infection. Analgesics and bed rest round out the regimen. Surgical drainage is the only recourse for pelvic abscess.

Penile cancer. Partial or total penectomy is the usual treatment for this rare condition. Radiation may be a helpful adjunct to surgery and is the primary treatment in inoperable cases.

Chemotherapy and hormone therapy offer limited results.

Peptic ulcer. Treatment aims to reduce acid production and muscle spasms through administration of an antacid, a histamine receptor antagonist like cimetidine, and an anticholinergic. Home care includes avoidance of foods that exacerbate symptoms, reduced stress, adequate rest, relaxation and exercise, and counseling if these changes don't reduce gastric turmoil. Surgery is necessary for recurrent ulcer, hemorrhage, perforation, or obstruction.

Perforated eardrum. Eardrum repair can be accomplished by tympanoplasty or myringoplasty, followed by ampicillin or penicillin to prevent infection.

Pericardial effusion. If fluid buildup proceeds to cardiac tamponade, pericardiocentesis can remove fluid and reduce the pressure.

Pericarditis. If infection exists, antibiotics form the first line of treatment, along with aspirin and corticosteroids. Severe, chronic pericarditis may warrant surgery to remove the scar tissue and constricted pericardium.

Peripheral neuritis. Treatment includes narcotic analgesics and anti-inflammatory drugs. Other measures include physical therapy to minimize respiratory problems, enteral and parenteral nutritional supplements, I.V. fluids, and frequent repositioning.

Peritonitis. Administer antibiotics for this emergency condition, combining either cefoxitin and an aminoglycoside or penicillin G, clindamycin, and an aminoglycoside. Give nothing by mouth, insert a nasogastric tube, and start I.V. fluids and electrolytes. Once the patient is stabilized, give an analgesic I.M. Drainage or surgery may still be necessary.

Peritonsillar abscess. Treatment includes penicillin and local irrigation with warm saline. Additional measures include surgical drainage and, at times, tonsillectomy.

Pernicious anemia. Parenteral administration of vitamin B_{12} corrects this condition.

Pertussis. Supportive therapy includes antimicrobials (such as erythromycin), corticosteroids, a mild sedative to decrease coughing, and oxygen to relieve dyspnea.

Pharyngitis. Ampicillin, penicillin, nystatin, and clotrimazole constitute the drugs of choice for this acute pharyngeal infection. Throat antiseptics, saline rinses, and aspirin promote comfort.

Phenylketonuria. Restrict the patient's intake of foods containing phenylalanine: milk, meat, nuts, cheese, eggs, fish, and breads. Give infants a formula containing minimal phenylalanine but normal levels of other amino acids. Suggest genetic counseling.

Pheochromocytoma. Surgery is the treatment of choice, preceded by administration of an alpha-adrenergic blocker like phenoxybenzamine and perhaps nitroprusside to reduce blood pressure. Long-term therapy with adrenergic blockers and metyrosine offers an alternate when surgery isn't possible.

Photosensitivity disorders. Treatment includes systemic and topical corticosteroids and antihistamines, avoidance of irritating clothing, gentle handling of affected areas, good hygiene, faithful use of sun blockers and other prescribed skin creams, and prompt reporting of unusual skin lesions.

Pilonidal disease. Antibiotics and frequent sitz baths form the first line of treatment for sacrococcygeal infections. Cyst or sinus tract excision may be necessary in recurrent cases.

Pituitary cancer. Pituitary tumors must be surgically removed. If the tumor can't be completely removed or is inoperable, the patient will need radiation therapy. Hormone replacement therapy is necessary postoperatively.

Pityriasis rosea. Treatment may involve antihistamines and emollients for pruritus, and topical corticosteroids for inflammation.

Placenta previa. Bed rest and possibly hospitalization should begin as the fetus nears maturity. Cesarean section should be performed if placental displacement exceeds 30% or the mother has heavy bleeding. If placental displacement doesn't exceed 30%, administration of I.V. oxytocin can stimulate labor; however, cesarean section should be performed if labor doesn't commence within 6 hours.

Plague. Massive doses of streptomycin should begin within 18 hours of onset. Tetracycline, chloramphenicol, and kanamycin are alternate choices. Corticosteroids will combat toxemia and shock.

Platelet function disorders. Depending on the cause, treatment may include platelet transfusions, corticosteroids, or plasma fractions.

Pleural effusion. Thoracentesis or chest tube insertion allows removal of excess fluid from the pleural space. Antimicrobials should be administered if infection is present.

Pleurisy. Treatment generally includes anti-inflammatory drugs, bed rest, analgesics, and sometimes an intercostal nerve block for severe pain. Treatment for chronic pleurisy includes surgical removal of the cortical tissue and thickened pleura. Thoracentesis will be necessary for patients with pleural effusion.

Pneumoconioses. No treatment exists for disorders caused by inhaling dust. High-dose corticosteroids may reduce symptoms.

Pneumonia. Uncomplicated pneumonia generally responds to antibiotics, bed rest, fluids, and frequent coughing. Complicated or nosocomial pneumonia requires aggressive I.V. therapy, oxygen, and antibiotics. Unresponsive hypoxemia secondary to pneumonia will need intubation and mechanical ventilation.

Pneumothorax. Invasive treatment isn't necessary unless pneumothorax diminishes lung capacity by more than 25%. In such cases, treatment includes insertion of a chest tube connected to underwater seal drainage.

Poisoning. General measures may include emergency resuscitation and support, prevention of further absorption, symptomatic and supportive care, and, if the source is known, use of an antidote. Induction of emesis (with syrup of ipecac), gastric lavage, or cathartics—such as magesium sulfate (epsom salts)—can prevent further absorption of certain poisons. However, if the poison is a corrosive acid or a petroleum product, or if the patient is unconscious or convulsive, nasogastric instillation of the appropriate antidote can neutralize it. Milk, magnesium salts, and activated charcoal are common antidotes.

If several hours have elapsed since ingestion, treatment involves diuresis by infusion of I.V. fluids. Severe poisoning necessitates dialysis. Skin areas contaminated by a poisonous substance require flushing with large amounts of water.

Poliomyelitis. No specific treatment exists. Supportive measures include bed rest and use of a foot board (until acute discomfort subsides). Hot, moist packs reduce muscle spasm, whereas analgesics relieve headache, back pain, and leg spasms. Long-term rehabilitation may be necessary for paralysis.

Polyarteritis. Corticosteroids and perhaps cytotoxic drugs halt or reverse the immune response believed to cause this disease. Plasmapheresis may also be performed.

Polycystic kidney disease. Treatment includes control of accompanying hypertension, prevention of infection, and administration of nonnephrotoxic antibiotics. End-stage renal disease requires dialysis. Family members should be screened and given genetic counseling.

Polycythemia vera. Phlebotomy lowers hematocrit to the normal range. If platelet and granulocyte counts are elevated, hemapheresis may be performed. Severe disease requires cytotoxic drugs.

Polymyositis. Supportive measures include corticosteroids and nonsteroidal anti-inflammatory drugs.

Portal hypertension. Bleeding varices require gastric lavage, esophagogastric tamponade, sclerotherapy, vitamin K injections, and blood transfusions. A portal-systemic shunt may divert blood from the liver into lower pressure systems, thus preventing variceal rupture.

Precocious puberty. Treatment may include surgery and radiation. For pseudoprecocious puberty in females resulting from granulosa cell tumors of the ovaries, choriocarcinomas, or an unknown cause, medroxyprogesterone and danazol inhibit ovarian estrogen production and ovulation. For pseudoprecocious puberty in males resulting from adrenal lesions, cortisone may slow symptoms. If the tumor is inaccessible or the cause is idiopathic, medroxyprogesterone may lower the levels of plasma gonadotropin.

Pregnancy-induced hypertension. Home management involves daily checks for edema, increased blood pressure, urine protein, and weight gain. Initial treatment calls for bed rest and a diet high in calcium and complex carbohydrates, moderate in protein, and low in fats. If the patient's condition worsens, she may need hospitalization with fetal monitoring, seizure precautions, sedatives, and regular assessment and diagnostic studies. If seizures occur, I.M. magnesium sulfate should be given. If diastolic pressure exceeds 110 mm Hg, I.V. hydralazine should be given. Severe hypertension calls for emergency delivery.

Premature ejaculation. Treatment calls for sex therapy, which may involve teaching the squeeze technique or Sernan's technique to the patient and his partner.

Premature labor. Labor that begins before 37 weeks gestation requires magnesium sulfate I.V. If this proves ineffective, treatment may involve ritodrine I.V. to inhibit uterine contractility, bed rest in the left lateral position to reduce frequency and intensity of contractions, and I.V. fluids to provide hydration and possibly decrease release of antidiuretic hormone and oxytocin from the posterior pituitary gland. Corticosteroids, such as betamethasone, may delay labor 24 to 48 hours to allow fetal lung maturation.

Premature membrane rupture. If spontaneous labor and delivery don't occur within 24 hours, induction of labor with oxytocin is usually required. If oxytocin is ineffective, cesarean delivery may be necessary.

Premature nodal contraction. An extra beat that arises in the atrioventricular junctional tissue requires no treatment.

Premature ventricular contractions. Drug therapy includes lidocaine, procainamide, quinidine, or disopyramide.

Premenopausal bleeding abnormalities. Deviation from the normal menstrual cycle before menopause may include *oligomenorrhea* (infrequent bleeding); *polymenorrhea* (frequent bleeding); *menorrhagia* (excessive bleeding); *hypomenorrhea* (deficient bleeding); and *metrorrhagia* (bleeding between menses). If required, treatment depends on the type and cause of bleeding. For example, hormonal therapy may induce ovulation, surgery may be used to excise cervical polyps or uterine leiomyomas, and anti-inflammatory drugs help reduce blood loss in menorrhagia.

Premenstrual syndrome. A detailed history and daily log of symptoms and mood fluctuations spanning several cycles help plan treatment. Appropriate measures may include drug therapy to relieve depression, irritability, headache, and edema; daily exercise; avoidance of alcohol; and a diet low in sodium, sugar, and caffeine. It should include natural diuretics.

Prenatal syphilis. Treatment consists of aqueous penicillin G procaine, given I.M. or I.V.

Proctitis. Treatment consists of frequent cleansing, sitz baths, and application of warm packs and ointments. Incision and drainage may be necessary for infection.

Progressive systemic sclerosis. This multisystem disorder is characterized by inflammatory, vascular, and fibrotic changes of the skin (scleroderma) and internal organs. Palliative therapy with immunosuppressants, corticosteroids, colchicine, and D-pencillamine may soften the fibrotic skin. Agents that block the renin-angiotensin system, such as propranolol, clonidine, and minoxidil, may stabilize or reverse renal failure. Captopril, which inhibits angiotensin-converting enzyme, may help with renal compromise, and diuretics and digitalis treat cardiac complications.

Prostatic cancer. Prostatectomy cures Stage A cancer. Stage B with diffuse gland involvement calls for radical prostatectomy. In Stages C and D (advanced disease), radical prostatectomy doesn't prolong survival, so radiation therapy and internal radium implants with radioactive iodine are the primary treatments. Other treatment in advanced disease includes androgen deprivation therapy with surgical castration or estrogen administration to decrease pain. Chemotherapy may also be used.

Prostatitis. In an acute episode, treatment calls for an appropriate antimicrobial. Adjunctive measures include warm sitz baths, stool softeners, and analgesics. In chronic prostatitis, effective treatment may include therapy with co-trimoxazole, warm sitz baths, prostatic massage, transurethral resection of the prostate, or total prostatectomy. However, antimicrobials don't penetrate the prostate very well, and prostatic massage, although useful for chronic prostatitis, may be associated with septicemia if it's performed in acute episodes of prostatitis.

Protein-calorie malnutrition. Treatment focuses on the underlying disorder and delivery of quality protein and other essential nutrients to correct dietary deficiencies.

Pruritus ani. This requires exacting perianal care, sitz baths, ointments, diarrhea control.

Pseudomembranous enterocolitis. Resulting from a necrolytic toxin, this colitis causes severe dehydration. If mild, it responds to cholestyramine. Other drugs, such as vancomycin, metronidazole, or bacitracin, kill the organism.

Pseudomonas infections. Gentamicin or tobramycin combined with a penicillin helps treat this gram-negative infection. Localized infection requires debridement and drainage and topical application of colistimethate and polymyxin B.

Psoriasis. Psoriasis requires topical agents—corticosteroids, tar preparations, and keratolytics—to slow cell proliferation and normalize keratinization. Ultraviolet light therapy may prove beneficial. Etretinate and methotrexate may help severe refractory psoriasis.

Puerperal infection. This acute febrile infection requires penicillin or erythromycin, bed rest, analgesics, and, if necessary, antipyretics and anticoagulants.

Pulmonary edema. Treatment aims to relieve hypoxemia, retard venous return, and improve cardiac function. In acute pulmonary edema, it includes morphine to reduce anxiety and promote adrenergic vasoconstriction in the arteries and veins, diuretics to decrease circulating blood volume, nitroprusside to decrease left ventricular work load, and aminophylline to decrease bronchoconstriction. Other measures include oxygen therapy, Fowler's position, and rotating tourniquets applied to the extremities.

Pulmonary embolism. Treatment consists of I.V. heparin, oxygen therapy to reverse hypoxemia, and, in some patients, streptokinase or other thromboembolytic agents to speed clot lysis. Surgical ligation of the inferior vena cava or insertion of filters or umbrellas is reserved for patients who can't take anticoagulants or are prone to recurrent emboli.

Pulmonary hypertension. This elevation of pulmonary vascular pressure requires oxygen therapy to prevent continued vasoconstriction secondary to hypoxemia. Treatment also includes vasodilators and anticoagulants. Of course an important goal of treatment is correction of the underlying disorder.

Pulmonary infarction. No direct therapy exists. Instead, the focus is on prevention, early recognition, and treatment of pulmonary emboli.

Pyelonephritis. In the acute form, treatment centers on administration of antibiotics, bed rest, adequate fluids, and periodic urine reculturing for 6 months. In chronic pyelonephritis, treatment calls for aggressive antibiotic therapy and assessment for obstructive uropathy, which contributes to the disease and requires surgical correction. In children, low-dose maintenance antibiotics may be used to prevent infection.

R

Rabies. The bite requires immediate cleansing and flushing with soap and water. Passive immunization with rabies immune globulin and active immunization with human diploid cell vaccine should be given in five I.M. injections over 30 days. Tetanus prophylaxis and antibacterial treatment may also be necessary. Wound closure with sutures is delayed.

Radiation exposure. Incurred through inhalation, ingestion, or direct contact, radiation exposure requires initial decontamination (removal of clothing, bathing of the patient and his wounds, and flushing of all orifices), complete evaluation of the injury, antiemetics to control nausea and vomiting, rehydration, prophylactic antibiotics, and, if convulsions occur, sedatives. Transfusions of plasma, platelets, and RBCs may be necessary. In extreme cases, bone marrow transplant may be needed, too.

Rape trauma syndrome. Treatment consists of physical care of injuries sustained during the rape and counseling for the patient and immediate family, spouse, or partner.

Raynaud's disease. This condition requires drug therapy to inhibit sympathetic activity. Patients should also keep the extremities warm and avoid smoking.

Rectal polyps. The most common treatment is surgical removal.

Rectal prolapse. Prolapsed rectal tissue requires surgical repair.

Relapsing fever. In this acute infection caused by a spirochete, treatment calls for tetracycline to eliminate louse infestation and I.V. fluids and electrolytes.

Renal calculi. Current treatment includes percutaneous ultrasonic lithotripsy, extracorporeal shock wave lithotripsy, or, in an attempt to dissolve the stone, medication administered via a nephrostomy tube. If these measures can't be used, pyelolithotomy, nephrolithotomy, or nephrectomy may be necessary. Symptomatic treatment includes analgesics, antibiotics, and increased fluids.

Renal failure. *Acute renal failure* requires fluid restriction to 500 ml daily, appropriate carbohydrate intake, and antibiotics, if needed. Dialysis may be necessary while awaiting the return of renal function.

In *chronic renal failure*, dietary measures aim to decrease metabolic wastes by reducing the intake of protein and preventing the catabolism of existing protein stores. Such a diet also restricts potassium and phosphorus. If hyperkalemia does occur, cation exchange resins may promote potassium excretion. Aluminum hydroxide promotes excretion of phosphorus. Further treatment may involve dialysis or kidney transplant.

Renal tubular acidosis. For proximal tubule acidosis, treatment calls for bicarbonate replacement and diuretics. Distal tubular acidosis also necessitates bicarbonate replacement and may include replacement of fluids and electrolytes, especially potassium.

Renal vein thrombosis and infarction. Resulting from an ascending thrombus, an inflammatory lesion, or disseminated malignancy, this disorder requires anticoagulant therapy and careful monitoring of fluid and electrolyte balance.

Renovascular hypertension. Conservative treatment using antihypertensives hasn't been successful in this disorder. Other treatments include dilation of the involved renal artery by percutaneous transluminal renal angioplasty and surgery, such as renal artery bypass or endarterectomy, to restore adequate circulation and control hypertension. As a last resort, unilateral nephrectomy may be performed.

Respiratory acidosis. Treatment requires correction of the underlying cause.

Respiratory alkalosis. If anxiety is the cause, treatment may be as simple as rebreathing carbon dioxide from a paper bag. In acute pulmonary conditions, adequate oxygen therapy frequently reverses respiratory alkalosis. In other conditions, treating the underlying cause resolves the problem.

Respiratory syncytial virus infection. In this viral disease, symptomatic treatment includes decongestants, cough medicine, increased fluids, antipyretics, and analgesics.

Restrictive cardiomyopathy. Treatment of the underlying infiltrative disease may lead to improvement. However, in extensive disease, a heart transplant may be the only option.

Retinal detachment. Rhegmatogenous detachments require surgery to close the breaks in the sensory retina and drain the subretinal fluid. Cryotherapy or laser surgery may be used to repair tears, scleral buckling to reattach the retina. Serous detachments, separations without a hole or break in the sensory retina, usually resolve and the retina reattaches spontaneously. Drainage of the subretinal fluid may also be necessary.

Reye's syndrome. Treatment focuses on reversing metabolic problems and controlling intracranial pressure. It includes administration of lactulose to lower ammonia levels, insulin to control hyperglycemia, vitamin K to treat hypoprothrombinemia, osmotic diuretics such as mannitol, and hyperventilation to help maintain normal levels of intracranial pressure. Prophylactic treatment may include anticonvulsants. In severe disease, barbiturate coma may help manage intractable, increased intracranial pressure.

Rheumatic fever. Treatment aims to eradicate the infection, relieve symptoms, and prevent recurrence. It includes bed rest, analgesics and aspirin, oral or I.V. prednisone (to treat carditis), and penicillin. To prevent recurrence, patients receive monthly injections of penicillin G benzathine I.M.

Rheumatic heart disease. Resulting from rheumatic fever and marked by myocarditis or valvular heart disease, this disorder requires monthly injections of penicillin G benzathine I.M. Persistent congestive heart failure may require valve surgery or replacement.

Rheumatoid arthritis. The mainstays of treatment, nonsteroidal anti-inflammatory drugs, aspirin, and low-dose corticosteroids aim to decrease inflammation. Gold compounds, auranofin, and D-penicillamine constitute second line therapy intended to induce remission. Cytotoxic immunosuppressants (such as azathioprine and cyclophosphamide), lymphocytapheresis, and physical therapy prove helpful for some patients.

Rocky Mountain spotted fever. Treatment for this disease, which is spread by infected ticks, includes careful removal of the tick, antipyretics, and administration of an antibiotic such as tetracycline or chloramphenicol until 3 days after fever subsides. Additional measures include close monitoring of fluid and electrolyte balance and, if pulmonary complications arise, oxygen therapy and respiratory support.

Rosacea. To mediate this chronic skin eruption, patients should avoid any activity that causes flushing and vasodilation—for example, ingestion of hot or spicy foods, tea, coffee, or alcohol; exposure to sunlight or temperature extremes; and emotional stress. They should also receive a topical medication containing sulfur or benzoyl peroxide, and perhaps a systemic antibiotic.

Roseola infantum. Symptomatic treatment of this acute viral illness includes acetaminophen and tepid sponge baths to help reduce fever.

Rubella. Treatment for this febrile disease calls for acetaminophen to reduce fever, and isolation until the fever subsides.

Rubeola. For this acute, highly contagious viral infection, treatment includes respiratory isolation during the communicable period, bed rest, fluids, and acetaminophen for fever. Providing sunglasses or darkening the patient's room helps relieve photophobia.

S

Salmonellosis. Treatment for this bacterial infection includes fluids and bed rest. Infants or patients with debilitating illness or continued high fever should receive an antibiotic, such as ampicillin or amoxicillin, chloramphenicol, or co-trimoxazole.

Sarcoidosis. If asymptomatic, patients with this multisystem disorder require no treatment. If symptomatic, they should be treated with systemic or topical corticosteroids. Patients with hypercalcemia should follow a low-calcium diet, eliminate vitamin D, and apply chloroquine or hydroxychloroquine to reduce skin effects.

Scabies. Treatment includes application of gamma benzene hexachloride cream for a period of 8 to 12 hours, with retreatment at 1 week to kill ova.

Schistosomal dermatitis (swimmer's or clam digger's itch). Local and systemic antipruritics provide comfort until skin lesions resolve spontaneously in a few days.

Schistosomiasis. Praziquantel, taken orally with meals, is the treatment of choice for blood flukes. Niridazole, available from the Centers for Disease Control, is the treatment of second choice. For both regimens, retreatment may be necessary in 3 to 6 months.

Schizophrenic disorders. The acute phase requires antipsychotic drugs. After the acute phase, treatment includes psychotherapy, milieu therapy, and antipsychotic drugs.

Scoliosis. In mild cases of this spinal curvature, stretching exercises can prevent further bending. In moderate curvature, a brace can prevent worsening of the condition. In severe curvature, cast application may be necessary, followed by spinal fusion.

Seborrheic dermatitis. Treatment includes frequent washing with selenium sulfide or zinc pyrithione shampoo plus nightly application of keratolytic agents, such as salicylic acid or Baker's P&S Liquid, under occlusion. Further treatment includes fluorinated corticosteroids to reduce inflammation on hairless areas.

Second-degree heart block. Mobitz type I heart block generally needs no treatment. However, Mobitz type II block may need temporary or permanent ventricular pacing to reduce the risk of complete blockage.

Seizure disorders. Treatment includes osmotic diuretics, a corticosteroid such as dexamethasone, a nutritious diet, adequate sleep, and reduced alcohol consumption. For generalized tonic-clonic and complex partial seizures, it also may include phenobarbital, phenytoin, carbamazepine, or primidone. For absence seizures, it may involve valproic acid, clonazepam, or ethosuximde. For status epilepticus, emergency treatment includes diazepam, phenobarbital, and phenytoin.

If seizures fail to respond to drug therapy, surgery may be necessary. It may include excision of the epileptic foci, stereotactic ablation and resection of the corpus callosum, or implantation of a cerebellar stimulator to indirectly inhibit motor function.

Septal deviation. Antibiotics, analgesics, and decongestants can help reduce symptoms. Surgery offers the only permanent correction.

Septal perforation. Surgery can correct the defect, if necessary.

Septic arthritis. Surgical drainage forms the first line of treatment for an infected joint, along with parenteral and intraarticular antibiotics, and codeine or propoxyphene for pain. A splint or traction may be used to immobilize the limb. For severe infections, joint reconstruction may be necessary; however, joint replacement is controversial at this time.

Septicemia. Treatment of choice calls for a drug specific to the organism cultured from the patient's blood.

Septic shock. Treatment includes immediate transfusions of whole blood or plasma extenders to increase volume, along with an aminoglycoside and penicillin or a cephalosporin. Chloramphenicol is the drug of choice if the infection results from nonsporulating anaerobes. Additional measures include pulmonary artery catheterization to monitor pulmonary capillary wedge pressure (it should reach 14 to 18 mm Hg), mechanical ventilation if the patient is hypoxic, insertion of an indwelling (Foley) catheter to measure urine output, and administration of a vasopressor, such as dopamine, if shock doesn't abate after fluid infusion. I.V. bicarbonate may be given to correct acidosis, and I.V. corticosteroids to improve perfusion and increase cardiac output.

Severe combined immunodeficiency syndrome. Bone marrow transplants have been successful, as have fetal thymus and liver transplants to a lesser degree. Immune globulin infusions may be helpful. Strict protective isolation is mandatory.

Shigellosis. To treat this acute intestinal infection, promptly infuse electrolyte replacements, as ordered. Also administer organism-specific antibiotics; co-trimoxazole, ampicillin, tetracycline, and chloramphenicol are employed in some severe cases. Instruct the patient to follow a low-residue diet and avoid antidiarrheal drugs since they reduce intestinal motility.

Sickle-cell anemia. In this severe inherited anemia, treatment is supportive and conservative. It includes administration of folic acid (to prevent worsening anemia) and pneumococcal vaccine. Analgesics relieve pain in vaso-occlusive crisis. Blood transfusions, though of limited value, prevent vaso-occlusive crisis.

Sideroblastic anemia. Patients who have this abnormal hemoglobin synthesis often respond poorly to treatment, although some may respond to folic acid and pyridoxine (vitamin B_6). When the condition becomes severe, patients may need blood transfusions; however, they run the risk of iron toxicity.

Sinoatrial arrest or block. Since the atrioventricular node assumes the role of pacemaker in the absence of atrial activity, treatment usually isn't necessary.

Sinus bradycardia. The condition requires no treatment unless the patient becomes hypotensive. In this case, atropine and isoproterenol can boost heart rate.

Sinusitis. Antibiotics are the primary treatment. Phenylephrine and ephedrine can reduce stuffiness and runny nose; acetaminophen or codeine can relieve pain; local applications of moist heat may ameliorate pain and congestion. If sinusitis persists, maxillary sinus irrigation is the next step, along with allergy testing. Corticosteroids, epinephrine, surgical reconstruction of the nasal passage, or invasive sinus drainage may be needed in severe sinusitis.

Sinus tachycardia. Treatment aims to eliminate the underlying cause (such as use of amphetamines, coffee, or tobacco). A beta-adrenergic blocker and a calcium channel blocker should be given to patients who've had recent M.I.s.

Sjögren's syndrome. Therapy for this collagen disorder is largely supportive, including nonsteroidal anti-inflammatory drugs to reduce joint inflammation. Drugs that dry the mouth, such as atropine, should be avoided.

Skin cancer. Surgery, the treatment of choice for basal cell carcinoma, may include simple excision, currettage and desiccation, cryosurgery, or Moh's micrographic approach. Local excision is the preferred treatment for squamous cell carcinoma; however, chemotherapy may be indicated if metastasis is present.

Sleep apnea. Treatment of mild conditions includes supplemental oxygen, avoidance of alcohol near bedtime, and protriptyline. Nasal continuous positive airway pressure (CPAP) can improve sleep quality dramatically and reverse daytime symptoms. Dramatic measures may include surgery or tracheostomy.

Sleep disorders. To treat insomnia, encourage activities that promote relaxation near bedtime. Suggest deep breathing, a back massage, a foot soak, or a warm bath. Take steps to relieve any pain. To treat hypersomnia and narcolepsy, help the patient develop a rhythmic day-night cycle by increasing sensory stimulation during the day and reducing it at night.

Snakebite. Emergency treatment of a poisonous snakebite involves keeping the patient still and placing the affected limb below the level of the heart in order to prevent the rapid assimilation of venom into the patient's circulatory system. A constricting band placed above the fang marks or just above the first proximal joint may delay effects of the venom until after completion of antivenin administration. Besides antivenin administration, treatment may include tetanus toxoid, broad-spectrum antibiotics, and analgesics.

Somatoform disorders. For physical symptoms without physical cause, treatment generally includes psychotherapy, behavior therapy, and sometimes antidepressants.

Spina bifida. Spina bifida occulta usually needs no treatment. However, spina bifida with a meningocele or myelomeningocele requires surgery to repair the protruding sac. Surgery should take place as soon as possible after birth.

Spinal cord injury. Injury to the cervical area calls for immediate immobilization with sandbags on both sides of the patient's head, a plaster cast, hard cervical collar, or skeletal traction with skull tongs or a halo device. A stable lumbar or dorsal fracture requires that the patient receive bed rest on a firm support (such as a bed board), analgesics, and muscle relaxants until the injury heals (usually in 10 to 12 weeks).

At that point, treatment should include exercises to strengthen the patient's back muscles and a back brace or corset to provide support while he's walking. An unstable dorsal or lumbar fracture requires a plaster cast, turning frame, and, in severe cases, a laminectomy and spinal fusion. A patient with a compression injury may require neurosurgery to relieve the pressure, as opposed to an orthopedic technique. Surface wounds will need tetanus prophylaxis unless the patient has had a recent immunization for tetanus.

Spinal cord tumors. Treatment varies. Intradural and extramedullary tumors, for instance, require surgery. Intramedullary gliomas demand laminectomy, decompression, and radiation. Extradural tumors require radiation.

Sporotrichosis. For the *cutaneous lymphatic form* of this fungal infection, treatment includes application of a saturated potassium iodide solution to be continued 1 to 2 months after the lesions heal. Hot compresses help relieve pain; some lesions may need excision or drainage.

For the *disseminated form*, amphotericin B should be given for several weeks.

Sprains. Treatment includes restoring alignment of the bones and joint space; immobilizing the joint with a bandage, tape, or plaster cast; and applying ice to reduce swelling and compression to minimize bleeding. A gauntlet bandage, which prevents nonunion of possible carpal and navicular fractures by immobilizing the thumb, is the preferred wrap for a sprained wrist. Additional measures include elevating the limb whenever possible and performing appropriate joint exercises after a prescribed period of immobilization.

Staphylococcal infections. Recurrent local infections should be treated with bacitracin, neomycin, or polysporin ointment applied twice daily for 2 weeks plus hot compresses to reduce pain. Systemic infections call for treatment with penicillinase-resistant penicillins, such as nafcillin or methicillin. If the patient is allergic to penicillin, he may be treated with a cephalosporin or vancomycin.

Staphylococcal scalded skin syndrome. This dermal infection generally responds to I.V. administration of a penicillinase-resistant penicillin, such as nafcillin, plus application of cool, sterile saline compresses.

Stasis dermatitis. Treatment for this vascular disease of the lower legs aims to reduce high venous pressure through bed rest, elevation of the affected limb, and elastic bandages or support stockings. If the skin is open and weeping, the regimen should include aluminum acetate compresses and corticosteroid ointments. If the infection recurs, treatment includes systemic antibiotics.

Status asthmaticus. A patient suffering a prolonged asthma attack will need oxygen, I.V.

aminophylline, I.V. fluids, corticosteroids, nebulizer treatment, a bronchodilator such as metaproterenol or isoetharine, and perhaps intubation and mechanical ventilation.

Stomatitis. This inflammation of the buccal mucosa should be treated with good oral hygiene, a nonirritating diet, topical anesthetic rinses to relieve pain, and antibiotic or antifungal drugs to fight infective organisms.

Strabismic amblyopia. Treatment of "lazy eye" includes patching the normal eye and prescribing glasses. Correction of more serious strabismus requires surgery on the eye muscles, followed by postoperative eye exercises, glasses, and sometimes further surgery.

Streptococcal infection. Penicillin, the drug of choice for this infection, can be administered P.O., I.M., or I.V., depending on the infection site. Erythromycin or another broad-spectrum antibiotic can be substituted for patients allergic to penicillin.

Strongyloidiasis. To treat this parasitic infection of the duodenum and jejunum, give thiabendazole as ordered for 2 to 3 days. Replace protein, fluids, and blood as necessary.

Stye. This local infection of the eyelid will generally resolve with hot compresses applied 3 or 4 times daily, a sulfonamide or antibiotic eye drop, and, occasionally, a systemic antibiotic. A persistent stye may require drainage.

Subdural hematoma. Treatment includes surgical removal of the blood clot via a burr hole. If the clot can't be completely aspirated in this way, creation of a bone flap will facilitate evacuation.

Syndrome of inappropriate antidiuretic hormone secretion (SIADH). Characterized by hyponatremia, this disorder should be treated with fluid restriction (800 to 1,000 ml daily), I.V. saline as necessary in more severe cases, and furosemide to prevent congestive heart failure.

Syphilis. Treatment of choice is penicillin, penicillin G benzathine, or aqueous penicillin G procaine, administered I.M. Alternate treatment includes tetracycline (except in pregnant women) or erythromycin.

T

Taeniasis. The treatment of choice for tapeworm is oral, chewable niclosamide, available from the Centers for Disease Control. A second course of treatment may be necessary based on the condition of stool specimens after 3 to 5 weeks.

Tay-Sachs disease. This rare lipid storage disease has no cure and is generally fatal by age 5. Supportive treatment includes tube feeding

696

to provide supplemental nutrients, good skin care to prevent decubiti, suctioning and postural drainage to reduce pharyngeal secretions, and counseling to help the family.

Tendinitis. Treatment aims to relieve the pain of this inflammation by immobilizing the joint with a cast, splint, or sling; delivering systemic analgesics as ordered; giving local injections of anesthetic or corticosteroids; applying hot or cold compresses; and evaluating ultrasound studies.

Testicular cancer. Treatment generally involves some combination of surgery, radiation, and chemotherapy, depending on the staging and cell types involved. Chemotherapeutic drugs include chlorambucil, methotrexate, and dactinomycin. Hormone replacement may be necessary, especially after bilateral orchiectomy. A combination of bleomycin, vinblastine, and cisplatin may prolong survival.

Testicular torsion. Initial treatment includes gentle twisting of the testis in the opposite direction. If this fails, prompt surgery must be performed, either to fix both testes to the scrotal walls or to remove the necrosed testis. Cosmetic treatment may include a testicular implant.

Tetanus. To prevent this bacterial infection, tetanus immune globulin (TIG) or tetanus antitoxin must be given within 72 hours of a puncture wound (if the patient hasn't been immunized in the previous 5 years). If tetanus develops, treatment includes airway maintenance and administration of a muscle relaxant such as I.M. or I.V. diazepam, high-dose I.V. penicillin, and a neuromuscular blocker for continued muscle contractions.

Tetralogy of Fallot. Cardiopulmonary bypass surgery is the treatment of choice to correct this congenital heart anomaly; it should be preceded by administration of morphine and oxygen and by maintenance of the knee-chest position. Propranolol may prevent cyanotic spells. In lieu of complete correction, palliative surgical techniques may be used to join the subclavian artery to the pulmonary artery (Blalock-Taussig), the descending aorta to the pulmonary artery (Potts-Smith-Gibson), or the ascending aorta to the right pulmonary artery (Waterston).

Thalassemia. Thalassemia minor and thalassemia intermedia usually need no treatment. Thalassemia major requires transfusions of packed RBCs to raise hemoglobin levels, slow subcutaneous injections of deferoxamine or other iron chelation agent, and perhaps splenectomy or bone marrow transplant.

Third-degree atrioventricular block. Treatment includes isoproterenol, atropine, and cor-

ticosteroids (if the cause is inflammatory). In chronic cases, treatment includes a permanent ventricular pacemaker.

Thoracic aneurysm. For an aneurysm of 10 cm or more, surgical resection with a Dacron or Teflon graft is the treatment of choice, particularly if the patient has symptoms. Emergency surgery is necessary to close a dissecting aneurysm, along with such stabilizing measures as nitroprusside, propranolol, oxygen, narcotic analgesics, and whole blood transfusions.

Thrombocytopenia. For this deficiency of circulating platelets, treatment aims to increase the platelet count and decrease bleeding. It calls for discontinuing anticoagulant drugs whenever possible and administering corticosteroids. Treatment for severe hemorrhage may include platelet transfusions.

Thrombophlebitis. Treatment aims to prevent thrombus formation and to relieve pain. In superficial conditions, the regimen may include elevation of the feet, warm compresses and soaks, antiembolism stockings, and anti-inflammatory drugs. In severe conditions, it shifts to analgesics, anticoagulants, surgical insertion of an intracaval filter, or vessel ligation.

Thrombotic thrombocytopenic purpura. Plasmapheresis, the treatment of choice, may be used with corticosteroids and antiplatelet drugs.

Thyroid cancer. Thyroid adenomas and carcinomas call for partial or complete removal of the thyroid gland and sometimes the lymph nodes. They may also require external radiation, either alone or with surgery. At times, these neoplasms respond to chemotherapy with doxorubicin. After thyroidectomy, the patient will need thyroid hormone replacements.

Thyroiditis. Aspirin generally relieves the pain and inflammation of subacute, nonsuppurative thyroiditis. In severe thyroiditis, 10 mg of prednisone should be given three times daily for 1 to 2 weeks. In lymphocytic thyroiditis, propranolol should be given to control cardiovascular symptoms. In Riedel's thyroiditis, partial thyroidectomy must be performed to relieve tracheal pressure.

Thyroid storm. Treatment for this hyperthyroid crisis includes maintaining a patent airway, administering I.V. fluids to support blood volume, and giving antithyroid drugs, such as propylthiouracil and iodide, to block further thyroid hormone release. Additional measures include high-dose corticosteroids to inhibit conversion of T_3 and T_4, propranolol to control tachycardia and other sympathetic effects, and cooling blankets and nonsalicylate antipyretics to battle hyperthermia.

Tinea versicolor. Treatment for this superficial fungal infection includes daily scrubbing of the lesions for several weeks plus application of a topical antifungal, such as selenium sulfide shampoo, 25% sodium thiosulfate, 3% to 6% salicylic acid cream or ointment, haloprogin, or tolnaftate. The regimen may also call for an oral antifungal, such as griseofulvin or ketoconazole. Additional steps include washing all clothes, towels, and bed linens in hot water.

Tonsillitis. Viral tonsillitis requires bed rest, fluids, and aspirin or acetaminophen. Bacterial tonsillitis generally responds to penicillin G (erythromycin or another broad spectrum drug for allergic patients). Chronic, recurrent infection requires tonsillectomy.

Torticollis. Initial treatment for wryneck may include application of heat, massage, biofeedback, muscle relaxants, analgesics, or cervical traction. When necessary, surgery can interrupt innervation of the spinal accessory nerve on the affected side, either at the extrapyramidal tracts of the brain or at the spinal cord.

Toxic shock syndrome. Treatment includes an I.V. beta-lactamase–resistant antibiotic, such as methicillin, oxacillin, or nafcillin, and saline or colloid fluid replacement to reverse shock.

Toxoplasmosis. Pyrimethamine combined with sulfadiazine should be administered for approximately 4 weeks during the acute stage of this protozoal infection. Folinic acid (leucovorin calcium) may be added as needed to control pyrimethamine's side effects.

Tracheoesophageal fistula. Immediate surgical closure is generally necessary. Tracheal intubation and a low-pressure cuff placed below the fistula can reduce the risk of aspiration while the fistula heals.

Trachoma. Topical or oral tetracycline or erythromycin, plus sulfonamides, should be given for 3 to 4 weeks. In chronic trachoma, doxycycline may be taken once daily for 40 days.

Transient ischemic attack (TIA). Warfarin represents the treatment of choice. If contraindicated, antiplatelet therapy with aspirin or sometimes dipyridamole offers an alternative. Endarterectomy or cerebral microvascular bypass may be performed as well.

Transposition of the great vessels. Treatment for this congenital heart defect involves immediate atrial balloon septostomy followed by digoxin and diuretics until the patient can undergo tolerate surgical correction.

Trichinosis. Thiabenzadole is the drug of choice for treating the intestinal stage of this parasitic infection. Corticosteroids may be needed if the infection worsens and comes to involve the CNS.

Trichomoniasis. Metronidazole, the drug of choice for this protozoal infection of the genitourinary tract, may be prescribed as a single oral dose or as several smaller doses taken over 7 days. The drug must be taken by both sexual partners.

Trigeminal neuralgia (tic douloureux). Palliative treatment includes such drugs as carbamazepine, phenytoin P.O., and occasionally propranolol. Surgical treatment includes temporary interruption of the cranial nerve via alcohol injections or trichloroethylene, avulsion of peripheral nerve branches, and rhizotomy.

Tuberculosis. Typically, tuberculosis responds to 9 to 18 months of therapy with isoniazid (INH) or rifampin combined with ethambutol. Atypical or intractable tuberculosis may require capreomycin, streptomycin, pyrazinamide, cycloserine, or para-aminosalicylate.

Turner's syndrome. This gonadal dysgenesis calls for treatment with progesterone, estrogen, and pituitary growth hormone to promote growth before the epiphyses close. The syndrome causes untreatable infertility.

U

Ulcerative colitis. Treatment includes the anti-inflammatory drug sulfasalazine, adrenal corticosteroids, anticholinergics, and an antidiarrheal drug, such as diphenoxylate or codeine. Other measures include I.V. fluid and electrolyte replacements and blood transfusions. Treatment for severe colitis involves elective colectomy with ileostomy.

Undescended testes. Occasionally, chorionic gonadotropin may stimulate descent. Failing that, orchiopexy is the surgery of choice to seat the testes in the scrotum.

Urinary tract infection. Antibiotic therapy can prove effective after culture and sensitivity studies identify the microorganism. Preventive measures include wiping the perineum from front to back, increasing fluids, making frequent stops to void when traveling, and voiding after intercourse.

Urticaria. Treatment aims to identify and eliminate trigger factors. Antihistamines, such as diphenhydramine, provide symptomatic relief.

Uterine cancer. Low-grade *sarcoma* demands radical hysterectomy and bilateral salpingo-oophorectomy. Metastatic or recurrent sarcoma may require chemotherapy with doxorubicin or dacarbazine, perhaps combined with cyclophosphamide, vincristine, or dactinomycin. Radiation may be used adjunctively.

Endometrial *carcinoma* requires surgical excision and radiation. If recurrent or unresponsive, it calls for progesterone or, in some cases, chemotherapy with doxorubicin, cyclophosphamide, or fluorouracil.

Uterine leiomyoma (fibroid, myoma). If the patient is of childbearing age, myomectomy is the treatment of choice. Hysterectomy may be performed when leiomyomas are extensive or the patient has passed childbearing age.

Uveitis. To reduce ocular inflammation, give local and systemic cortisone, as ordered. To reduce photophobia, ocular congestion, and pain, administer atropine 1% drops and scopolamine 2% drops. Start appropriate antimicrobials if culture results are positive.

V

Vaginal cancer. Radiation, the treatment of choice, is usually given externally at first, then internally if necessary. Surgical procedures include vaginectomy, abdominal hysterectomy, bilateral salpingo-oophorectomy, and pelvic lymphadenectomy; however, surgery is usually recommended only when the tumor is extensive enough to require exenteration.

Vaginismus. If no physical cause can be detected for vaginal muscle spasms, the patient may respond to sex education, relaxation and deep-breathing techniques, sensate focus exercises, and digital and instrument dilatation. Psychotherapy is sometimes helpful.

Valvular heart disease. Depending on the extent and severity of disease, treatment may involve conservative measures, surgery, or both. Conservative measures include a low-sodium diet, diuretics, digoxin for heart failure, and, in acute disease, oxygen. Surgical procedures include commissurotomy to widen the mitral valve, valvuloplasty, and valve replacement. Postoperative measures include anticoagulants to prevent thrombus formation and prophylactic antibiotics.

Varicella. Acetaminophen is the drug of choice for reducing fever. Diphenhydramine or another antipruritic can help control itching, along with topical aids such as bicarbonate of soda and calamine lotion. Isolation is crucial until all vesicles and most of the scabs have resolved (about 1 week after the rash appears).

Varicose veins. Antiembolism stockings, elevation of the feet, and exercise comprise the treatments of choice for mild to moderate varicose veins. Ligation and stripping of the saphenous veins or injection of a sclerosing agent are treatments of choice for severe varicosities.

Variola. This infection has been officially eradicated worldwide. However, if a patient were to develop it, he would require analgesics, antipruritics, I.V. fluids, and antimicrobials.

Vasculitis. When this vascular inflammation results from a toxin or a drug reaction, treatment consists of avoiding the causative agent. When it's related to a systemic disease, treatment includes administration of a corticosteroid, such as prednisone, or an immunosuppressant, such as azathioprine.

Vascular retinopathy. Therapy differs with the type of retinopathy and the underlying disease. For *central retinal artery occlusion*, treatment includes inhalation of 95% oxygen–5% carbon dioxide, global massage to dislodge the embolus, anticoagulants, and sometimes an anterior chamber tap or acetazolamide. Treatment for *central retinal vein occlusion* includes anticoagulants and possibly enucleation. For *diabetic retinopathy*, laser photocoagulation can be performed even though it may not halt progressive changes. For *hypertensive retinopathy*, antihypertensive drugs should be given to lower blood pressure.

Ventricular aneurysm. Surgical resection represents the treatment of choice for this outpouching of the ventricle wall. Other measures may include drug therapy (such as antiarrhythmics, cardiotonic glycosides, diuretics, and anticoagulants) to control ventricular arrhythmias, congestive heart failure, and emboli.

Ventricular fibrillation. Defibrillation must be performed immediately to prevent death from this arrhythmia.

Ventricular septal defect. Surgical closure of the opening ranges from a small suture for a minor defect to a patch graft for a large one. Preoperative therapy includes a low-sodium diet, diuretics, digoxin, and antibiotics.

Ventricular standstill. Atropine, epinephrine, or isoproterenol can help stimulate ventricular activity. CPR and a temporary or permanent pacemaker may be necessary.

Ventricular tachycardia. Cardioversion followed by administration of lidocaine, procainamide, or bretylium is the treatment of choice. Surgery may be needed when ventricular tachycardia resists drug therapy.

Vesicoureteral reflux. Initial treatment for urine backflow includes an organism-specific antibiotic. If infections recur, as they often do, treatment eventually involves surgery to repair obstructions or reimplant the ureters.

Vincent's angina. Therapy for this pharyngeal infection should include oral penicillin or erythromycin, hourly mouthwashes with hydrogen peroxide and warm water, a soft diet, and abstention from smoking.

Vitamin A deficiency. Acute deficiency requires large doses of oral vitamin A, treatment of any underlying disease, and increased consumption of foods containing carotene and retinol. These include yellow and orange vegetables, such as carrots and pumpkin, fish liver oil, liver, egg yolks, and fortified milk.

Vitamin B-complex deficiency. Treatment for this deficiency includes consumption of a B-complex concentrate and foods naturally high in B vitamins.

Vitamin B₁ (thiamine) deficiency. Mild deficiency can be corrected by increasing thiamine-rich foods, such as wheat germ, pork, liver, egg yolks, dry beans, and whole grain breads and cereals. Severe deficiency requires oral thiamine.

Vitamin B₂ (riboflavin) deficiency. Treatment includes increased consumption of organ meats, eggs, and green leafy vegetables; severe deficiency requires oral and I.M. riboflavin.

Vitamin B₃ (niacin or nicotinic acid) deficiency. This deficit responds to a dietary regimen that favors niacin- and tryptophan-rich foods, such as organ meats, fish, poultry, peanuts, and peanut butter; severe deficit requires administration of nicotinic acid or nicotinamide.

Vitamin B₆ (pyridoxine) deficiency. Increased consumption of wheat germ, pork, whole grain cereals, potatoes, bananas, and oatmeal can help correct this deficiency.

Vitamin B₁₂ (cobalamin) deficiency. Treatment includes I.M. vitamin B₁₂ injections, oral supplements, treatment of any related disorders (stress, chronic fever, renal disease, cancer), and increased consumption of liver, kidney, eggs, milk, cheese, and fish.

Vitamin C (ascorbic acid) deficiency. A diet rich in citrus fruits, tomatoes, peppers, strawberries, and potatoes will reverse this deficiency. Oral supplements are available for those who can't or won't follow dietary guidelines.

Vitamin D (calciferol) deficiency. Treatment consists of added consumption of vitamin D–fortified products, such as milk and butter, and use of vitamin D supplements. For congenital metabolic anomalies, treatment should include an active metabolite of vitamin D or a synthetic analog, either of which will bypass the defect.

Vitamin E (tocopherol) deficiency. Foods high in vitamin E include cereal germs, green vegetables, egg yolks, milk, butter, meat, nuts, and vegetable oils. Treatment calls for emphasis on these foods and for natural and synthetic supplements.

Vitamin K-complex deficiency. To reverse this shortage, patients should eat more green, leafy vegetables, wheat bran, cheese, egg yolks, and liver. I.M. supplements may be necessary.

Vitiligo. No cure exists for this loss of skin pigmentation. Temporary repigmentation may be accomplished with systemic and topical psoralen (methoxsalen and trioxsalen) combined with ultraviolet A (UVA) light treatments.

Volvulus. An intestine twisted 180° requires surgical repair.

Von Willebrand's disease. This hereditary bleeding disorder requires treatment with cryoprecipitate or fresh-frozen plasma.

Vulval cancer. Simple or radical vulvectomy is the treatment of choice; the amount of resection depends on the extent of the tumor. Secondary treatment includes fluorouracil and, for an inoperable or recurrent tumor, radiation therapy.

Vulvovaginitis. Clotrimazole and miconazole are the drugs of choice for treating infections caused by *Candida albicans*. Metronidazole is the first choice for *Trichomonas vaginalis* infections and bacterial vaginosis. Estrogen cream helps treat atrophic vaginitis. Other measures include warm sitz baths (15 minutes long, 3 to 4 times daily), use of mild unscented soaps and creams, proper wiping of the perineum (gently, from front to back), washing hands after toileting, use of cotton-crotch underwear, and avoidance of tight-fitting pants.

W-Y

Warts. Several treatments exist, including electrodesiccation and curettage, cryosurgery, acid therapy, and keratolytics.

Wilson's disease. To reduce the excessive copper levels characteristic of this disease, the patient should avoid eating copper-rich foods, such as liver, kidney, oysters, chocolate, nuts, cereal, dried fruits, and poultry. He may also take penicillamine; this drug binds with copper, promoting its excretion in the urine.

Z

Zinc deficiency. The primary treatment is a dietary shift toward foods high in zinc, including meat, liver, wheat germ, and nuts. Treatment must also address any underlying disease.

Zollinger-Ellison syndrome. Characterized by gastrin-secreting tumors and peptic ulcers, this disorder calls for use of a histamine-receptor antagonist, such as cimetidine. However, if drug therapy can't control the syndrome, vagotomy and pyloroplasty may be necessary.

Index

Boldface page numbers indicate major entries; i refers to an illustration, t to a table.

Boldface page numbers indicate major entries; i refers to an illustration, t to a table.

Boldface page numbers indicate major entries; i refers to an illustration, t to a table.

Boldface page numbers indicate major entries; i refers to an illustration, t to a table.

Drug excretion, 5
Drug-induced erection, **386, 389**
  patient-teaching aid for, 387-388i
Drug interactions, 5-6
Drug overdose, treatment of, 647
Drug selection, 2-4
Drug therapy, 2-7
  for cancer, **458-476**
  for cardiovascular dysfunction, **24-53**
  for endocrine dysfunction, **398-414**
  for GI dysfunction, **140-150**
  for hematologic and immune dysfunction, **436-443**
  for infection, **482-495**
  for mental and emotional problems, **630-641**
  modification of, 6-7
  for musculoskeletal dysfunction, **280-285**
  for neurologic dysfunction, **238-253**
  for nutritional and metabolic dysfunction, **194-202**
  for pain, **604-615**
  patient-teaching aid for, 7, 8-9
  for renal and urologic dysfunction, **310-312**
  for respiratory dysfunction, **100-108**
  for sexual dysfunction, **386-389**
  for skin dysfunction, **558-566**
  for trauma, **586-588**
  for visual dysfunction, **500-506**
Drug toxicity, 5-6
  in the elderly, 6-7
Drug withdrawal, 646, 647
Dulcolax. See Bisacodyl.
Duracillin. See Penicillin G procaine.
Dyclonine, 611
Dynapen. See Dicloxacillin.
Dyphylline, 600
Dysfunctional uterine bleeding, 675
Dysmenorrhea, 675
Dyspareunia, 675

E

Ear canal benign tumor, 675
Ear disorders, treatment of, 533, **535-539, 552-553**
Eardrum perforation, repair of, 535
Ear irrigation, 653-654
Eating disorders, 675
Echothiophate, 500

ECT. See Electroconvulsive therapy.
Ectopic pregnancy, 675
Edlich tube, 184i
Elavil. See Amitriptyline.
Elective surgery, 11
Electrical bone growth stimulators, 301, 302t
Electric shock, 675
Electrocautery, for endometrial implant removal, 376t
Electroconvulsive therapy, **648-649**
Electrodesiccation, 654
Electrolyte imbalance, 225t, 227
  postoperative, 20
Embolectomy, 75i. See also Vascular repair.
Embolization, of arteriovenous malformations, **271-272**
Emergency surgery, 11
Emollient therapeutic bath, 581t
Emotional problems. See Mental and emotional problems, treatment of.
Empyema, 675
Enalapril, 27-28
Encainide, 47t
Encephalitis, 675
Encephalocele, 675
Endocarditis, 675
Endocrine dysfunction, treatment of, **397-433**
Endometriosis, 676
Endoscopic retrograde sphincterotomy, **188-190**
Endoscopy, for GI dysfunction, 188-190
Enteral nutrition, **223-224, 226**
  complications of, 225t
Enterobacterial infections, 676
Enterobiasis, 676
Enucleation, **524-525, 528**
Ephedrine, 505, 534
Epicardial pacemaker, 78
Epicondylitis, 676
Epidermolysis bullosa, 676
Epididymectomy, 654
Epididymitis, 676
Epidural hematoma, 676
  aspiration 258-259
Epidural nerve block, 612-613t, 615
Epiglottitis, 676
Epikeratophakia, 507
Epinephrine, 41, 42-43t, 44, 102, 441-443, 442-443i, 503, 586, 587t
Epinephryl, 503
Epistaxis, 676
Erectile dysfunction, 676
Ergot alkaloids, **244-245**
Ergotamine tartrate, 244

Erythrityl tetranitrate, 36
Erythroblastosis fetalis, 676
Erythromycins, **488-489**
Escharotomy, 654
Esophageal atresia, 676
Esophageal bougienage, 654
Esophageal cancer, 676
Esophageal diverticula, 676
Esophageal surgeries, **150-153**
  types of, 152i
Esophageal tubes, 186i
Esophagectomy, 151, 152i
Esophagitis, corrosive, 673
Esophagogastric tamponade, **185, 187-188**
Esophagogastrostomy, 152i, 153
Esophagomyotomy, 151, 152i
Estradiol, 362, 363, 474
Estrogens, **362-364, 474-475**
Estrone, 474
ESWL. See Extracorporeal shock-wave lithotripsy.
Ethacrynic acid, 34-35t
Ethambutol, 654
Ethinyl estradiol, 362, 474
Ethmoidectomy, **539-540**
Ethosuximide, 242-243t
Ethotoin, 241-242
Ethyl chloride, 611
Etidocaine, 613
Etoposide, 465i, 472
Etretinate, 564
Ewald tube, 184i
Exchange transfusion, **451-453**
Exercise(s)
  effect of, on carbohydrate needs, 416-417t
  isometric, 657
  Kegel, 657
  in musculoskeletal dysfunction, **299-306**
  for neck and shoulders, after radical neck dissection, 551i
  postoperative, 20
Exfoliative dermatitis, 676
Exophthalmos, 676
Expectorants, 108
Extended insulin zinc suspension (Ultralente), 401t
Extended radical mastectomy, 369, 370
Extender for metered-dose inhaler, 106i
External fixation, 289i
External nasolacrimal massage, 654
External radiation therapy, 477, 478, 479
External sphincter relaxants, **311-312**

Gynecologic dysfunction. *See* Obstetric and gynecologic dysfunction.

H

Halazepam, 630, 631
Halcinonide cream, 559t
Haldol. *See* Haloperidol.
Hallux valgus, 679
Haloperidol, 632
Haloprogin, 562
Hammer toe, 679
H-BIG. *See* Hepatitis B immune globulin.
Headaches, 478t, 679
Health, restoration of, as treatment goal, 2
Hearing aids, **552-553**
Hearing loss, 679
Heart defects, congenital, repair of, **69-72**
Heart-lung machine, 64-65i
Heart rate, postoperative assessment of, 16
Heart transplant, **53-58**
Heat cramps, 679
Heat exhaustion, 679
Heatstroke, 679
Hematologic and immune dysfunction, treatment of, **435-455**
Hemin, 655-656
Hemipelvectomy, 286
Hemodialysis, **338-339**, 339i, **341-342**
access sites for, 340i
Hemoperfusion, 656
Hemophilia, 679-680
Hemophilus influenza, 680
Hemorrhage, 174t, 424, 548, 617
Hemorrhoidectomy, **166-168**
Hemorrhoid reduction, 656
Hemorrhoids, 680
Hemothorax, 680
Heparin, 49, 50i, 51
Hepatectomy, subtotal, 175
Hepatic encephalopathy, 680
Hepatic failure, 174t
Hepatitis, 680
Hepatitis B immune globulin, 656
Hepatorenal syndrome, 680
Hereditary angioedema, 680
Hereditary hemorrhagic telangiectasia, 680
Hereditary spherocytosis, 680
Hernia repair, **153-154**
Herniated disk, 680
Hernioplasty, 153
Herniorrhaphy, 153
Herpangina, 680
Herpes simplex, 680
Herpes zoster, 680
Heterograft, 575t
Hiatal hernia, 680

High-carbohydrate diet, 656
High-density lipoprotein, 209
High-fiber diet, 205-207
High-flow oxygen system, 126, 127
High-frequency ventilation, 117, 118t
High-potassium diet, 656
High-protein diet, 207, 208
Hip replacement, 294-296
Hirschsprung's disease, 680
Histamine-receptor antagonists, **141-143**
Histoplasmosis, 680
Hodgkin's disease, 680
Homatropine, 503
Homograft, 575t
Hookworm disease, 680
Horizontal supraglottic laryngectomy, 546i
Human chorionic gonadotropin, 364, 365i
Humidification treatments, **128-129, 131**
Humidifiers, types of, 130-131t
Humulin L, 401t
Humulin N, 400t
Humulin R, 400t
Huntington's disease, 680
Hyaline membrane disease, 680
Hydantoin anticonvulsants, **241-244**
Hydatidiform mole, 680
Hydralazine, 28-29
Hydrocele, aspiration of, 335i
Hydrocelectomy, **334-336**
Hydrocephalus, 680
Hydrochlorothiazide, 34-35t
Hydrocortisone, 252, 281, 398, 440t, 505
Hydrocortisone valerate ointment, 559t
Hydromorphone, 606
Hydronephrosis, 681
Hydroxyamphetamine, 503
Hydroxyprogesterone, 361
Hydroxyzine, 609
Hyperaldosteronism, 681
Hyperalimentation, intravenous, **226-228**
Hyperbaric oxygenation, 656
Hyperbilirubinemia, 681
Hypercalcemia, 681
Hyperchloremia, 681
Hyperemesis gravidarum, 681
Hyperglycemia, 225, 227
Hyperkalemia, 681
Hyperlipoproteinemia, 681
Hypermagnesemia, 681
Hyperosmolar laxatives, 146-147t, 148
Hyperparathyroidism, 681
Hyperphosphatemia, 681
Hyperpituitarism, 681

Hypersplenism, 681
Hypertension, 681
Hypertensive crisis, 681
Hyperthyroidism, 681
Hypervitaminosis A, 681-682
Hypervitaminosis D, 682
Hypocalcemia, 424, 682
Hypochloremia, 682
Hypoglycemia, 227, 682
Hypogonadism, 682
Hypokalemia, 682
Hypomagnesemia, 682
Hypoparathyroidism, 682
diet for, 422
Hypophosphatemia, 682
Hypophysectomy, **418-420**
Hypoplastic anemia, 667-668
Hypotension, 274t
Hypothermia, 682
Hypothyroidism, 682
Hypovolemia
as complication of transfusion, 446-447t
as postoperative complication, 14
Hypovolemic shock, 682
as complication of fracture, 291
as complication of liver transplant, 174t
irreversible, prevention of, 600i
Hysterectomy, **373-375**
types of, 373
Hyzyd. *See* Isoniazid.

I

Ibuprofen, 280, 360, 604
Iced gastric lavage, **182-183, 185**
Ice massage, 624
I & D. *See* Incision and drainage.
Idiopathic hypertrophic subaortic stenosis, 682
Idiopathic thrombocytopenic purpura, 682
IL-2. *See* Interleukin-2.
Ileal conduit, **319-320**, 321i, **322-323**
Imipramine, 637, 639i
Immobilization, **303, 306**
types of, 304-305t
Immune dysfunction. *See* Hematologic and immune dysfunction, treatment of.
Immunoglobulin A deficiency, 682
Immunosuppressants, 316, **437, 439**
Impetigo, 682
Implantable insulin pumps, 406i
Implosion therapy, 644
Inactive colon, 682

Boldface page numbers indicate major entries; i refers to an illustration, t to a table.

708

Incentive spirometry, **131-133**
Incision and drainage, **496**
Inclusion conjunctivitis, 682
Inderal. *See* Propranolol.
Indocin. *See* Indomethacin.
Indomethacin, 280, 604
Indwelling catheterization, 354, 356
Infection
  nosocomial, 481
  patient-teaching aid for avoidance of, 438
  treatment of, **481-497**
Infectious mononucleosis, 682
Infectious myringitis, 682
Inferior vena cava, surgical interruption of, 75i. *See also* Vascular repair.
Infertility, 682-683
Inflatable penile prosthesis, 390, 391i, 392
Influenza, 683
Inguinal hernia, 683
Inhalation therapy, **116-133**
Inhaled corticosteroids, **105, 107**
Inotropic drugs, 41-44
Insulatard NPH, 400t
Insulin infusion, continuous
  subcutaneous, **405, 407-409**
  complications of, 407
Insulin injection
  subcutaneous, **399-401, 404-405**
Insulin preparations, 400-401t
Insulin pump, 406i, 408
Insulin zinc suspension (lente), 401t
Intake/output, postoperative assessment of, 16, 17, 20
Interferons, **475-476**
Interleukin-2, 656
Intermediate-acting insulins, 400-401t
Intermittent catheterization, 354
Intermittent positive-pressure breathing, **122-123**
Intermittent ventilation
  demand, 121
  mandatory, 117, 121
Internal fixation, **288-289, 291**
  methods of, 290i
Internal radiation therapy, 477, 478-479
Interpositional reconstruction, 295
Intestinal lymphangiectasis, 683
Intestinal obstruction, 683
Intraaortic balloon counterpulsation, **81-83, 85**
Intraaortic balloon pump, 82i
  timing, 84i
Intraarticular injection, 282i

Intracapsular cataract extraction, 508-509i
Intracranial hematoma, aspiration of, **258-259, 261**
Intracranial pressure, increased, 260
  barbiturate coma, as treatment for, 273, 275
Intrauterine intraperitoneal transfusion, 656
Intravenous hyperalimentation, **226-228**
Intravenous insulin infusion, 404
Intrinsic pathway of clot formation, 50i
Intubation, in gastrointestinal dysfunction, **180-188**
Intussusception, 683
In vivo fertilization, **381-383**
Iodine 131 administration, **431, 433**
  patient-teaching aid for precautions after, 432i
Iodine deficiency, 683
Iodism, 413
Ionescu-Shiley valve, 67i
Ipecac syrup, 656-657
Ipodate, 413
Iridectomy, **513-515**
  use of laser in, 529
Iron, oral/parenteral, 200
Iron deficiency anemia, 683
Iron lung, 119t
Irrigation of wound, 577, 578
Irritable bowel syndrome, 683
Islet cell transplant, 657
Isocarboxazid, 634, 639i
Isoetharine, 101
Isoflurophate, 500
Isometric exercises, 657
Isoniazid (INH), 494-496t
Isophane insulin suspension (NPH), 400t
Isophane (NPH) 70%, regular insulin 30%, 401t
Isopropamide iodide, 143
Isoproterenol, 41, 42-43t, 101
Isosorbide, 36,502
Isotretinoin, 564
Isoxsuprine, 366
Isuprel. *See* Isoproterenol.

J

Jarvik 7 artificial heart, 55i
Jenamicin. *See* Gentamicin.
Jejunoileal bypass, 657
Johnson extractor, in calculi basketing, 347i
Joint replacement, **294-296**
  reconstruction alternatives to, 295
Joint resection, 295
Juvenile rheumatoid arthritis, 683

K

Kanamycin, 487
Kaolin and pectin mixtures, 145
Kaopectate, 145
Kegel exercises, 657
Keratitis, 683
Keratoconus, 683
Keratolytic agents, 657
Keratomileusis, 507
Keratoplasty, **510, 512-513**
Keratotomy, radial, **507-508**
Ketoconazole, 657
Kidney cancer, 683
Kidney transplant, **314-316, 317i, 318-319**
  rejection, management of, 318
  success rate of, 315
Klinefelter's syndrome, 683
Knee replacement, 294-296
Kock ileostomy, 158, 161
Kwell. *See* Lindane.
Kyphosis, 683

L

Labyrinthectomy, 657
Labyrinthitis, 683
Lactose intolerance, 222i
  diet to relieve symptoms of, **221, 223**
Lactose-reduced diet, **221, 223**
Lactulose-induced catharsis, 657
Lamellar (partial thickness) keratoplasty, 512, 513
Laminectomy, **292-294**
  alternatives to, 293
Lanoxin. *See* Digoxin.
Laparoscopy, **375, 377**
  in endometrial implant removal, 376t
Laparotomy, **375, 377**
  in endometrial implant removal, 376t
Laryngeal cancer, 683
Laryngectomy, **545-549**
  complications of, 548
  types of, 546-547i
Laryngitis, 683
Laryngofissure, 545, 547i
Laryngoscopy, 545
Laser neurosurgery, 657-658
Laser stapedectomy, 537-538
Laser surgery
  for ophthalmic disorders, **528-530**
  safety precautions during, 529
  for skin lesions, **569-571**
Lasix. *See* Furosemide.
Laxatives, **145-149**
Lead, 77
Legg-Calvé-Perthes disease, 683

Boldface page numbers indicate major entries; i refers to an illustration, t to a table.

Boldface page numbers indicate major entries; i refers to an illustration, t to a table.

Boldface page numbers indicate major entries; i refers to an illustration, t to a table.

Boldface page numbers indicate major entries; i refers to an illustration, t to a table.

Boldface page numbers indicate major entries; i refers to an illustration, t to a table.

Boldface page numbers indicate major entries; i refers to an illustration, t to a table.